European Family Therapy Ass

Founding Editors

Maria Borcsa
University of Applied Sciences Nordhausen, Nordhausen, Germany

Peter Stratton
University of Leeds, Leeds, West Yorkshire, UK

This series offers contributions from the European Family Therapy Association's community of senior authors and experienced editors. It brings together state-of-the-art contributions on crucial issues in family therapy in Europe with a focus on systemic family therapy. The topics alternate between those that make research findings accessible and of immediate value to practitioners and those that cover clinical areas. This series is essential reading for family therapists, counselors, and social workers across the globe.

More information about this series at http://www.springer.com/series/13797

Matthias Ochs • Maria Borcsa
Jochen Schweitzer

Editors

Systemic Research in Individual, Couple, and Family Therapy and Counseling

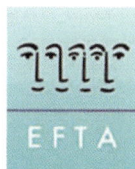

Springer

Editors
Matthias Ochs
Fulda University of Applied Sciences
Fulda, Germany

Maria Borcsa 🆔
University of Applied Sciences Nordhausen
Nordhausen, Germany

Jochen Schweitzer
University Clinic of Heidelberg
Heidelberg, Germany

ISSN 2569-877X   ISSN 2569-8796   (electronic)
European Family Therapy Association Series
ISBN 978-3-030-36562-2   ISBN 978-3-030-36560-8   (eBook)
https://doi.org/10.1007/978-3-030-36560-8

This Springer imprint is published by the registered company Springer Nature Switzerland AG
The registered company address is: Gewerbestrasse 11, 6330 Cham, Switzerland

Foreword

The European Family Therapy Association and the Heidelberg Systemic Research Conferences

The European Family Therapy Association (EFTA) was established in 1990, integrating today 32 national organizations of family therapy all over Europe (EFTA-NFTO), plus the so-called foreign members from Canada, Brazil, Chile, Israel, Senegal and the USA, with 136 training institutes (EFTA-TIC) and 1100 individual members (EFTA-CIM). EFTA is an international association dedicated to scientific purposes. It is an independent and strictly nonprofitmaking association (Borcsa, 2017).

EFTA's involvement with the Heidelberg systemic research conferences started in 2009. Maria Borcsa, then chair of EFTA's Chamber of National Family Therapy Organisations (NFTO) and representative of the two German systemic associations in EFTA, convened a European meeting in Leipzig. The presidents of the two German associations, Cornelia Oestereich (for Systemische Gesellschaft (SG)) and Jochen Schweitzer (for Deutsche Gesellschaft für Systemische Therapie, Beratung und Familientherapie (DGSF)), were present to welcome all delegates. A scientific event had become a good tradition during these assemblies.

After that meeting, Jochen Schweitzer wrote to Peter Stratton:

> We met in Leipzig on a Friday evening in June (Your wife and grandson were there, too) and talked briefly about your work with SCORE. I want to invite you to come as a presenter to a conference called "Systemic research in therapy, education and organizational development". You will meet approx. 150 highly motivated researchers and practitioner-researchers.
>
> I would like you to participate in a two-hour symposium on "systemic research and the promotion of systemic research in Great Britain". I believe we Germans can learn a lot from you British folks in particular in that respect. (…) And we ask you to do a research methodology workshop on "developing the SCORE" in the afternoon of that same day. (…).

At the following 2010 Heidelberg conference, Peter duly presented on SCORE as "a collaborative endeavour of European systemic therapists" (Stratton, Bland, Janes, & Lask, 2010), the German version of SCORE was translated and introduced by Maria (Borcsa & Schelenhaus, 2011). SCORE, an indicator of family functioning and therapeutic change, is both a purpose-built measure of therapeutic progress and an indicator of quality of life within the family and has become freely available on the EFTA website in more than 20 languages: http://www.europeanfamilytherapy.eu/efta-community-news (see also chapter "The Idiographic Voice in a Nomothetic World: Why Client Feedback is Essential to Our Professional Knowledge" in this book).

Subsequently, the EFTA Board recognized the work of Alan Carr and Peter Stratton by an EFTA Award for their contributions to family therapy research (Carr & Stratton, 2017). This prize was not the sole indication that the role of research within EFTA had increased during the years.

At the start of the presidency of Arlene Vetere (2004–2010), an NFTO Research Support Group and a wider "Research Task Force" were established with Peter Stratton (chair), Mina Polemi Todoulou and Nevena Čalovska Hercog as members. Their mission was to survey existing research in EFTA's training institutes, national organizations and individual members and to promote more (outcome) research throughout the organization. The EFTA Research Committee was formally constituted in 2010 with Peter Stratton as chair. Arlene's strong support for research was continued by the two subsequent EFTA presidents, Kyriaki Polychroni (2010–2013) and Maria Borcsa (2013–2017). For more details on the development of EFTA and the role of research, see Borcsa, Hanks and Vetere (2013) and Borcsa and Stratton (2016).

EFTA was fortunate to have a succession of leaders who supported research and put EFTA in a strong position for its members of EFTA to become regular contributors to the Heidelberg conferences. In 2014, EFTA formally became a participating organization and the conference developed into a European Systemic Research Conference, correspondingly with active participation of the authors: Maria Borcsa gave a keynote speech on "The State of Implementation of Systemic Therapy in the National Health Care Systems in Different European Countries" (Borcsa, 2016) and organized an EFTA Research Group Symposium on "Qualitative Research in Couple and Family Therapy: Multiple Perspectives" (Borcsa & Rober, 2016). Peter Stratton presented a keynote on "Researching the Effectiveness of Systemic Therapy Within Europe", a discussion panel "Evidence-Based Systemic Research and Practice" and a workshop "Knowing What We Are Trying to Achieve: Assessing Therapeutic Progress Through Quality of Life in the Family System – The SCORE Index of Family Functioning and Change".

In 2017, the scope was widened even further, and the conference became the International Systemic Research Conference "Linking Systemic Research and Practice". Besides other associations, EFTA functioned again as a participating organization, helping to promote the conference all over Europe and beyond. Rodolfo de Bernart represented EFTA as then new president, and numerous EFTA members participated in various formats.

The triumphant International Systemic Research Conference 2017 has unhappily transpired to be the last of the series in Heidelberg. This is a great sadness for all of us in EFTA who have enjoyed the conferences, the wonderful city of Heidelberg and especially the professional organization and the hospitality of Jochen Schweitzer, Matthias Ochs and their teams; we wish to express our unlimited gratitude!

In showing our recognition, we, Maria and Peter as EFTA book series' founding editors, are pleased to introduce major contributions of this conference to the reader.

We dedicate this volume in memoriam Rodolfo de Bernart, who sadly died after a serious illness in February 2019.

Institute of Social Medicine,   Maria Borcsa
Rehabilitation Sciences and Healthcare Research
University of Applied Sciences Nordhausen
Nordhausen, Germany

Leeds Institute of Health Sciences (LIHS)   Peter Stratton
University of Leeds
Leeds, UK

References

Borcsa, M. (2017). European Family Therapy Association. In J. Lebow, A. Chambers, D. Breunlin (Eds.), *Encyclopedia of Couple and Family Therapy.* Cham: Springer. https://doi.org/10.1007/978-3-319-15877-8_613-3

Borcsa, M. (2016). Systemische (Familien-)Therapie und staatliche Gesundheitssysteme in Europa. Ein Überblick. *Familiendynamik, 41*(1), 24–33.

Borcsa, M. & Rober, P. (Eds.) (2016). *Research Perspectives in Couple Therapy. Discursive Qualitative Methods.* Cham: Springer.

Borcsa, M., Hanks, H., & Vetere, A. (2013). The development of family therapy and systemic practice in Europe: Some reflections and concerns. *Contemporary Family Therapy, 35*(2), 342–348.

Borcsa, M., & Stratton, P. (2016) From origins and originality - family therapy and the European idea. In M. Borcsa and P. Stratton (Eds.). *Origins and Originality in Family Therapy and Systemic Practice* (pp. 1–10). Cham: Springer.

Borcsa, M. & Schelenhaus, S. (2011). Der Fragebogen zur Erfassung der Wirksamkeit von Systemischer Therapie SCORE 15. Ein Werkstattbericht. *Systeme, 25*(2), 137–140.

Carr, A. & Stratton, P. (2017). The SCORE family assessment questionnaire: A decade of progress. *Family Process, 56,* 285–301. https://doi.org/10.1111/famp.12280

Stratton, P, Bland, J., Janes, E. & Lask, J. (2010). Developing a practicable outcome measure for systemic family therapy: The SCORE. *Journal of Family Therapy, 32,* 232–258.

Contents

Contributors

Corina Aguilar-Raab Institute of Medical Psychology, Center of Psychosocial Medicine, Heidelberg University Hospital, Heidelberg, Germany

Eia Asen Anna Freud National Centre for Children and Families, University College London, London, UK

Petra Bauer Institute of Educational Sciences, Department of Social Pedagogy, Tübingen University, Tübingen, Germany

Maria Borcsa Institute of Social Medicine, Rehabilitation Sciences and Healthcare Research, University of Applied Sciences Nordhausen, Nordhausen, Germany

Alan Carr School of Psychology, University College Dublin, and Clanwilliam Institute Dublin, Dublin, Ireland

Ashley Collette Royal Roads University, Victoria, BC, Canada

Eva Deslypere Institute for Family and Sexuality Studies (IFSS), Department of Neurosciences in the School of Medicine KU Leuven, Leuven, Belgium

Mona DeKoven Fishbane Chicago Center for Family Health, Chicago, IL, USA

Peter Fonagy Anna Freud National Centre for Children and Families, University College London, London, UK

Peter Fraenkel The City College of The City University of New York, New York, NY, USA

Andrea Goll-Kopka School of Social Science and Law, SRH University Heidelberg, Heidelberg, Germany

Leslie Greenberg Faculty of Health, York University in Toronto, Toronto, ON, Canada

Tommi Härkänen Finnish Institute for Health and Welfare, Helsinki, Finland

Markus W. Haun Department of General Internal Medicine and Psychosomatics, Heidelberg University, Heidelberg, Germany

Erkki Heinonen Finnish Institute for Health and Welfare, Helsinki, Finland

Lucie Hornová Psychologická ambulance, Rychnov nad Kněžnou, Czech Republic

Jukka Kaartinen Department of Psychology, University of Jyväskylä, Jyväskylä, Finland

Paul Knekt Finnish Institute for Health and Welfare, Helsinki, Finland

Virpi-Liisa Kykyri Department of Psychology, University of Jyväskylä, Jyväskylä, Finland
Faculty of Social Sciences/Psychology, University of Tampere, Tampere, Finland

Aarno Laitila Department of Psychology, University of Jyväskylä, Jyväskylä, Finland

Glenn Larner Riley Street Practice, Sydney, NSW, Australia

Jay L. Lebow Family Institute at Northwestern University, Evanston, IL, USA

Gilbert M. D. Lemmens Department of Psychiatry, Ghent University Hospital, Ghent, Belgium
Department of Head and Skin – Psychiatry and Medical Psychology, Ghent University, Ghent, Belgium

Olavi Lindfors Finnish Institute for Health and Welfare, Helsinki, Finland

Timo Maljanen Social Insurance Institution, Helsinki, Finland

Sheila McNamee University of New Hampshire, Durham, NH, USA
Taos Institute, Chagrin Falls, OH, USA

Philip Messent Association of Family Therapy and Systemic Practice, Warrington, UK

Petra Nyman-Salonen Department of Psychology, University of Jyväskylä, Jyväskylä, Finland

Matthias Ochs Department of Social Work, Fulda University of Applied Sciences, Fulda, Germany

Markku Penttonen Department of Psychology, University of Jyväskylä, Jyväskylä, Finland

Mario Pfammatter University Hospital of Psychiatry and Psychotherapy, University of Bern, Bern, Switzerland

Martin Pinquart Department of Psychology, Philipps University, Marburg, Germany

Fabian Ramseyer Department of Clinical Psychology and Psychotherapy, University of Bern, Bern, Switzerland

Peter Rober Institute for Family and Sexuality Studies (IFSS), Department of Neurosciences in the School of Medicine KU Leuven, Leuven, Belgium

Luigi Schepisi Centro di Studi e di Applicazione della Psicologia Relazionale, Prato, Italy

Günter Schiepek Institute of Synergetics and Psychotherapy Research, University Hospital for Psychiatry, Psychotherapy and Psychosomatics, Paracelsus Medical University, Salzburg, Austria

Jochen Schweitzer Institute of Medical Psychology, Center of Psychosocial Medicine, Heidelberg University Hospital, Heidelberg, Germany

Jaakko Seikkula Department of Psychology, University of Jyväskylä, Jyväskylä, Finland

Reenee Singh Association of Family Therapy and Systemic Practice, Warrington & Child and Family Practice, London, UK

Chelsea Spencer School of Family Studies and Human Services, Kansas State University, Manhattan, KS, USA

Sandra M. Stith School of Family Studies and Human Services, Kansas State University, Manhattan, KS, USA

Peter Stratton Leeds Institute of Health Sciences (LIHS), University of Leeds, Leeds, UK

Terje Tilden Modum Bad, Vikersund, Norway

Anu Tourunen The Gerontology Research Center, Faculty of Sport and Health Sciences, University of Jyväskylä, Jyväskylä, Finland

Valeri Tsatsishvili Faculty of Information Technology, University of Jyväskylä, Jyväskylä, Finland

Wolfgang Tschacher University Hospital of Psychiatry and Psychotherapy, University of Bern, Bern, Switzerland

Freiburg Institute for Advanced Studies (FRIAS), Albert-Ludwigs-Universität Freiburg, Freiburg, Germany

Eleftheria Tseliou Laboratory of Psychology, Department of Early Childhood Education, University of Thessaly, Volos, Greece

Michael Ungar Canada Research Chair in Child, Family and Community Resilience, Dalhousie University, Halifax, NS, Canada

Berta Vall Faculty of Psychology, Education, and Sport Sciences, Blanquerna, Ramon Llull University, Barcelona, Spain

Gaëlle Vanhee Department of Experimental Clinical and Health Psychology, Ghent University, Ghent, Belgium

Justine Van Lawick Lorentzhuis, Centrum voor systeemtherapie, opleiding en consultatie, Haarlem, The Netherlands

Lesley L. Verhofstadt Department of Experimental Clinical and Health Psychology, Ghent University, Ghent, Belgium

Esa Virtala Finnish Institute for Health and Welfare, Helsinki, Finland

Margreet Visser Children's Trauma Center, Kenter Youthcare, Haarlem, The Netherlands

Marc Weinhardt School of Professional Studies, Darmstadt Protestant University of Applied Sciences, Darmstadt, Germany

Julika Zwack Institute of Medical Psychology, Center of Psychosocial Medicine, Heidelberg University Hospital, Heidelberg, Germany

About the Editors

Matthias Ochs is a professor of Psychology and Counselling at the Department of Social Work, Fulda University of Applied Sciences, Germany. He is also a diploma psychologist, a psychological psychotherapist (licensed by German Psychotherapy Law), a Gestalt therapist, a family therapist and a certified teacher for systemic therapy/counselling. His Diploma and PhD theses were honoured with research awards. He was co-president of the two International Systemic Research Conferences in Heidelberg (2014 and 2017); vice president of the German Association for Systemic Therapy, Counselling and Family Therapy (DGSF); member of the General Board of the European Family Therapy Association (EFTA); and professorial member of the PhD Centre Social Work of the Official Hessian Universities of Applied Sciences. With Jochen Schweitzer, he edited a German systemic research textbook. His current special research interests are unwanted side effects and negative events in systemic therapy/counselling, systems theory/practice regarding inter-professional/inter-institutional cooperation and networks, systemic practitioner research, dialogical-systemic practice and the interrelation of social work and psychotherapy.

Maria Borcsa, PhD, is professor of Clinical Psychology at the University of Applied Sciences in Nordhausen (UASN), Germany, licensed psychological psychotherapist (CBT), family therapist, trainer and supervisor. She is founding member of the Institute of Social Medicine, Health Care Research and Rehabilitation Sciences at UASN; coeditor of the scientific journals *Systeme* (2001–2014) and *Psychotherapie im Dialog* (2007–2019); member of the Editorial Board of the journals *Testing, Psychometrics, Methodology in Applied Psychology* and *Contemporary Family Therapy*; advisory editor of *Family Process*; associate editor of *Encyclopedia of Couple and Family Therapy*; and founding editor of the EFTA Family Therapy book series. She has been board member of the Systemic Society (Systemische Gesellschaft) German Association for Systemic Therapy, Counselling and Family Therapy (2005–2011) and European Family Therapy Association (EFTA) (2007–2016), chair of the Chamber of National Family Therapy Organizations of

EFTA (2010–2013) and president of EFTA (2013–2016). Her research interests focus on qualitative methods in mental health and on globalized families. In 2019, she received an award from the European Family Therapy Association for her excellence in the research field of family therapy and systemic practice.

Jochen Schweitzer is associate professor of Medical Psychology and Psychotherapy at Heidelberg University Medical School and head of its Division of Organizational Psychology in Medicine. He gained his Diploma in Psychology from the University of Giessen in 1978, his doctorate in Social Sciences from the University of Tübingen in 1986 and his habilitation in Medical Psychology and Psychotherapy from Heidelberg University in 1995. In 2002, he co-founded and then co-chaired the Helm Stierlin Institute for Systemic Training in Heidelberg. His primary interests include family therapy in medicine, psychiatry and juvenile services, organizational consultation in non-for-profit institutions and political contexts of psychosocial practice, for example with refugees or poor clients. Among his major projects have been the implementation of family systems psychiatry (SYMPA) in German Hospitals and the Heidelberg Systemic Research Conferences from 1998 to 2017, serving as president (2007–2013) of the German Association for Systemic Therapy, Counselling and Family Therapy (DGSF) and gradually with many others helping to introduce systemic therapy into evidence-based medicine and health insurance coverage in Germany between 2003 and 2018. His work was honoured by awards from the American Family Therapy Academy in 2016 and the European Family Therapy Association in 2019.

The Heidelberg Systemic Research Conferences: Their History, Goals and Outcomes

Jochen Schweitzer and Matthias Ochs

A Brief History

The Heidelberg Systemic Research Conferences started at the Department of Medical Psychology at the Heidelberg University Hospital in 1998 – as a place for exchanging ideas and approaches for scientists, practitioners and students, interested in the question, what it means to do research in a systemic way. The conference restarted 2004 after a 6-year pause and then took place as a German language conference biannually until 2012. It finally turned into a larger European conference in 2014 and into an international conference in 2017 (www.ISR2017.com). Jochen Schweitzer initiated and then directed all conferences from 1998 to 2017; Matthias Ochs joined him as conference co-president in 2010.

All conferences had three major goals:

- We wanted to represent systemic research approaches on psychotherapy and counselling (including coaching, supervision and team development) in the fields of medicine, education, social work and organizations/management. Systems theory (dynamical and sociological systems theory) and/or constructivism (especially social constructionism) had inspired these practices, they had spread into all these fields of application, and we wanted to support that "dissemination" of the systemic approach by providing a regular platform for further scientific "professionalization" via research and ongoing theoretical discourses.

J. Schweitzer (✉)
Institute of Medical Psychology, Center of Psychosocial Medicine, Heidelberg University Hospital, Heidelberg, Germany
e-mail: Jochen.Schweitzer-Rothers@med.uni-heidelberg.de

M. Ochs
Department of Social Work, Fulda University of Applied Sciences, Fulda, Germany

© Springer Nature Switzerland AG 2020
M. Ochs et al. (eds.), *Systemic Research in Individual, Couple, and Family Therapy and Counseling*, European Family Therapy Association Series,
https://doi.org/10.1007/978-3-030-36560-8_1

1

- We wanted to help "linking practice with research" – which became the continuous subtitle of the conference. Therefore, we encouraged practitioners to bring to the conferences their research-related ideas, interests, projects, questions and impulses– and to do "practitioner research". Once there, we wanted to connect them to senior and junior researchers (e.g. Bachelor, Masters and PhD students).
- We wanted to stimulate the discourse on what exactly differentiates "systemic" from "non-systemic" research and what theories and research methods are more or less appropriately called "systemic".

Attendance grew from 150 in 1998 to 500 participants in 2017. This research conference will now possibly move to another location. This turning point makes it interesting to look back on the motivations, the history, the format and the possible outcomes of these Heidelberg systemic research conferences.

The Start: Why and How It Began in 1998

The late 1990s formed a transitional period in systemic research. There had been much research in the early American development of family therapy – e.g. the Palo Alto Group in the 1950s and the investigations of Murray Bowen, Lyman Wynne and Helm Stierlin et al. at the US National Institutes of Mental Health in the 1960s or of Salvador Minuchin's research on families of the slums and on psychosomatic families in the 1970s.

In the German language countries, many systemic research activities developed in the 1970s and 1980s in the Heidelberg University Department of Psychoanalytic Basic Research and Family Therapy (Helm Stierlin, Michael Wirsching, Inge Rücker-Embden-Jonasch, Fritz. B. Simon, Arnold Retzer, Gunthard Weber, Gunter Schmidt, Jochen Schweitzer), with projects on systemic therapy for patients with cancer, psychosis and eating disorders. Research on couple therapy had a focus in Zürich (Jürg Willi, Josef Duss von Werdt, Rosmarie Welter-Enderlin), Multigenerational Family Therapy in Göttingen (Eckart Sperling, Almuth Massing, Günther Reich). The year 1990 saw the start of the so-called Herbst Akademie (Autumn Academy), an annual or biannual meeting, dedicated to the study of self-organization processes in psychology and social sciences, under the paradigm of the theory of dynamical systems (especially synergetics); pioneers then were Günther Schiepek, Ewald Johannes Brunner, Jürgen Kriz and Wolfgang Tschacher.

However, systemic research activities in the German language countries declined between mid-1980 and mid-1990, for several reasons:

- The perspectives of radical constructivism and of second-order cybernetics made it questionable to research what "really happened" in families or in family therapies. If the construction of reality solely relied on the perspective of an observer, it seemed to no longer make sense to search for an objective understanding of social realities. This epistemological debate was sometimes criticized as "epistobabel" but certainly diminished the popularity of empirical research in the systemic context.

- The systemic approach as a set of very practical psychosocial attitudes and tools had become quite popular and fascinating among psychosocial, medical and organizational practitioners. That generated a rapidly growing "training market", mostly outside university contexts in private institutes. In those years, training in systemic therapy was great fun and experienced a great boom, and to train systemic therapists/counsellors became much more rewarding than researching, experientially as well as financially. The "experienced evidence" of systemic practice work seemed so strong, that no need was felt for additional "scientific evidence". (Of course, this practice research gap can be observed in many other approaches of counselling and therapy: for practitioners, research feels boring and irrelevant; for scientists, practice feels "built on sand", theoretically and empirically).
- Systemic practice and training flourished mainly outside universities and other research oriented contexts. This situation had negative implications for systemic research: there were only very view university professorships with an explicit systemic orientation, and so the possibilities of running research projects, graduate colleges or doing bachelor/ master thesis, PhDs or habilitations with a clear systemic stance were very limited. This, in turn, had adverse effects on supporting systemic junior researchers.

Motivations for and styles of doing research changed in the midst of the 1990s. The so-called "neoliberal economies" had reached the health and social services sector. Quality and cost management became a topic. Esthetic fascination by therapies counted less; figures and statistics demonstrating "quality" started to count more. In the medical field, "evidence-based medicine" called for facts and figures on the efficacy and effectiveness of what providers do. Psychotherapy was about to become regulated. In Germany, the "Psychotherapeutengesetz" (psychotherapy regulation law) was expected to become effective in 1999 – and it was expected to leave systemic therapy outside the domains of "acknowledged" treatments. At German language universities, those psychiatric pioneers that had established family therapy and social psychiatry research institutes at medical departments in the late 1960s and early 1970s – H.E. Richter, H. Strotzka, E. Sperling, H. Stierlin, L. Kaufmann, L. Ciompi, J. Willi and a few others – had already retired or were about to retire. It was expected that their work would often not be continued in the same universities.

So there was a very vivid, lively, growing field of systemic practitioners, trainers and theorists on the one hand and a shrinking research field. Both were at the same time confronted with the new challenges of the "evidence-based" philosophy and of "regulation by science", in which the old virtues of action research and theory development by practice observation were in danger to become outdated. However the systemic field started to react. One response was some sort of systematic knowledge management by the writing of first "teaching books of systemic therapy" by e.g. Kurt Ludewig (1992), Arist von Schlippe and Jochen Schweitzer (1996) and Klaus Mücke (2003). Another response was that the – at that time – three German systemic associations asked Günter Schiepek in 1995 to collect and present all available knowledge on empirical process and outcome research about systemic therapy (Schiepek, 1999). Unfortunately, that endeavour failed to win the approval of a then newly established "ʿScientific Approval Board for Psychotherapy" of the German Psychotherapy Law in 1998. (According to the German Psychotherapy Law, the purpose of this board is to give the health administration recommendations concerning the licensing of psychotherapeutic methods and approaches for trainings. The board consists of six medical and six psychological psychotherapists.)

It was in this context that Jochen Schweitzer decided early in 1997 to organize a rather experimental conference. Networking should substitute structures, excitement should substitute thoroughness, and experimental conference designs should complement classical formats of lectures, posters and workshops. Experimental forms included a talk show and a plenary research consultation of a PhD candidate by three professors of very divergent theoretical orientations (Professor of Social Work Maja Heiner, Professor for Microsociology Bruno Hildenbrand, Professor for Psychoanalytical Family Therapy Manfred Cierpka). These formats tried to combine the interest of the systemic field in innovative, experimental and reflexive settings with the research topic.

Networking by Conferencing: The German Language Conferences, 2004 Until 2012

The 2004 conference restarted biannually, now with a somewhat more "mainstream" conference format, but still with strong experimental features. Now, internationally known and mostly Anglo-American keynote speakers were invited and came – among them José Szapocznik, Bill Pinsof, Russell Crane, Chuck Borduin, Guy Diamond, Peter Fraenkel, Eia Asen, Peter Stratton and Charlotte Burck. German-speaking keynote speakers included those with a strong focus on systems theory (Helmuth Willke, Dirk Baecker, Jürgen Kriz), on empirical methods of a more quantitative (Günther Schiepek, Wolfgang Tschacher, Ewald Johannes Brunner) or a more qualitative nature (Michael Buchholz, Bruno Hildenbrand) and scientist practitioners (Arist von Schlippe, Johannes Ruegg-Stürm, Rolf Arnold, Julika Zwack).

The 2004 conference became quite important for the next decade of systemic research in Germany. The so-called expertise group (consisted of Kirsten von Sydow, Stefan Beher, Rüdiger Retzlaff, Jochen Schweitzer) met by happenstance on this conference and started to cooperate collecting the evidence for the positive outcome of systemic psychotherapy (von Sydow et al., 2007). This cooperation was very successful, because it led, in 2008, to the scientific acknowledgment of systemic therapy by the same council (the Scientific Approval Board for Psychotherapy), which had disapproved of the first attempt 10 years earlier. This acknowledgment had professional legal effects in that sense, that it was now allowed by the health administration to do trainings in systemic psychotherapy for treating mental illnesses; it had no effects regarding the funding of systemic psychotherapy by the public health insurances.

Besides this, the "German language only" conference years from 2004 to 2012 bore some other important "fruits":

- They encouraged practitioners to do "practitioner research" via a PhD path.
- They allowed a lot of networking for junior and senior researchers, students and research- interested practitioners in the systemic field.
- They stimulated the discourse between different systemic theoretical orientation (e.g. sociological systems theory, dynamical systems and social constructionism), different research approaches (e.g. quantitative, qualitative, process and outcome oriented, critical rationalism and constructivist research) and different fields of application (see above).
- They made systemic research observable by the professional, discipline and social political environments (e.g. we invited chairs, presidents and experts from non-systemic associations and organizations for welcome words and discussion panels).
- In cooperation with the two German Systemic Associations DGSF (Deutsche Gesellschaft für Systemische Therapie, Beratung und Familientherapie) and SG (Systemische Gesellschaft), we launched in 2008 a German Internet platform for systemic research: www.systemisch-forschen.de.
- In 2012 we (Matthias Ochs, Jochen Schweitzer) published a German edited textbook on systemic research "Handbuch Forschung für Systemiker" (textbook of systemic research) (Ochs & Schweitzer, 2012) that tried to represent the diverse perspectives and approaches on what systemic research could be – as they were presented at the conferences in those years.
- In 2012 we did a thematically oriented conference on "research on rituals" with colleagues, such as Jan Weinhold, Bruno Hildenbrand, Guni Leila Baxa, Gunthard Weber, Diana Drexler and Christina Hunger, that were partially active in the so-called Heidelberg DFG Sonderforschungsbereich "Ritualdynamik" – a complex inter- and multidisciplinary research network located at the Heidelberg University and funded by the German Research Foundation (DFG Deutsche Forschungsgemeinschaft) with the aim to study the multidimensionality of structures and dynamics of rituals (www.ritualdynamik.de).

Going Big: The European Conference 2014 and the International Conference 2017

Meanwhile, our European and international systemic research networks grew, which made us consider to "go bigger". Therefore, in 2014 we established a European systemic research conference, with similar goals and a similar mission. Of course, this was only possible with strong European cooperation partners: Maria Borcsa, then president of the European Family Therapy Association (EFTA), and Peter Stratton, then chair of the research committee of EFTA, who supported us heavily regarding that project. This support helped us to connect more strongly with European research colleagues and their excellent work, such as Jakko Seikkula

(Finland), Peter Rober (Belgium), Rolf Sundet (Norway), Terje Tilden (Norway), Gilbert Lemmens (Belgium), Gail Simon (UK), Bogdan de Barbaro (Poland), Laura Fruggeri (Italy), Elefteria Tseliou (Greece) and many others. Since funding of systemic therapies by health insurances was and still is an important topic in several European countries, we also used the 2014 conference to discuss the cost effectiveness of treating families vs. individuals in medical mental health (Crane & Christenson, 2014) and the integration of systemic psychotherapy in the official psychotherapeutic care system in European countries (Borcsa, 2016). The conference attracted 300 participants from roundabout 20 European countries and North America. It was, in the view of most participants, a great success, so we developed the idea to broaden the perspective also outside of Europe.

The 2017 conference attracted 500 participants from 29 countries, among them 130 from non-German-speaking European countries, 30 from Asia and 20 from the American continent. This time, a major focus was on the discussion with other than explicitly "systemic" schools of psychotherapy. Keynote speakers like Peter Fonagy (psychodynamic therapy), Lesley Greenberg (emotion-focused therapy) and Bruce Wampold (generic factors research) symbolized this "psychotherapy in dialogue" approach. Relational neurobiology, with reference to couple therapy applications (Mona Fishbane, Beate Ditzen), was included for the first time in the conference. Also we "pick up" the mindfulness movement in psychotherapy and counselling and its applications to social contexts (Diane Gehart, Corina Raab). Wider political topics became discussed, most prominently refugee aid (Renos Papadopoulos), collective trauma (Michal Shamai), the resilience of young people worldwide (Michael Ungar), family and intimate violence (Sandra Stith, Justine van Lawick, Margreet Visser) and the populistic turn in politics worldwide (Sheila McNamee, Susan McDaniel). Instant electronic feedback to therapists and clients, a topic already opened in 2006 and meanwhile quite well-developed, was demonstrated (Bill Pinsof, Günter Schiepek, Terje Tilden and others), instructed and critically discussed. We could win most of the abovementioned colleagues to contribute to this present editor book that documents some of the most interesting contributions to the Heidelberg Systemic Research Conference in 2017 and is also for us some kind of completion of our activities in the context of the Heidelberg Systemic Research Conference.

So What? An Attempt to Look Back on Process and Outcome of These Conferences

As a personal conclusion, we can say that these conferences, although their preparation involved tremendous labour, were fun to organize and to participate in. It was possible to create an atmosphere of curiosity, stimulation, cooperation and friendliness. A lot of cooperation started here or was intensified. Quite a number of systemic practitioners were encouraged by the conferences to do a master thesis or a PhD thesis with a systemic focus. Several research instruments later became quite practical and are today used widely in clinical and organizational evaluations. Many junior researchers later reported these conferences to be their "moment of initiation". Contacts with invited psychotherapy leaders (e.g. all of the three presidents of the German Psychotherapy Chamber and several professors of psychiatry, psychosomatic and clinical psychology) certainly helped to create a favourable climate for the professionalization of systemic therapy in Germany.

However, some conflicts implicit in the conference's conception were never really solved, and some goals were not really achieved until today:

1. It has remained open, whether there are "genuinely systemic" research methods that can be clearly differentiated from "non-systemic" methods (we discussed that topic, e.g. in Schweitzer & Ochs, 2012; Ochs, 2013).
2. The conference has primarily become a psychotherapy conference – the involvement of organizational researchers remained much weaker, and the involvement of social work and education researchers remained very weak.
3. Within the psychotherapy communities of various countries, it is generally recognized today that systemic therapy and consultation have a strong theoretical and empirical basis. However, their representation in the big research-active universities and powerful research institutions is still weak as of now. This may and we hope will change during the next 10 years. There is a much brighter picture at the Universities of Applied Sciences, where systemic thinking seems well-established today. (Matthias Ochs, e.g., is supervising systemic oriented PhDs as a full professorial member at the Promotion Centre of Social Work in Hessen/Germany.)

At the point of writing this manuscript, it is not yet clear if this conference will continue in the future, in Heidelberg or elsewhere. In both cases, we hope the many inspiring collective experiences of many people made during these eight conferences will live on in new ventures and activities, no matter where and when.

Acknowledgements The success of the Heidelberg systemic research conferences has always heavily relied on our cooperation and support partners. We particularly want to thank Rolf Verres and Beate Ditzen (former and current directors of the Institute of Medical Psychology); to Susanne Richter, Susanne Metzger, Ibolya Kurucz, Antonia Drews and Marieke Born (the conference secretaries during the various phases); and to the systemic associations and organizations that supported us, in particular to DGSF, SG, EFTA, lately also the American Family Therapy Association (AFTA), the International Family Therapy Association (IFTA), the Chinese Association of Mental Health and the Chinese-German Association for Psychotherapy (DCAP). Finally, we thank the German Research Foundation (DFG) and the Heidehof Foundation for their continuous financial support.

References

Borcsa, M. (2016). Systemische (Familien-)Therapie und staatliche Gesundheitssysteme in Europa. Ein Überblick. *Familiendynamik, 41*(1), 24–33.

Crane, D. R., & Christenson, J. (2014). A summary report of cost-effectiveness: Recognizing the value of family therapy in health care. In J. Hodgson, A. Lamson, T. Mendenhall, & D. R. Crane (Eds.), *Medical family therapy: Advanced applications* (pp. 419–436). Cham, Switzerland: Springer International Publishing. https://doi.org/10.1007/978-3-319-03482-9_22

Ludewig, K. (1992). *Systemische Therapie. Grundlagen klinischer Theorie und Praxis*. Stuttgart: Klett-Cotta.

Mücke, K. (2003). *Probleme sind Lösungen: Systemische Beratung und Psychotherapie – ein pragmatischer Ansatz – Lehr- und Lernbuch*. Potsdam: ÖkoSysteme-Verlag.

Ochs, M. (2013). Pluralität und Diversi(vi)tät systemischer Forschung. *Familiendynamik, 38*(1), 4–11.

Ochs, M., & Schweitzer, J. (Eds.). (2012). *Handbuch Forschung für Systemiker*. Göttingen: Vandenhoeck & Ruprecht.

Schiepek, G. (1999). *Die Grundlagen der Systemischen Therapie. Theorie – Praxis – Forschung*. Göttingen: Vandenhoeck & Ruprecht.

Schweitzer, J., & Ochs, M. (2012). "Forschung für Systemiker" oder "Systemisch Forschen"? – Unser Buchtitel als erkenntnistheoretisches Problem und forschungspraktische Herausforderung. In M. Ochs & J. Schweitzer (Eds.), *Handbuch Forschung für Systemiker* (pp. 17–32). Göttingen: Vandenhoeck & Ruprecht.

von Schlippe, A., & Schweitzer, J. (1996). *Lehrbuch der systemischen Therapie und Beratung*. Vandenhoek & Ruprecht: Göttingen.

von Sydow, K., Beher, S., Retzlaff, R., & Schweitzer-Rothers, J. (2007). *Die Wirksamkeit Systemischer Therapie/Familientherapie*. Göttingen: Hogrefe.

Part I
Innovations in Systemic Research Paradigms

Contributions of Systemic Research to the Development of Psychotherapy

Günter Schiepek

Challenges of Contemporary Psychotherapy

Compared with its early decades at the beginning of the twenty-first century, psychotherapy has less urgent needs to legitimate its effectiveness in general but is confronted with other challenges concerning the development of the profession, the question of how research should be realized and how the effectiveness of treatments can be optimized. Other challenges concern the development and dissemination of psychotherapy in health-care systems and the understanding of the mechanisms of change. The points I will bring up for discussion refer to our knowledge on the field as represented in contemporary conferences and textbooks (e.g., Duncan, Miller, Wampold, & Hubble, 2010; Lambert, 2013; Wampold & Imel, 2015):

1. Psychotherapy works on the average, but not for every client. There is a considerable number of nonresponders, deteriorations, or not sustainable effects. One of the consequences could be optimized and tailored treatments for the individual.
2. Psychotherapy works, but we do not know how, or in other words, we have many concepts on this (each therapeutic confession has its own), but no approved and generalizable models, may it be on the level of neurobiological or psychological mechanisms (Kazdin, 2009).

G. Schiepek (✉)
Institute of Synergetics and Psychotherapy Research, University Hospital for Psychiatry, Psychotherapy and Psychosomatics, Paracelsus Medical University, Salzburg, Austria
e-mail: guenter.schiepek@ccsys.de

© Springer Nature Switzerland AG 2020
M. Ochs et al. (eds.), *Systemic Research in Individual, Couple, and Family Therapy and Counseling*, European Family Therapy Association Series, https://doi.org/10.1007/978-3-030-36560-8_2

3. We have acquired an accumulated knowledge on the ingredients or factors (e.g., common factors) contributing to the effects of psychotherapy, but not on how they interact. The development of models which could explain change dynamics is at its very beginning.
4. We cannot predict the trajectories of change, and we cannot predict if and when therapeutic crises will appear.
5. Interventions or treatment techniques have only a small impact on the outcome. This may have consequences for how we conceptualize psychotherapy.
6. Discontinuous jumps to the better or to the worse appear, but the jumps often are independent of interventions. Existing linear models cannot explain this; the phenomenon has the status of empirical "anomalies."
7. There are many approaches in psychotherapy (maybe several hundreds), but no unifying paradigm.
8. Research data often are not produced in real-world practice but are collected in artificial settings (e.g., RCTs in the setting of university hospitals). Practice-based research in realistic settings of health care should create ecologically valid and generalizable results.

Systemic research has to be judged by if and how it contributes to meet these challenges. Independent on how we may define systemic research, any step on this way requires that the term "systemic" will not be reduced to research on a psychotherapeutic school (e.g., systemic therapy) or on a specific setting (e.g., family therapy). We define *systemic research* as a *theoretical and methodological approach to measure, analyze, and model the structures and functioning of complex dynamic systems at a biological, mental, and/or social level*. Examples of complex systems may be brains, physiological systems (e.g., endocrine or immune networks), cognitions and emotions, communication and social interaction, health-care systems, and others. The methods to be applied should cover a wide range of approaches, qualitative and quantitative, idiographic (focused on the individual) and nomothetic ones (focused on generalizable models and theories) (see Schiepek, 2012 in Schweitzer & Ochs, 2012).

Principles of self-organization and basic features of nonlinear dynamics are independent of contexts and of the substrate of the concrete system we are concerned with. Self-organization and nonlinear dynamics are ubiquitous phenomena occurring at different spatial and time scales. One example is the relationship between the connectome of the brain (neural network structures) and its functional connectivity dynamics (Hansen, Battaglia, Spiegler, Deco, & Jirsa, 2015; Ritter, Schirner, McIntosh, & Jirsa, 2013); another is the mental or behavioral change dynamics during psychotherapy. In this general sense, the systemic approach is a meta-theoretical or paradigmatic framework for multi-methods research. Systemic research and complexity science are characterized by transdisciplinarity and by a structuralistic view on theories (Haken & Schiepek, 2006; Stegmüller, 1973). However, in clinical contexts (psychotherapy), in counseling, and in organizational development, systemic research often adopts the criteria of practice-based and participative procedures and of ecological validity. Data should be produced in real-world settings by active cooperation with subjects, may it be practitioners, clients, or members of social networks (see Seikkula, this volume). One approach fulfilling these criteria is Internet-based real-time monitoring of change dynamics in everyday routine practice.

Combining Practice and Research by Monitoring Change Dynamics

Since many years and in diversified clinical contexts, practitioners have used therapy feedback for continuous cooperative process control of change processes (Schiepek, Eckert, Aas, Wallot, & Wallot, 2015; Tilden & Wampold, 2017). The technical device for realizing real-time monitoring and feedback procedures is the Synergetic Navigation System (SNS), an Internet-based tool for the continuous assessment of change processes by self-related or interpersonal ratings of the included subjects (e.g., clients, coaches, family, or team members). Continuous assessments create time series data which is the raw material for any further analysis.

Systems like human or social networks are characterized by their ever-changing dynamics – pattern formation and pattern transitions (Haken & Schiepek, 2006). In consequence, feedback systems have to mirror these dynamics by the option of performing frequent (e.g., daily) assessments and by applying methods of nonlinear time series analysis on the data. Given the fact that nonlinear and chaotic processes are complex, unpredictable, and specific in each case, these features have to be represented by feedback systems. Individual dynamics do not follow any standard track or expected response curve (Schiepek, Gelo, Viol, Kratzer, Orsucci, et al. 2020).

The Synergetic Navigation System

The Synergetic Navigation System (SNS) is a highly flexible and generic Internet-based service for data acquisition, time series analysis, and visualization of outcome and process data as well as analysis of results. It allows for the implementation of various questionnaires or coding systems. Data can be entered and results can be checked by most web-compatible devices, including PCs, notebooks, tablets, or smartphones (ubiquitous computing). Also an SNS app is available.

The sampling rate of the data acquisition (time sampling, event sampling) is up to free choice (e.g., pre-post, weekly, session-related, once per day, higher frequencies). Using the questionnaire editor of the SNS, outcome or personal process questionnaires can be created. Comment fields for text entry and scales for quantitative measures can be combined. Global indicators of change processes can be defined by a "traffic lights" editor. The system does not expect standard tracks.

Outcomes are visualized by histograms, and processes are visualized by time series graphs. Different sizes and alignments of the diagrams can be chosen. If necessary, all diagram fields can be configured independently. The selected item configurations can be saved. When selected again subsequently, the changes automatically are activated and show the current stage of a client's development. When the cursor is moved over the graph of a time series, it displays the value, the entry date, and the diary entry of each data point.

The available analysis and visualization tools:

- Visualization of time series
- Superposition of time series (even if the time series are only partially overlapping or were recorded with different sampling rates, e.g., once per day and once per session)
- Color-coded visualization of the values of one or many time series in a diagram
- Calculation of the dynamic complexity in a running window
- Color-coded visualization of the synchronized dynamic complexities of many time series (complexity resonance diagram)
- Dynamic correlation pattern analysis
- Colored Recurrence Plots

A further option is to assess interpersonal relations by a dynamic interaction matrix tool for dyads (e.g., in couples therapy), families, groups, teams, or organizations.

Interested users can get into contact with the Center of Complex Systems for using this web service. License fees are 780 Euro/year for an outpatient psychotherapy office; see www.ccsys.de. There is an international and transdisciplinary SNS network/community of users and also a professional user group at the German Society of Systemic Therapy and Family Therapy (DGSF).

Hospitals and institutions using the SNS (selection):

- University Hospital of Psychiatry, Psychotherapy, and Psychosomatics, Salzburg, Austria (Dept. of Psychotherapy, Dept. for Crisis Intervention and Suicide Prevention, Day Treatment Centre of Psychosomatics, Institute of Clinical Psychology)
- University Hospital of Child and Adolescent Psychiatry/Psychotherapy, Salzburg, Austria
- Klinikum Grieskirchen-Wels, Dept. of Psychotherapy, Dept. of Adolescent Psychosomatics, Grieskirchen, Austria
- University Hospital of Lower Austria, Psychiatric Day Treatment Centre, Tulln, Austria
- Psychosomatic Clinic St. Irmingard, Prien am Chiemsee, Germany
- Clinic for Psychosomatics (Chiemseewinkel), Seebruck am Chiemsee, Germany

- Psychosomatic Clinic Bad Zwischenahn, Germany
- Rottal-Inn-Kliniken, Simbach am Inn, Germany
- Health Center sysTelios, Siedelsbrunn, Germany
- Christophsbad Hospital, Dept. of Psychiatry and Psychotherapy, Göppingen, Germany
- Marienhospital, Papenburg, Germany
- Center for Training in Psychotherapy, Bielefeld, Germany
- Erzbischöfliches Jugendamt Munich, Germany
- Johanna Kirchner Haus, AWO, Marktbreit, Germany
- Universität Heidelberg, Institute of Counseling Research, Heidelberg, Germany
- MEDIAN Klinik Odenwald, Breuberg, Germany
- Psychiatric Hospital Münsterlingen, Thurgau, Switzerland
- Behavioural Science Institute, Radboud University Nijmegen, Netherlands
- Interacting Minds Centre, Aarhus University, Denmark
- South Denmark University, Center for Human Interactivity, Odense, Denmark
- Psychiatric Hospital Bronderslev, Denmark
- Others

The Identification of Order Transitions: Converging Evidence from Different Methods

From the perspective of self-organization and nonlinear dynamics, an important aim of doing feedback on change processes is to get early warning signals on upcoming order transitions. Periods of critical instability preceding such transitions are often sensitive to minor interventions, personal decisions, or new and encouraging activities. These periods are critical moments which in the ancient Greek mythology were called "kairos" (see the *generic principles* of Synergetics; Schiepek et al., 2015). Critical instabilities can be decisive for developments to the better, e.g., sudden gains, or to the worse, e.g., sudden losses or even suicidal states (Fartacek, Schiepek, Kunrath, Fartacek, & Plöderl, 2016).

The simplest way to identify precursors of order transitions is the inspection of raw data time series by the naked eye. Given some experience in pattern recognition, this provides a first visual impression, which can be consensually validated by the oral reports and the electronic diaries of the client. Figure 1 shows some examples of order transitions as presented by the diagrams shown in the SNS. In many cases critical instabilities can be identified before an order transition occurs (Fig. 1a); in other cases, a transient deterioration may be a precursor (Fig. 1b,c).

A next step is the presentation of the factor dynamics. Factors are subscales of a process questionnaire combining information from several items. In the SNS, the

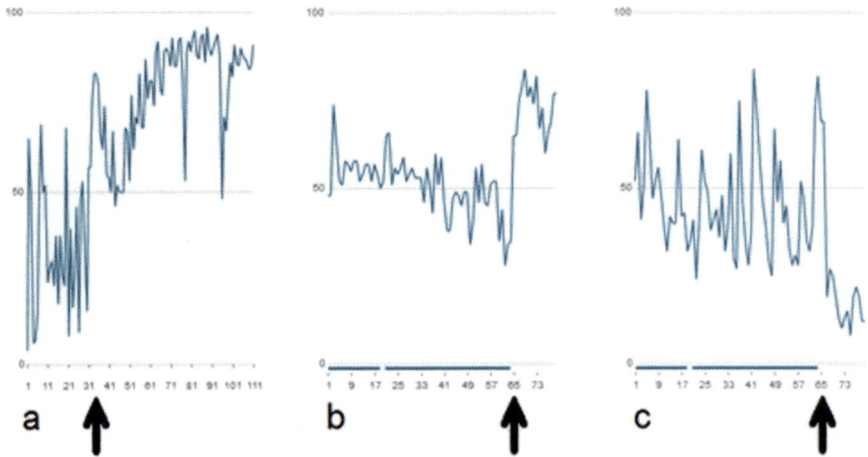

Fig. 1 Time series of items (raw data) of the Therapy Process Questionnaire (TPQ, Schiepek, Stöger-Schmidinger, Kronberger, Aichhorn, Kratzer, Heinz, Viol, Lichtwarck-Aschoff, & Schöller, 2019a). (**a**) "Today I felt joy," (**b**) "Today I felt intended to change my problems," (**c**) "Experienced intensity of problems and symptoms" (time series (**b**) and (**c**) are taken from the same client, see also Figs. 2b,c, 4a, 8, and 12). (**a**) shows a critical instability before the transition (comp. Figs. 2a, 4b, and 6), (**b**) and (**c**) show a transition after a short period of deterioration. The arrows indicate significant order transitions

items which contribute to a factor are averaged and z-transformed (Fig. 2). In many cases, the z-transformed factor dynamics gives a more pronounced picture on the processual Gestalt than the time series of each particular item. Figure 3 shows an example of a client diagnosed with "dissociative identity disorder" (for a detailed description of this case, see Schiepek, Stöger-Schmidinger, Aichhorn, Schöller, & Aas, 2016a). The time series of the raw data are quite noisy and fluctuating (Fig. 3a), whereas the factor dynamics shows a much clearer Gestalt with one dominating order transition (Fig. 3b) (see the "short case illustration" below). The SNS also allows for the superposition of several time series in a diagram, which creates an optimized picture of critical instabilities and order transitions (Fig. 2a).

Colored raw data diagrams transform the values of all included time series as given by the items of a process questionnaire into rainbow colors. These diagrams create a synopsis of the evolutionary pattern of multiple time series (Fig. 4).

Short Case Illustration

The case of Mrs. A. diagnosed with "dissociative identity disorder" and "Borderline Personality Disorder" was before therapy and through the first half of the therapy marked by a pattern of roughly daily interchanging ego states. At a certain point of the therapy (marked as time point number 1 in Figs. 5 and 9), this alternating pattern disappeared. Then, the client had abolished her previous goal to soon enter the first labor market again, which she

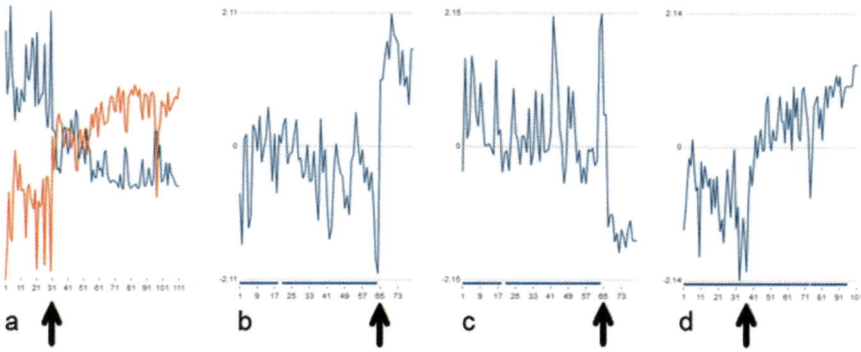

Fig. 2 Time series of factors of the TPQ. (**a**) Two factors superimposed: "Problem and symptom severity" (blue) and "self-awareness/body experience" (red; same client as in Figs. 1a and 4b). (**b**) "Therapeutic progress/confidence/self-efficacy," (c) "problem and symptom severity." (**b**) and (**c**) refer to the same client as Figs. 1b,c, 4a, 8, 10, and 12, (**d**) "therapeutic progress/confidence/self-efficacy" (another client). The arrows indicate significant order transitions

described as a great relief. An attractive job offer by a friend had triggered days of ambivalent feelings, ambiguity, and inner conflicts (critical fluctuations before the order transition). Instead of her earlier behavior of allowing others to "whip her into" new situations, she was capable to allow herself of turning down the offer. She experienced this decision as big liberation, listening to her inner voice. A process enabled by previous work on traumata and states, in which the creation of an idiographic system model and thereby the better understanding of mechanics of her state dynamics played a major role (e.g., understanding the relation between as disturbing experienced voices and incidences of traumatizing violence in earlier relationships).

Mrs. A's record in her SNS-based electronic diary at this order transition said: "…I have the feeling of being myself again (…) the last couple of days were unpleasant and painful. (…) Decisions for the time after the hospital stay have been made, that are better for me. I want to make peace with myself, which not always works out, but is so important!! Because the last years I always tried and worked on myself to find work again, but always felt so much stress and pressure (…) and that is not how things work!! My switches are set differently (…), in order to have some room for peace and let the stress go and to think about, what I really want to do and what I could work. (…) I will not surrender, to nothing and nobody!!"

This pattern transition can be seen in the item's and factor's time series (comp. Fig. 3 and 5). Also the mutually exclusive correlation pattern of the personality states (items of factors I and II, see Fig. 5a and 11a) disappeared almost immediately after the order transition (Fig. 5a and 11b). All this information was integrated to the ongoing therapy, clarifying the change in terms of state dynamics and related cognitions and emotions, for both therapist and client.

Accompanied was this crisis and the resolution thereof by an increase of depression and stress scores (assessed by the weekly administered DASS-21), followed by a drop to low scores on these attributes just at the order transition (Fig. 9a). Figure 9b shows an increased inter-item-synchronization during the state-driven pattern before the first order transition (pathological oversynchronization), which disappeared after the order transition (flag 1) (this case is presented in detail in Schiepek, Stöger-Schmidinger, Aichhorn, Schöller, & Aas, 2016a).

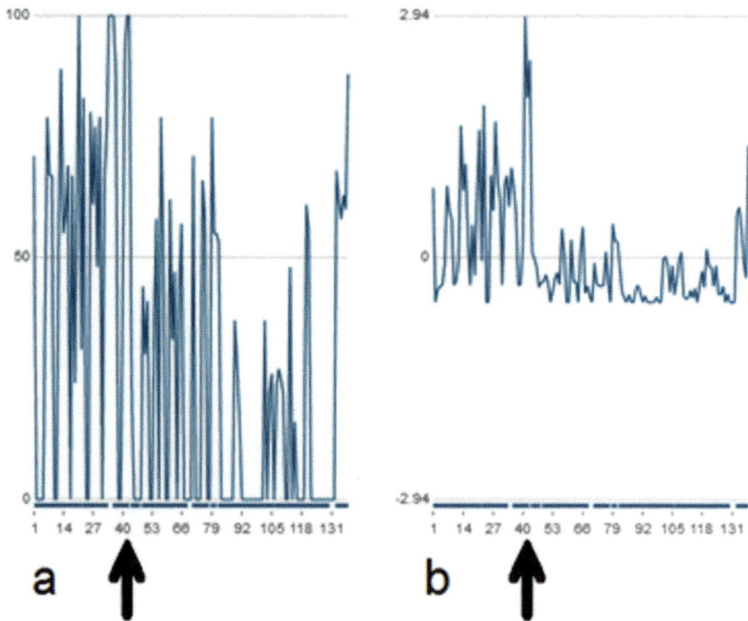

Fig. 3 (**a**) Time series of the item "Today I experienced stress." (**b**) Time series of the factor "stress and coping with stress" (individualized questionnaire). The items of this factor correspond to a child-related ego state of a client diagnosed with "dissociative identity disorder" (see also Figs. 5, 9, and 11, which refer to the same client). The arrows indicate the dominating order transition

Pattern transitions appear not only in changed mean levels of a time series but also in their variability, rhythms, frequency distribution, complexity, or other dynamic features. The option of a superposition of time series in a diagram (Fig. 2a) or the visualization of colored raw data diagrams can show such synchronized or anti-synchronized rhythms in multiple time series (Fig. 5a). In some cases, order transitions are characterized by the emergence or submergence of synchronized rhythms.

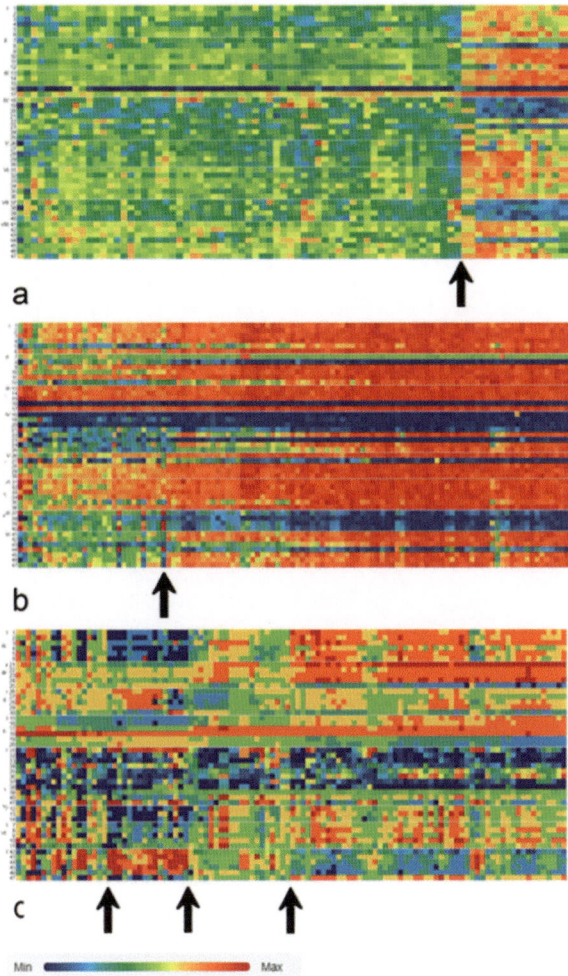

Fig. 4 Color-coded raw data diagrams. The arrows indicate significant transitions. (**a**) Same client as in Figs. 1b,c, 2b,c, 8, 10, and 12; (**b**) same client as in Figs. 1a, 2a, and 6. X-axis: time (days)

A common precursor of order transitions is critical instability (Haken, 2004; Haken & Schiepek, 2006). In the SNS this is represented by the measure of dynamic complexity, which combines the amplitude, the frequency, and the distribution of the values of a signal over the available range of a scale. All three features (amplitude, frequency, and distribution) are calculated within a gliding window which runs over the time series (given daily measures the usual window width is 7 days) (Haken & Schiepek, 2006; Schiepek & Strunk, 2010). The evolution of dynamic complexity can be presented as time series (Fig. 6) or as colored complexity resonance diagrams (Fig. 7). In the resonance diagrams, vertical columns or sudden changes of complexity over many items indicate order transitions. Another way of

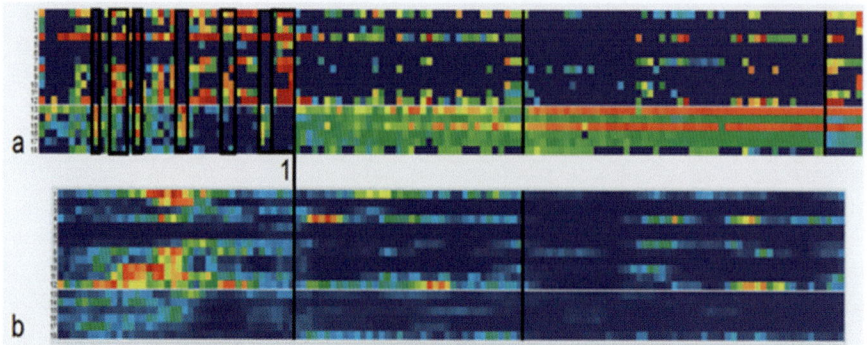

Fig. 5 (a) Color-coded raw data diagram of a client diagnosed with "dissociative identity disorder" (individualized questionnaire). X-axis: time (days). Blue colors represent low intensities, yellow to red colors represent high intensities of the ratings. The vertical line (1) indicates the most significant order transition of this therapy. Before the first transition, an alternating pattern between the items corresponding to two ego states can be identified. Black frames underline periods of alternating item scores and manifestations of states. Items 1 to 12 correspond to a "child state", shown above the thin white line in the diagram; items 13 to 18 correspond to an "adult state", shown under the thin white line. (b) Complexity resonance diagram of this client's change process. The cluster of high dynamic complexity occurs especially in the items of the "child state" before the order transition occurs (at 1), corresponding to the intensely fluctuating and mutually exclusive states. The x-axis is time (days) or, to be more precise, the number of overlapping running windows (window width: 7 days)

representing dynamic complexity is not to include all complexity values from all items and to transform them into colors, but to calibrate the complexity values within each time series. The ten highest complexity values of an item's time series are transformed into gray steps (from black corresponding to the highest to a bright gray as the lowest complexity value, all others are white). This procedure is more sensitive to low complexity values and shows the synchronization of intra-item calibrated complexity in a gray-step diagram (Fig. 8).

In some cases, the weekly assessed symptom or stress intensity may indicate an upcoming order transition. In the example presented in Fig. 9a, the intensities of depression and stress are increased just before the order transition takes place. After this transition, the values are significantly reduced. In routine practice, depression, anxiety, and stress are assessed once per week by the short form of the Depression Anxiety Stress Scales (DASS-21; Lovibond & Lovibond, 1995).

Another precursor of order transitions is increased synchronization of emotions and cognitions, as represented by the items of a process questionnaire. In the SNS, the absolute (sign-independent) values of inter-item correlations of a questionnaire are averaged within a moving window and presented as averaged correlation strengths over time. This is a measure of coherence (in terms of Synergetics: "enslaving") of the dynamics (Figs. 9b and 10). The changes of all inter-item correlations are presented in a sequence of correlation matrices with color-coded correlations (from −1 [dark red] over 0 [white] to +1 [dark green]). The correlation

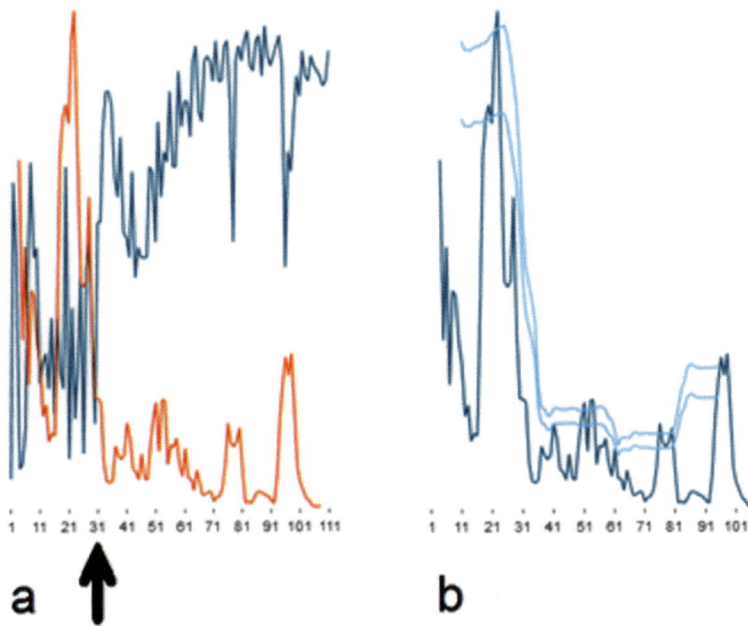

Fig. 6 (a) Dynamic complexity (red) of the time series "Today I felt joy" (blue, see Fig. 1a). In the SNS diagrams, the dynamic complexity curve (red) can be superimposed onto the time series of raw data or factors. The complexity peak precedes the order transition. (b) Over the dynamic complexity (blue line), dynamic confidence intervals are calculated in a running window (95% and 99%, bright blue lines). The width of the running window for the calculation is 21

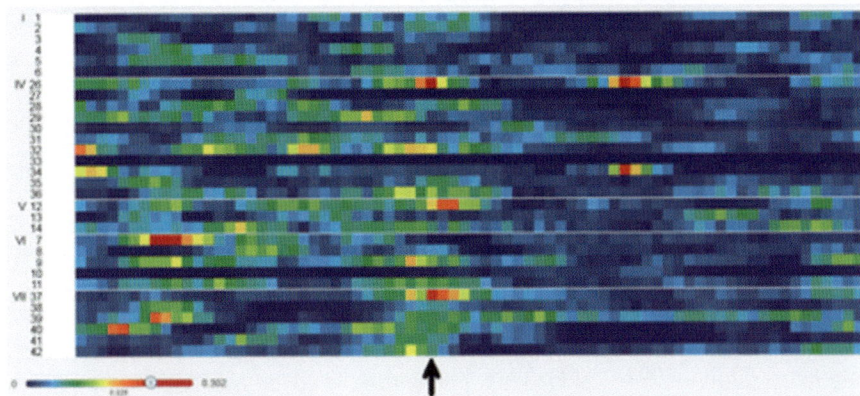

Fig. 7 Complexity resonance diagram. The dynamic complexity is calculated in overlapping running windows (window width = 7 days). Each line corresponds to an item of the process questionnaire (TPQ, factors II, III, VIII not shown). The maximum score of the dynamic complexity is depicted by a full red pixel, while all other values are graded according to that maximum (red = high, yellow = medium, blue = low complexity). The order transition is marked by the arrow. The x-axis is time (days) or, to be more precise, the number of overlapping running windows

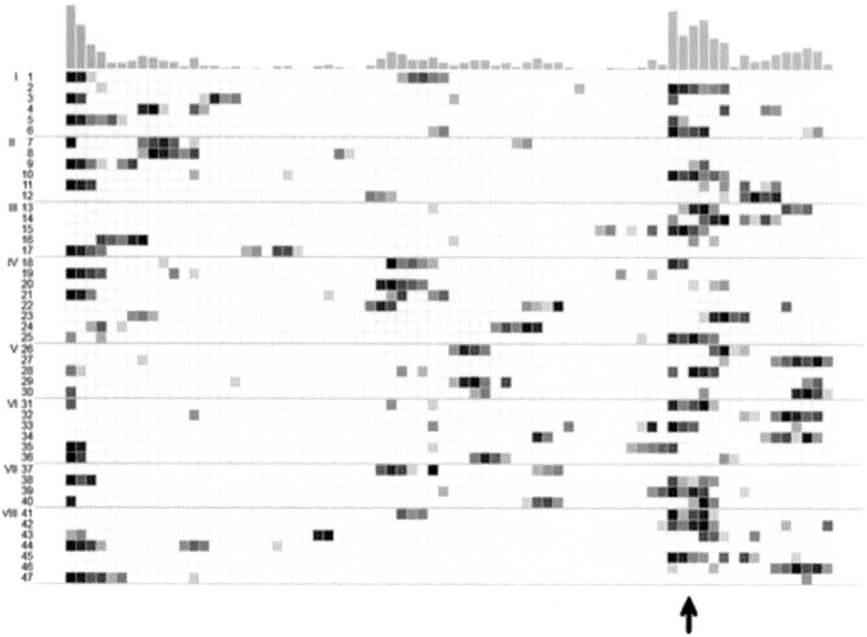

Fig. 8 Complexity resonance diagram, based on an intra-item calibration of the dynamic complexity. Each line corresponds to an item of the TPQ. The ten highest complexity values of each item are coded by gray steps. The arrow indicates the order transition (same client as in Figs. 1b,c, 2b,c, 4a, 10, 12). The x-axis is time (days) or, to be more precise, the number of overlapping running windows (window width: 7 days)

matrices are calculated within a running window (the window width is up to free choice, here: 7). A marker can be dragged along the time points to display the change of synchronization patterns over time. The local increase of the absolute inter-item synchronization together with a more pronounced correlation pattern of the matrices in many cases corresponds to a qualitative change of the correlation pattern. Figure 11 illustrates this pattern transition in the case of the client diagnosed with "dissociative identity disorder." Before the first-order transition, the correlation matrix represents the alternating ego states (high positive *intra*-state correlations of cognitions and emotions [green], high negative *inter*-state correlations [red]) which is dissolved after the order transition.

A method which identifies recurrent patterns within a time series in a time×time diagram is Recurrence Plots (Eckmann, Oliffson Kamphorst, & Ruelle, 1987; Webber & Zbilut, 1994). Snippets of a longer time series are embedded in a phase space with time-delay coordinates. Each snippet represents a vector point in the phase space (with each measurement point represented on an axis). The Euclidean distances between the vector points can be binary coded according to a selected threshold or, alternatively, the distances can be directly color-coded. By this means, recurrent patterns and their transients (e.g., periods of critical instability) become apparent. Usually, Recurrence Plots and CRDs show complementary patterns:

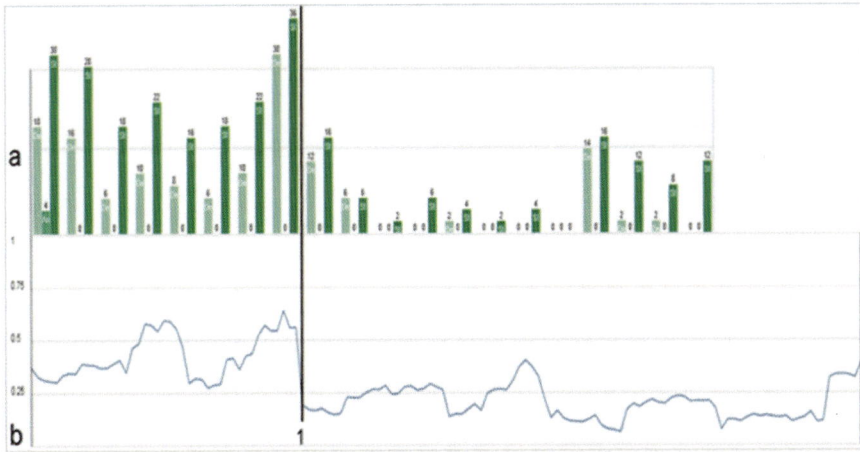

Fig. 9 (**a**) Intensity of depression (light green columns), anxiety (except for the first week always at 0), and stress (dark green columns), assessed once per week by the DASS-21 (Lovibond & Lovibond, 1995). Just before the order transition (vertical line), the values are increased; after it the values decrease immediately to a lower level. (**b**) Averaged inter-item correlation calculated in a running window of 7 measurement points. The first part of the process is characterized by a pathological oversynchronization with the maximum just before the order transition (vertical line, same client as in Figs. 3, 5, and 11)

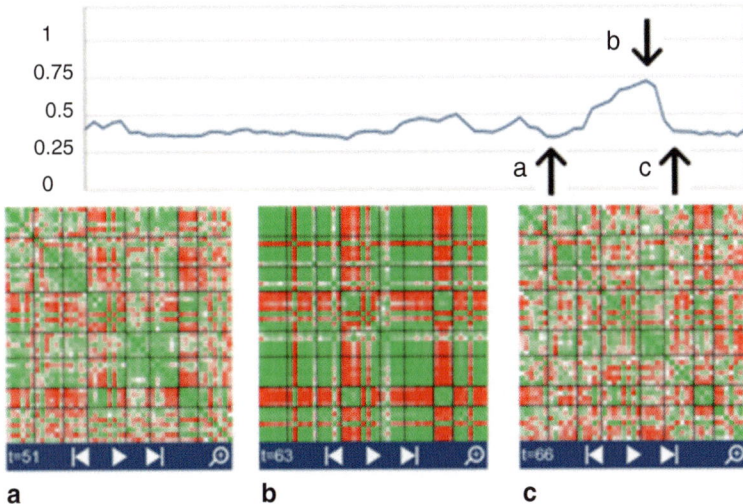

Fig. 10 Locally increased inter-item synchronization during the period of an order transition (arrow at **b**). The inter-item correlation matrices show an intensified and more pronounced pattern during the order transition compared to the matrices before and after the transition (**a** before, **b** during, **c** after). Each cell of the matrices depicts the correlation of a respective item with another item on a gradual green (positive correlation values, $0 < r < 1$) or red (negative correlation values, $-1 < r < 0$) scale (white cells correspond to a correlation of 0) (same client as in Figs. 1b,c, 2b,c, 4a, 8)

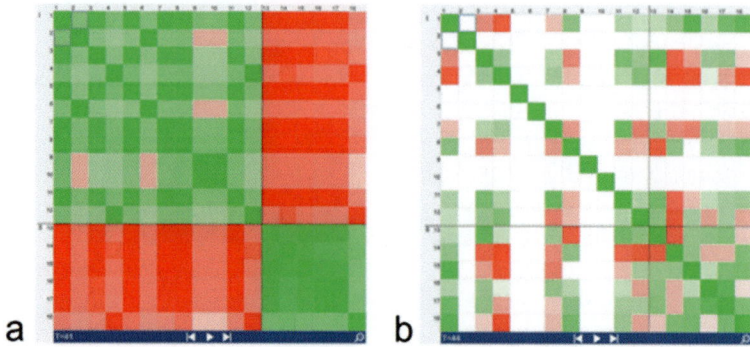

Fig. 11 (**a**) Color-coded inter-item correlation pattern characterizing the first third of the monitoring period (before the vertical line in Figs. 5 and 9). The black lines differentiate the items of factor I ("child state") and factor II ("adult state"). The left matrix ($t = 41$–47) is characterized by high positive within-factor item correlations (green colors) and negative between-factor item correlations (red colors). (**b**) Only some days later ($t = 49$–56), but after the main transition of the therapy (occurring at the vertical line in Figs. 5 and 9), this pattern dissolved. The change of correlation patterns concurs with the client's reports of increasing integration of her separate ego states throughout the therapeutic process

transient periods (yellow to red colors; out-of-attractor dynamics) correspond to periods of critical instabilities and, hence, increased dynamic complexity, whereas recurrent periods (turquoise to blue) represent more or less stable quasi-attractors. Figure 12 illustrates the transition from one stable pattern to another (blue rectangles), with a short transient period in between (yellow to orange pixels).

Besides the transition markers which are technically implemented in the SNS, there are others, like increased local frequencies, as identified by the wavelet-based method of time-frequency distributions (Cohen, 1989; see Haken & Schiepek, 2006, pp. 402ff.) or change points which can be identified by the method of change point analysis (James & Matteson, 2014). It should be noted that the coincidence of more than one transition marker or precursor is needed to identify an order transition (Schiepek et al., in review).

Dynamic Patterns of Interpersonal Systems

In order to assess interpersonal dynamics as they are realized in couple therapy, family therapy, or team development projects, the SNS offers two options: The first is to superimpose the time series of several persons (e.g., family or team members) in one and the same diagram. By this the processes of more than one person can directly be compared. For example, the experienced well-being or stress of the family members can be shown in superimposed time series. The other option is based on the assessment of sent or received communications by all involved members of a social system – a method which is called *dynamic interaction matrices* (Schiepek et al., 2015). In a first step, the dimensions on which this "sending" and "receiving" is experienced

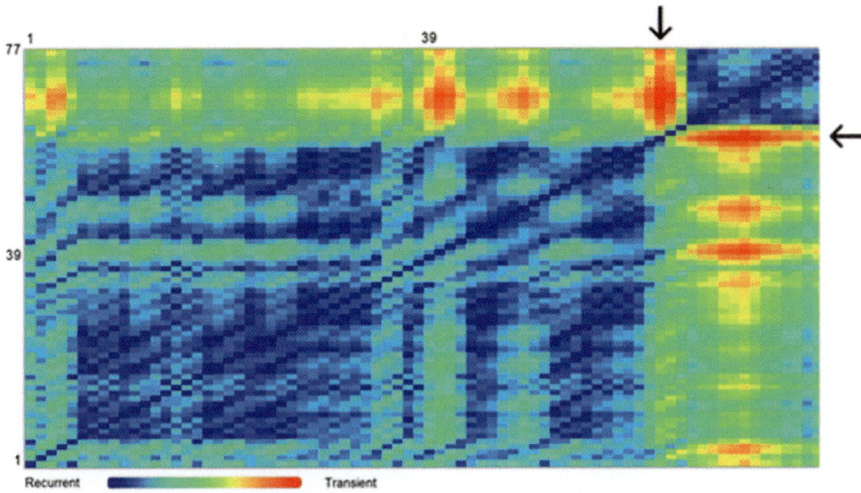

Fig. 12 Recurrence Plot. The arrows show a short transient period (coded by yellow to red colors) between two more stable quasi-attractors (compare Figs. 1b,c, 2b,c, 4a, and 8)

have to be defined, e.g., support, information flow, or stress. The questionnaire asks for the intensity of sending the defined quality (e.g., support) from one person to all others (arrows) and also for the intensity of receiving this quality from all other persons (counter-arrows, i.e., the space around the arrows in the cells). When all persons involved in the communication process during a defined period (e.g., a family therapy session) have rated their exchange, the results are presented by an interaction matrix, with the persons as senders arranged in lines and the persons as receivers arranged in columns (Fig. 13). The numbers in the lines at the right border of the matrices and under the columns at the bottom of the matrices represent the sum or the average of all arrows in a line (sent by one person) or the sum or average of all arrows in a column (sent to a person). The second number represents the perceived intensity of received communication (counter-arrows from one person as perceived by all others in lines, counter-arrows from all others as perceived by one person in columns).

Usually interaction matrices are assessed repeatedly, e.g., after every therapy session, every week, or every month (e.g., in a longer process of organizational dynamics). The sequence of such matrices can be visualized in the diagram wizard of the SNS by dragging a flag along a time series which represents the relation of sending (intensity of all arrows) and receiving (intensity of all counter-arrows). Methods like the interaction matrix which can be scaled up to 100 or more persons or the option of comparing the dynamics of many persons by time series diagrams can be used for the monitoring of change processes in organizations, interconnected teams, or other interpersonal networks. Current developments of the SNS concern the option of introducing not only time series from one and the same process questionnaire (intra-individual assessment) into raw data diagrams or complexity resonance diagrams but from different persons (inter-individual assessment). Here the lines would represent persons corresponding to different teams or departments of an organization. The SNS is on the way to get a powerful monitoring tool for change dynamics in organizations.

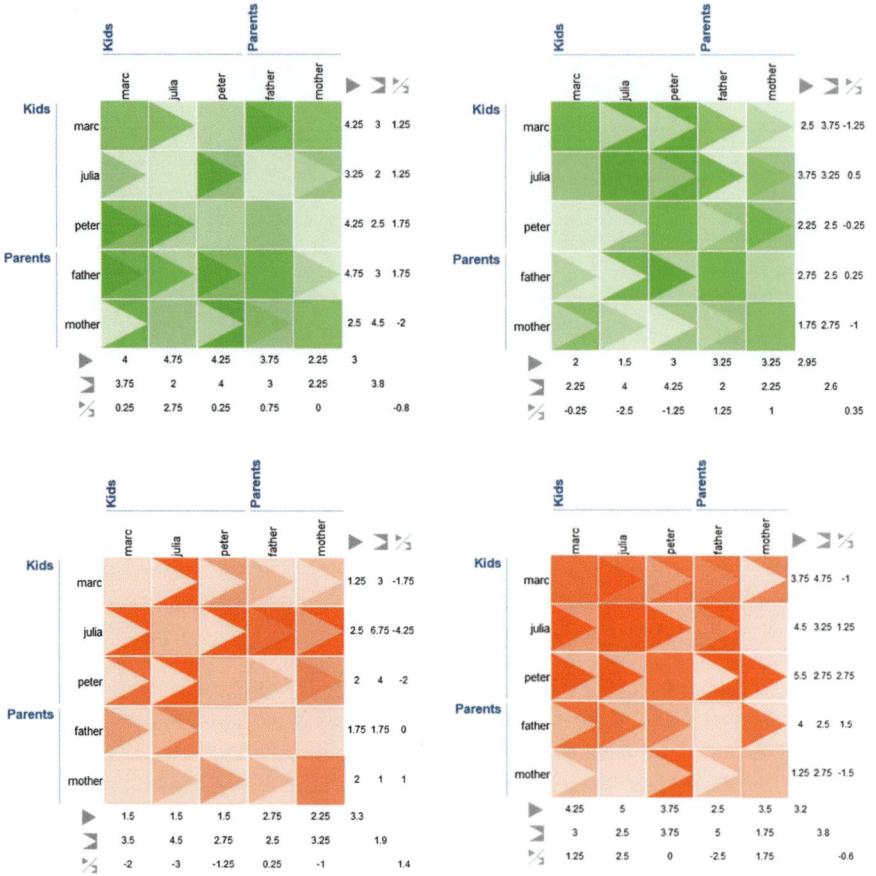

Fig. 13 Snapshots from a sequence of interaction matrices taken from 20 family therapy sessions. The matrices refer to session 8 (left) and session 17 (right). Upper part (green colors): The family members (father, mother, and the kids Marc, Julia and Peter) rated the intensities of sending (arrows) and receiving (counter-arrows in the cells) "support" to and from each other. Lower part (red colors): sending and receiving "stress"

Criteria of a Systemic Monitoring and Feedback Approach on Change Dynamics

Feedback procedures are able to capture the nonlinear features of human dynamics. Ten years of experience with the Synergetic Navigation System allowed for a deep insight into these features in many cases (e.g., Heinzel, Tominschek, & Schiepek, 2014; Schiepek, Tominschek, & Heinzel, 2014; Schiepek et al. 2016b). Actually, a data set of about 1.100 valid cases is available from different treatment centers. This continuously increasing data base opens the door to the investigation of many research questions and to a further validation of the mostly used process questionnaire (Therapy Process Questionnaire, TPQ; Schiepek et al., 2019a). In times of upcoming doubts on research results based on smaller (RCT) samples, it is important for quantitative and qualitative psychotherapy science to enter the world of big data. Perhaps more important is the option to combine big data with the individualization of measures and treatment procedures (e.g., Fisher, 2015; Fisher & Bosley, 2015; Schiepek et al., 2015).

Compared to other approaches in psychotherapy feedback, systemic concepts make a difference in practice as well as in technology. Most of the existing approaches focus on outcome and are far from any high-frequency assessment of change dynamics. Usually data are taken only at therapy sessions. In consequence, they cannot identify nonlinear features of change processes (e.g., order transitions, critical instabilities) and expect linear standard tracks of change dynamics. In contrast to this, the following criteria should be respected within a systemic monitoring approach:

- The theoretical framework is given by systemic theories like Synergetics, chaos theory, and complexity science.
- In order to identify the core concepts of systemic theories, e.g., dynamic patterns and pattern transitions, critical instabilities, or synchronization, it is necessary to assess processes and to visualize the processes by time series.
- The implemented linear and nonlinear methods of time series analysis should be able to identify important features of complex, nonlinear dynamics and self-organization.
- Sampling rates should be up to free choice, may it be event sampling or time sampling. In clinical practice, the preferred sampling rate is once per day. This is not imposed by the system, but is a decision of clinicians.
- Flexibility should exist concerning the applied questionnaires. In the SNS, standardized or individualized questionnaires – which are developed together with the client – can be used and combined. Of course, also process and outcome measures can be used and combined.
- Assessment of therapy outcome can be done in different ways: At rare time points – e.g., pre, post, follow-up – primary and secondary outcomes can be assessed. Based on high-frequency measurements, changing dynamic patterns of behavior, cognitions, and emotions can be identified. An example would be the transition of emotional instability of a borderline personality disorder to a more stable pattern of emotion processing.
- It should be possible to assess interpersonal patterns. In the SNS, this can be realized by dynamic interaction matrices or by superimposed time series from different persons.
- Individualized and client-specific procedures in psychotherapy and counseling should be facilitated by monitoring systems. Personalized procedures are based on the option of using individualized questionnaires and by mirroring individual dynamic patterns.

Understanding the Mechanisms of Change

The Investigation of Order Transitions

High-frequency monitoring of change dynamics provides the data base for understanding the mechanisms of change in psychotherapy and counseling. Especially from Synergetics and chaos theory hypotheses can be derived which are up for empirical proof. One hypothesis is that phase-transition-like phenomena (order transitions) characterize the short-term as well as the long-term evolution of cognitive, affective, and social networks. In order to investigate these phenomena in psychotherapy, we used the data from daily self-assessments of 18 clients diagnosed with obsessive-compulsive disorder (OCD; ICD diagnosis, F42; average age, 32.2 years, SD = 9.6; 9 female, 9 male) (Heinzel et al., 2014; Schiepek et al., 2014). The therapies were realized in a day-treatment center in Munich. Mean duration of treatment was 61 days (SD = 12.5, range from 37 to 88 days). Exposure with response prevention (ERP) was the most important intervention of the therapy. ERP is a therapeutic procedure where clients are confronted with symptom-provoking stimuli but abstain from performing compulsive rituals (e.g., cleaning). Every day, clients completed the Therapy Process Questionnaire (TPQ) and two times per week the Yale-Brown Obsessive Compulsive Scale (Y-BOCS), a self-assessment scale for obsessions and compulsions (Goodman et al., 1989). In order to compare individual change dynamics to ERP, we related the individual symptom severity trajectories to the onset of ERP.

The measure of dynamic complexity was calculated for the items of the TPQ in a running window (window width: 7 days). The time series of each client reveals increased dynamic complexity of the subscales and most of the items of the TPQ just before or during sudden changes, which were characterized by the steepest decrease gradient of the Y-BOCS scores. Significant decrease of symptom severity takes place before (!) the most important therapeutic intervention (ERP) has started. Figure 14 illustrates the mean z-transformed complexity signal of the change processes of all clients. Besides a complexity peak at the beginning of the treatment, which may be interpreted as an initial instability period representing individual ambiguity and varying degrees of working intensity, the most important peak occurred 3 days before the steepest gradient of symptom reduction was realized and about 7 days before ERP (flooding) onset (T(17) = 2.48, p = 0.026). In terms of Synergetics, this corresponds to the assumed critical instabilities accompanying order transitions of a self-organizing process.

Another study investigated order transitions of brain activity related to subjective experiences of clients during their psychotherapy process (Schiepek et al., 2013). Repeated fMRI scans were related to the degree of stability or instability of the ongoing dynamics (measured by the dynamic complexity of daily TPQ-ratings). The time series of dynamic complexity were averaged over the items of the TPQ, and the maxima of these dynamics were used as an indicator of the most intensive fluctuation periods and the discontinuous transition(s) during the therapies. Three or four fMRI scans were realized during each of the psychotherapy processes of nine clients and

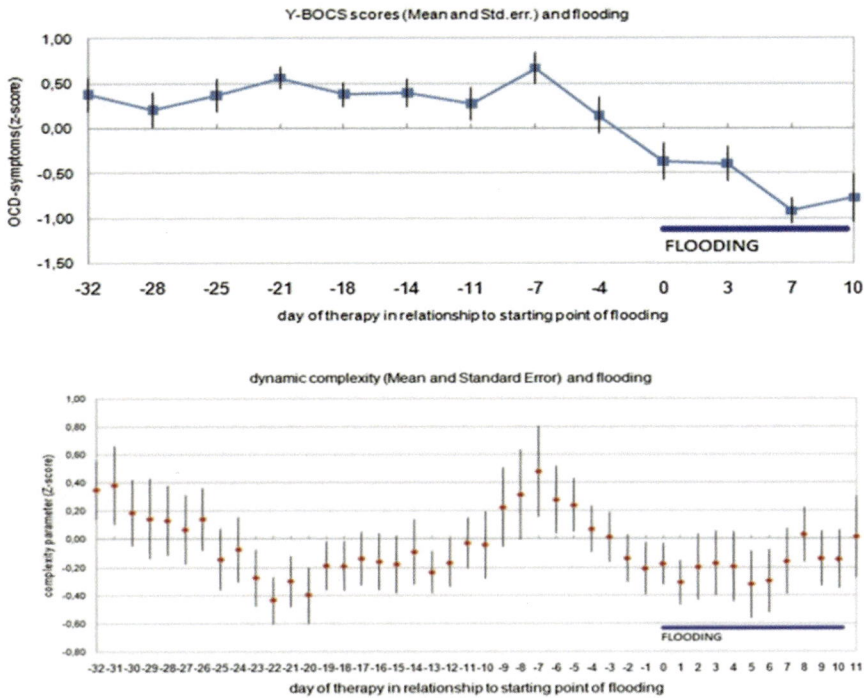

Fig. 14 Mean course of symptom severity (Y-BOCS, z-transformed) (upper part of the Figure), and mean course of the dynamic complexity of the TPQ (z-transformed) (lower part of the Figure), normalized in relation to the beginning of ERP. Vertical bars: standard error. The figure aggregates the dynamics of all 18 clients. For each client, the individual ERP onset was defined at $t = 0$, and the trajectories of the total Y-BOCS scores were related to this event. In 72% of the 18 cases, the steepest gradient of symptom change was located before ERP onset. The figure illustrates that the mean trajectory of the z-transformed individual total scores of the Y-BOCS has its steepest change gradient before ERP starts ($t = -4$ days), and symptom severity reaches a significantly reduced level at the day of ERP onset at $t = 0$ (T(17) = 3.07; $p = 0.007$). The averaged dynamic complexity reaches a maximum value at about 7 days before ERP (flooding) starts

compared to the scans of nine healthy controls. The study included clients with obsessive-compulsive disorder (OCD) of the washing/contamination fear subtype (DSM IV, 300.3), without comorbid psychiatric or somatic diagnoses. All clients except of one were drug naïve. Clients were matched to healthy controls. The visual stimulation paradigm of the fMRI scans used individualized symptom provoking, disgust provoking, and neutral pictures. The disgust and the neutral pictures were taken from the International Affective Picture System, whereas the client-specific OCD-related pictures were photographed in the home setting of the clients. Here we refer on the contrast of individualized symptom-provoking pictures vs. neutral pictures.

Eight brain regions (ROIs) were identified that are important in OCD-related neuronal processing: the anterior and the medial cingulate cortex as well as the supplementary motor area (CC/SMA), the dorsolateral prefrontal cortex (DLPFC) right and left, the insular cortex right and left, the parietal cortex right and left, and the cuneus.

When interscan intervals including order transitions (OT) were compared to intervals without (no) order transitions (NOT), the changes of the number of significant voxels for the contrast between individualized symptom-provoking pictures and neutral pictures show increased BOLD responses during OT in all relevant brain regions. The healthy controls received no therapy so that any distinction between intervals with and without order transitions has no importance. In healthy subjects functional changes were averaged across all interscan intervals (ISI). Figure 15 illustrates the changes in significant voxels averaged for each of the eight brain areas of OT and NOT of the clients and of interstimulus intervals (ISI) of the controls. Activation rates and change rates were significantly higher for clients compared to controls.

The differences between order transition intervals (OT) of the clients (mean voxel number difference: 7480, SD: 6835) and non-order-transition intervals (NOT) of clients (mean voxel number difference: 1900, SD: 1968) reached significance. In addition, the number of activated voxels differenced significantly between order transition intervals of clients and the interscan intervals (ISI) of the controls, whereas the differences between the NOT intervals of clients and the ISI intervals of the controls were quite similar. For each of the eight brain regions, pronounced differences occurred between OT and NOT and even more clearly for OT vs. ISI, but not for NOT vs. ISI. The most pronounced differences were realized in the CC/SMA, the DLPFC left, the DLPFC right, and the insula right. The differences in the area of the cuneus and the left parietal cortex did not reach significance because of large confidence intervals of the NOT number voxel differences. The high individual variability is partly the result of distinctly differing change patterns in clients as well as therapy processes.

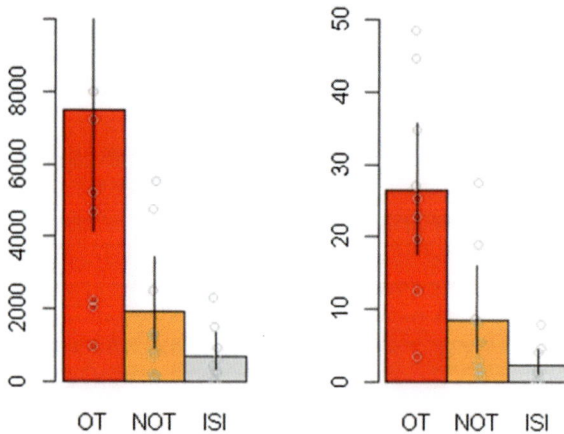

Fig. 15 Differences of significant voxels (averaged over subjects) between fMRI scans. OT (red): Differences between scans before and after an order transition occurred; NOT (yellow): Differences between scans where no order transition occurred (non-order transitions); ISI (gray): interscan intervals of fMRI scans of healthy controls. 95% confidence intervals of the means (vertical lines) were bootstrapped with R's boot.ci function using 10,000 resamples and the "bca" type of confidence intervals

An additional result concerned the intercorrelations of the involved brain areas. When comparing correlations before and after order transitions, the difference is striking, independent of where the order transitions were located in the course of therapy. The mean intercorrelation of the brain areas changed from 0.73 (SD: 0.09) to 0.33 (SD: 0.33) (p of the difference < 0.001). In addition to the decline in correlation, a differentiation of intercorrelations occurred which is reflected in an increase in variation (standard deviation of the intercorrelations increased from 0.09 to 0.33). This could be taken as an indicator of a decreased (pathological) network synchronization of OCD-specific brain areas.

To conclude: Most clients showed clearly recognizable order transitions in different brain areas. Changes in the activity of brain areas outside of order transitions were considerably weaker, similar to the differences between fMRI scans of the healthy controls which did not undergo psychotherapy and by this did not experience any significant dynamic changes. The strong connection between cognitive-affective order transitions and BOLD responses reversely validate the operationalization of order transitions by the maximum of dynamic complexity of the time series gained from daily self-assessments by the Synergetic Navigation System.

Modeling the Mechanisms and Dynamics of Psychotherapeutic Change

Like all other fields of research, systemic research tries to combine empirical studies with theoretical modeling. Conjectures and hypotheses are based on theoretical models of the systems under investigation. Because of its focus on complexity and dynamics, modeling plays an outstanding role in systemic research. The *explanandum* not only is the outcome of change processes but the process itself. We have to explain the mechanisms behind the dynamics of nonlinear systems, what needs for a qualitative modeling of the involved variables and parameters *and* for mathematical formalizations. In a next step, computer-based simulations of the processes can be realized ("experimentum in silico"). One example for theoretical systems research (*computational systems psychology*) is the modeling of client-related mechanisms of change. We developed a model which is based on profound knowledge in cognitive, emotional, and motivational psychology, psychopathology, and research on common factors of psychotherapy (described elsewhere, see Schiepek et al., 2017; Schöller et al., 2018). It includes five variables which are connected by 16 functions (Fig. 16a, b). The functions are represented in mathematical terms, which are integrated into five coupled nonlinear equations (one for each variable). The graphs in the coordinate planes of Fig. 16b (x-axis, input variable; y-axis, output variable) illustrate how the shape of each respective function depends on the parameter values. The full range of the variables is covered by the functions defining the influence of other variables, that is, there are no arbitrary segmentations or thresholds, which would have been introduced from the beginning. Thresholds and discontinuous jumps of the dynamics are emerging from the dynamics and not forced by specific predefined assumptions.

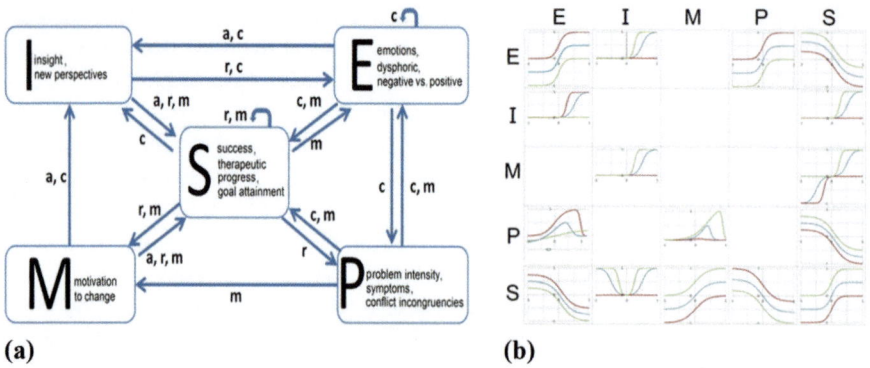

(a)   (b)

Fig. 16 A client-centered theoretical model of psychotherapeutic change. (**a**) The structure of the model illustrates the dependencies between the variables and the parameters of the system. (**b**) The matrix represents the 16 functions of the model (for a detailed description, see Schiepek et al., 2017). The variables noted on the left of the matrix (lines) represent the input; the variables noted at the top (columns) represent the output. Each function is represented by a graph in a coordinate system (x-axis, input; y-axis: output). Green function graphs correspond to the maximum of the respective control parameter(s) (= 1), red graphs to the minimum of the parameter(s) (= 0). Blue graphs represent an in-between state (0 < parameter value <1)

The model includes the following variables and parameters:

(E) Emotions. This bidimensional variable represents dysphoric emotions (e.g., anxiety, grief, shame, guilt, and anger) at the upper end of the dimension (positive values of E) and positive emotional experiences (e.g., joy, self-esteem, happiness) at the lower end (negative values of E). This definition of polarity is based upon the results of a factor analysis of the TPQ (factor "dysphoric affectivity")

(P) Problem and stress intensity, symptom severity, experienced conflicts, or incongruence

(M) Motivation for change, readiness for the engagement in therapy-related activities and experiences

(I) Insight, getting new perspectives on personal problems, motivation, cognition, or behavior (clarification perspective in terms of Grawe.)

(S) Success, therapeutic progress, goal attainment, and confidece in a successful therapy course.

The parameters of the model mediate the interactions between variables. Depending on their values, the effect of one variable on another is intensified or reduced, activated, or inhibited. Formally, parameters modify the functions which define the relationship of the variables to each other:

(*a*) Working alliance, capability to enter a trustful cooperation with the therapist, quality of the therapeutic relationship, and interpersonal trust. This parameter signifies the disposition to engage in a trustful relationship (attachment disposition) and also resembles the realized quality of the therapeutic alliance.

(*c*) Cognitive competencies, capacities for mentalization and emotion regulation, and mental skills in self-reflection.

(*r*) Behavioral resources and skills for problem-solving.

(*m*) Motivation for change as a trait, self-efficacy, hopefulness, and reward expectation.

The model reproduces some basic features of human change dynamics, as chaoticity (Fig. 17), sensitive dependency of the dynamics on initial conditions, minor interventions, and parameter values, order transitions (sudden changes), time sensitivity of interventions, impact of dispositions and competencies on the course of psychotherapy, and others (Schiepek et al., 2017). One important development of the model is the evolution of parameters (competencies or traits of a client) depending on the variables (state dynamics). The model realizes a circular causality of the parameters (traits) on the variables (states) and of the variables on the parameters (Schöller et al., 2018). Parameters are changing at a slower time scale, but in principle, a co-evolutive loop is realized between variables and parameters. Figures 18 and 19 illustrate the dependency of the processes on interventions. Figure 18 shows how dynamic noise can trigger order transitions if a self-organized threshold is reached or fails to create an order transition below this threshold. Figure 19 illustrates some long-term dynamics after intensive continuous interventions on all variables (e.g., a hospital stay for inpatient psychotherapy), including a rebound effect after release from treatment and a long-term evolution to stable effects when external emotion regulation (e.g., anxiety-reducing drugs) is stopped.

Further steps are model testing by using empirical data from the SNS (Schöller, Viol, Goditsch, Aichhorn, Hütt, & Schiepek, 2019) and the integration of data-driven computer simulations of individual processes into therapy feedback and treatment control.

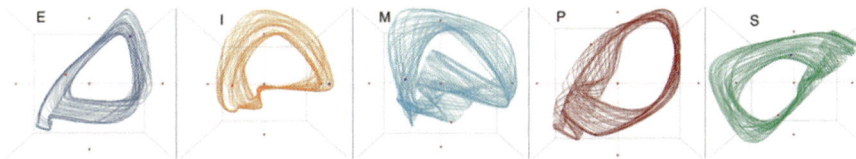

Fig. 17 The attractors of the variables E, P, M, I, S in a chaotic regime. *a*: 0.400; *c*: 0.675; *r*: 0.740; *m*: 0.475. Initial conditions of the simulation run: E: 0.99; P: 0.57; M: −0.34; I: 0.01; S: −0.32. Three-dimensional time delay embedding with $\tau = 1$. The attractors are based on 413 valid iterations (the last iterations from a simulation run of 5000 iterations) splined by the Excel standard spline function

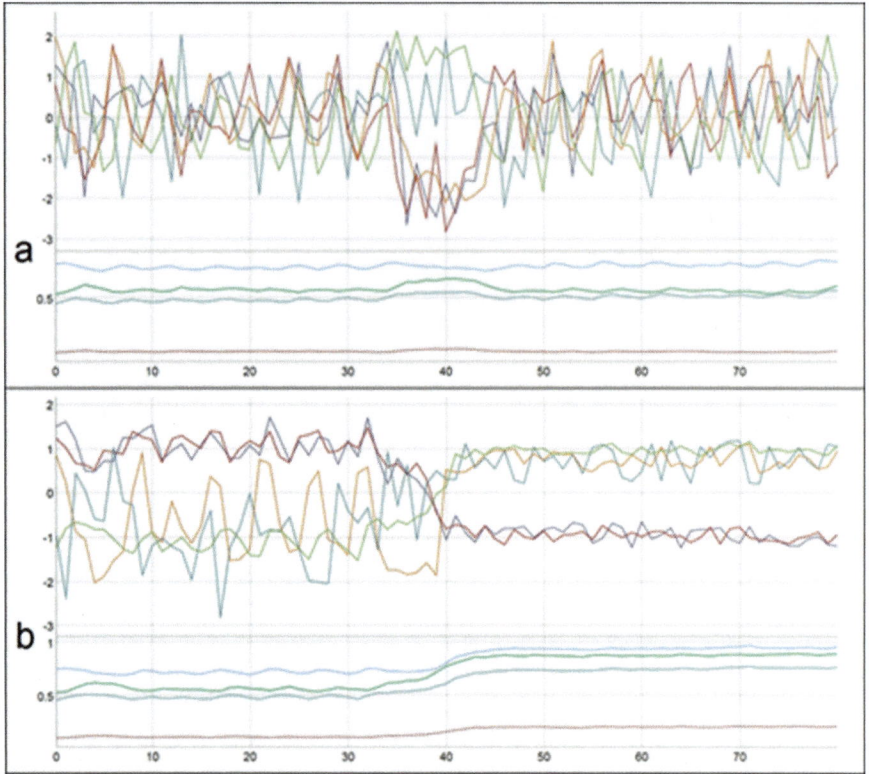

Fig. 18 Two realizations of dynamic noise (same amplitude and distribution of random numbers) applied on two realizations of simulation runs (**a** and **b**). Parameters: *a*: red; *m*: green; *c*: bright blue; *r*: dark blue. In both cases, the initial values of variables and parameters are identical: E: 97.6; P: 61.5; M: 7.5; I: 100; S: − 40.7. *a*: 0.10; *c*: 0.75; *r*: 0.46; *m*: 0.53. Dynamic noise 10% on E and P, 5% on M, I, and S, continuously. Data: (**a**) Direct access to simulation, Download CSV-file, (**b**) Direct access to simulation, Download CSV-file

Can Systemic Research Meet the Challenges of the Profession?

Coming back to the beginning, we refer to the challenges which were outlined in the introductory paragraph of this article. After presenting some ways of doing systemic research, it may be evident that at least some of the challenges can be met by the available methods and practice-related research strategies:

1. Deteriorations or precursors of dropouts can be identified in time by the process-related data and the analysis methods implemented in the SNS. Systemic methods of case formulation (Schiepek et al., 2015, 2016a) – which are beyond the scope of this article – provide the background for client-specific, tailored therapy concepts and for individualized questionnaires by which the monitoring of change processes can be optimized.

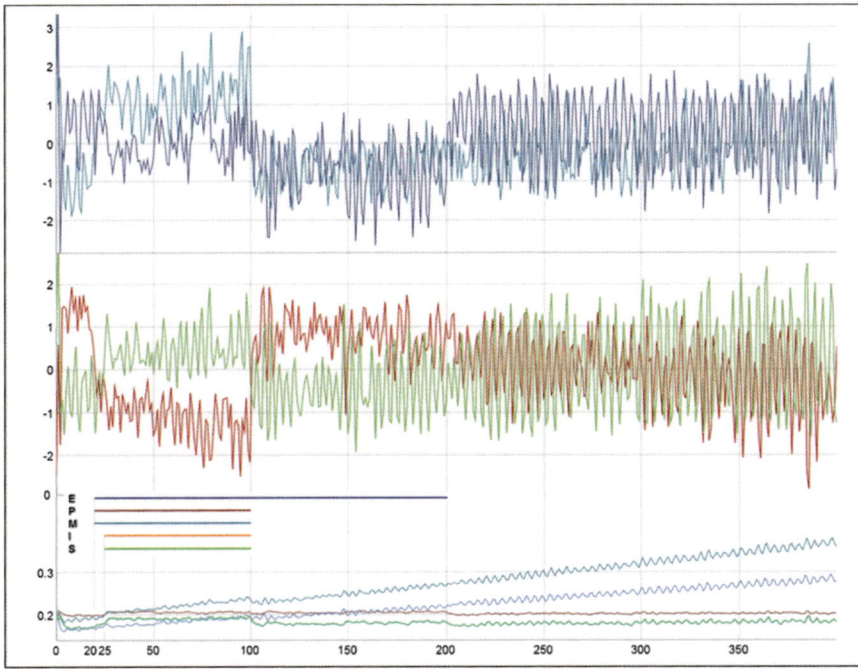

Fig. 19 Simulation run from $t = 1$ to $t = 400$. Assumed that one iteration corresponds to one measurement per day, 400 iterations represent a period of about 1 year and 1 month. Interventions on E, P, and M start at $t = 20$, interventions on I and S at $t = 25$ (+5% on M, + 10% on S and I, −10% on E and P). Except for E, all interventions end at $t = 100$, the intervention on E continues to $t = 200$. Effects of the interventions on all variables are to be seen but also a distinct rebound effect in S and M (decreases) and P (increase). The continued intervention (−10%) until $t = 200$ on E reduces stressful emotions but also the motivation to change (M) (upper part of the figure). After this period, M and S increase, and P decreases. It seems that a long-term recovery and self-healing process can only start if negative emotions no longer are suppressed, that is, the self-organizing effect onto another stable attractor can only take place if the system can follow its own unrestricted dynamics. Initial values of variables and parameters: E: 97.6; P: 61.5; M: 7.5; I: 100; S: −40.7; *a, c, r, m*: 0.20. Dynamic noise, 2%, continuously. (Data: Direct access to simulation, Download CSV-file)

2. Internet-based e-MentalHealth technologies like the SNS create a guiding thread across different segments of health care, like outpatient and inpatient psychotherapy. Clients can be monitored before, during, and after hospital stay and different professional health-care providers can use one and the same monitoring procedure, independent of the setting. This will contribute to the sustainability of treatment effects.
3. Complexity science, especially Synergetics and chaos theory, helps to understand the functioning of complex, self-organizing systems like brains, cognitive-emotional dynamics, and social networks. Beyond the meta-theoretical and paradigmatic framework for systemic research and practice, the development of concrete theories and models on the mechanisms of psychotherapy has started. These models integrate the knowledge of the ingredients and factors contributing

to the effects of psychotherapy (Schiepek et al., 2017; Schöller et al., 2018). The new transdisciplinary field of computational systems psychology opens the way to data-driven computer simulations of human change processes, which can be linked with real-time monitoring for the optimization and control of professional work.

4. The fact that we can neither predict the long-range trajectories of change nor the points in time when therapeutic crises will appear is an essential quality of non-linear systems. Another consequence of nonlinearity is that interventions only have a small impact on the outcome. Indeed, this has consequences for how we have to conceptualize human change processes. Psychotherapy or counseling is not the manualized administration of treatment techniques but the support of self-organizing processes, which are conceptualized by the generic principles and driven by feedback on the processes.

5. Indeed, the fact that discontinuous jumps to the better or to the worse usually are independent of specific interventions cannot be explained by linear models, but by nonlinear models. These models including computer simulations based on such models gave rise to quite sophisticated concepts of "interventions" which are far beyond the idea of simply "disturbing" systems or "disrupting" patterns (Schiepek, Schöller, Carl, Aichhorn, & Lichtwarck-Aschoff, 2019b).

6. The meta-theoretical framework of nonlinear complex systems and computational systems psychology together with specific concretizations in theory development, empirical research, and feedback-driven practice create a new unifying paradigm in psychotherapy. As we know, paradigms are not exclusive in psychology, but a useful general frame for understanding and optimizing the profession.

7. Computer-assisted and Internet-based monitoring of human change processes has opened the way for practice-based research in realistic settings of health care and creates more ecologically valid and generalizable results than RCTs in research settings ever can provide.

Summary: Systemic research – as outlined in this article – can meet some important challenges of psychotherapy and hopefully will contribute to the development of our profession.

References

Cohen, L. (1989). Time-frequency distributions – A review. *Proceedings of the IEEE, 77*, 941–981.

Duncan, B., Miller, S., Wampold, B., & Hubble, M. (2010). *The heart and soul of change* (2nd ed.). Washington, D.C.: APA.

Eckmann, J. P., Oliffson Kamphorst, S., & Ruelle, D. (1987). Recurrence plots of dynamical systems. *Europhysics Letters, 4*, 973–977.

Fartacek, C., Schiepek, G., Kunrath, S., Fartacek, R., & Plöderl, M. (2016). Real-time monitoring of nonlinear suicidal dynamics: Methodology and a demonstrative case report. *Frontiers in Psychology for Clinical Settings, 7*, 130. (1-14). https://doi.org/10.3389/fpsyg.2016.00130

Fisher, A. J. (2015). Toward a dynamic model of psychological assessment: Implications for personalized care. *Journal of Consulting and Clinical Psychology, 83*, 825–836.

Fisher, A. J., & Bosley, H. G. (2015). Personalized assessment and treatment of depression. *Current Opinion in Psychology, 4*, 67–74.

Goodman, W. K., Price, L. H., Rasmussen, S. A., Mazure, C., Fleischmann, R. L., Hill, C. L., … Charney, D. S. (1989). The Yale-Brown obsessive compulsive scale. I. Development, use, and reliability. *Archives of General Psychiatry, 46*, 1006–1011.

Haken, H. (2004). *Synergetics. Introduction and advanced topics*. Berlin: Springer.

Haken, H., & Schiepek, G. (2006). *Synergetik in der Psychologie [Synergetics in Psychology]* (2nd ed. 2010). Göttingen: Hogrefe.

Hansen, E. C. A., Battaglia, D., Spiegler, A., Deco, G., & Jirsa, V. K. (2015). Functional connectivity dynamics: Modeling the switching behavior of the resting state. *NeuroImage, 105*, 525–535.

Heinzel, S., Tominschek, I., & Schiepek, G. (2014). Dynamic patterns in psychotherapy – discontinuous changes and critical instabilities during the treatment of obsessive compulsive disorder. *Nonlinear Dynamics, Psychology, and Life Sciences, 18*, 155–176.

James, N. A., & Matteson, D. S. (2014). ecp: An R package for nonparametric multiple change point analysis of multivariate data. *Journal of Statistical Software, 62*(7).

Kazdin, A. E. (2009). Understanding how and why psychotherapy leads to change. *Psychotherapy Research, 19*, 418–428. https://doi.org/10.1080/10503300802448899

Lambert, M. J. (Ed.). (2013). *Bergin and Garfield's handbook of psychotherapy and behavior change* (6th ed.). New York, NY: Wiley.

Lovibond, S. H., & Lovibond, P. F. (1995). *Manual for the depression anxiety stress scales*. Sydney: Psychology Foundation.

Ochs, M., & Schweitzer, J. (Hrsg.) (1995). *Handbuch Forschung für Systemiker*. Göttingen: Vandenhoeck & Ruprecht.

Ochs, M. & Schweitzer, J. (Hrsg.) (2012). *Handbuch Forschung für Systemiker*. Göttingen: Vandenhoeck & Ruprecht.

Ritter, P., Schirner, M., McIntosh, A. R., & Jirsa, V. K. (2013). The virtual brain integrates computational modeling and multimodal neuroimaging. *Brain Connectivity, 3*, 121–145.

Schiepek, G. (2012). Systemische Forschung – ein Methodenüberblick *[Systemic research – an overview on methods]*. In M. Ochs & J. Schweitzer (Eds.), *Handbuch Forschung für Systemiker* (pp. 33–68). Göttingen: Vandenhoeck & Ruprecht.

Schiepek, G., Schöller, H., de Felice, G., Steffensen, S.V., Skaalum Bloch, M., Fartacek, C., … Viol. K. (in review). Convergent validation of methods for the identification of phase transitions in time series of empirical and model systems. *Frontiers in Psychology for Clinical Settings*.

Schiepek, G., Eckert, H., Aas, B., Wallot, S., & Wallot, A. (2015). *Integrative psychotherapy. A feedback-driven dynamic systems approach*. Boston, MA: Hogrefe International Publishing.

Schiepek, G., Stöger-Schmidinger, B., Aichhorn, W., Schöller, H., & Aas, B. (2016a). Systemic case formulation, individualized process monitoring, and state dynamics in a case of dissociative identity disorder. *Frontiers in Psychology for Clinical Settings, 7*, 1545. https://doi.org/10.3389/fpsyg.2016.01545

Schiepek, G., Aichhorn, W., Gruber, M., Strunk, G., Bachler, E., & Aas, B. (2016b). Real-time monitoring of psychotherapeutic processes: concept and compliance. *Frontiers in Psychology for Clinical Settings, 7*, 604. https://doi.org/10.3389/fpsyg.2016.00604

Schiepek, G., & Strunk, G. (2010). The identification of critical fluctuations and phase transitions in short term and coarse-grained time series – A method for the real-time monitoring of human change processes. *Biological Cybernetics, 102*, 197–207.

Schiepek, G., Tominschek, I., Heinzel, S., Aigner, M., Dold, M., Unger, A., … Karch, S. (2013). Discontinuous patterns of brain activation in the psychotherapy process of obsessive compulsive disorder: converging results from repeated fMRI and daily self-reports. *PloS ONE, 8*(8), e71863

Schiepek, G., Tominschek, I., & Heinzel, S. (2014). Self-organization in psychotherapy – testing the synergetic model of change processes. *Frontiers in Psychology for Clinical Settings, 5*(1089). https://doi.org/10.3389/fpsyg.2014.01089

Schiepek, G., Viol, K., Aichhorn, W., Hütt, M. T., Sungler, K., Pincus, D., & Schöller, H. (2017). Psychotherapy is chaotic—(not only) in a computational world. *Frontiers in Psychology for Clinical Settings, 8*, 379. https://doi.org/10.3389/fpsyg.2017.00379

Schiepek, G., Stöger-Schmidinger, B., Kronberger, H., Aichhorn, W., Kratzer, L., Heinz, P., … Schöller, H. (2019a). The Therapy Process Questionnaire. Factor analysis and psychometric properties of a multidimensional self-rating scale for high-frequency monitoring of psychotherapeutic processes. *Clinical Psychology & Psychotherapy, 26*, 586–602. https://doi.org/10.1002/cpp.2384

Schiepek, G., Schöller, H., Carl, R., Aichhorn, W. & Lichtwarck-Aschoff, A. (2019b). A nonlinear dynamic systems approach to psychological interventions. In E.S. Kunnen, N.M.P. de Ruiter, B.F. Jeronimus, & M.A.E. van der Gaag (Eds.), Psychosocial Development in Adolescence: Insights from the Dynamic Systems Approach (pp. 51-68). New York: Routledge.

Schiepek, G., Gelo, O., Viol, K., Kratzer, L., Orsucci, F., de Felice, G., … Schöller, H. (2020). Complex individual pathways or standard tracks? A data-based discussion on the trajectories of change in psychotherapy. *Counselling & Psychotherapy Research.* https://doi.org/10.1002/capr.12300

Schöller, H., Viol, K., Aichhorn, W., Hütt, M.T., & Schiepek, G. (2018). Personality development in psychotherapy: a synergetic model of state-trait dynamics. *Cognitive Neurodynamics, 12* (5), 441–459. https://doi.org/10.1007/s11571-018-9488-y

Schöller, H., Viol, K., Goditsch, H., Aichhorn, W., Hütt, M.T., & Schiepek, G. (2019). A nonlinear dynamic systems model of psychotherapy: first steps toward validation and the role of external input. *Nonlinear Dynamics in Psychology and the Life Sciences, 23* (1), 79–112.

Stegmüller, W. (1973). *Theorienstrukturen und Theoriendynamik.* Heidelberg/Berlin: Springer.

Tilden, T., & Wampold, B. E. (Eds.). (2017). *Routine outcome monitoring in couple and family therapy* (European Family Therapy Association Series). Berlin/Heidelberg: Springer International.

Wampold, B. E., & Imel, Z. E. (2015). *The great psychotherapy debate: The evidence for what makes psychotherapy work* (2nd ed.). New York, NY: Routledge.

Webber, C. L., & Zbilut, J. P. (1994). Dynamical assessment of physiological systems and states using recurrence plot strategies. *Journal of Applied Physiology, 76*, 965–973.

The Social Present in Psychotherapy: Duration of Nowness in Therapeutic Interaction

Wolfgang Tschacher, Fabian Ramseyer, and Mario Pfammatter

Introduction

Let us start with a definition of psychotherapy: Psychotherapy is a social practice that causes or triggers a learning process of a client or, in systemic approaches, of a multipersonal system. The goal of this practice is to facilitate changes of experiencing and/or behavior in the client(s) that are instrumental in alleviating their symptoms and problems. To attain its goals, psychotherapy presupposes the application of interventions, which are commonly performed by a therapist.

All the elements of this definition are subject to research, and many questions in psychotherapy research are actually open questions: What types of interventions are there? What is the unit that interventions are aimed at – the client, or the client's social system, or the client's experiences or behavior? How essential is the relationship between client and therapist? In this chapter, we shall list some assumptions that we think are helpful to answer such questions and then propose a novel concept, the social present.

The first assumption, *embodiment*, originates from a broad recent discussion in psychology and cognitive science. This discussion has shown the importance of the

W. Tschacher (✉)
University Hospital of Psychiatry and Psychotherapy, University of Bern, Bern, Switzerland

Freiburg Institute for Advanced Studies (FRIAS), Albert-Ludwigs-Universität Freiburg, Freiburg, Germany
e-mail: wolfgang.tschacher@upd.unibe.ch

F. Ramseyer
Department of Clinical Psychology and Psychotherapy, University of Bern, Bern, Switzerland
e-mail: fabian.ramseyer@psy.unibe.ch

M. Pfammatter
University Hospital of Psychiatry and Psychotherapy, University of Bern, Bern, Switzerland

© Springer Nature Switzerland AG 2020
M. Ochs et al. (eds.), *Systemic Research in Individual, Couple, and Family Therapy and Counseling*, European Family Therapy Association Series,
https://doi.org/10.1007/978-3-030-36560-8_3

body for virtually all mental processes. Embodiment is defined as the conviction that mental processes are influenced by bodily variables and vice versa; thus, the relationship between mind and body is characterized by a fundamental bidirectionality. "Implications of embodiment" (Tschacher & Bergomi, 2011) are that these bidirectional influences between mental states and bodily states must be considered throughout psychology and thus also in psychotherapy. Psychotherapy is not only a "talking cure" or a training for the restructuring of cognitive beliefs, but psychotherapy also and importantly involves the body – nonverbal behavior, posture, and physiological arousal are factors that are closely connected to mental variables. Bodily parameters are not just an expression of the mind, but they may in turn shape and control the mind. The same is true for psychopathological conditions: the cognitivistic concept of mental disorders must be criticized as one-sided and misguided. This is true for schizophrenia spectrum disorder, which is characterized by many psychomotor abnormalities (Tschacher, Giersch, & Friston, 2017; Walther, Ramseyer, Horn, Strik, & Tschacher, 2014), so that schizophrenia may be best considered a disembodiment disorder (Fuchs & Schlimme, 2009; Martin, Koch, Hirjak, & Fuchs, 2016). Affects and emotions are likewise based on a specific embodiment (Michalak et al., 2009), and symptoms of depression can be enhanced or even generated by the way we move and position our bodies. This embodied stance is consistent with the introduction of mindfulness into cognitive-behavioral psychotherapy and mentalization into dynamic psychotherapy, and it is certainly consistent with systemic therapy approaches (Ochs & Schweitzer, 2012). Thus, the new emphasis on embodied cognition signals a turning away from the "computer metaphor" of mind that has been the foundation of cognitive psychology for decades. Mind is not a device for digital information processing.

A second assumption is that we must put *process over cross-section* in methodology and philosophy. In our view, it does not make much sense to neglect time as a variable when all topics of interest – psychotherapy, social interaction, and therapeutic alliance – are obviously processes unfolding in time (Salvatore & Tschacher, 2012) instead of frozen states. Yet in the reality of psychological research, this neglect of addressing the process quality of psychotherapy is pervasive. Academic research is still heavily biased toward cross-sectional designs. We however assume that the application of time series analysis is overdue and mandatory (Tschacher & Ramseyer, 2009; Ramseyer, Kupper, Caspar, Znoj, & Tschacher, 2014).

Notwithstanding the so-called replication crisis presently discussed in psychotherapy outcome research (Hengartner, 2017), the issue of the effectiveness of psychotherapy is settled to a large degree. The results of thousands of outcome studies have shown that the effect sizes of the principal forms of psychotherapy are moderate to large when compared to untreated or waiting list controls (Lambert, 2013) and small to moderate when compared to treatment-as-usual control groups (Cuijpers et al., 2016). We therefore assume thirdly that the time has come to explore what it is that makes psychotherapy effective (Pfammatter & Tschacher, 2012). This type of process research should depict the dynamics of the *here-and-now* of therapeutic interaction. We should turn to the careful observation of the very situation in which therapeutic changes occur.

In short, we claim that psychotherapy should be viewed as embodied, processual, and situated. In this chapter, we will therefore cover what we think are promising steps toward such a perspective. We will in the next section discuss a "minimal model" of psychotherapy, namely, the interaction system of therapist and client. We will describe the systems-theoretical underpinnings of this model. In Sect. 3, we will continue and explain the methods that can be used to explore the minimal model. We will focus on time series that are sufficiently fine-grained to cover the very moment in which therapist and client communicate and to directly address the here-and-now of therapeutic interaction. In Sect. 4, preliminary findings will be presented.

A Minimal Model of Psychotherapy

We wish to model in detail what happens in the therapeutic setting and in the therapeutic relationship. Our model of psychotherapy is "minimal" insofar as we restrict the model to its bare essentials and for the time being disregard the specifics of psychotherapeutic schools with their philosophies and conventions. Systems theory, seen as a structural science, is an appropriate vantage point for establishing a basic model of therapeutic interaction.

The psychotherapy system in its totality is always highly complex because when we consider all the variables that can influence the therapeutic situation, we end up with a huge number of variables. In the minimal model, however, we are dealing with just two variables, namely, the temporal sequences of a therapist's and a client's individual states. Thus we have to consider a two-dimensional system, which can be represented by two differential equations because these variables will change in time. Here we will not formulate this system in mathematical terms (see Tschacher & Haken, 2019) but describe its properties in natural language.

First, we believe that psychotherapeutic processes are always a mixture of stochastic and deterministic influences. "Stochastic" means that random inputs from outside the system must be considered; there is a constant influx of randomness that cannot be foreseen but must be acknowledged in any phase of treatment. "Deterministic" influences are those inputs that have a directed influence. Obviously, in the context of psychotherapy, interventions and therapeutic techniques can represent such deterministic inputs. When we consider the canon of ingredients and mechanisms that are currently discussed in psychotherapy research (Wampold, Imel, & Flückiger, 2018; Tschacher, Junghan, & Pfammatter, 2014), we see a multifaceted picture of interventions, ranging from unspecific contextual factors of intervention (e.g., good alliance between therapist and client) to quite specific techniques (e.g., the family constellations technique). All interventions have their own profile of stochastic and/or deterministic effects, where the specific techniques are commonly the more deterministic interventions. Wampold's contextual factors (in the discussion usually termed "common factors"), on the other hand, often deal with the modulation of stochastic inputs acting on the client.

Our goal is to represent both *stochastic* and *deterministic* inputs in a systems-theoretical framework; thus we have to realize the limitations of most popular methodological approaches. On one hand, conventional social science statistics constitute the very basis of psychotherapy research but suffer from the shortcoming of a strong reliance on statistical null hypothesis testing and the neglect of dynamics. Dynamical systems theory and chaos theory, on the other hand, are partially insufficient because they are purely deterministic theories albeit dynamical theories. The framework of synergetics (Haken, 1977) offers a systems theory that explicitly addresses both types of modeling, stochastic and deterministic. This can be realized by using the mathematical model of the Fokker-Planck equation, which describes the probability of some state variable x depending on time t. This equation is a stochastic differential equation, which has two components, a stochastic and a deterministic term. The mathematical *ansatz* of the Fokker-Planck equation can be used to discuss psychotherapy processes in principle; while it is quite formal and abstract, it is not biased toward one type of process.

Second, we are usually dealing with asymptotic *stability*, i.e., equilibrium behavior. Concretely, this means that the processes we observe are stationary and therefore remain in the bounds of a subclass of values of the state variables. In terms of dynamical systems theory, this is the hallmark of behavior within the basin of an attractor. Such stability over time can be either negative or beneficial – affective disorders can be represented by an attractor in the aversive range of emotionality; healthy functioning may be represented by stability in the agreeable range of emotionality. At any rate, it is necessary to use a theory that can encompass equilibrium behavior and that predicts forces that will pull behavior back into its attractor if the system state has been displaced before.

Third, we are interested in the *coupling* between people. Coupling is a technical term in systems theory that describes how two processes become mutually connected. Especially in psychotherapy, the coupling between therapist and client is the focus of interaction because a therapist's interventions can only have a grip on the client's problems when the two are somehow linked. Coupling in psychotherapy is the basis for common factors such as the therapeutic relationship, alliance, goal consensus, transference relationship, and many more (Tschacher et al., 2014). We will in the next section define therapeutic presence as the time during which therapist and client are significantly coupled.

Fourth, we are interested in observing the here-and-now of therapeutic encounters directly. Indirect assessments are common ground in psychology – the use of questionnaires allows the insight into self-reported experience, but usually this is a subjective aggregation over many experiences, for example, over an entire session. Even ecological assessments and experience sampling cannot give an account of what happens in the very moment of psychotherapy because sampling necessarily disrupts the therapeutic moment. Thus we have to resort to other kinds of data and analyze observational data instead of self-report. The psychology of time says that the "now," i.e., the moment of conscious experience, extends over a few seconds (Fraisse, 1984; Wittmann, 2011). The "now" can be derived from a variety of temporal estimation tasks in psychophysics, from dwell times of bistable gestalt stimuli, or, indirectly, from the durations of verses in poetry and melody lines in music (Tschacher, Ramseyer, & Bergomi, 2013). Therefore, to assess and explore such durations, we need observational variables that can be measured at least with frequency 1 Hz or higher. *Fine-grained time series* are a necessary premise for addressing the social present of psychotherapy, that time span in which therapy is actually situated.

Methods to Assess the Minimal Model of Psychotherapy

Social embodiment has been a topic of phenomenological philosophy decades before the phenomenon was analyzed in psychology: Merleau-Ponty's (1945) *intercorporéité* means that my interaction partner is first of all perceived and assessed on the basis of his/her body expression, and this expression will have a bodily impact on myself prior to my cognitive reflections. Intercorporeal resonance (Fuchs, 2010) was thus recognized in phenomenology as a basis of embodied communication. The phenomenological method for studying intercorporeality was philosophical reflection and introspection.

Social psychology was later among the scientific fields to study the relevance of embodiment in the context of interaction by quantitative empirical observations. It was found repeatedly in experiments and systematic observations that, for instance, emotional processes do not only get expressed as facial expressions, but the same emotions can also be caused by prescribed activations of face muscles. Body variables such as postures can affect attitudes and appraisals. One conclusion from such findings was that embodiment has profound implications for social interaction and communication because attitudes and emotional appraisals are essential elements of social behavior. A concept coined in this line of research is the chameleon effect (Chartrand & Bargh, 1999), a kind of social mimicry of nonverbal behavior in communicative situations. As soon as one interaction partner observes the behavior of the other, the probability of the respective behavior in himself/herself is involuntarily increased. Walkers in a group, for instance, tend to synchronize their gait. Further examples are the alignments of body postures of people in close conversations (Grammer, Kruck, & Magnusson, 1998). In interacting humans, motor synchrony arises spontaneously, often escaping the awareness of the individuals involved in such resonance.

In developmental studies, social synchronization processes were also examined at different levels (Feldman, 2007). Meltzoff and Moore (1983) found synchronized behaviors to occur even in newborn infants, who tend to mimic caregivers' behavior (e.g., facial behavior such as sticking out of the tongue). Isabella and Belsky (1991) showed that interactional synchrony of mother and child was associated with attachment styles. Reciprocal and temporally attuned interaction behavior – i.e., synchronized interaction – was higher in secure attachment.

Nonverbal synchrony can be computed based on several observables: on physiological signals such as skin conductance or cardiac parameters (e.g., Karvonen,

Kykyri, Kaartinen, Penttonen, & Seikkula, 2016; Coutinho et al., 2019), on prosodic variables such as voice loudness and pitch, and on variables of motor behavior, i.e., body movement. The latter operationalization of synchrony as movement synchrony has specifically proved valuable to study social interactions in the here-and-now. Movement synchrony was studied in most of the studies cited above.

Recently, we adopted a methodology by which movement can be recorded objectively and quite economically – Motion Energy Analysis (MEA, Ramseyer & Tschacher, 2011). MEA was inspired by the approach of Grammer, Honda, Schmitt, & Jütte (1999), who operationalized the extent of body movement via video analysis – movement was derived from the number of pixel changes in certain "regions of interest" in video recordings. One of us (FR) wrote a software application (www. psync.ch), which reads out the movement in selected regions of interest of digital videos that, for example, depict psychotherapy sessions. The result of MEA is one time series per region of interest. The time series are fine-grained because digital video formats consist of between 25 to 60 frames per second, which results in time series of 25 to 60 MEA data points per second (i.e., 25 to 60 Hz). Hence, this operationalization conforms with the demands of the minimal model mentioned before because it yields embodied, processual, and situated data streams.

How can we derive nonverbal synchrony and the social present from such time series? We apply windowed cross-correlation together with surrogate tests (Moulder, Boker, Ramseyer, & Tschacher, 2018). Since we compute *su*rrogate *sy*nchrony, we may use the abbreviation SUSY for this methodological step (Tschacher & Meier, 2019). Let us assume that we have defined two regions of interest in MEA, each of which contains the movement of one participant, e.g., therapist and client (Fig. 1). Then SUSY estimates the degree of correlated movement of both participants by using simultaneous as well as time-lagged correlations between their movement streams. The number of time lags determines a moving window; within this window (our default value is ten seconds), all cross-correlation coefficients are computed and aggregated. In the case of 30 Hz data

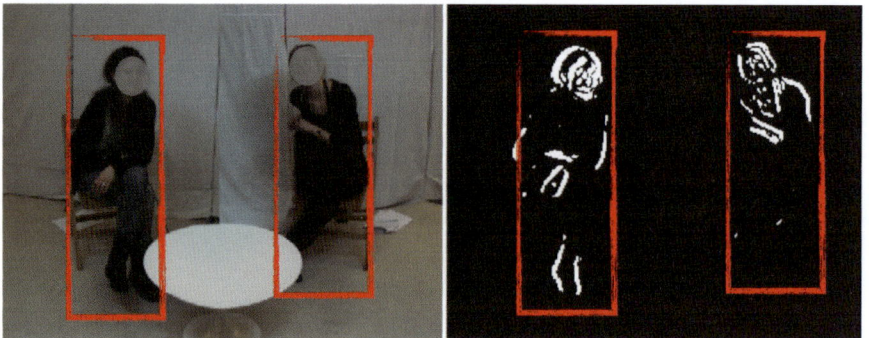

Fig. 1 The principle of Motion Energy Analysis (MEA). All pixel changes within the original video recording (left panel) of an interaction scene are highlighted (right panel). The rectangles delimit the respective regions of interest

and a 10 seconds window, this means $10 \times 30 + 1 = 301$ correlations ("+1" because of the correlation at lag = 0). From these (cross-)correlations, we can compute the mean of all cross-correlations using their absolute values and plot the cross-correlations against the different lags (Fig. 2).

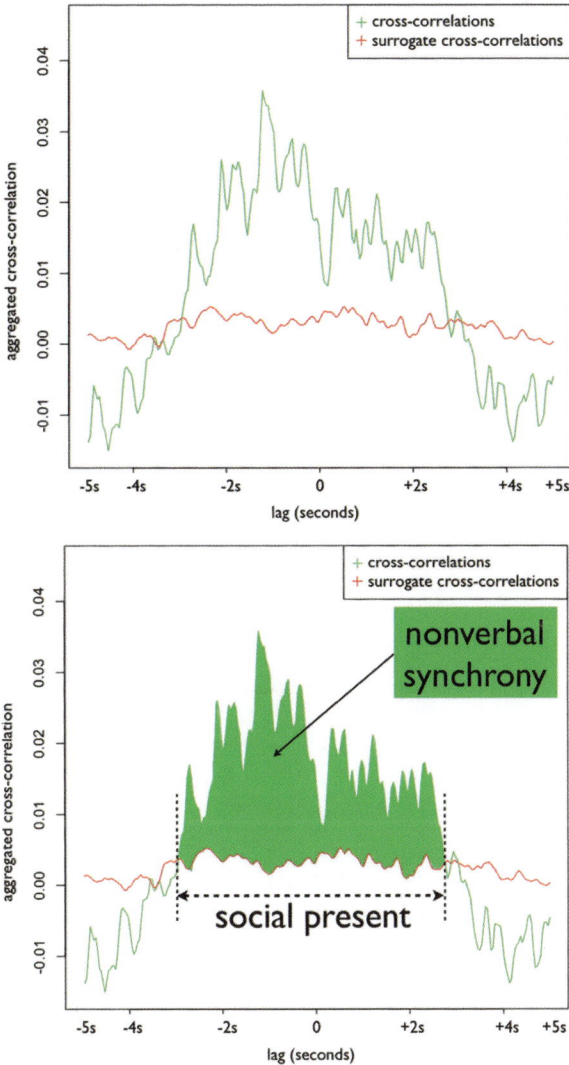

Fig. 2 The principle of surrogate synchrony (SUSY). Upper panel: The raw data are 10 minutes of interaction of two individuals such as shown in Fig. 1. The green graph depicts the cross-correlations as a function of the respective lag. The red graph does the same for the average of all surrogate time series, representing pseudosynchrony. Lower panel: Significant synchrony is found when the green graph exceeds the red graph. The duration of significant synchrony (here approximately six seconds) is called social present. The area under the curve is defined as nonverbal synchrony

SUSY then assesses the significance of this synchrony measure. The surrogate method is applied by randomly shuffling the genuine movement time series and then computing the synchrony of shuffled (i.e., surrogate) data. For details of the surrogate step, see Moulder et al. (2018) or Ramseyer and Tschacher (2010). Comparing genuine synchrony to shuffled "pseudosynchronies" allows proof of existence and, if present, estimating the magnitude of genuine movement coordination.

The comparison of genuine synchrony with pseudosynchrony delivers two quantities, *nonverbal synchrony* and the *social present*. This can be illustrated by the example shown in Fig. 2: Nonverbal synchrony is the area under the green graph, whereas social present is the time during which the green graph exceeds the red graph. Nonverbal synchrony can be expressed by an effect size statistic, the social present by a temporal duration (in seconds).

There are quite a number of different methodological options for synchrony computation. One may apply windowed cross-correlation such as we do in SUSY, but it is also feasible to apply wavelet analysis, i.e., analysis in the frequency domain (Fujiwara & Daibo, 2016). Some researchers do not use the cross-correlations directly but the correlations of piece-wise slopes of the time series and then compute a "concordance index" from these (Karvonen et al., 2016). We have applied sensitivity analyses of the various possible parameter settings in SUSY (Ramseyer & Tschacher, 2016), finding that different parameters give moderately different results, which is however a common finding in statistics. Schoenherr et al. (2019) have recently discussed the pros and cons of the different approaches. We cannot go into more detail here, but certainly more studies are needed that compare the different algorithms of synchrony detection. Thus we have to choose one of several algorithms to compute synchrony and have to make the decision whether we base the computation on cross-correlation or on frequency/wavelets.

In the following overview of findings, we have relied on movement synchrony, mostly measured by MEA, and have always used windowed cross-correlation and surrogate synchrony, SUSY.

Findings on the Social Present of Psychotherapy

As mentioned, the social synchrony that characterizes the here-and-now of the therapeutic setting can be expressed by two quantities, by the extent of synchrony and by the duration of synchrony. The former quantity has been studied in the majority of applications to psychotherapy (Altmann, 2013; Ramseyer & Tschacher, 2011, 2014; Paulick et al., 2018; Lozza et al., 2018). The latter quantity, duration of synchrony, is a way to illustrate the social present or nowness. It constitutes an emerging field in embodiment research, and only very limited published evidence is available at this moment (Table 1).

The measure of the social present was introduced in a paper on the subjective present in psychopathology (Tschacher et al., 2013). In this paper, we reported on

Table 1 Studies of social present available until 2018. WCC, windowed cross-correlation; SUSY, surrogate synchrony determination; MEA, Motion Energy Analysis

Type of interaction	Sample	Method	Covariates	Duration of "nowness"	Reference
Conversations between non-acquainted healthy individuals	51 dyads, $n = 153$ conversations	MEA: Whole body SUSY	–	Mean 5.7 s	Tschacher et al. (2013)
Conversations between non-acquainted healthy individuals	84 dyads, $n = 420$ conversations	MEA: Whole body SUSY	Sex, avoidant attachment, openness for experiences	Mean 6.0 s	Tschacher, Ramseyer, and Koole (2018)
Dyadic psychotherapy in a single case	1 dyad, $n = 27$ sessions	Actigraphy: Wrist sensors SUSY	Phase of therapy	Mean 6.0 s; Initial 6.0 s; Final 8.0 s	Ramseyer and Tschacher (2016)
Dyadic psychotherapy	84 dyads, $n = 104$ sessions	MEA: Whole body SUSY	Self-efficacy	Mean 5.75 s	Unpublished (cf. Ramseyer and Tschacher, 2011)
Dyadic psychotherapy	142 dyads, $n = 284$ sessions	MEA: Whole body Windowed cross-correlation	Depression (HSCL)	–	Schwartz, Paulick, Deisenhofer, and Lutz (2017)

various studies in which we explored the individual present moment and one additional study, where we explored the socially shared present by introducing the procedure as illustrated by Fig. 2. We applied this procedure to a dataset of 51 dyads of unacquainted healthy participants from the Stanford study (Ramseyer & Horowitz, in preparation). All dyads interacted in three prescribed conversations of six minutes duration each. It was found that the mean social present in this student sample was 5.7 seconds. No covariates of the social present were analyzed.

The first comprehensive study of the social present was conducted in a sample of 84 unacquainted dyads (Tschacher, Ramseyer, & Koole, 2018). The 168 participants performed dyadic conversational interactions in five runs of five minutes each. The social present in this study had an overall duration of 6.0 seconds. The social present was found associated with task-related variables: competitive conversations had the longest duration, a fun task the shortest duration, and the cooperative tasks ranged in-between the other task affordances. The duration of the social present varied significantly with personality: longer present was found when participants had higher openness for new experiences (a "Big Five" trait of the Five Factor Personality Inventory, NEO-FFI, Borkenau & Ostendorf, 1991) and low narcissistic inclinations (IIP, Inventory of Interpersonal Problems, Horowitz, Strauss, & Kordy, 1994). Individuals with a tendency toward avoidant attachment (Measure of Attachment

Qualities, MAQ, Carver, 1997) were also involved in conversations with longer social present. Male-male dyads had longer social present than female-female dyads. The results of this study showed that the social present was not a good-or-bad issue. It was further found that although the social present was significantly correlated with the extent of synchrony, both measures were connected with covariates in a diverging way. Thus, the social present and synchrony are qualitatively different indicators of embodied interaction.

We computed the social present in a psychotherapy course with 27 sessions, where hand movements of both therapist and patient were monitored by actigraphy sensors attached to the wrists (Ramseyer & Tschacher, 2016; the data were originally monitored in the "Vitaport study" on sociophysiology: Tschacher & Brunner, 1995). Forty minutes of each session were analyzed. The mean social present in this psychotherapy course was again 6 seconds. In a comparison of the initial 10 sessions with the final 10 sessions, several changes across the therapy course were identified: The strength of synchrony increased from $Z = 0.129$ to $Z = 0.143$ [$T(9) = 2.23$; $p = 0.053$], and a shift from the patient being (subconsciously) "imitated" by the therapist (pacing) toward the patient imitating the therapist is visible ("leading" higher synchrony at negative lags). Additionally, the social present appears to be extended from around 6 seconds in the initial phase toward roughly 8 seconds in the final phase of therapy (see Fig. 3 for details).

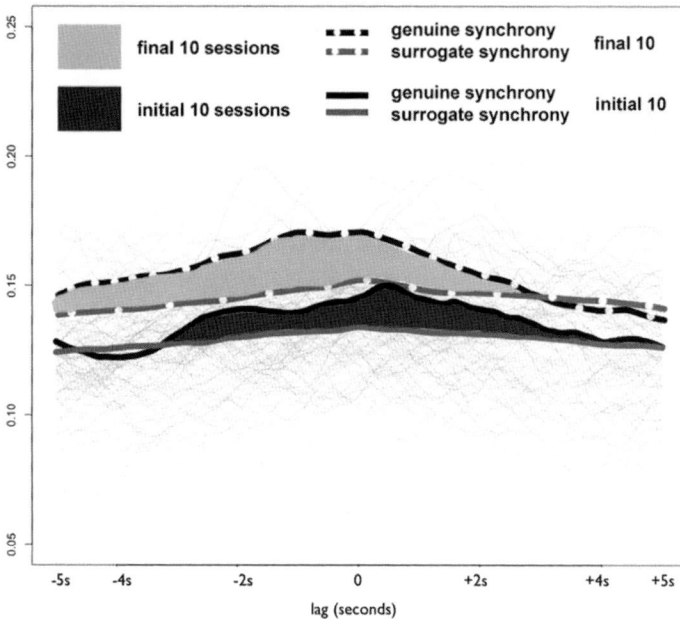

Fig. 3 Comparison of social present at initial stage of therapy (first ten sessions, dark gray) versus final stage of therapy (last ten sessions, light gray). Ordinate, synchrony Z values

We further reanalyzed the data of a psychotherapy process study of 104 sessions of cognitive-behavioral psychotherapy, a random selection that included 70 different patients (Ramseyer & Tschacher, 2011). The raw data of this study were MEA assessments of whole-body movement in 15-minute sections of the respective treatments. These sections were taken randomly from the initial third and the final third of the therapy courses. The mean social present in this sample was 5.75 seconds. There was no clear association of the social present with overall outcome, but longer durations of the present were linked with higher self-efficacy of the patients in the respective session (using items of the patients' session reports as a measure of self-efficacy).

Schwartz et al. (2017) studied a large sample of 142 outpatients undergoing treatment with cognitive-behavioral psychotherapy, following the same procedure as Ramseyer and Tschacher (2011) – 15 min sections were taken from the initial and final third of the respective therapies, and movement synchrony was monitored using MEA. The authors focused on the changes of the social present from sessions earlier to later in the course of psychotherapy. A decrease of the social present was associated with lower depression at the end of treatment, however only in patients who were high in initial depression. This finding may suggest that a reduced social present represents a patient's (healthy) detachment, and prolonged present may indicate psychomotor retardation in affective disorders.

The state of research in this field is currently still provisional; it is in need of conventions and standards that all researchers can agree upon. Only a standardized procedure in SUSY will allow a comparison of the absolute nowness durations between datasets. Currently, it is therefore unclear whether the social present durations increase in the course of psychotherapy (Ramseyer & Tschacher, 2016), decrease (Schwartz et al., 2017), or remain constant (Ramseyer & Tschacher, 2011).

Conclusions for Psychotherapy

The "here-and-now" of psychotherapy is considered to be of high significance, especially in humanistic psychotherapy and mindfulness-based psychotherapy approaches. Whenever the therapeutic relationship is acknowledged as a core factor of psychotherapy, such as in client-centered psychotherapy (Pascual-Leone & Greenberg, 2007) or dialogical family therapy (Seikkula, 2008), the present moment of psychotherapy must be a focus of attention as it characterizes the here-and-now (Stern, 2004). The present moment in psychotherapy is also highly relevant for other common change factors such as problem activation (Gassmann & Grawe, 2006) or corrective emotional experience (Castonguay & Hill, 2012), as they unfold their therapeutic impact in the here-and-now. In this theoretical view, the therapeutic presence (Geller & Porges, 2014) is a prerequisite of change. Experiencing, consciousness, and mindfulness – all these can, by definition, only occur in the present moment.

Nevertheless, in terms of empirical research, not much is known about this present moment in psychotherapy settings. We have therefore constructed a quantitative method that complements the phenomenological view of the therapeutic situation. We suggested a novel data-driven approach to study the here-and-now of psychotherapy by time series analysis of a "minimal model" of psychotherapy. This analysis uses cross-correlations and surrogate tests to define the social present as the duration of nonverbal synchronization of two interacting individuals, such as therapist and client. The methodology relies on fine-grained process data that describe the therapeutic encounter via body movement or physiological recordings. It directly addresses the coupling between therapist and client, i.e., their alliance, which is the core of such encounters. And additionally, it recognizes this coupling as a stable dynamical phenomenon, namely, the ongoing synchronization of the two individuals.

Preliminary findings have suggested that the resulting measure of the social present may be linked with some aspects of personality and with task affordances in healthy participants engaged in conversations. In psychotherapy data, we found an association with an important common factor of therapy process, the client's self-efficacy, and thus maybe also with therapy outcome. The mean duration of the social present was approximately six seconds when synchrony computation and surrogate testing were performed with default parameters. We are wondering whether it is more than mere coincidence that this duration is roughly twice the duration of individual nowness. This of course does not imply that the duration of the present increases linearly with the number of interacting people. At this stage of research, both synchrony and the social present are defined for dyadic systems only.

We consider these results as promising beginnings of a new field of psychotherapy process research that address a previously unstudied phenomenon. More studies are obviously needed to confirm the alleged significance of the social present in psychotherapy. Future studies should compare the data-driven situated approach proposed in the present chapter to phenomenological ratings performed by clients and therapists. Questionnaire measures – the Therapeutic Presence Inventory for therapists (TPI-T) and clients (TPI-C) – are already available (Geller, Greenberg, & Watson, 2010). This will provide an opportunity to connect the experiences of therapeutic presence with the time series measures we have introduced. The distant goal of such research is obviously the translation of findings into therapeutic practice – how shall we shape the therapist-client encounter in the present moment in order to optimize therapeutic effects?

References

Altmann, U. (2013). *Synchronisation nonverbalen Verhaltens. Weiterentwicklung und Anwendung zeitreihenanalytischer Identifikationsverfahren.* Berlin: Springer.

Borkenau, P., & Ostendorf, F. (1991). Ein Fragebogen zur Erfassung fünf robuster Persönlichkeitsfaktoren [a questionnaire to assess five robust personality factors]. *Diagnostica, 37,* 29–41.

Carver, C. S. (1997). Adult attachment and personality: Converging evidence and a new measure. *Personality and Social Psychology Bulletin, 23*, 865–883.

Castonguay, L. G., & Hill, C. E. (Eds.). (2012). *Transformation in psychotherapy: Corrective experiences across cognitive behavioral, humanistic, and psychodynamic approaches.* Washington, D.C.: American Psychological Association.

Chartrand, T. L., & Bargh, J. A. (1999). The chameleon effect: The perception-behavior link and social interaction. *Journal of Personality and Social Psychology, 76*, 893–910.

Coutinho, J. F., Oliveira-Silva, P., Fernandes, E., Gonçalves, O. F., Correia, D., Perrone McGovern, K., & Tschacher, W. (2019). Psychophysiological synchrony during verbal interaction in romantic relationships. *Family Process, 58*, 716-733.

Cuijpers, P., Cristea, I. A., Karyotaki, E., Reijnders, M., Marcus, J. H., & Huibers, M. J. H. (2016). How effective are cognitive behavior therapies for major depression and anxiety disorders? A meta-analytic update of the evidence. *World Psychiatry, 15*, 245–258.

Feldman, R. (2007). Parent-infant synchrony: Biological foundations and developmental outcomes. *Current Directions in Psychological Science, 16*, 340–345.

Fraisse, P. (1984). Perception and estimation of time. *Annual Review of Psychology, 35*, 1–36.

Fuchs, T. (2010). *Das Gehirn – ein Beziehungsorgan. Eine phänomenologisch-ökologische Konzeption.* Kohlhammer: Stuttgart.

Fuchs, T., & Schlimme, J. E. (2009). Embodiment and psychopathology: A phenomenological perspective. *Current Opinion in Psychiatry, 22*, 570–575.

Fujiwara, K., & Daibo, I. (2016). Evaluating interpersonal synchrony: Wavelet transform toward an unstructured conversation. *Frontiers in Psychology, 7*, 516.

Gassmann, D., & Grawe, K. (2006). General change mechanisms: The relation between problem activation and resource activation in successful and unsuccessful therapeutic interactions. *Clinical Psychology and Psychotherapy, 13*, 1–11.

Geller, S. M., Greenberg, L. S., & Watson, J. C. (2010). Therapist and client perceptions of therapeutic presence: The development of a measure. *Psychotherapy Research, 20*, 599–610.

Geller, S. M., & Porges, S. W. (2014). Therapeutic presence: Neurophysiological mechanisms mediating feeling safe in therapeutic relationships. *Journal of Psychotherapy Integration, 24*, 178–192.

Grammer, K., Honda, R., Schmitt, A., & Jütte, A. (1999). Fuzziness of nonverbal courtship communication unblurred by motion energy detection. *Journal of Personality and Social Psychology, 77*, 487–508.

Grammer, K., Kruck, K. B., & Magnusson, M. S. (1998). The courtship dance: Patterns of nonverbal synchronization in opposite-sex encounters. *Journal of Nonverbal Behavior, 22*, 3–29.

Haken, H. (1977). *Synergetics – An introduction. Nonequilibrium phase-transitions and self-organization in physics, chemistry and biology.* Berlin: Springer.

Hengartner, M. P. (2017). Raising awareness for the replication crisis in clinical psychology by focusing on inconsistencies in psychotherapy research: How much can we rely on published findings from efficacy trials? *Frontiers in Psychology, 9*, 256.

Horowitz, L. M., Strauss, B., & Kordy, H. (1994). *IIP-D. Inventar zur Erfassung interpersonaler Probleme – Deutsche version [IIP-D. Inventory of interpersonal problems – German version].* Beltz: Weinheim.

Isabella, R. A., & Belsky, J. (1991). Interactional synchrony and the origins of infant-mother attachment: A replication study. *Child Development, 62*, 373–384.

Karvonen, A., Kykyri, V.-L., Kaartinen, J., Penttonen, M., & Seikkula, J. (2016). Sympathetic nervous system synchrony in couple therapy. *Journal of Marital and Family Therapy, 42*, 383–395.

Lambert, M. J. (Ed.) (2013). *Bergin and Garfield's Handbook of Psychotherapy and Behavior Change* (6 ed.). New York: Wiley.

Lozza, N., Spoerri, C., Ehlert, U., Kesselring, M., Hubmann, P., Tschacher, W., & La Marca, R. (2018). Nonverbal synchrony and complementarity in unacquainted same-sex dyads: A comparison in a competitive context. *Journal of Nonverbal Behavior, 42*, 179-197.

Martin, L. A., Koch, S. C., Hirjak, D., & Fuchs, T. (2016). Overcoming disembodiment: The effect of movement therapy on negative symptoms in schizophrenia-a Multicenter randomized controlled trial. *Frontiers in Psychology, 7*, 483.

Meltzoff, A. N., & Moore, M. K. (1983). Newborn infants imitate adult facial gestures. *Child Development, 54*, 702–709.

Merleau-Ponty, M. (1945). *Phénomènologie de la perception*. Paris: Editions Gallimard.

Michalak, J., Troje, N. F., Fischer, J., Vollmar, P., Heidenreich, T., & Schulte, D. (2009). Embodiment of sadness and depression – Gait patterns associated with dysphoric mood. *Psychosomatic Medicine, 71*, 580–587.

Moulder, R. G., Boker, S. M., Ramseyer, F., & Tschacher, W. (2018). Determining synchrony between behavioral time series: An application of surrogate data generation for establishing falsifiable null-hypotheses. *Psychological Methods, 23*, 757–773.

Ochs, M., & Schweitzer, J. (Eds.). (2012). *Handbuch Forschung für Systemiker*. Göttingen: Vandenhoeck & Ruprecht.

Pascual-Leone, A., & Greenberg, L. S. (2007). Emotional processing in experiential therapy: Why "the only way out is through". *Journal of Consulting and Clinical Psychology, 75*, 875–887.

Paulick, J., Deisenhofer, A.-K., Ramseyer, F., Tschacher, W., Rubel, J., & Lutz, W. (2018). Nonverbal synchrony: A new approach to understand psychotherapeutic processes and drop-out. *Journal of Psychotherapy Integration, 28*, 367–384.

Pfammatter, M., & Tschacher, W. (2012). Wirkfaktoren der Psychotherapie – eine Übersicht und Standortbestimmung. *Zeitschrift für Psychiatrie, Psychologie und Psychotherapie, 60*, 67–76.

Ramseyer, F., Kupper, Z., Caspar, F., Znoj, H., & Tschacher, W. (2014). Time-Series Panel Analysis (TSPA) – Multivariate modeling of temporal associations in psychotherapy process. *Journal of Consulting and Clinical Psychology, 82*, 828–838.

Ramseyer, F., & Tschacher, W. (2010). Nonverbal synchrony or random coincidence? How to tell the difference. In A. Esposito, N. Campbell, C. Vogel, A. Hussain, & A. Nijholt (Eds.), *Development of multimodal interfaces: Active listening and synchrony* (pp. 182–196). Berlin: Springer.

Ramseyer, F., & Tschacher, W. (2011). Nonverbal synchrony in psychotherapy: Coordinated body movement reflects relationship quality and outcome. *Journal of Consulting and Clinical Psychology, 79*, 284–295.

Ramseyer, F., & Tschacher, W. (2014). Nonverbal synchrony of head- and body-movement in psychotherapy: Different signals have different associations with outcome. *Frontiers in Psychology, 5*, 979.

Ramseyer, F., & Tschacher, W. (2016). Movement coordination in psychotherapy: Synchrony of hand movements is associated with session outcome. A single-case study. *Nonlinear Dynamics Psychology and Life Sciences, 20*, 145–166.

Salvatore, S., & Tschacher, W. (2012). Time dependency of psychotherapeutic exchanges: The contribution of the theory of dynamic systems in analyzing process. *Frontiers in Psychology, 3*, 253, 1–14.

Schwartz, B., Paulick, J., Deisenhofer, A.-K., & Lutz, W. (2017). The change in social present over the course of psychotherapy, and its relation to outcome. Paper presented at the conference of the Society of Psychotherapy Research (SPR), Oxford, September 2017.

Seikkula, J. (2008). Inner and outer voices in the present moment of family and network therapy. *Journal of Family Therapy, 30*, 478–491.

Stern, D. N. (2004). *The present moment in psychotherapy and everyday life*. New York, NY: Norton.

Schoenherr, D., Worrack, S., Dittmann, J., Strauss, B. M., Rubel, J., Schwartz, B., … Altmann, U. (2019). Quantification of nonverbal synchronization using time series analysis methods: Overview and examination of construct validity. *Behavior Research Methods, 51*, 361–383.

Tschacher, W., & Bergomi, C. (Eds.). (2011). *The implications of embodiment: Cognition and communication*. Exeter: Imprint Academic.

Tschacher, W., & Brunner, E. J. (1995). Empirische Studien zur Dynamik von Gruppen aus der Sicht der Selbstorganisationstheorie. *Zeitschrift für Sozialpsychologie, 26*, 78–91.

Tschacher, W., Giersch, A., & Friston, K. J. (2017). Embodiment and schizophrenia: A review of implications and applications. *Schizophrenia Bulletin, 43*, 745–753.

Tschacher, W., & Haken, H. (2019). *The process of psychotherapy – Causation and chance*. Cham: Springer.

Tschacher, W., Junghan, U., & Pfammatter, M. (2014). Towards a taxonomy of common factors in psychotherapy – Results of an expert survey. *Clinical Psychology & Psychotherapy, 21*, 82–96.

Tschacher, W., & Ramseyer, F. (2009). Modeling psychotherapy process by time-series panel analysis (TSPA). *Psychotherapy Research, 19*, 469–481.

Tschacher, W., Ramseyer, F., & Bergomi, C. (2013). The subjective present and its modulation in clinical contexts. *Timing & Time Perception, 1*, 239–259.

Tschacher, W., Ramseyer, F., & Koole, S. L. (2018). Sharing the now in the social present: Duration of nonverbal synchrony is linked with personality. *Journal of Personality, 86*, 129–138.

Tschacher, W. & Meier, D. (2019). Physiological synchrony in psychotherapy sessions. *Psychotherapy Research*.

Walther, S., Ramseyer, F., Horn, H., Strik, W., & Tschacher, W. (2014). Less structured movement patterns predict severity of positive syndrome, excitement, and disorganization. *Schizophrenia Bulletin, 40*, 585–591.

Wampold, B. E., Imel, Z. E., & Flückiger, C. (2018). *Die Psychotherapie-Debatte*. Bern: Hogrefe. (engl: Wampold & Imel (2015). The great psychotherapy debate).

Wittmann, M. (2011). Moments in time. *Frontiers in Integrative Neuroscience, 5*, 66.

Significant Moments in a Couple Therapy Session: Towards the Integration of Different Modalities of Analysis

Petra Nyman-Salonen, Berta Vall, Aarno Laitila, Maria Borcsa (iD),
Markku Penttonen, Anu Tourunen, Virpi-Liisa Kykyri, Jukka Kaartinen,
Valeri Tsatsishvili, and Jaakko Seikkula

Introduction

In recent years, research in the social sciences has taken an affective turn. Hence, in attaching meanings to phenomena, it is considered necessary to take into account emotions, affects and feelings, as well as spoken content (Cromby, 2012). Here, we present a case study on the significant moments of a single couple therapy session, our aim having been to integrate information gained from (i) the verbal dialogue and the therapeutic process, (ii) personal autonomic nervous system responses (skin conductance responses, i.e. SCRs) and (iii) observed nonverbal synchronization behaviour. After the session, all the participants were individually interviewed. Their personal accounts were viewed as giving meaning to their embodied reactions.

P. Nyman-Salonen (✉) · A. Laitila · M. Penttonen · J. Kaartinen · J. Seikkula
Department of Psychology, University of Jyväskylä, Jyväskylä, Finland
e-mail: petra.nyman-salonen@jyu.fi

B. Vall
Faculty of Psychology, Education, and Sport Sciences, Blanquerna, Ramon Llull University,
Barcelona, Spain

M. Borcsa
Institute of Social Medicine, Rehabilitation Sciences and Healthcare Research,
University of Applied Sciences Nordhausen, Nordhausen, Germany

A. Tourunen
The Gerontology Research Center, Faculty of Sport and Health Sciences,
University of Jyväskylä, Jyväskylä, Finland

V.-L. Kykyri
Department of Psychology, University of Jyväskylä, Jyväskylä, Finland

Faculty of Social Sciences/Psychology, University of Tampere, Tampere, Finland

V. Tsatsishvili
Faculty of Information Technology, University of Jyväskylä, Jyväskylä, Finland

© Springer Nature Switzerland AG 2020
M. Ochs et al. (eds.), *Systemic Research in Individual, Couple, and Family Therapy and Counseling*, European Family Therapy Association Series,
https://doi.org/10.1007/978-3-030-36560-8_4

In this case study, we wished to discover what the embodied reactions of the participants might indicate concerning the therapy process, notably whether the data obtained from the different modalities were intertwined or independent from each other, i.e. whether they complemented each other or told different stories of a given moment. We also wanted to see if the differing roles of therapists and clients in the therapy situation were reflected in their autonomic nervous system responses and in their nonverbal synchronization behaviour.

The data used in this study were collected in the project *Relational Mind in Events of Change in Multiactor Therapeutic Dialogues.* The project has aimed to increase our understanding of attunement and of the embodied quality of dialogues in couple therapy (Seikkula, Karvonen, Kykyri, Kaartinen, & Penttonen, 2015). The project was situated at the University of Jyväskylä, where data were gathered from 12 couple therapy cases. In all the cases, the autonomic nervous system responses of both the therapists and the couple were measured, usually in the second and sixth sessions. After the measurement sessions, the participants were individually interviewed, using the *Stimulated Recall Interview* method (hereafter SRI), which employs video clips to prompt recall of the participants' thoughts and feelings and bodily sensations at certain moments in the therapy session. The project has international collaborators at the Aristotle University in Thessaloniki, at the Nordhausen University of Applied Sciences and at the Masaryk University in Brno, where additional data from psychotherapy cases has been collected.

In this chapter, we first present the research methods applied, indicating the type of information they provide. Thereafter, we give an overview of the session under study, referring to information provided by the methods applied. Finally, we integrate the information gained, concentrating on the four clips that were selected to the SRIs.

The Analysis of the Dialogue

In psychotherapy research the dialogue plays a crucial role, not just because it is the main communication tool but also because it connects the participants to each other. In this study the Dialogical Investigations of Happenings of Change (DIHC) method was used for organizing the session into thematic entities (Seikkula, Laitila, & Rober, 2012). DIHC focuses on the quality of the dialogue; so in addition to looking at the verbal content, it focuses on how things are said and how they are responded to (Olson, Laitila, Rober, & Seikkula, 2012). Therefore, with DIHC it is possible to differentiate dialogical and monological dialogue in psychotherapy conversations. Dialogical dialogue refers to dialogue in which participants include, within their speech, ideas previously mentioned by other participants; moreover, utterances are expressed so that they allow the other participants to respond. The presence of dialogical dialogue in the therapy process has been related to the outcome of the therapeutic process (Räsänen, Holma, & Seikkula, 2012; Vall, Seikkula, Laitila, Holma, & Botella, 2014). In addition, DIHC is used to analyse the dominances in the dialogue, for instance, interactional dominance (i.e. who regulates the speech turns). The use of the method provides a good base for analysing the embodied reactions of the participants by focusing on the thematic entities.

Autonomic Nervous System Responses: Skin Conductance Responses (SCRs)

In this study, electrodermal activity (EDA) was recorded to track arousal, as indicated by changes in sympathetic nervous system (SNS) activity. Increases in SNS activation are related to the increased physiological arousal that accompanies preparation for action and emotions causing an increase in action tendency (Boucsein, 2012; Kreibig, 2010). In particular, rapid changes in EDA – measured as skin conductance responses (SCRs) – are thought to be a direct measure of SNS activity (Benedek & Kaernbach, 2010). In this case study, the SCRs were chosen because of the interest in looking at how aroused each participant was in the session.

In previous studies on SNS activity in psychotherapy, the client's arousal level has been shown to rise at moments of confrontation (Olson & Claiborn, 1990), when one's identity is blamed (Päivinen et al., 2016) and when the therapist is empathic towards the client (Finset, Stensrud, Holt, Verheul, & Bensing, 2011). It has been suggested that an increase in autonomic arousal could be a sign of active emotional engagement (del Piccolo & Finset, 2017). The client's electrodermal arousal decreases when the clinician uses affective communication (Sep, van Osch, van Vliet, Smets, & Bensing, 2014). In couple therapy, the participants' arousal levels can thus reflect emotions, emotional engagement and preparation for action.

Nonverbal Synchronization

During interaction, people tend to implicitly synchronize their nonverbal behaviour, i.e. gestures, postures and tone of voice. This adaption has several functions, including that of making the dialogue smoother by regulating turns and creating a mutual connection. This tendency has been related to increases in liking (Chartrand & Bargh, 1999) and rapport (Lakens & Stel, 2011). It has been suggested as a mechanism for emotionally attuning to the other person, facilitating an understanding of the other person's emotions (Stel & van den Bos, 2010).

In psychotherapy, the synchronization of postures has been seen as an external sign of rapport (Sharpley, Halat, Rabinowicz, Weiland, & Stafford, 2001; Trout & Rosenfeld, 1980) and as a sign of the therapist being attuned to the client (Davis & Hadiks, 1994; Raingruber, 2001).

Within psychotherapy, therapists and clients nod frequently. Therapists nod their heads when displaying and maintaining affiliation with clients (Muntigl, Knight, & Watkins, 2012). During dialogue, the listeners' head nods are important in creating moment-by-moment collaboration (Bavelas, Coates, & Johnson, 2000). The head nods are interpreted as expressing a wish for the speaker to continue talking, as well as expressing understanding (Stivers, 2008).

Another commonly occurring movement in therapy is self-touching. These movements, also called displacement behaviours, have been related to heightened arousal and are thought to act as self-soothing movements (Troisi, 2002). In the present study, the nonverbal synchronization of postures and movements were analysed.

Inner Dialogue Captured by the Stimulated Recall Interview (SRI)

The SRI is a video-assisted method for investigating what people recall concerning their own inner thoughts and emotions in an event in which they participated (Kagan, Krathwohl, & Miller, 1963). In the field of psychotherapy research, SRIs have been used to study the therapists' and clients' inner dialogues. The clients use the SRI to gain insight about themselves, whereas the therapists use the SRIs to elaborate on therapeutic strategies and to manage the therapeutic process (Rober, Elliott, Buysse, Loots, & De Corte, 2008; Vall et al., 2018). SRIs offer insight into information that is usually hidden when one looks only at transcripts of the session. In the present study, the information from the SRIs was used to gain an understanding of the embodied reactions of the participants during the therapy session.

In this case study, we aimed to integrate the information from these aforementioned research methods to gain a fuller understanding of a couple therapy session, especially the participants' embodied reactions in relation to the dialogue and the therapeutic process.

Method

The data for this study were gathered within the Relational Mind research project (Seikkula et al., 2015) at the University of Jyväskylä Psychotherapy Training and Research Centre. The couple therapy was non-manualized and employed narrative, dialogical and reflective therapeutic approaches. Two therapists were present. The sessions were video-recorded. The participants' autonomic nervous system (ANS) reactions (i.e. heart rate, electrodermal activity and respiration) were collected from both the couple and the therapists in the second and sixth sessions. After the ANS sessions, SRIs were conducted with the participants individually. Thus, video clips from the session were shown to the participants, who were asked to recall their thoughts, feelings and bodily sensations at the corresponding moment during the session.

The video clips were chosen by the researcher to represent four significant moments of therapy. They were chosen on the basis of (i) visible emotional expression, (ii) a notable change in the interaction and (iii) visible synchrony between participants in the ANS measurements (EDA, respiration). The participants gave their informed written consent for the use of the data, and the Ethical Committee of the University of Jyväskylä had approved the research.

The Case

The session analysed for this study came from a couple therapy with Tom and Mary (pseudonyms). The couple had been referred to couple therapy by Mary's therapist. Mary had suffered from depression after their child Eva (pseudonym) was born. Tom and Mary came to therapy, wanting to learn how to better communicate with each other and to explore their feelings of disconnectedness. The session was the second session of the therapy. Within it, ANS reactions were measured and SRIs were conducted. The two therapists were experienced couple and family therapists (both male).

Research Procedure

The various research methods were first applied separately. The Dialogical Investigations of Happenings of Change (DIHC) method was conducted by Berta Vall (BV) and Aarno Laitila (AL), and the extraction of the SCRs was conducted by Valeri Tsatsishvili and Markku Penttonen. The analysis of observing nonverbal synchronization of body postures and movements was done by Petra Nyman-Salonen (PNS), and the SRIs were analysed by Maria Borcsa.

Integration of the information from the different analyses was conducted by focusing on the clips selected for the SRIs. First, we started by looking at the dialogue and the therapy process in the session, in conjunction with the embodied reactions of each participant (SCRs and nonverbal synchronization). The integration analysis was conducted by PNS, BV and AL.

Thereafter, the analysis was conducted starting from the individual information that the participants shared in the SRIs, which was looked upon as information concerning individual emotions or personal stances towards the topic spoken of in the therapy session. The individual emotions and thoughts were then related to the individual's arousal level and nonverbal synchronization behaviours, as well as to the actual dialogue in the session and the therapy process.

Dialogical Investigations of Happenings of Change (DIHC)

The session transcripts were investigated using the three steps of DIHC (Seikkula et al., 2012). Step 1 divides the session into thematic entities called *Topical Episodes* (TEs), within which the same topic is spoken about. Step 2 explores the quality of the therapeutic conversation as either dialogical or monological and the dominance present in the dialogue, differentiating among (i) quantitative (who speaks the most), (ii) semantic (who regulates the topics that are spoken of) and (iii) interactional dominance (who regulates the turns). Step 3 involves a detailed analysis of the data, in which the Narrative Processes Coding System (NPCS) is applied (Angus et al., 2012; Angus, Levitt, & Hardtke, 1999; Laitila, Aaltonen, Wahlström, & Angus, 2005). There are three *modes* in the model, namely, (i) *External mode* (E) (accounts and descriptions of events that can be both real and imagined and answering the question 'what'), (ii) *Internal mode* (I) (descriptions of experiences or feelings,) and (iii) *Reflexive mode* (R) (referring to meaning-making and to reflecting on meanings). The TEs comprised entities in relation to which the information from the other research methods were examined.

Electrodermal Activity: Skin Conductance Responses (SCRs)

Electrodermal activity was recorded using two electrodes attached to the palm of the participant's nondominant hand. Skin conductance was obtained via a GSR sensor, an amplifier, a data acquisition unit (ExG 16) and a data acquisition programme (all from Brain Products, Germany).

SCRs, representing phasic changes of EDA related to movement-by-movement changes in SNS activity, were extracted with Ledalab, a Matlab-based software package designed for skin conductance analysis (Benedek & Kaernbach, 2010). Subsequently, the SCRs from each participant were resampled to 1 Hz and z-scored. For each participant, the arousal level during the TE was expressed as the average SCR amplitude within the TE. The extraction method used in this study has been used in a case study conducted by Laitila et al. (2019). Here, the term *arousal level* is used to refer to the participants' skin conductance responses.

In this case study, the arousal level was interpreted in a qualitative manner. Thus, arousal levels with a value near to 0 indicated a level near to that participant's average arousal in the session. When the SCR was greater than 0.3, it was classified as *high arousal*. Arousal between 0.1 and 0.3 was classified as *some arousal*. Values close to 0 were classified as *average arousal*, values of −0.1 to −0.3 were classified as *low arousal*, and values of less than −0.3 were classified as *very low arousal*.

Observing Nonverbal Synchrony (ONS)

The nonverbal synchronization of postures and movements was analysed via a method created by Nyman-Salonen (submitted). The nonverbal synchronization behaviour of the participants was observed continuously using the Noldus Observer programme. Posture-synchronization occurred when two or more participants were in a similar posture (either a mirror image or congruent), and movement-synchronization occurred when someone mimicked another's movement within 3 seconds. The synchronized movements were either head movements, arm movements (usually displacement behaviour, meaning touching of the head or face), leg movements (mostly shifts in leg positions), torso movements and hand movements (mostly displacement behaviours).

SRIs

The researcher had selected four episodes for participants to view in the SRIs. The participants viewed these clips from the session individually and recalled the thoughts and emotions they had had at these particular moments in the session.

Results

Overview of the Session

We begin with the dialogical analysis for the complete session under study, showing the division of the session into *topical episodes* (TEs) (Table 1). These are used in presenting the results for the individual SCRs (Fig. 1) and for the nonverbal synchronizations (Figs. 2 and 3).

Table 1 Topical episodes in the session. The clips chosen for the SRIs occurred in TEs 12, 14 and 16–18 (shaded)

TE	Content	TE	Content
1	Wife's return, relation daughter	11	Ideal mother vs. mother-as-she-is
2	Husband doubts about job	12	Reason for therapy–disconnection (SRI 1)
3	Aside to wife's trip abroad	13	What was different before child?
4	Argument about where to live	14	The conversation here and now (SRI 2)
5	Job man, living on another city	15	Man holding back in therapy and life
6	Both work oriented	16	Reasons for disconnecting (SRI 3)
7	Evaluation consequences of move	17	Not "natural mother"–guilt (SRI 4)
8	How would it be without Eva?	18	Acceptance of others (SRI 4)
9	Father–child relation; third wheel	19	Role models
10	Positions as parents		

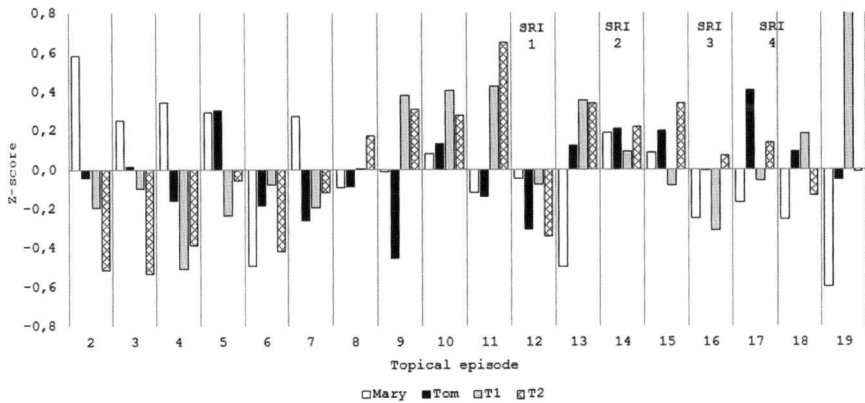

Fig. 1 Skin conductance responses for each participant, in relation to their average in the session per TE. A zero value refers to each participant's average during the session

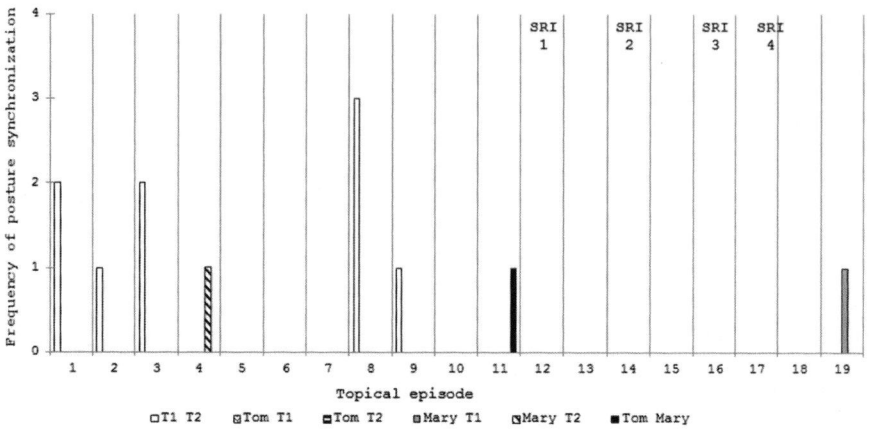

Fig. 2 Posture-synchronization per dyad in each TE

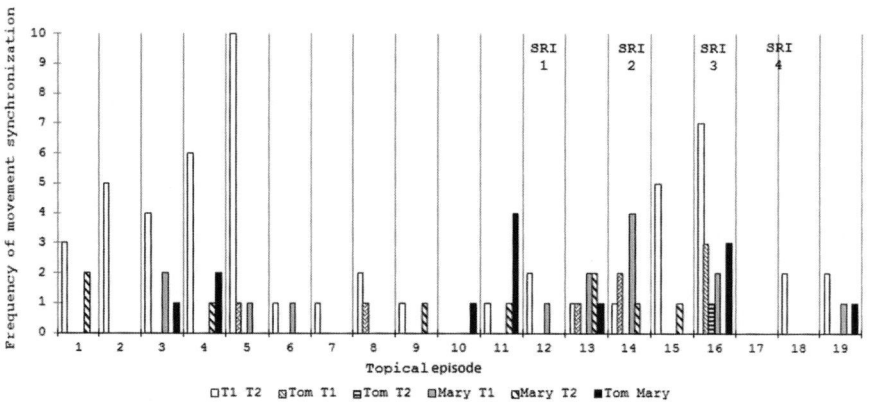

Fig. 3 Movement-synchronization per dyad in each TE

The Dialogue

Table 1 presents the topical episodes and the title that was given to each of them denoting the topic under conversation. The session as a whole was strongly dialogical, meaning that the clients were engaged in talking to each other. Initially, they mainly talked about their job issues (TEs 2, 3, 4, 5 and 7), with utterances expressing a reflective mode. However, Mary was already talking about her emotions in those moments. In the central part of the session (TEs 1, 8, 9, 10, 11, 13, 17, 18, 19), the conversation moved towards issues of motherhood and parenthood. In these moments, Tom started to talk about his emotions for the first time in the session. At the end of the session, the reason for being in therapy was discussed, which was related to the couple's feelings of disconnection (TEs 6, 12, 14, 15, 16). Within these moments, most of the participants talked emotionally, though in conjunction with external and reflective talk. This meant that they were jointly engaging in meaning-construction processes.

In terms of dominance, it seemed that the couple talked to each other and were actively involved in the session, presenting dominance equally (regarding who talks more, who regulates what is talked about and who regulates the turns). Primarily, it was the therapists who regulated the discussion (in 17 TEs out of 19), and the therapists also chose the topics of the conversation (in 12 TEs). In general terms, there was a natural exchange among participants.[1]

Electrodermal Activity as Manifested SCRs

Figure 1 presents the skin conductance responses for each participant in relation to their average in the session per TE. The results are presented from TE 2 onwards, because TE 1 was omitted due to technical difficulties in recording the EDA. At the beginning of the session (TEs 2, 3, 4 and 7), Mary was more aroused, whereas the other participants were less aroused. Apart from TE5, Tom's arousal was more evident later in the session, most notably in TE17. The therapists were more activated towards the middle and the end of the session: therapist 1 (hereafter T1) was aroused during TEs 9, 10, 11, 13, 18 and 19, while therapist 2 (hereafter T2) was aroused during TEs 9, 10, 11, 13, 14 and 15. In TE5 only the couple were aroused.

The Nonverbal Synchronization of Body Postures and Movements

Figures 2 and 3 present the dyadic nonverbal synchronization patterns in the session. Posture-synchronization occurred 12 times, with 9 of these instances occurring between the therapists. In TE 11, Mary and Tom were in posture-synchrony. There was no posture-synchronization within the episodes chosen for the SRIs.

All the participants were synchronized to each other's movements. The therapists were the most active (81 and 71) and then Mary (42) and Tom the least (26). Tom was more synchronized with Mary (13) than with the therapists (8), and Mary was more synchronized with the therapists (23) than with Tom (13).

Most of the synchronized movements in the session were head movements (81), i.e. head nods. The therapist-dyad were synchronized the most (49), followed by T2 and Mary (8), then Mary and Tom (7), T1 and Tom (6) and then other dyads or triads. Displacement behaviour synchronization occurred 21 times (arm movements 11 times and hand movements 10 times).

At the beginning of the session, the therapists showed most synchrony (both in postures and head movements). Towards the end of the session, there was a rise in the frequency of synchronized movements between all the participants, until TE 17, when all movement synchronization stopped.[2] There was no difference in the amount of movement synchrony between the TEs selected for the SRIs and the other TEs.

---

[1] Exhaustive explanation of the DIHC results is beyond the scope of this chapter.

[2] This chapter is necessarily limited in scope; hence, not all the results obtained via this method are presented here.

Integration of the Information from the Different Research Methods Based on the Participants' Inner Dialogues (Information from the SRIs)

The results here are presented separately for each SRI clip.[3] First of all, we present information on what happened *within the session* in the SRI clip shown to the participants. This includes the dialogue and the participants' arousal levels plus their nonverbal synchronization behaviour that were analysed for the corresponding TE (for an overview of these, see Figs. 1, 2 and 3). Thereafter, we present the participants' *individual SRI accounts*. Here we seek to integrate their personal account to the embodied reactions with the dialogue and therapy process. Finally, a summary of the results for each clip is given.

SRI Clip 1 (TE12)

The clip was chosen for the SRI because of visible emotion (crying, laughter) and the theme (motherhood) and also because of Tom's noticeable movements and his EDA that decreased concurrently with that of T1. This clip occurred in the middle part of TE12 ('reasons for therapy – disconnection').

Within the session Mary did most of the talking (quantitative dominance), stating that she and Tom were disconnected and that they tried to talk to each other but lacked the necessary skills. Mary said she felt that Tom was still processing something, whereas Tom responded that he did not know what that might be. Mary reflected on her struggle of becoming a mother and of Tom just being a 'natural father'. Within the session the therapists regulated the conversation (interactional dominance). In analysing the therapeutic process, in this episode the therapists were preparing the ground for discussing the reason for therapy (disconnection).

Within the session (TE12), all the participants had low arousal levels, especially Tom, and T2 had very low arousal (compared to their own personal arousal level means in the session) (see Fig. 1). The only synchronized movements in this clip were head movements between the therapists (T1 and T2) and between T1 and Mary (see Fig. 3).

Individual thoughts and emotions When Mary watched the video clip from the session, she shed tears. She said she had felt frustrated in the session because Tom had not been willing to address something – he was holding back, which meant that she had to bring up the difficult conversations they had had. She said she had been sad in the session because of them being disconnected. Mary's feelings of frustra-

---

[3]The length of the SRI clips differed from the length of the TEs. In some instances the SRI clips contained segments from one TE or covered more than one TE.

tion were not visible in her arousal level in the session; however, her description of sadness would be in line with her low arousal level.

In the SRI, Tom said he had felt an unpleasant feeling in the session but simultaneously felt that they were getting somewhere, as in starting to make sense of their difficulties. Tom's SCR indicated very low arousal at this moment in the session. This could reflect a feeling that he had no need to react: he felt that they were getting somewhere in the therapy and that he could just let matters evolve. Tom was left outside the nonverbal synchronization in this episode.

In the SRI, T1 said that within the session he had been very pleased when Mary said that Tom was holding back, because it was the first critical comment on their relationship. This stance was also seen in the session, where T1 was nodding along with Mary. T1's arousal had been near to his average. He stated in the SRI that he had been somewhat annoyed at Tom in the session, because he talked so rationally and unemotionally, but his feelings of frustration didn't affect his arousal level.

In the SRI, T2 commented that during the session he had felt interest when Mary said she felt disconnected with Tom. However, T2's arousal level had been very low at that juncture, which could reflect that he felt it unnecessary to react or intervene in the therapeutic situation.

Summary At this moment the concurrent nods of the therapists during the session accorded with their comments in the SRI. Both said that they had felt that the topic was important. T1 had felt empathy with Mary's stance, and he nodded with her in the therapy, whereas Tom was 'left outside' the nonverbal synchronization. T2 also mentioned having been interested in Mary's point of view, but this did not appear in his nonverbal synchronization behaviour.

One reason for choosing the clip to SRI was the concurrent decreasing arousal levels of T1 and Tom. However, the SRI provided no definite explanation for this. One might have expected the decreasing arousal levels to reflect empathy between T1 and Tom. However, T1's account in the SRI conflicted with this interpretation. He had been annoyed with Tom and had empathized with Mary's situation.

SRI Clip 2 (TE14)

The clip was chosen for the second SRI clip because of the theme (man holding back) and visible laughter (Tom) and the EDA responses of T2, Tom and T1. This episode occurred within TE14 ('the conversation here and now').

Within the session T2 asked if Mary and Tom felt connected during the therapy session. Mary answered that she had shown her emotions and talked about their issues. However, as she saw it, Tom was holding back. Tom answered, mentioning that after the previous session Mary had said to him 'I hope next week they pick on you'. However, they both indicated that the therapy had led them to do things differently in their everyday life, in terms of talking more. In the session, it was Mary who talked the most, though both she and Tom regulated the discussion. The therapists were not active.

When analysing the therapeutic process, we viewed this point as an ambivalent moment in the therapy. There were two parallel processes going on: the couple were talking to each other (being very dialogical). However, although Mary raised the matter of Tom holding back, the theme was avoided thereafter by both Mary and Tom.

During the session (TE12), the SCRs of all the participants indicated some arousal, except for T1 who remained close to his average arousal level. T2 introduced the theme, which could be seen as a reason for his arousal (see Fig. 1). All the participants were involved in movement-synchronization behaviour with each other, and there were some synchronized displacement behaviours, between T1 and Mary and between T1 and Tom (see Fig. 3).

Individual thoughts and emotions In the subsequent SRI, Mary said that she had felt uncomfortable in the session throughout the clip chosen for the SRI, because she felt Tom was making her defend herself. She thought Tom had shifted attention towards her after they had talked about him holding back. This surprised her. She said that she had felt many emotions, first surprise and in the end joy. The emotions could be seen in her SCR, which indicated some arousal. Another possible source to it was the fact that Mary and Tom were regulating the conversation, with no co-regulation on the part of the therapists. Mary's arousal might also have been connected to her doing displacement behaviours with T1.

In the SRI, Tom said that he had found it interesting that Mary said he was holding back. He was taken aback by her comment and felt that he needed to talk about it with her. In the actual session (TE 14), Tom's SCR indicated some arousal. This could be related to his feeling of surprise at Mary's comment or to the co-regulation of the conversation. Tom's arousal level could also be connected to him doing displacement behaviours in the session which T1 synchronized to.

In the SRI, T1 said he had felt pleased that Mary was showing her emotions in the session. He wondered if Mary was protecting Tom by showing her emotions, so that Tom did not have to show his. T1 felt that Mary's comment regarding Tom holding back contained a lot of truth, since he did not observe an emotional reaction from Tom. Within the episode, T1 had nodded along with T2 and did displacement behaviours with both Mary and Tom. This could reflect T1's endeavour to feel his way into their emotions (a bodily contagion process used as therapeutic empathy). T1 had not been highly aroused during this episode; it seemed that he was able to let the discussion take its course.

In his SRI, T2 said that the theme talked about in the session was very important. He had considered asking more about the topic. He was thus preparing for an action, which might be seen in his arousal level, as his SCR indicated some arousal. In the actual session, T2 followed the nodding of Mary and T1. This could have been a signal to the others that he felt the topic under discussion was important and that he was listening.

Summary At this moment, all the participants were aroused in the actual session. This could reflect the way in which the couple talked together and regulated the discussion while avoiding genuine exploration of the theme of Tom holding back. T2 was aroused, possibly because he was preparing for an intervention. T1 was less aroused, although he was synchronized to both Mary's and Tom's displacement behaviour.

SRI Clip 3 (TE16)

The episode was selected for the SRI because of the theme (heart of our disconnectedness), Mary crying and the long silences. Clip 3 covered a moment mid-way through TE16 ('reasons for disconnecting').

Within the session Mary talked about her realization that they had had such completely different experiences of their child's first year. For Tom it had been the best time of his life, whereas for her it was very different, i.e. a struggle. They had been a strong unit previously, but their different experiences of the time after the birth of their daughter was the heart of the disconnectedness. She said that Tom had never made her feel bad about her struggles: he had only once said that it was the best time of his life, to which Tom answered that he knew how that would have made her feel. From the point of view of the overall therapeutic process, this episode was a significant moment: within it, Tom and Mary talked about the issue of being in therapy. Within the session Mary did most of the actual talking; however, Tom had chosen the topic, with T2 regulating it.

In the actual session (TE 16), Mary had had low arousal, and T1 very low arousal, whereas Tom and T2 had been averagely aroused (see Fig. 1). In this particular clip, there was considerable movement-synchronization (the highest amount per episode in the session as a whole). All the participants were synchronized in their movements, and very importantly, the couple was synchronized to each other (see Fig. 3).

Individual thoughts and emotions In the SRI, Mary said that the episode was a moment of insight in the therapy. She felt sadness because of their separate experiences. Within the session she was crying; moreover, her arousal was low. In the session, Mary was synchronized to Tom and T1 in their head nods and displacement behaviours. She also nodded simultaneously with Tom. The displacement behaviours that might have been thought to reflect arousal did not, in fact, show in Mary's arousal level. The head nods could be related to her signalling the importance of the topic under discussion.

Tom indicated the importance of the topic in his SRI, saying that this was the main issue they were dealing with. At this moment within the session, he had nodded together with each therapist separately and also with Mary. Tom said he had felt sad in the therapy session, but he now felt it even more in the SRI situation. He reflected on feelings of guilt for enjoying life with the baby while being aware of how it impacted on Mary. His arousal level within the episode had been near to his average for the session. This could reflect the combination of feeling sad and a feeling of important issues being discussed. Importantly Tom's arousal level had not been high, even though he did displacement behaviours. Interestingly, Tom showed more feelings in the SRI situation than in the therapy session itself. It seemed as if the context (being alone with the interviewer) allowed him to experience (and share) emotions.

In the SRI, T1 reflected on the couple's history: they had been such a strong unit before, and now felt disconnected. He also recognized his own unease at Tom having words for everything, without very much emotion. T1's SCR had indicated very low arousal, which could reflect that he did not need to react in the situation; thus, his frustration with Tom's rational talk was not seen in his arousal level. Within the episode, T1 had been nonverbally synchronized with all other participants and equally to Tom and Mary. He also nodded frequently with T2, expressing the importance of the topic.

In the SRI, T2 said that he had seen the topic as very important: it lay at the heart of the couple's disconnection. He said that he had been very interested in Mary's point of view and had wanted to know more about Mary's feelings. His interest could be seen in his head-nodding behaviour.

Summary In this moment Tom and Mary were nonverbally synchronized to each other in the actual session. It was the only episode chosen for the SRIs in which this occurred. It appeared to signal an embodied connection between them. The other participants were also involved in the nonverbal synchronization behaviour. This could signal the importance of the topic, with everyone actively collaborating in the discussion. When they discussed a significant issue, there was considerable movement-synchronization between everyone, but not a particularly high level of arousal in all the participants. The displacement behaviours were not accompanied by high arousal.

SRI Clip 4 (TE17 to TE18)

The clip was selected for the SRI because of the theme (gender roles), the couple's laughter, and it was chosen by the researcher to end the SRI situation with a less stressful episode. The clip was from the middle of TE17 ('not "natural mother" – guilt') to the end of TE18 ('acceptance of others').

Within the session The topic primarily concerned Tom's role as a father and their untraditional parental roles, within which Tom did much of the caring for Eva – something that had been very similar in Tom's family of origin. Mary and Tom did most of the talking. Mary and T2 regulated the discussion and introduced the topics. From the perspective of the therapeutic process, this was a moment where not so much intensive therapy work was done.

Within the session (TE17 and TE18), Mary's arousal had been below her average, whereas Tom had moved from very high arousal to an arousal level near his average of the session. T2 had moved in the same direction as Tom, from having had some arousal to low arousal. By contrast, T1's arousal went in the opposite direction: he first had low arousal, and then his arousal level rose (see Fig. 1).

In this clip (TE 17 and 18), there was a very low frequency of nonverbal synchronization in the actual session, with only the therapists nodding together (on two occasions) (see Fig. 3).

Individual thoughts and emotions In the SRI, Mary indicated that this clip was not as emotionally strong as the others had been. Her low arousal level confirmed this.

For his part, Tom observed that he looked more relaxed in the clip. However, as he recalled the session, he had not in fact felt so relaxed at this point. His recollection seemed to be closer to reality, since in the session he had shown high arousal (in TE17), which then decreased (in TE18).

T1 said that he thought the topics towards the end of the session had been increasingly interesting and important. T1 was anxious because of the important topics coming up and because he knew he would have to end the session earlier than expected. Within the session T1's arousal level was rising, which could relate to his feeling of unease.

T2 did not recall any specific emotion during the clip. He had felt curious about the couple's roles and Tom's family of origin. In his SRI he commented that the couple's situation was like a puzzle, becoming piece by piece more complete. This could possibly be seen in his arousal levels, which had gone in the same direction as Tom's, i.e. decreased.

Summary This moment was not a significant moment in therapy. This was also seen in the lower arousal levels of the participants during the actual session. Only T1 was aroused, and this was possibly related to his feelings of distress of having to end the session prematurely.

Summary of the Findings from the SRIs in Combination with the Findings on Autonomic Nervous System Arousal and Nonverbal Synchronization

In general terms, the analysis of the SRI conversations revealed the complexity of the embodied reactions, in that (for instance) when a participant had high arousal, it did not always mean that the discussion was particularly emotional or difficult. The differing roles of the therapists and the clients were also visible in their embodied reactions. The therapists were more active in synchronizing nonverbally to others. It could be that the therapists were using nonverbal synchronization to further the dialogue and to signal the importance of the topic under discussion but also as a therapeutic tool to understand the clients' experiences. In the SRIs the therapists were more empathic towards Mary's point of view, but this was not seen in their embodied reactions (SCR and nonverbal synchronization).

It also seemed that the different embodied reactions of the participants were not in a linear relation to each other, meaning that when there was much movement-synchronization, there were no concurrent or consecutive higher or lower arousal levels among the participants. It would thus seem that the different embodied reactions (SCRs and nonverbal synchronization) within the session could have had different and independent functions within the therapy process. For example, the level of arousal was not directly connected to the emotional load of the dialogue or to the felt importance of it. When participants stated that the topic was important for them, they weren't highly aroused at that moment in the session.

Discussion

In this case study, we wanted to know what the embodied reactions of the participants might indicate concerning the therapy process. We discovered that they were not easy to interpret. Earlier research on the autonomic nervous system responses has shown that many factors affect the arousal level of the participants in psychotherapy. We reached a similar conclusion. We discovered that the arousal patterns differed in different moments of the therapy process. As the therapists were preparing the ground for discussing the couple's reason for coming to therapy, all participants had low arousal. But in an ambivalent moment, where the couple avoided discussing the issue of Tom holding back, all participants were aroused. This could reflect them all being activated by the situation, as if interested in seeing how it would unfold, which was in line with earlier research indicating that active emotional engagement in the therapeutic process increases arousal (del Piccolo & Finset, 2017). But within a significant moment in the session where the issue of why the couple was in therapy was discussed, all participants had low arousal. This could be interpreted as a feeling of relief in the participants, which would be in line with earlier research suggesting that relief is accompanied by lower arousal levels (Kreibig, 2010). As for the qualities of dialogue (dialogicity, dominance and narrative mode), it did not seem that they were directly related to the arousal levels or nonverbal synchronies among the participants.

As for the combination of the arousal levels and nonverbal synchronization behaviour, our study suggests that the arousal level and the nonverbal synchronization behaviours contribute to the therapeutic situation in different ways. Autonomic nervous system activity occurs 'under the skin', whereas synchronized nonverbal behaviour is visible to all participants in the session. Thus, nonverbal behaviour can implicitly impact the therapeutic situation. In our case study, one of the therapists interpreted Tom as more rational. The implicit nonverbal synchronization patterns in this session might have contributed to this interpretation. In the session Tom was mostly synchronized to Mary, whereas Mary was more synchronized to the therapists. Thus, Mary was more connected to the therapists at the embodied level, whereas Tom was not. This might induce the therapist to interpret Tom as more distant.

It was notable that in the present therapy process, the therapists used their bodies differently. Thus, one therapist was involved mainly in the regulation of the dialogue, through the use of head nods, whereas the other therapist showed more contagion from the couple's displacement behaviour, which could be seen as a way of feeling his way into the client's arousal.

When considering the nonverbal synchronization behaviour of the participants in relation to the therapeutic process, one finding was that within all the moments chosen for the SRIs, there was no posture-synchronization. This was no surprise, since earlier research suggests that posture-synchronization is related to moments of high rapport (Trout & Rosenfeld, 1980). The lack of posture-synchronization in these moments could be a reflection of a choice of moments to the SRIs that contained emotionally loaded or therapeutically interesting topics, in preference to situations where there was high rapport between the participants.

As for movement-synchrony, all the SRI clips showed head movement synchrony between participants. In the clips that were therapeutically more interesting, i.e. ambivalent or significant, there were more head nods between participants. This was in line with earlier research showing that head nods could be seen as a way of furthering the dialogue (Stivers, 2008) or marking interest in the topic discussed.

When one strives to integrate information from different research methods, straightforward conclusions are hard to make. Linear or correlational ways of thinking are challenged. It is too simplistic to think that arousal would rise as the emotional load of the dialogue, or the amount of nonverbal synchronization behaviour increases. The relations between the different modalities (i.e. autonomic nervous system responses, nonverbal synchronization and the dialogue) are by no means constant. They change depending on the therapeutic process and the challenge it forces the participants to face, their position or their role regarding the topic. The individual reactions of each participant can be seen as impacting on the dialogue, but they can also be a reaction to the dialogue or to each individual's personal agenda in the situation.

The individual agendas in the session could be accessed with the SRIs. It is a useful method to gain insight into the participants' inner thoughts and feelings during the session. The SRI is a valuable method because it narrows the gap between clinicians and researchers and promotes practice-oriented research (see Vall et al., 2018).

By using this kind of mixed-method procedure, it is possible to broaden our understanding of the therapeutic process and especially the impact the participants' embodied reactions have on it. Based on this study, further research combining the dialogue with embodied reactions is needed to clarify the functions of the different modalities.

References

Angus, L., Levitt, H., & Hardtke, K. (1999). The narrative processes coding system: Research applications and implications for psychotherapy practice. *Journal of Clinical Psychology, 55,* 1255–1270.

Angus, L., Lewin, J., Boritz, T., Bryntwick, E., Carpenter, N., Watson-Gaze, J., & Greenberg, L. (2012). Narrative processes coding system: A dialectical constructivist approach to assessing client change processes in emotion-focused therapy of depression. *Research in Psychotherapy: Psychopathology, Process and Outcome, 15*(2), 54–61.

Bavelas, J. B., Coates, L., & Johnson, T. (2000). Listeners as co-narrators. *Journal of Personality and Social Psychology, 79*(6), 941–952.

Benedek, M., & Kaernbach, C. (2010). A continuous measure of phasic electrodermal activity. *Journal of Neuroscience Methods, 190*(1), 80–91.

Boucsein, W. (2012). *Electrodermal activity.* New York, NY: Springer Science + Business Media.

Chartrand, T. L., & Bargh, J. A. (1999). The chameleon effect: The perception-behavior link and social interaction. *Journal of Personality and Social Psychology, 76*(6), 893–910.

Cromby, J. (2012). Feeling the way: Qualitative research and the affective turn. *Qualitative Research in Psychology, Special Issue on Qualitative Clinical Research, 9*(1), 88–98.

Davis, M., & Hadiks, D. (1994). Nonverbal aspects of therapist attunement. *Journal of Clinical Psychology, 50*(3), 393–405.

Del Piccolo, L., & Finset, A. (2017). Patients' autonomic activation during clinical interaction: A review of empirical studies. *Patient Education and Counseling, 101*(2), 195–208.

Finset, A., Stensrud, T. L., Holt, E., Verheul, W., & Bensing, J. (2011). Electrodermal activity in response to empathic statements in clinical interviews with fibromyalgia patients. *Patient Education and Counseling, 82*(3), 355–360.

Kagan, N., Krathwohl, D. R., & Miller, R. (1963). Stimulated recall in therapy using video tape: A case study. *Journal of Counseling Psychology, 10*(3), 237–243.

Kreibig, S. D. (2010). Autonomic nervous system activity in emotion: A review. *Biological Psychology, 84*(3), 394–421.

Laitila, A., Aaltonen, J., Wahlström, J., & Angus, L. (2005). Narrative process modes as a bridging concept for the theory, research, and clinical practice of systemic therapy. *Journal of Family Therapy, 27*(3), 202–216.

Laitila, A., Vall, B., Penttonen, M., Karvonen, A., Kykyri, V.-L., Kaartinen, J., … Seikkula, J. (2019). The added value of studying embodied responses in couple therapy research: A case study. *Family Process, 58,* 685–697.

Lakens, D., & Stel, M. (2011). If they move in sync, they must feel in sync: Movement synchrony leads to attributions of rapport and entitativity. *Social Cognition, 29*(1), 1–14.

Muntigl, P., Knight, N., & Watkins, A. (2012). Working to keep aligned in psychotherapy. Using nods as a dialogic resource to display affiliation. *Language and Dialogue, 2*(1), 9–27.

Nyman-Salonen, P., Tourunen, A., Kykyri, V.-L., Penttonen, M., Kaartinen, J., & Seikkula, J. (submitted). Observing nonverbal synchrony in couple therapy— studying implicit posture and movement synchrony in psychotherapy.

Olson, D. H., & Claiborn, C. D. (1990). Interpretation and arousal in the counseling process. *Journal of Counseling Psychology, 37*(2), 131–137.

Olson, M. E., Laitila, A., Rober, P., & Seikkula, J. (2012). The shift from monologue to dialogue in a couple therapy session: Dialogical investigation of change from the therapists' point of view. *Family Process, 51*(3), 420–435.

Päivinen, H., Holma, J., Karvonen, A., Kykyri, V.-L., Tsatsishvili, V., Kaartinen, J., … Seikkula, J. (2016). Affective arousal during blaming in couple therapy: Combining analyses of verbal discourse and physiological responses in two case studies. *Contemporary Family Therapy, 38*(4), 373–384.

Raingruber, B. J. (2001). Settling into and moving in a climate of care: Styles and patterns of inter-action between nurse psychotherapists and clients. *Perspectives in Psychiatric Care, 37*(1), 15–27.

Räsänen, E., Holma, J., & Seikkula, J. (2012). Dialogical views on partner abuser treatment: Balancing confrontation and support. *Journal of Family Violence, 27*(4), 357–368.

Rober, P., Elliott, R., Buysse, A., Loots, G., & De Corte, K. (2008). What's on the therapist's mind? A grounded theory analysis of family therapist reflections during individual therapy sessions. *Psychotherapy Research, 18*(1), 48–57.

Seikkula, J., Karvonen, A., Kykyri, V.-L., Kaartinen, J., & Penttonen, M. (2015). The embodied attunement of therapists and a couple within dialogical psychotherapy: An introduction to the Relational Mind research project. *Family Process, 54*(4), 703–715.

Seikkula, J., Laitila, A., & Rober, P. (2012). Making sense of multi-actor dialogues in family therapy and network meetings. *Journal of Marital and Family Therapy, 38*(4), 667–687.

Sep, M. S. C., van Osch, M., van Vliet, L. M., Smets, E. M. A., & Bensing, J. M. (2014). The power of clinicians' affective communication: How reassurance about non-abandonment can reduce patients' physiological arousal and increase information recall in bad news consultations. An experimental study using analogue patients. *Patient Education and Counseling, 95*, 45–52.

Sharpley, C. F., Halat, J., Rabinowicz, T., Weiland, B., & Stafford, J. (2001). Standard posture, postural mirroring and client-perceived rapport. *Counseling Psychology Quarterly, 14*(4), 267–280.

Stel, M., & van den Bos, K. (2010). Mimicry as a tool for understanding the emotions of others. In A. J. Spink, F. Grieco, O. E. Krips, L. W. S. Loijens, L. P. J. J. Noldus, & P. H. Zimmerman (Eds.), *Proceedings of measuring behavior: 7th international conference on Methods and Techniques in Behavioral Research 2010* (pp. 114–117). Wageningen, The Netherlands.

Stivers, T. (2008). Stance, alignment, and affiliation during storytelling: When nodding is a token of affiliation. *Research on Language & Social Interaction, 41*(1), 31–57.

Troisi, A. (2002). Displacement activities as a behavioral measure of stress in nonhuman primates and human subjects. *Stress, 5*(1), 47–54.

Trout, D. L., & Rosenfeld, H. M. (1980). The effect of postural lean and body congruence on the judgment of psychotherapeutic rapport. *Journal of Nonverbal Behavior, 4*(3), 176–190.

Vall, B., Seikkula, J., Laitila, A., Holma, J., & Botella, L. (2014). Increasing Responsibility, Safety, and Trust Through a Dialogical Approach: A Case Study in Couple Therapy for Psychological Abusive Behavior. *Journal of Family Psychotherapy, 25*(4), 275–299.

Vall, B., Laitila, A., Borcsa, M., Kykyri, V.-L., Karvonen, A., Kaartinen, J., … Seikkula, J. (2018). Stimulated recall interviews: How can the research interview contribute to new therapeutic practices? *Revista Argentina de Clínica Psicológica, XXVII*(2), 274–293.

Collaborative Family Program Development: Research Methods That Investigate and Foster Resilience and Engagement in Marginalized Communities

Peter Fraenkel

Introduction

This chapter presents the ten-step Collaborative Family Program Development model (CFPD; Fraenkel, 2006a, 2007a, 2007b) for engaging disempowered and socioculturally and economically marginalized families as experts in teaching researchers about their unique challenges and in creating and evaluating community-based programs to serve families' needs and to foster family resilience. Programs and interventions for marginalized families and communities are typically created and evaluated by academics or social service professionals from their "expert position," relying heavily on quantitative assessments, and based on what is already known about the community's challenges primarily from other experts' research. But this approach fails to incorporate members' detailed expertise on their own lives, the unique qualities of the specific community, and community members' ideas about what would make a program useful. As a result, these expert-driven community-based programs fail to enroll many families, or result in high attrition, because the programs do not recognize families' self-perceived needs and the constraints they face in attending a program – such as timing, location, and cost. In contrast, the approach described in this chapter reverses the typical hierarchy between professional psychologist/researcher and the families who are recipients of programs, such that the psychologist –typically in the role of expert – instead becomes the learner and the family is viewed as the expert on their own lives and

P. Fraenkel (✉)
The City College of The City University of New York, New York, NY, USA

© Springer Nature Switzerland AG 2020   75
M. Ochs et al. (eds.), *Systemic Research in Individual, Couple, and Family Therapy and Counseling*, European Family Therapy Association Series,
https://doi.org/10.1007/978-3-030-36560-8_5

program needs. The research and program development approach described here is paradigmatically and methodologically similar to participatory action research (Chevalier & Buckles, 2019), cooperative inquiry (Reason & Heron, 1995), and contemporary qualitative social justice and evaluation research that engages multiple perspectives and all stakeholders and, therefore, is interdisciplinary (Charmaz, Thornberg, & Keane, 2018; Dahler-Larsen, 2018; Reitinger, 2008).

The approach will be illustrated by a program called Fresh Start for Families (Fraenkel, 2006b; Fraenkel, Hameline, & Shannon, 2009), a 6- to 8-week multiple family discussion group (MFDG) created, conducted, and evaluated by the author and his students at The City College of New York and the Ackerman Institute for the Family, in collaboration with families and frontline workers, to serve families living in homeless shelters, including a shelter for families that had specifically escaped domestic violence. However, the emphasis of the chapter is to articulate details of the methodology, rather than to describe in detail the significant plight of homeless families in the United States, with the idea that the program development methods can readily be utilized to create and evaluate programs for families facing other sorts of challenges besides homelessness – for instance, adjustment to a new country after immigration (Fraenkel, Shannon, & Diaz Alarcon, 2009), chronic drug and alcohol abuse, reintegration of a parent who had been incarcerated, or severe mental illness. Indeed, the CFPD model can be utilized for creating and evaluating programs for families of all levels of socioeconomic, educational, and cultural privilege, but the emphasis here is on the method's empowering effects for multi-stressed families (Madsen, 2007) whose opinions about their lives and needs are frequently overlooked, because it is often implicitly assumed that they are at least somewhat to blame for their challenging circumstances.

Expert-Driven Versus Collaboratively - Created Family Programs: A Brief Review

The usual model followed by psychologists to develop a program bases it upon expert knowledge about families accumulated largely through large sample quantitative methodologies. The program is then implemented based upon psychologists' and other professional stakeholders' judgments about the program's optimal location/setting, timing (meeting schedule, frequency, length of sessions), content and activities, and other processes. And the program's impact is then evaluated, usually only in a pre-/post-/follow-up framework, using standardized instruments to assess target mental health and other desired outcomes. Based on the Institute of Medicine model (Institute of Medicine, 2003; Mrazek & Haggerty, 1994), and known in the fields of prevention-intervention science more informally as the "top-down" approach, it has, in the terse assessment of eminent American developmental psychologist/community health interventionist Kenneth Dodge, "not succeeded" (Dodge, 2018, p. 1118). Dodge writes: "…psychologists often assume that progress moves unidirectionally from laboratory science to small randomized controlled efficacy trials to community-based effectiveness trials to impact through community-wide scaling up" (p. 1118). Dodge lists several factors leading to failure of these programs (and by way of introducing the CFPD approach and the resulting Fresh Start program, the present author describes how the CFPD and Fresh Start program evaded each of these failure factors):

1. "Scale-up failures," due largely to a lack of match between the children and families who participate in laboratory-based interventions and others in actual communities, wherein the former subgroup are often more economically advantaged and better functioning and, thus, able to come to a lab on a regular basis, versus the latter subgroup in the same community, who are less advantaged and less well-functioning and who therefore do not benefit from the same interventions, whereas the better functioning families don't need as much intervention in the first place. Given the limits of grants, per child funding for scale-up in the community also typically gets reduced, which negatively impacts fidelity to the original, usually more extensive intervention.

   In contrast, the basic research on challenges faced by homeless families leading to creation of the Fresh Start for Families program developed through the CFPD approach was conducted entirely on site, as was the program itself, in the community where the families lived – namely, in the shelters. There was therefore no accidental selection bias in accessing families for the research or ensuing program and no struggle around transportation or other issues (e.g., obtaining childcare for infants and toddlers) for families to participate – the program came to them, rather than requiring that they come to the program.

2. "Poor incentives," meaning that grant limitations often result in only short-term, partial implementation of programs, resulting in no long-term support of families to achieve desired outcomes. When the government or other institutional funding source (and perhaps the researcher himself or herself) advertises success, this may inadvertently lead policy makers to conclude that a problem has been solved, resulting in decremental funding for future, long-term, potentially more effective programs. A parallel process occurs often in large-scale international aid interventions on material challenges – for instance, when a bridge is built in a rural area that does not yet have complete roads on either side, or, in one extreme notable case, when hundreds of refrigerators were shipped to a remote area of the Sudanese desert that had no electricity, and the refrigerators were used instead as protective places to sleep in to avoid bites from desert insects (Hancock, 1989).

   In contrast to the types of multi-million dollar grants usually sought from the federal government for community interventions from the National Institute of Mental Health (NIMH) or similar federal granting agencies (SAMSHA, NIDA), the Fresh Start for Families program was operated for 14 consecutive years with a director (the present author) and staff of 10 doctoral- and masters-level graduate students on a limited but sustainable series of small grants from private foundations and small federal, state, and city grants, with a typical yearly budget of about $220,000. This allowed the kind of flexibility, creativity, and changes of course needed to adapt to the fluctuating real-life conditions experienced by families.

3. "Family context matters": As Dodge (2018) writes, "By starting in a university laboratory, psychologists sometimes develop interventions without sufficient regard to a young child and family's working and community context…many programs to improve a child's parenting have not kept pace with trends in family ecology and are therefore constrained in their ability to achieve population impact." (p. 1119). For example, without conferring with families about their daily routines, researcher-interventionists may attempt to launch a program in the late afternoon, when parents are still at work or when they have just returned from work and need to gather children from childcare, prepare meals, and supervise homework.

   In contrast, the detailed interviews conducted through the CFPD approach specifically asked families to identify factors that might limit their ability to engage in the program and asked for recommendations about such issues as what time of the day to hold program sessions. Based on consistent parent input, it was decided to serve dinner at the start of each weekly early evening meeting (the program met from 18:00 to 19:30 hours once a week, for 8 weeks), because parents said they wouldn't be able to come otherwise, as their responsible commitment was to feed their children.

4. "Peer context matters": without ascertaining the academic and social functioning of an intervention-targeted child's peers, the negative impact of a less-well-functioning peer group may override any potential beneficial effects of the intervention. This finding speaks to the need to implement the same intervention for all members of a community, so that the entire peer group of children and families benefit and can support one another directly, or indirectly, through observing one another's progress.

   In contrast, the format of the Fresh Start program was a multiple family discussion group, with 6–8 families in each group, with some activities conducted with all families present together in the room and some activities in separate kids/teens groups and parents' groups (Fraenkel, 2007a, 2007b; Fraenkel & Shannon, 1999). This multimodal approach allowed for fostering of mutual support among the kids/teens across ages 5 through 18, opportunities for parents to discuss parenting and other adult issues without kids present, and among the families as a whole.

5. "Resource context matters": Top-down programs typically do not consider that the resources families need to improve through the program's interventions are scarce and not equally distributed – resources such as employment, housing, food, childcare, and so on. An employment and permanent housing program for homeless parents is likely to fail when jobs and apartments are not available to all program participants.

   In contrast, because the program was developed and implemented as a service within the homeless family shelter, it was linked to other services provided to families, such as job training and placement, permanent housing search specialists, social services (assistance with welfare benefits, court cases around child custody and child welfare), mental health referrals, and recreational services. In the early stages of program development, staff members of the shelter from all levels of the employment hierarchy (from shelter director to security guards and cleaning staff) were interviewed to ascertain their sense of the challenges families faced, families' strengths, what families most needed in a program, what would facilitate and what would block their participation, and how the program could best complement their professional efforts to support the families.

Reed (2015) elegantly summarizes the spirit and general methodological approach of the "bottom-up," collaborative, or as he terms it, "community-engaged" approach to program evaluation that mirrors well the CFPD approach. He traces the history of this approach to the challenges posed to positivism by critical theory (see review by Kincheloe, McLaren, Steinberg, & Monzo, 2018), postmodern thinking (Foucault, 1980), and the liberation psychology of Paulo Freire (1968/2000). He writes:

> Theories of community-engaged research emerged from within this tradition as an approach to research conducted in community contexts, and encouraged the development of collaborative strategies for advancing community wellbeing, in so doing seeking to foster and support partnerships between 'researchers' and 'researched' characterized by two-way learning built on a commitment to knowledge exchange and mutual respect and recognition. (pp. 118–119)

Reed argues that engaging community members as collaborators in program evaluation (and by easy extension, the earlier stages of program development and implementation) provides clear benefits, especially that (a) the research process itself – alongside the actual programs being studied – leads to emancipation/empowerment rather than enforcing continued social control and marginalization and (b) treating participants with the respect due to them creates greater trust, which results in better quality, more valid, illuminative data, minimizing the tendency of oppressed groups to tell researchers what they think the researchers want to hear.

Although the literature on collaborative program development/evaluation methods has grown since the present author's original (2006a) publication on the CFPD approach, Reed notes that community-engaged research is far from the dominant approach – a point clearly noted by Dodge (2018) as well, in his plea for combining bottom-up with top-down interventions. Reed writes, "The current literature on community engagement is emergent rather than established, and the frameworks that do exist are varied in quality, detail, scope and applicability" (p. 122).

The Effects of Homelessness on Families

There is a growing incidence of homeless families in the United States, particularly in urban areas. New York City reports the highest rates in the nation: In November 2016, there were 16,000 families – 48,000 people – sleeping in shelters, 14% more than in January of 2014 (Routhier, 2017). Although the rates of families in shelters are alarmingly high, even more concerning is the case of San Bernardino, California, which has a warmer year-round climate than New York and where many homeless families are literally living outdoors – in cars, in parks, and so on (Lobo, 2018). The following summary of effects of homelessness on families is taken verbatim and with permission from a dissertation (Lobo, 2018, pp. 4–6) on which the present author served as a committee member[1]:

> Homelessness impacts families and family life in multiple ways. The instability, stress and potentially traumatic experiences associated with homelessness impacts all members of the household (Bassuk, 2010; Moore & McArthur, 2011). In children, this often results in decreased physical health (Markos & Lima, 2003), poor academic performance (Bassuk, 2010; Fetherman & Burke, 2015; Perlman & Fantuzzo, 2010), and significant mental health challenges leading to behavioral issues (Grant, Gracy, Goldsmith, Shapiro, & Redlener, 2013; Park, Metraux, Culhane, & Mandell, 2012; Piehler et al., 2014; Ziol-Guest & McKenna, 2014) and other long-term consequences such as increased risk for incarceration (Fowler, Henry, & Marcal, 2015) and suicide (Cleverley & Kidd, 2011). Adults in homeless families also face numerous stressors and mental health issues, including potential impact of past trauma and abuse (L. Anderson, Stuttafod, & Vostanis, 2006; Anooshian, 2005; Barrow & Lawinski, 2009), the stressors of parenting and meeting children's needs while homeless (Hilton & Trella, 2014; Holtrop, McNeil, & McWey, 2015; McNeil Smith, Holtrop, & Reynolds, 2015; Swick et al., 2014), and their own mental health challenges, often including depression (Bassuk & Beardslee, 2014; Park, Ostler, & Fertig, 2015; Toy, Tripodis, Yang, Cook, & Garg, 2016). Additionally, families as a whole face difficult transitions and stressors while experiencing homelessness. These may include temporary separations of family members (Barrow & Lawinski, 2009), limited social networks to access for support (Howard, Cartwright, & Barajas, 2009), and challenges in maintaining family rituals and routines (Mayberry, Shinn, Benton, & Wise, 2014). Parenting processes and parent-child relationships are also significantly affected (Holtrop et al., 2015; Schulz, 2009; Swick et al., 2014), with higher levels of conflict (Park et al., 2015; Swick, 2008) and the focus on meeting physical needs leaving emotional needs for children neglected. (Hilton & Trella, 2014)

This quite recent review of the devastating concomitants and effects of homelessness unfortunately mirrors the one published a decade ago by the present author (Fraenkel & Carmichael, 2008).

Steps in the Collaborative Family Program Development Approach: Application to Families in Homeless Shelters

Table 1 lists the 10 steps of the CFPD. Given that this section illustrates how the CFPD approach was utilized in creating what became the Fresh Start for Families program, it will shift from third person ("the present author") into first person ("I", "we", "us", "our") grammar as the story is told.

---

[1] Listing the original references summarized in this review would lead this chapter to exceed page limits.

Table 1 Steps in the Collaborative Family Program Development model

1. Initiating the project, forming the collaborative professional relationships, and engaging cultural consultants
2. Intensive interviewing of family members
3. Intensive interviewing of agency professionals
4. Phrase-by-phrase qualitative coding
5. Creating program formats and contents and writing an initial manual
6. Piloting of the group with session-by-session evaluations by participants
7. Revising the program and manual
8. Intensive interviewing of families for each subsequent group cycle
9. Evaluating the effectiveness in comparison or randomized designs
10. Disseminating and adapting the program to other settings

Step 1: Initiating the Project, Forming the Collaborative Professional Relationships, and Engaging Cultural Consultants

A project may be initiated by a professional researcher/program developer interested in a particular problem in a community; by a mental health, social service, religious, or other professional working with a particular community; or by members of the community itself, who may seek guidance in creating the program from a professional researcher/program developer. Initial meetings will center on answering, at least preliminarily, a number of key questions:

Passion and purpose Do members of the potential collaborative partnership have enough passion and sense of common purpose to sustain the joint effort of researching a problem and build a program? Far from being dispassionate scientists seeking solely to advance knowledge, applied social science researchers, like professionals working with the community and community members themselves, generally care deeply about the communities they engage with to study problems and design interventions. First meetings among stakeholders can and should be passionate affairs, with opportunities for all to express their interests, concerns, and desires about the problems facing the community. Members of the emerging partnership should be invited to express these passions, either in their role as a professional, as a person, or both, as is warranted and comfortable for them. Often, these passions are revealed as people share accounts of how they came to be interested in or involved with the problem, the challenges they've faced, and the fantasies they've held about how best to address it. As in psychotherapy, self-help, and other working groups, the interactive processes that occur in collaborative partnerships provide psychosocial benefits to their members, which in turn contribute to the energy needed to fulfill project goals. Each member's passion is validated and even amplified by hearing others with similar as well as different but related passions about the target problems. Identifying overlapping passions and goals builds a sense of group cohesion, a sense of no longer being alone with one's concerns but rather part of a community dedicated to making a difference. The relational, emotional, intellectual, and pragmatic benefits of sharing and linking passions and purposes in these initial meetings are crucial as the group commits to embark on a path of joint endeavor that will inevitably be strewn with roadblocks.

In addition to increasing group cohesion and strengthening collective emotional resilience for the tasks that lie ahead by sharing personal/professional passions, one of the principles of the CFPD approach is to ground all aspects of the program in the narratives of families and other persons (including ourselves) involved in the program, so that the program is relevant to the "local knowledge" (Geertz, 1983) and needs of the persons for whom it is designed. In this way, following Reason and Heron (1995), "practical knowledge" (how to do something – like conduct research and a program) and "propositional knowledge" (beliefs and theories about the social-psychological conditions the program is designed to address and about the nature of the program's potential impact) need to be grounded in "experiential knowledge" ("direct encounter face-to-face with persons, places, or things" [p. 123]). Thus, sharing respective passions and their sources in professional and personal histories is an important first step in the collaborative program development process.

In our case, our program for families that are homeless in transition from welfare to work began when an agency (HELP USA) requested assistance from a family therapy training and research institute (Ackerman). The representatives of these two institutions (Tom Hameline, Ph.D., and myself, respectively) spoke emotionally about our shared concerns for poor families. Tom spoke of the new challenges these families and the agencies that served them faced following enactment of the 1996 Personal Responsibility and Work Opportunity Reconciliation Act. Agencies across the country that served poor families were scrambling to develop programs to assist parents to develop "job readiness" skills (such as the ability to search effectively for employment, interviewing skills, good work habits and attitudes, and so on) and to find employment. An agency's success in meeting welfare-to-work goals affected their funding and capacity to provide services. HELP's ability to continue to provide housing was dependent on meeting welfare-to-work goals.

HELP found that although shelter residents were repeatedly reminded, by on-site case managers, welfare agency workers, and employment specialists that they needed to obtain employment and that their welfare benefits would end, few residents were engaging in the job programs. Although 65–70% of those who completed the 1-week readiness program and got placed in employment still had their jobs 6 months later, by 1 year, less than 50% remained employed. These outcomes mirrored those obtained nationally: One review indicated that although national welfare rolls decreased and more persons previously on welfare obtained employment, job loss was common: 25% stopped work within the first 3 months, 50% were not working within 1 year, and periods between jobs were often long (Strawn & Martinson, 2000). Existing employment skills and placement programs tended to be created solely by experts with little input from recipients. The guiding premise of such programs is that persons on welfare lack positive work attitudes and skills and need to learn them and/or lack adequate motivation and must be challenged forcefully. Neither type of program addressed the challenges related to the changes necessary in family life when a parent makes the transition from welfare to work that Tom was hearing about from speaking with case workers, employment specialists, and participants in the employment programs at HELP.

In addition to urgent issues about families' and the agency's survival, Tom brought a passion for creating coordinated services, and I brought an abiding interest in how families create and sustain family time (Fraenkel, 2001) and how they balance work and family responsibilities (Fraenkel & Capstick, 2012), which had not been explored extensively in poor families and families of color. I also brought an interest in collaborative approaches to intervention, developed over 8 years in work with sexually abused children and their families (Sheinberg & Fraenkel, 2001), and in qualitative study of family members' perceptions of what was useful about the therapy (Fraenkel et al., 1998). Having witnessed the powerful impact of providing families opportunities to take charge of their therapy and to comment about it in some detail, I responded to Tom's casting the main problem as parents' lack of "engagement" in work programs by suggesting a collaborative approach to research and program development featuring qualitative interviews. The interviews would focus on what families see as the challenges they face and what they wanted in a program to serve their needs.

The fundamental premise of treating families as experts who could inform us in building and evaluating the program made good sense to all the participants in the process: to Tom and his colleagues at HELP USA, to the staff of the shelter whom we met with to obtain their guidance and assistance, to me and my students as the main conductors of the research and program, to senior colleagues of color whom I engaged as mentors (see below), and, most important, to the participant families. Having the research and program development practices make good sense to all strengthened everyone's commitment to the project. Thus, having the fundamental premise of one's approach to program development hold a certain "face validity" is one important way to address the issue of "engagement" for all involved.

Multiple perspectives Do the persons assembled in the collaborative team represent a diverse enough range of ideas, skills, and goals? Just as qualitative research seeks out diversity in experiences about the phenomenon of study in order to build an inclusive, comprehensive theory, a well-functioning collaborative team requires diverse contributions. Hearing different passions, concerns, and goals issuing from members' differing perspectives and sources of expertise also lends members a sense that they are part of an emerging team, that they will not need to solve all the problems or seek out all relevant information themselves (thereby decreasing the sense of overwhelm that can discourage change efforts), and that they stand to learn something from one another. An open discussion of the range of possible goals for the project at the beginning also allows for a sense of inclusiveness of all members' concerns and for thoughtful planning, so that foci that could have been addressed are not discovered after most of the data are collected, and allows the group to prioritize and sequence goals realistically.

Although the point of the collaborative approach is to include and even prioritize the perspective of persons who will participate in the program, in many cases, especially when working with communities that represent multi-stressed, vulnerable populations, early meetings will be solely among professionals (e.g., researchers and agency directors). This is because of the need to decide whether a project and partnership is even feasible before involving members of the community, and because of various legal or institutional regulations regarding confidentiality and researcher access to community members. However, in the CFPD model, community members are involved in the project as soon as these conditions are met, so that the project does not develop without their contributions.

Following the initial meeting between Tom and me, the next meeting included HELP's regional director, the director of the shelter where Tom thought the research and program might best take place, and the director of social services for that shelter. These professionals, all of whom had master's degrees in social work and exposure to family systems theory and community research, were quite excited about the possibility of a program to help parents move into the workforce, as they too shared a concern, and some frustration, about the inconsistent attendance of the parents in job readiness, training, and placement programs, especially given the specter of the new welfare time limits. Importantly, these professionals were all African-American or Afro-Caribbean, and their years of experience in the field enabled them to serve as senior mentors to me. They did not voice concerns about the idea of developing the program through collaborative research in terms of the race or ethnicity of the residents. Rather, they responded enthusiastically to the stance of approaching families as experts and were cautiously optimistic about the potential for this stance to engage resident families.

Expert cultural knowledge Do members of the team include persons who can provide insider knowledge about the cultures of the communities of the persons who will participate in the program? Although the CFPD model's guiding premise of "families as the experts" and the correspondingly respectful approach to interviewing increase the likelihood that program participants will speak openly about their cultural beliefs and traditions, about the impact on their lives of racism, sexism, ethnicism, classism, and other oppressive societal practices, and about the adequacy and sensitivity of the research methods and program in addressing these themes, there are a number of forces that may restrict participants from speaking fully on these topics.

First, no matter how friendly and collaborative the interview, there remains an implicit hierarchy and power differential between an interviewer, who, even if of the same racial and ethnic background as the interviewee, will be of a higher social class and educational level. The hierarchy is likely to be even greater when interviewers and program developers are white and participating families are persons of color. Second, interviewees may be gracious and forgiving when questions are worded in ways that are linguistically awkward or even unwittingly insensitive from a cultural perspective or when program elements don't have the best cultural fit. Unfortunately, their graciousness may limit the degree of critical feedback to program developers that might greatly improve the research and program. Third, one of the major beliefs in most communities of color, at least in the United States, is that one does not share intimate details of family problems with outsiders (Boyd-Franklin, 2006; Falicov, 2015). This may apply particularly to the intimate details about experiences of oppression, which often carry painful, highly charged, and incompletely metabolized emotions. Fourth, the pernicious effects of internalized racism (Watson, 2019) and internalized classism (Walsh, 2019) may extend to interview and program participants silencing their anguish and well-deserved rage about these forms of social injustice, blaming themselves instead for failing to overcome adversity in the manner of the great American myth of the rugged individual (Walsh, 2019). Fifth, although there are outstanding examples of oppressed persons who have written and spoken eloquently about their experiences, most persons struggling with multiple sources of marginalization and limited resources may not have been afforded the luxury to research and reflect on the larger social forces that silence them. As a result, senior social scientists and interventionists who have to some degree focused their professional efforts on issues of race, ethnicity, class, gender, and other dimensions of difference which they also inhabit as persons provide a unique and crucial resource for program developers who need cultural consultation.

Importantly, it is not sufficient to include a multiracial, multiethnic, and multiclass team if the director of the project is white and educationally and economically privileged and all other members of the team are students or junior colleagues. For instance, in my experience, despite engaging bright, clinically sensitive, advanced, and outspoken students of color as team members from the beginning, and despite my attempts to engage them to evaluate critically our interview protocol, they lodged few critiques that focused on the appropriateness of the language of questions from a cultural point of view. Only when I conveyed, repeatedly, my concern that we needed to do better at providing an opportunity for participants to talk about their experiences of oppression did they begin to offer suggestions about adding new questions and revising old ones. My attention to these issues was heightened by conversations with senior colleagues of color.

For all these reasons and more, it is essential that program developers obtain ongoing cultural consultation and mentoring from persons senior to him or her who can provide expert and insider information (Tamasese & Waldegrave, 1993). This is especially necessary when program developers inhabit locations on dimensions of difference such as race, ethnicity, education, and class that afford them more privilege than the persons who will participate in the program.

In our case, Patricia Gray, M.S.W., who was the shelter director, a senior social service professional, and a woman of color, agreed to consult with the research team on an ongoing basis in shaping the research methods and procedures, including reviewing the interview questions in terms suitability of language for the shelter population. She also consulted with us on the creation of the program. One useful suggestion that would not have occurred to us was to hold a graduation ceremony at the end of the group program, complete with diplomas, speeches, and dinner. She noted that a graduation ceremony – commonly included in programs offered in social service contexts – would be a meaningful incentive to stay in the program, both for the adult residents who had completed high school and remembered the event with pride and for those who had not but longed to do so. Children would enjoy it as well, and it might provide them an incentive to stay in school so that they could experience those graduations. Interestingly, I realized from my initial critical reaction to her suggestion that this idea would not have occurred to me for two reasons. First, possibly as a result of my own educational privileges, I thought it might seem patronizing to hold a graduation for an 8-week group. Second, the program is not conducted as a psychoeducational course, but rather as a discussion and support group in which the families are the experts. We wanted to distinguish our program from the typically more hierarchical training programs offered.

However, Pat Gray turned out to be absolutely on target. The graduations were extremely moving experiences, with graduates dressing in their finest clothes, inviting family members living outside the shelter, and offering powerful accounts of the impact of the group in their lives as well as inspiring à cappella songs from the African-American popular and spiritual traditions. Importantly, a number of graduates referred to the program as the "Ackerman class," and most spoke of what they learned, and yet they were the instructors. Several noted with much emotion that this was their first graduation and that it inspired them to complete their high school degrees and go on to college – a lifelong dream. This is a good example of how it is critical to access and incorporate "insider knowledge" about the cultures of persons who will attend programs and of the institutions in which the programs will take place. It also illustrates the importance of forming collaborative teams of persons with different sorts of expertise that can complement and correct one another.

Roles What roles will each member of the team take in the project? The distribution of roles usually follows from the particular types of expertise and positions each member holds in their respective contexts. My area of expertise is family therapy, research, and program development: I took the lead in designing and conducting the research and implementing the program. Tom Hameline's area of expertise is the administration of social service programs; he took the lead in that area. Families offered their experiences, insights, and programmatic suggestions, as well as their time and energy to be in the program. Many of the key roles were filled by graduate students, who received funding, invaluable research and intervention experience, and in vivo training in "intersectional" or multicultural sensitivity (Johnson et al., 2010). Several students completed dissertations and master's theses based on the data collected in the project. Various agency staff members also fill critical roles: following up with families who do not show up for scheduled interviews, coordinating set-up, meals, and room scheduling, linking the family support program with the job readiness and placement program, and co-leading family groups.

Just as we needed to scale back our initial hopes that families might play an even more active role in the research, professionals also have their plates full. Unless someone expresses interest in serving a time-consuming new role, or has some of her or his other responsibilities scaled back, it is unlikely they will be able to follow through with research and programmatic responsibilities. We have had several occasions when the staff person assigned to assist us in coordinating meals and logistics suddenly was deployed to another site or accrued additional responsibilities, but did not want nor feel able to withdraw from the project – with the result that critical tasks did not get accomplished. Therefore, it is important to outline carefully the tasks and time commitments for each responsibility, to negotiate with supervisors from host institutions release from other responsibilities for participating staff (or provide additional salary), and to encourage project staff to recognize and discuss when they cannot fulfill their role.

Step 2: In-Depth Interviewing of Family Members

Collaborative, community-engaged approaches to research typically utilize qualitative methods (Charmaz, 2006), especially interviews, either alone or in combination with quantitative methods. The goal of qualitative research is to develop detailed, multilayered, "thick descriptions" (Geertz, 1983) of the nature and meaning of events, situations, and experiences from the point of those interviewed (the insider, or "emic," perspective). Qualitative methods rely upon the researcher's ability to socialize with the respondent or participant in such a way that the relationship feels comfortable enough that the participant feels free to reveal intimate details of her or his experience. This quality of relationship between researcher and participant is sought so that the participant is more rather than less likely to go beyond the pre-structured stimuli – for instance, to expand on the pre-set questions, or even suggest better or more important questions, and then answer them. All verbal and nonverbal behavior of the participant is noted and considered as potentially useful data, including comments made after the semistructured interview and formal video or audio-taping ends. In this approach, research is viewed as an inherently biased, socially constructed activity (Kidder & Fine, 1997); therefore, the qualitative researcher does not strive to control the interaction or data analysis so as to eliminate all biases but rather, through cultivating a curiosity about others' experiences and an enthusiasm for disconfirming their own views, poses open-ended questions that allow participants to share experiences that may disconfirm the researcher's preconceptions. These qualities of the researcher-community relationship may lead qualitative methods to be experienced as more inviting and less threatening for members of marginalized, oppressed communities than are traditional, quantitative methods.

In line with this emphasis on ascertaining the insider's viewpoint, the in-depth qualitative family interview is the heart of the CFPD approach. Through it, family members are explicitly engaged as experts on their experience and as consultants in constructing the program. For the Fresh Start program, the interview inquired into how families came to be in the shelter, how they coped with living in the shelter, their experiences with welfare and work, the challenges they faced or believed they would face as individuals and as a family as the parents moved into employment, their beliefs about family time and how this shifted or might shift with the transition into work, and what they recommended should be in a program to support them. For the families-with-teens program, we conducted a whole family interview as well as separate interviews with parents, each teen, and, when there were two teens, a conjoint interview with the siblings.

Interviews need to be at least 2 hours long, preferably 3-to-4 hours, so that neither interviewer nor interviewee feels rushed. This allows the interviewer to indulge her or his genuine curiosity about the family's experience and ideas without anxiety about "getting through the interview," and allows family members to respond fully and go "off the path" of the question, where they sometimes share their most spontaneous and heartfelt memories and opinions. A longer interview also necessitates breaks, during which informal conversation occurs around snacks. These informal conversations help to create a feeling of "hanging out" together, which, without creating a false intimacy, almost imperceptibly shifts the frame from a formal interview to a more authentic conversation in which the underlying roles of interviewer and interviewee are softened although not abandoned, thereby encouraging families to describe their experiences even more intimately.

Families were also asked to evaluate the interview process. Along with some useful suggestions for rephrasing questions, families invariably reported that they enjoyed it and seemed in no rush to end it. They often confused the program development research interview with the program itself. They often remarked spontaneously that this interview was the first time they had been asked to give an account of their experience of being homeless, of their positive qualities as a family and means of coping with adversity, or for input about programs. For instance, one African-American man – who reported frequent run-ins with police as a teenager, time in prison as an adult, and consequently, mistrust of "the system" – noted with a warm smile, "You got a lot of answers out of us that no one else could get out of us!" His female partner – viewed by some staff of the shelter as "uncooperative" – noted with an enthusiastic tone, "It's a good program – you definitely are on the right track with the questions."

Prior to the interview, families must first be contacted to inform them about the research and program that will follow and to obtain the adult family members' oral agreement to participate with their children. In our program, we randomly selected families from a roster and called them in their units. In order to increase the likelihood that families would be able to participate both in the research and in the 8-week group program, we selected only families who had been in the shelter 12 weeks or less. Random selection also increased the likelihood that we would obtain a more representative sample of families and associated experiences and ideas, rather than incurring the usual biases endemic to self-referral (in our case, biases could include being more or less motivated, more or less available due to employment or lack thereof, greater or lesser levels of coping, etc.).

We then scheduled a time to describe the study to the family in more detail and have each member sign age-appropriate informed consent forms. In addition to the usual guidelines about confidentiality, we emphasized that, barring information that raised our concern about possible harm to self or other, we would not disclose anything families tell us to professional staff of the shelter. With their permission, we might share with senior staff related general themes – for instance, complaints about the behavior of the shelter security guards or childcare workers – but would not link any particular comment to a particular family.

Among other things, included in this step was the information that we paid the family a small amount ($25) for their time in the interview and for completing questionnaires at three points ($25 for each point): following the interview, following completion of the group, and 1 year later. We also provided dinner on the night of the interview so that parents were able to participate into the early evening.

To facilitate families agreeing to participate in such extensive interviewing, it is recommended that they be seen in a setting that is most convenient and comfortable for them. This will vary depending on the community: some may prefer to be interviewed at home, in a community center, or other setting. In our case, all interviews occur in the shelters. Interviews were carried out in a comfortable, fairly quiet room in the social services wing of the shelters.

Step 3: In-Depth Interviewing of Community Professionals

Persons in a professional, service delivery role with members of the community offer unique perspectives that can powerfully shape the program. Whereas the initial planning meetings of Step 1 often involve professionals higher in an agency or institution's hierarchy, Step 3 involves interviewing professionals in all roles. Often, those lower in the hierarchy have more regular contact with the families served and so can provide the kind of detailed observations that provide a stimulus to creative program development. Interviewing these professionals also engages them as stakeholders and collaborators in mounting the program.

As informative as they can be, it is best to wait to interview professionals until one has had an opportunity to meet with several families and learn directly from them. This sequencing avoids inadvertently privileging the perspective of professionals, which often occurs in traditional program development. Sequencing the interviews this way also allows one to share with the professionals some of one's emerging observations and helps one to have referent experiences to help in understanding their comments.

In our work in the shelter, we interviewed the directors of all departments – childcare, employment, housing, social services, security, recreation, and maintenance, as well as workers at all levels of the hierarchy in these departments. In one focus group with these professionals at HELP's domestic violence shelter, a number of professionals described the frustrating experience of seeing women repeatedly miss appointments with them and respond in a belligerent or scattered manner when later reminded of these appointments. Asked for their opinions about what motivated this behavior, a number of the professionals spoke of the women's "low self-esteem." Further questioning led to the hypothesis that it was fear – remaining from the experience of battering and about taking next steps to locate housing and employment – that underlay low self-esteem and the women's resulting unproductive and uncooperative behavior. The importance of addressing fear and all the ways women strove to hide their fear resulted in one of the central activities of the group program which we called the Mask of Fear, in which women were given paper plates and arts and crafts materials and asked to create a mask that depicts the face they use to hide their fear and, on the other side, to depict the fear and other emotions they hide. The masks became a stimulus for further discussion of how the women handled their emotions and the relational resources available to them to express themselves and obtain soothing.

Just as families may experience the research interview as therapeutic, interviews of professionals may change their perspectives and practices. According to the director of the domestic violence shelter, the focus group conversation led to a profound shift in the culture of the shelter, with professionals' discussions about residents taking a more psychological and sympathetic tone. Remarkably, without any additional efforts to institutionalize it, this shift in professionals' ways of thinking and talking about the resident families was reportedly sustained years later.

Step 4: Phrase-by-Phrase Qualitative Coding of Interviews

In order to locate themes of challenge and resilience, and to capture families' and staff members' suggestions for the format and content of the program, we qualitatively coded the video or audiotapes (Charmaz, 2006). In qualitative coding, with each new participant's interview, there is the opportunity to create new codes. Codes are retained even if generated in response to only one participant – the data are not reduced to the most frequently used codes. Indeed, rather than being viewed as outliers that threaten to dispel an existing theory, unique responses are highly valued for the diversity they bring to building a truly inclusive theory that captures the lived complexity of the phenomenon under study.

In order to do justice to the richness of the information and feelings interviewees shared, codes were created for the smallest meaningful unit of speech, termed a "thought unit." On average, a thought unit is approximately a sentence in length, although when an interviewee's sentences are long and include multiple ideas, a thought unit may be as short as a phrase (in written text, a dominant or subordinate clause – e.g., the material up to or following a comma). This approach to qualitative coding can be compared to microanalytic quantitatively driven coding systems of couple interaction versus more global approaches (see Markman & Notarius, 1987).

Because of our need to transform qualitative data fairly quickly into program materials, we did not have time to transcribe the interviews prior to coding. Instead, we coded directly from the tapes, recording the precise time code for the beginning and end of each thought unit.

Step 5: Creating Program Formats and Contents and Writing an Initial Manual

The created program represents a "dialogue" between themes named by the potential participants and our knowledge base as professional program developers. Rather than being rigid templates for how to conduct a set of interventions, manuals, adapted over time, become the document that captures that dialogue and evolving story of the collaboration between professionals and families. In the CFPD model, the program materials and activities were potentially revised based on new themes learned from each new family interview. Of course, in order to conduct valid evaluations of the program in matched comparison or randomized clinical trials (see Step 9), the manual would need to be at least temporarily stabilized for the period of the evaluation.

In response to the numerous statements by families in research interviews that they felt put down and stigmatized because of their homeless status – and in response to several families' urgings that we include attention to the positive things about them – we adopted the practice of eliciting stories of pride used previously in the Ackerman sex abuse project (Sheinberg & Fraenkel, 2001) and created an exercise that involves families stating one thing they feel proud about in general and then, in a second round, something they feel proud about having to do with work. In response to the numerous negative effects of homelessness identified by families, we adapted the narrative practice of externalization (White, 1988) and created an activity in which families externalized the impact of homelessness. In response to teens' request for activities and not only discussion, we created a number of exercises that utilize the arts to express challenges and coping, as well as a "game show" activity in which parents guess what their teens view as challenging about being in the shelter.

One of the specific methods through which we directly linked coded themes from the research interviews with program materials and activities was through a "card sort" activity. We placed each of the coded challenges named by at least one family on a single 4″× 4″ card and over the 12 years of the program assembled a stack of over 100 cards. We had three separate sets of cards – one representing challenges facing families as a whole, one facing the adults in their role as workers and employees, and one for teens. In the third session of the 8-week multiple family group, each family was given the entire stack of family-as-a-whole cards and asked to sort them into three envelopes, in terms of the degree to which they have experienced these challenges affecting their family, from Not at all (1) to Somewhat (2) or Definitely (3). Families then rejoined the circle and were asked to select a card from envelope #1 (not at all a problem) to share with the group. Inevitably, a card/challenge that one family viewed as Not at All a Challenge was viewed as Somewhat or Definitely a Challenge by another family, and this led to lively group discussion, as one family shared coping skills and ideas with another family. Conversely, the stories shared by a family that had experienced struggle with a particular challenge helped families that had not yet experienced this challenge to anticipate how it might be a problem for them in the future.

Step 6: Piloting of the Group with Session-by-Session Evaluations by Participants

Families were invited to provide informal (oral) and more formal (written) feedback on the quality of their group experience and were reminded that they were helping to shape the program. We utilized an adaptation of a short evaluation form originally developed for research on the aforementioned family-based child sexual abuse treatment (Fraenkel et al., 1998). The scale asked family members to write a sentence in answer to the question, "What was the most important thing that happened or was said today?" They also rated the helpfulness of the group on a scale from 1 to 5 and were provided space to answer the question, "Was there anything you did not like about today's meeting? Or any suggestions you'd like to make for future meetings?"

Because all families who participated in group previously participated in the extensive family interview, they may have been more able to provide authentic critiques and suggestions on everything from logistics and formats to specific activities than if this had been the first time their opinions were being requested.

Step 7: Revising the Program and Manual

We utilized families' feedback, as well as the feedback provided by shelter staff and our own reflections on what worked and what didn't, to revise the program and manual periodically. For instance, one major change stimulated by families' evaluations was to revise the program to include time for parents to talk without children present. This necessitated obtaining (paid) after-hours assistance from the childcare service of the shelter. As another example, one intersession activity created on the suggestion of one group member (and with agreement of all other members) was for each family to think over the problems of another family between group and offer potential solutions in the following group session. This particular group member went beyond mere possible solutions and actually solved another family's long-standing difficulty finding permanent housing.

Step 8: Intensive Interviewing of Families for Each Subsequent Group Cycle

In a step that differs significantly from typical program development procedure (Dalton, Elias, & Wandersman, 2001), program development interviews were conducted with each new potential participant even after the program was created, and the program was revised as needed based on their comments. We maintained this time-consuming step because of our hypothesis that the interview experience was crucial to our high level of program engagement: Whereas the average rate of engagement in shelter-based programs at HELP at the time the program started was about 24%, 76% of the first 55 families we interviewed participated in the subsequent group cycle.

Step 9: Evaluating the Effectiveness of the Program in Matched Comparison or Randomized Designs

As Dodge (2018) realistically notes, "We are in an evidence-based era, so a system of care must provide interventions that have been proven to be effective through randomized controlled trials and other rigorous evaluation methods" (p. 1121). Ultimately, for scientific as well as funding purposes, collaboratively developed programs need to be subjected to rigorous matched comparison or randomized clinical designs to test their efficacy and effectiveness. Having obtained some quantitative, pre-post findings from the first 55 families suggesting that the Fresh Start program led to significant decreases in demoralization and in overall psychological distress for parents, we planned to conduct a randomized clinical trial of the program comparing it to a "no treatment" control. However, limits of access to enough families at any one time prevented us from carrying out this study. One challenge we anticipated if we had carried it out was how to maintain the collaborative atmosphere of the program while engaging in the more formal research endeavor of random assignment to treatments.

Step 10: Disseminating and Adapting the Program to Other Settings

Just as we interviewed each family for each new cycle of the program, we conducted entire new sets of interviews for each new shelter in the HELP USA agency that asked us to bring in the program, because each setting and its potential participants faced unique challenges and had unique sets of resources. This practice led to important changes (represented by separate manuals) in the content and format of the program we developed for families homeless due to domestic violence and for the program we developed for families with teenagers.

Summary

The Collaborative Family Program Development model provides a philosophy and set of associated practices that links rigorous research methods with contemporary family therapy sensibilities that enjoin professionals to view families as holding untapped strengths and considerable expertise on their problems as well as on what they need to overcome these problems. Engaging families as experts seems to lead them to engage more actively and regularly in programs, as these are designed with their input. As an older single mother of two teenagers who had a history of imprisonment and a long history of reliance on welfare noted emotionally at the end of a post-program follow-up interview 6 months after she had left the shelter, "You didn't treat us like we were clients – you treated us like we were friends, and that's what made the difference, and let me stop now or I'll start crying!" Her informal evaluative comment, and many others like it, encouraged our confidence that this approach to building and evaluating programs for families serves to foster a process of "rehumanizing" and "re-spiriting" families who all too often have felt dehumanized and dispirited by the many oppressive forces in their lives and in our society.

References

Boyd-Franklin, N. (2006). *Black families in therapy: Understanding the African American experience* (2nd ed.). New York, NY: Guilford Press.
Charmaz, K. (2006). *Constructing grounded theory: A practical guide through qualitative analysis*. London, UK: Sage Publications.
Charmaz, K., Thornberg, R., & Keane, E. (2018). Evolving grounded theory and social justice inquiry. In N. K. Denzin & Y. S. Lincoln (Eds.), *The Sage handbook of qualitative research* (5th ed., pp. 411–443). Thousand Oaks, CA: Sage Publications.
Chevalier, J. M., & Buckles, D. J. (2019). *Participatory action research: Theories and methods for engaged inquiry* (2nd ed.). New York, NY/London, UK: Routledge.
Dahler-Larsen, P. (2018). Qualitative evaluation: Methods, ethics, and politics with stakeholders. In N. K. Denzin & Y. S. Lincoln (Eds.), *The Sage handbook of qualitative research* (5th ed., pp. 867–886). Thousand Oaks, CA: Sage Publications.
Dalton, J. H., Elias, M. J., & Wandersman, A. (2001). *Community psychology: Linking individuals and communities*. Stamford, CT: Wadsworth.
Dodge, K. A. (2018). Towards population impact from early childhood psychological interventions. *American Psychologist, 73*, 1117–1129. https://doi.org/10.1037/amp0000393
Falicov, C. J. (2015). *Latino families in therapy: A guide to multicultural practice*. New York, NY: Guilford Press.
Foucault, M. (1980). *Power/knowledge: Selected interviews and other writings 1972–1977*. New York, NY: Vintage.

Fraenkel, P. (2001). The place of time in couple and family therapy. In K. J. Daly (Ed.), *Minding the time in family experience: Emerging perspectives and issues* (pp. 283–310). London, UK: JAI.

Fraenkel, P. (2006a). Engaging families as experts: Collaborative family program development. *Family Process, 45*, 237–257.

Fraenkel, P. (2006b). Fresh Start for Families: A collaboratively-built community-based program for families that are homeless. *AFTA Monographs, 1*, 14–19.

Fraenkel, P. (2007a). Groupes multifamiliaux pour familles sans domicile fixe (Multiple family discussion groups for families that are homeless). In S. Cook-Darzens (Ed.), *Thérapies multifamiliales, des groupes comme agents thérapeutiques. (Multiple family therapy: Groups as therapeutic agents)* (pp. 333–361). Éditions érès: Paris, France.

Fraenkel, P. (2007b). *Facing struggles, finding strengths: Six-session emotion regulation/reflective functioning (ERRF) Fresh Start for Families with pre-teens and teens program.* Unpublished manual, Ackerman Institute for the Family.

Fraenkel, P., & Capstick, C. (2012). Contemporary two-parent families: Navigating work and family challenges. In F. Walsh (Ed.), *Normal family processes: Growing diversity and complexity* (4th ed., pp. 78–101). New York, NY: Guilford Press.

Fraenkel, P., & Carmichael, C. (2008). Working with families that are homeless. In M. McGoldrick & K. Hardy (Eds.), *Revisioning family therapy* (2nd ed., pp. 389–400). New York, NY: Guilford Press.

Fraenkel, P., Hameline, T., & Shannon, M. (2009). Narrative and collaborative practices in work with families that are homeless. *Journal of Marital and Family Therapy, 35*, 325–342.

Fraenkel, P., Schoen, S., Perko, K., Mendelson, T., Kushner, S., & Islam, S. (1998). The family speaks: Family members' descriptions of therapy for sexual abuse. *Journal of Systemic Therapies, 17*, 39–60.

Fraenkel, P., & Shannon, M. (1999). *Multiple family discussion group manual: Family support from welfare to work program (Fresh Start for Families).* Unpublished manual, Ackerman Institute for the Family.

Fraenkel, P., Shannon, M., & Díaz Alarcón, L. (2009). The families are the experts: Collaborative methods of family program development in work with homeless families and poor immigrant families. In M. Andolfi & L. Calderón del la Barca (Eds.), *Working with marginalized families and communities: Professionals in the trenches* (pp. 105–107). Rome, Italy: Accademia di Psicoterapia della Famiglia.

Freire, P. (1968/2000). *Pedagogy of the oppressed* (30th anniversary ed.). New York, NY: Continuum.

Geertz, C. (1983). *Local knowledge: Further essays in interpretive anthropology.* New York, NY: Basic Books.

Hancock, G. (1989). *The lords of poverty: The power, prestige, and corruption of the international aid business.* New York, NY: The Atlantic Monthly Press.

Institute of Medicine, Committee on Assuring the Health of the Public in the 21st Century. (2003). *The future of the public's health in the 21st century.* Washington, DC: National Academies Press.

Johnson, D., Cabral, A., Mueller, B., Trub, L., Kruk, J., Upshur, E., ... Fraenkel, P. (2010). Training in intersectionality sensitivity: A community-based collaborative approach. *American Family Therapy Academy Monographs, 5*, 4–15.

Kidder, L. H., & Fine, M. (1997). Qualitative inquiry in psychology: A radical tradition. In D. Fox & I. Prilleltensky (Eds.), *Critical psychology: An introduction* (pp. 106–121). Thousand Oaks, CA: Sage Publications.

Kincheloe, J. L., McLaren, P., Steinberg, S. R., & Monzo, L. D. (2018). Critical pedagogy and qualitative research: Advancing the bricolage. In N. K. Denzin & Y. S. Lincoln (Eds.), *The Sage handbook of qualitative research* (5th ed., pp. 235–260). Thousand Oaks, CA: Sage Publications.

Lobo, E. S. (2018). *From homelessness toward self-sufficiency: A longitudinal study of families.* DAI-B 79/12(E), Dissertation Abstracts International, ProQuest Dissertations Publishing, Dissertation/thesis number 10830045, ProQuest document ID 2090807246.

Madsen, W. C. (2007). *Collaborative therapy with multi-stressed families* (2nd ed.). New York, NY: Guilford Press.

Markman, H. J., & Notarius, C. I. (1987). Coding marital and family interaction: Current status. In T. Jacobs (Ed.), *Family interaction and psychopathology: Theories, methods, and findings* (pp. 329–390). New York, NY: Plenum Press.

Mrazek, P. J., & Haggerty, R. J. (Eds.). (1994). *Reducing risks for mental disorders: Frontiers for preventive intervention research.* Washington, DC: National Academies Press.

Reason, P., & Heron, J. (1995). Co-operative inquiry. In J. A. Smith, R. Harré, & L. V. Langenhove (Eds.), *Rethinking methods in psychology* (pp. 122–142). Newbury Park, CA: Sage Publications.

Reed, R. (2015). Community-engaged research: Challenges and solutions. *Gateways: International Journal of Community Research and Engagement, 8,* 118–138.

Reitinger, E. (Ed.). (2008). *Transdisziplinäre Praxis. Forschen im Sozial- und Gesundheitswesen.* Heidelberg, Germany: Verlag für Systemische Forschung (218 S.).

Routhier, G. (2017). Homelessness in NYC: City and state must meet unprecedented scale of crisis with proven solutions. Briefing Paper, *Coalition for the Homeless.* Available online at: http://secure.coalitionforthehomeless.org/wp-content/uploads/2017/01/Family-Homelessness-1-2017_FINAL.pdf

Sheinberg, M., & Fraenkel, P. (2001). *The relational trauma of incest: A family-based approach to treatment.* New York, NY: Guilford Press.

Strawn, J., & Martinson, K. (2000). *Steady work and better jobs: How to help low-income parents sustain employment and advance in the workforce.* New York, NY: Manpower Demonstration Research Corporation.

Tamasese, K., & Waldegrave, C. (1993). Cultural and gender accountability in the "just therapy" approach. *Journal of Feminist Family Therapy, 5,* 29–45.

Walsh, F. (2019). Social class, rising inequality, and the American Dream. In M. M. McGoldrick & K. V. Hardy (Eds.), *Revisioning family therapy: Addressing diversity in clinical practice and training* (3rd ed.) (pp. 37–56). New York, NY: Guilford Press.

Watson, M. F. (2019). Facing the Black Shadow: Power from the inside out. In M. M. McGoldrick & K. V. Hardy (Eds.), *Revisioning family therapy: Addressing diversity in clinical practice and training* (3rd ed.) (pp. 200–2014). New York, NY: Guilford Press.

White, M. (1988). The externalizing of the problem and the re-authoring of lives and relationships. *Dulwich Centre Newsletter, Summer,* 3–21.

Resilience of Individuals, Families, Communities, and Environments: Mutually Dependent Protective Processes and Complex Systems

Ashley Collette and Michael Ungar

Introduction

Resilience in the psychological and social sciences has historically been conceptualized as an individual trait that offers protection against exposure to chronic and acute stress. It has focused almost exclusively on the individual as the unit of analysis, even though many of the factors associated with resilient outcomes (like social support) are not *within* the person. Fortunately, advances to the science of resilience and the methodologies that are being used are shifting the emphasis from individual capacities to the capacity of systems to overcome stress. Stemming in part from the challenges associated with measuring resilience over time in the context of a fast paced, complex, and globalized world, the discourse on resilience has evolved to one that conceptualizes resilience as the capacity of a dynamic system to be able to adapt successfully to events that threaten the function or development of that system. A systems-oriented understanding of resilience decenters the individual as the primary unit of analysis and shifts the focus to an examination of person-in-environment. Understood this way, the study of resilience becomes primarily focused on interdependent transactions between individual and context. An individual's response to stress is seen as something that takes place in the relational context of interactions with other humans and the surrounding social and physical ecology.

In this chapter we explore the development of the concept of resilience from individually focused invulnerability to an interactional, systemically complex

A. Collette
Royal Roads University, Victoria, BC, Canada

M. Ungar (✉)
Canada Research Chair in Child, Family and Community Resilience, Dalhousie University, Halifax, NS, Canada
e-mail: Michael.ungar@dal.ca

© Springer Nature Switzerland AG 2020
M. Ochs et al. (eds.), *Systemic Research in Individual, Couple, and Family Therapy and Counseling*, European Family Therapy Association Series,
https://doi.org/10.1007/978-3-030-36560-8_6

phenomenon with an emerging literature. We begin with a history of the concept of resilience, define resilience in terms of social and physical ecologies, provide evidence that resilience is the capacity of a dynamic system to adapt successfully, and offer two case illustrations that view resilience in a military context from a systems standpoint. We end the chapter with a discussion of the implications of a systemic understanding of resilience for interventions at individual and community levels, and for research on adaptation and transformation in stressed environments and other conditions of adversity.

History of Conceptualizing Resilience: Movement from Individuals to Complex Systems

The scientific study of resilience originated during the 1970s when a group of pioneering researchers discovered positive adaptations among children who had been labeled at risk of developing psychopathology (e.g., Murphy & Moriarty, 1976). Originally conceptualized as *those who beat the odds*, research in the area of resilience was dominated by a cultural ethos that exalted the robust individual (Wright, Masten, & Narayan, 2013). Historically, resilience has been defined as the ability of individuals to recover, or bounce back from, exposure to chronic and acute stress. The phenomenon has been overwhelmingly studied from a positivist epistemological standpoint, emphasizing a cause and effect relationship between variables, and a predetermined idea of health outcomes (Bottrell, 2009; Ungar, 2004).

Those who could pick themselves up by their own bootstraps were considered the epitome of resilience, and the study of the phenomenon focused almost solely on the individual as the locus of change. Children who beat the odds were seen at first as invulnerable to the effects of crisis. However, as research broadened across time and populations, investigators began to realize that given the right context, resilience was actually a normal and expected outcome (Masten, 2001). This was even more likely when individuals receive access to the resources they need to do well (Bonanno & Mancini, 2012; Ungar, 2013). By the 1980s, the discourse on resilience had shifted to conceptualize factors that either protect a person or put them at risk of suffering adverse effects as a result of a trauma or crisis (Rutter, 1987). Researchers set out to discover correlates that might predict positive outcomes in the presence of adversity or risk through the expanding use of longitudinal cohort studies which were able to distinguish those who developed successfully from those that experienced problems with mental health and social functioning despite common histories of exposure to risk (Garmezy & Rutter, 1983).

Although early resilience studies informed the discussion of *factors* associated with resilient outcomes, they provided limited insight with respect to the *processes* that might promote resilience. Definitions of resilience have broadened to acknowledge that there are intersecting factors and systems that contribute to resilience and that resilience may not be present across all domains of life at the same time due to its contextual, time-specific nature (Berger et al., 2011).

Most recently, research has shifted focus to better understanding the complex, systemic processes that shape resilient or pathological outcomes. The conversation on resilience shifted from a question of *what* to a question of *how* and broadened its perspective to include the ways in which individuals interact with many nested systems across time (Wright et al., 2013). Thus emerged a systems outlook on resilience, with one possible definition being, resilience refers to the capacity of a dynamic system to adapt successfully to disturbances that threaten the viability, the function, or the development of that system (Masten, 2014; Southwick, Bonanno, Masten, Panter-Brick, & Yehuda, 2014). A systems-oriented understanding of resilience decenters the individual as the singular unit of analysis and shifts the focus to an examination of the person x environment equation (Ungar, 2015c). The inquiry of resilience, then, focuses on interdependent transactions between individual and context. An individual's response to stress is seen as something that takes place in (and partially as an outcome of) the relational context of interactions with other humans and the surrounding social and physical ecology.

In keeping with this shift in perspective, a social ecological definition of resilience, developed by Ungar (2008), is as follows:

> In the context of exposure to significant adversity, resilience is both the capacity of individuals to navigate their way to the psychological, social, cultural, and physical resources that sustain their well being, and their capacity individually and collectively to negotiate for these resources to be provided and experienced in culturally meaningful ways. (Ungar, 2008, p. 225)

The dual processes of navigation and negotiation are important to consider in conceptualizing the mobilization of resilience from a social ecological standpoint. Indeed, both processes are critical to the development of interventions and best practices. Therefore, Ungar's definition not only posits that resilience is the capacity of individuals to navigate to resources that sustain them during a crisis, it also stipulates that individuals need to be empowered to affect the ways in which these resources are offered in culturally meaningful and attuned ways.

Within the literature on developmental psychology, we can find abundant evidence to support the notion that one's surrounding physical and social ecology potentiates resilience. By way of illustration, in a longitudinal study following 700 children on the island of Kauai from infancy through adulthood, Werner and Smith (2001) found that several key findings influence resilient outcomes over time, including individual characteristics (self-esteem and purpose in life), characteristics of families (maternal caregiving and extended family support), and the larger social context (adult role models that provide support). Defining resilience systemically, it would be an error to study only the individual as the locus of change without also studying the quality of the individual's social ecology. In order to understand causal mechanisms involved in heterogeneous responses to stress and adversity, we must ask whether changing an individual's physical and social ecology can increase the likelihood of resilience despite traits innate to the individual (Ungar, 2013).

As the understanding of processes and pathways that support resilience has developed, it has become possible for researchers to test practices and policies designed to foster resilience, first through theory-driven interventions and then through experimental designs (Luthar, 2006; Prince-Embury & Saklofske, 2013). Although the discourse on resilience has widened its scope, the focus is still largely on the study of resilience as displayed by the individual, even though the evidence suggests that positive outcomes are mostly the result of environments that increase the capacity of the individual to succeed (Ungar, 2011).

Shifting the Focus from Risk to Resilience

This change in focus from individual success to the concurrent success of multiple systems in sequence or concurrently reflects an equally systemic shift in our understanding of the risk factors which are the antecedents of physical and mental disorder. For example, in 2011, the World Health Organization (WHO) published a world report on disability, adopting the International Classification of Functioning, Disability and Health (ICF) as a conceptual framework for understanding the complex, contested, and multidimensional experience of disability (WHO, 2011). The WHO world report on disability states that at some point in a person's life, most people will experience at least one episode of impairment in one or more domains of functioning. Much like the evolution of resilience, the ICF defines disability as a condition that arises from the *interaction* of health conditions with environmental factors. Both the individual and the environment are important considerations within this critical model of understanding disability. Therefore, within the ICF, people with impairments are viewed as being disabled when the environment is not adapted to meet their particular health needs. Being disabled cannot be understood as a trait of the individual without also accounting for the capacity of the environment to account for the individual's needs and, discursively speaking, to label the individual's condition as either disabled or differently abled. In this sense, the risk to well-being originates within the individual's environment.

Turning our collective focus toward understanding the environmental factors that can be changed to support effective and meaningful participation in family, work and community settings helps us to identify solutions rather than diagnosing disorder. By way of example, the social functioning of a person with a hearing impairment is exponentially affected by the presence of a sign language interpreter or a community that shares the common experience of being "deaf." Likewise, the person in a wheelchair is less "disabled" (and indeed, more resilient) when communities and institutions provide buildings with accessible washrooms and elevators. Looking at the issue of disability ecologically helps us to locate the source of successful adaptation to being differently able-bodied within the person x environment interaction. Resilience is, arguably, dependent on the quality of the person's social and physical ecology, whether built or natural in quality (Brown, 2016; Ungar, 2018).

Defining Resilience in Terms of Social and Physical Ecologies

An ecological understanding of resilience is a contextualized one. While nature and nurture are both processes at play in determining the individual's resilience, nurture trumps nature when risk exposure is high, as individual solutions will seldom be adequate to cope with complex, multilevel environmental insults (Ungar, 2015b). Individual gains result from the congruence between an individual's needs and the capacity of an individual or group's environment to facilitate growth. Defining resilience in terms of social and physical ecologies means conceptualizing success under stress as a process and not a quality of any single system or part thereof. It suggests that resilience is something that operates across the lifespan of an individual – before, during, and after adverse life experiences (Rutter, 2013) – and it means conceptualizing an individual's capacity for resilience as something that is potentiated by a person's ecology instead of as a genotypic or phenotypic trait.

Ungar (2011) suggests the following principles as guides to understanding resilience from a social ecological lens: *Decentrality* (social and physical ecology first, interaction between environment and person second, and the individual him or herself third when investigating resilience), *complexity* (not expecting a resilient person to be resilient at all times, under all circumstances), *atypicality* (resilience related qualities are contextual in that in some cases a behavior may be considered resilient and in other cases not), and *cultural relativity* (positive growth is culturally embedded).

Individual and ecological positions on resilience are not antagonistic; instead, they emphasize different aspects of a complex phenomenon (Ungar, 2013). For example, the capacity of youth to access social supports depends both on individual traits such as attachment to a caregiver or adult equivalent (Sroufe, Egeland, Carlson, & Collings, 2005; Werner & Smith, 2001) and environmental factors (such as whether or not social supports are offered in culturally meaningful ways) that allow for such access. The problem lies not in whether resilience is within a person or the environment but instead in the lack of detailed analysis of the capacity of the environment to facilitate (or inhibit) opportunities for psychological resilience and growth. Achieving this level of analysis typically requires transdisciplinary approaches to resilience research (Brown, 2016; Masten, 2014) that facilitate gathering data at multiple systemic levels (biological, interpersonal, social, environmental, etc.) in order to understand how the resilience of one system influences the resilience of other co-occurring systems (Ungar, 2018). To do this, research teams have had to agree on a common set of outcomes that may result from any number of protective factors and processes. For example, studies of school children's success in the classroom and emotional and physical health can be attributed to individual cognitive patterns of children, child-teacher interactions, and the physical environment of the school and its surrounding playgrounds (DiClemente et al., 2018; Theokas & Lerner, 2006), as well as a myriad of other aspects of the multiple peer, family, and community systems with which a child interacts.

Evidence that Resilience Is the Capacity of a Dynamic System to Adapt Successfully

Several longitudinal studies within developmental psychology provide a starting point from which to understand resilience as the capacity of a dynamic system to adapt successfully. These studies emphasize the importance of studying resilience over time and across multiple levels of analysis (e.g., individuals, families, communities). They expose the problematic nature of conceptualizing illness or struggle as the opposite of resilience, instead placing it as part of a contextualized longitudinal process that may, or may not, result in a desirable outcome (Zautra, Hall, & Murray, 2010). Within the context of human development over the lifespan, a review of longitudinal studies supports the notion that an individual's functioning is a product of individual capacity for resilience, in relation to the person's cumulative past history and current life circumstance at any one point in time (Supkoff, Puig, & Sroufe, 2013; Ungar, 2015a).

The Minnesota Longitudinal Study of Risk and Adaptation (MLSRA; Sroufe, Egeland, Carlson, & Collings, 2005) provides an example of one of the most in-depth continuous studies of human development ever accomplished (Supkoff et al., 2013). Starting in 1975, this study has followed a poverty sample of over 180 children of first-time mothers receiving care from the Minneapolis Public Health Clinic between 1975 and 1977. As with other investigators of resilience within a developmental and longitudinal context, Sroufe et al. (2005) found that a child's surroundings account in part for resilient outcomes. For example, changes in life stress and social support were two variables found repeatedly to account for positive changes in functioning. The MLSRA also found, as with other developmental studies, that an early history of positive adaptation due to consistent and supportive care by a secure adult is a powerful and enduring influence on adaptation throughout the developmental trajectory and increases the probability that an individual will use social support later in life (see also, Werner, 2012).

Longitudinal studies of adaptation throughout the lifecycle also show evidence that there are opportunities for positive adaptation despite adverse childhood experiences that become available during adulthood. For example, the Kauai Longitudinal Study (Werner & Smith, 2001) monitored the impact of biological and psychosocial risk factors, stressful life events, and protective factors on the development of children born in 1955 in Kauai, a Hawaiian island. Individuals from this study were exposed to risk factors including chronic poverty, perinatal complications, parental psychopathology, and family discord. When researchers followed up with this cohort in their adult years, they found that individuals experienced a second chance to rebound toward a positive outcome through engagement with protective processes such as adult education, voluntary military service, active participation in a church community, and a supportive friend or marital partner (Werner, 2012; Werner & Smith, 2001). If inquiry into pathways to positive adaptations to adversity is stopped prematurely, we may miss the opportunity to see struggle as a part of the process of navigation toward resilience that can take decades to be realized.

Case Illustrations: Military Personnel and Their Many Possible Pathways to Resilience

It is not surprising that military personnel and their families have long been a focus for the study of resilience given the stress they experience. Recent work on military deployment (Anderson, Amanor-Boadu, Stith, & Foster, 2013) is expanding our understanding of the unique patterns of individual and family coping that follow exposure to exceptional forms of risk. Interestingly, this work has been one of the most contextualized areas of resilience research, with many of the studies of soldier resilience integrating a focus on external factors like institutional culture, leadership, family relationships, and post-deployment supports (Lee, 2011). This complexity in the study of resilience dates as far back as Hill's (1949) ABCX model of family adjustment which built on research with 135 Iowa military families with a father who had returned from war. Hill showed that a stressor interacts with a family's resources and the meaning they attribute to a potential crisis. These attributions shape whether interactions between risk and resources produce a positive or negative outcome. Much later, McCubbin and his colleagues (McCubbin & McCubbin, 2013; McCubbin & Patterson, 1983) also explored military families and resilience, contending that resilience should be understood in relation to people's cultures and the diverse meaning systems that influence attributions and access to resources of both a social nature, like friends, and material nature, like housing.

While all military personnel experience adversity by the nature of their role as service members, it is as yet unclear exactly which individual and ecological factors are most likely to prevent mental illness associated with warfare such as post-traumatic stress disorder (PTSD) and family dysfunction. At best, evidence is accumulating for a complex explanation for a soldier's resilience and the resilience of those in her or his family. The following two case illustrations highlight the diversity of pathways available to soldiers coping with potentially traumatizing events encountered during deployment and the period of adjustment afterward.

Case Illustration 1 Sergeant Steven Slack[1] was an infantry sergeant with the Canadian Armed Forces (CAF). During his career, he deployed on three operations of 6–8 months duration, one to Kosovo (1999–2000) and two to Afghanistan (2003–2004 and 2010). Although he went through periods of adjustment following all of his deployments, it was upon his return from his final deployment to Afghanistan that he started to notice that he was no longer able to perform his duties as he had always been able to in his work environment. His wife started to notice that there was something different about him as well. Finally, it was his desire to provide a good example to soldiers more junior to him that motivated his help seeking behavior. He found the courage to seek mental health support from the services offered to current serving members of the CAF. His wife (a serving member herself) also

---

[1] Pseudonyms have been used for case illustrations.

sought help. When Sgt Slack sought help, he was posted to the Joint Personnel Support Unit (JPSU), a unit intended to help members recovering from illness or injury who either return to active duty or transition to civilian life. Despite these efforts to deal with possible post-traumatic stress, Sgt Slack's wife moved out of the family home when she no longer felt able to support her spouse. Sgt Slack reflects back now on his experience, stating that it was the loss of the group he had deployed with, his unit's support net, and his wife that caused him to significantly deteriorate almost to the point of suicide.

Sgt Slack attributes his recovery to another soldier from the Operational Stress Injury Social Support (OSISS) group who reached out to him to tell him that he was not alone, that there were many soldiers who had struggled like he was struggling. This mentor from OSISS supported Sgt Slack in navigating the complicated health supports available to him. With Sgt Slack in treatment, his wife rejoined her husband. Sgt Slack was even able to return to active duty. He subsequently finished his long career with the CAF, and he and his wife have purchased a piece of land in Central America where they are currently building a retreat center for members and veterans of the forces to find community and a place for recovery with one another.

Case Illustration 2 Captain Nathalie Greene is a nurse in the CAF in her 12th year of service. Thus far in her career, she has completed two 6-month overseas operations, both to Afghanistan (2008 and 2011). She has also supported many domestic operations and exercises. She has worked in both military leadership and clinical roles throughout her career as a CAF officer and has been geographically located at different bases across Canada. In reflecting on the challenges inherent in her work as a serving member of the CAF, Captain Greene identified that what she finds most challenging about her service in the forces is providing healthcare within a highly politicized environment. She highlighted that the greatest effect on her personal mental health has not come from the challenges of providing healthcare to individual soldiers, but instead her work environment. For example, she stated that on her first tour of duty in Afghanistan, she was negatively affected by the lack of support that she felt from her superior commanders. She stated that due to a lack of team support, she returned home with a lot of anger and experienced symptoms of depression for a few years following her return home to Canada.

Despite this setback, Captain Greene has found meaning in her CAF service. When asked what keeps her healthy and functioning in her work environment, she highlighted the importance of having people around her who support one another as a close family would. She attributes her resilience partially to the meaning she finds in mentoring junior members, and stated that she has learned many things due to her negative experiences at the beginning of her career. She also attributes a good portion of her well-being to the support she receives from her family, and the spiritual community in which she grew up.

The Many Resources Required for Resilience

Both case studies highlight what we know about resilience, whether among military members or other people who experience high levels of stress. A focus on resilience shifts our attention from the dominant discourse of disorder to the coping strategies *and resources* which maintain well-being during periods of adversity. An Internet search of trauma and CAF members, however, reveals a cultural bias toward disordered language and the diagnostic negative consequences that have, in some cases, resulted from individuals' struggles with traumatic events (CBC, 2015; Galloway, 2016; Steeves, 2016). And yet there are many pathways on which individuals find themselves resulting in resilience and growth. Clearly, the issue is complex and cannot be simplified into diagnostic criteria that remove an individual from the systems within which they negotiate for mental health-supporting resources. Power relations and issues of social justice, for example, shape the experience of trauma (American Psychiatric Association, 2013). Trauma, by its very nature contributes to feelings of powerlessness as individuals struggle with intrusive thoughts, depressive mood, and hyper vigilance.

The problems facing CAF members that threaten their resilience are partly structural. Upon signing for service, they commit to what is known as unlimited liability, meaning that they can be ordered to conduct necessary military operations at any time. CAF members are often moved geographically across the country on short notice and sent on exercises and operations that take them away from their family for prolonged periods of time. Depending on the member's rank and position within the CAF, there are varying degrees of influence over the policies that greatly affect the member's life. It may be true that CAF members have power to exercise their rights; however, this idea becomes exponentially more complicated when seen from the view of unlimited liability. The concepts of *choice* and *empowerment* become complicated for the service member.

There is increasing evidence to support the idea that trauma not only affects the individual who has directly experienced the traumatic event but that there is a cost to those who support the trauma survivor (Crawford, Brown, Kvangarsnes, & Gilbert, 2014; Crawford, Gilbert, Gilbert, Gale, & Harvey, 2013; Hernandez-Wolfe, Killian, Engstrom, & Gangsei, 2015; Killian, 2008). Compassion fatigue, burnout, and vicarious traumatization are all areas of particular interest in understanding resilience systemically. Said differently, if we are to provide adequate and sustainable support for those who have been directly affected by potentially traumatic events, there is evidence that we must simultaneously support those surrounding the individual in order for our interventions to have any positive effect.

Thus, themes from the resilience literature are evident in the two case studies. While both soldiers were exposed to potentially traumatizing events, the resources available to them from their environments, and the meaningfulness of these resources to each of them, varied based on each of their lived experience, culture, gender, and other contextual factors. While these two case illustrations are clinical anecdotes, they highlight the complexity of the pathways to resilience and the need to account as much for the contextual factors that shape resilience as individual characteristics.

Implications of a Systemic Understanding of Resilience for Interventions

The study of systemic resilience can contribute to the social sciences in meaningful and sustainable ways by informing program and policy development. In the same way that the WHO (2011) makes the argument that accessibility to social environments is a key component of creating opportunity for meaningful participation in society, a social ecological view of resilience allows us to open areas of opportunity for individuals to find pathways to resilience in the face of crisis and challenge.

To better understand these complex patterns to resilience, it can be useful to consider the principle of equifinality (Ungar, 2011). Equifinality means that in open systems, a given end-state can be reached through many possible means. Explained contextually, if resilience is the capacity of a dynamic system to adapt successfully to disturbances that threaten its viability, function, or the development of that system, then employing the principle of equifinality means that interventions will support multiple pathways to a common outcome, most typically success amid adversity. Indeed, research shows that many life trajectories can become acceptable pathways to a number of outcomes we associate with resilience (Masten & Wright, 2010; Ungar, 2015a). For military members, this could mean redeployment or disengagement from active duty. Both outcomes can be signs of success depending on the meaning the member attaches to his or her experience and the sense of fulfillment that follows.

Implications of a Systemic Understanding of Resilience for Research

Defining resilience in terms of social and physical ecologies is much like turning a pair of binoculars around and looking at the world in the inverse direction. To understand resilience comprehensively from a social ecological standpoint, we must *first* explore *the context* in which individuals experience adversity, and *then* explore the *qualities of the individual*. Individual responses to adversity take place in the context of interactions with other human beings and their surrounding environments (resources, cultures, communities). This calls for different ways to study the phenomenon of resilience that must include looking at the experience of individuals and groups from a systems point of view, where "linear cause and effect analysis is replaced by observing patterns of interaction that mutually influence each other" (Coghlan & Brannick, 2010, p. 94).

Conducting research on resilience that is able to account for the social and physical ecologies that shape developmental outcomes that are experienced as positive requires a methodologically diverse toolbox. This includes, first, the need for mixed methods, with qualitative studies critical to either identifying a population's preferred coping strategies (which can then be assessed quantitatively for their frequency across the population as a whole) or interpreting findings from quantitative studies where results show differences by context (e.g., differences in patterns of resilience based on gender, race, ability or class, or the intersection of several of these social locations) (Ungar, 2008).

Second, resilience research that is able to account for contextual variation tends to be systemically complex, identifying protective factors and processes at multiple scales within a single system, or multiple systems (Folke, 2016). In practice this means that understanding a soldier's ability to withstand potentially traumatizing events also means studying the functioning of the soldier's family to see if their capacity to communicate and look after instrumental tasks like childrearing has a positive impact on a soldier's mental well-being.

Third, whether research is qualitative or quantitative, patterns of resilience are easier to understand in context when historical and longitudinal data are collected. Qualitatively, repeated interviews over time to track change phenomologically and historical narratives that detail adaptations and transformations as social conditions change, both help researchers understand the reciprocity between individuals and their environments (Panter-Brick, 2015). Likewise, quantitatively, longitudinal research provides the statistical advantage of more powerful means for analysis and the ability to identify the factors and processes which account for the most variance in positive outcomes. Disaggregating data into subpopulations over time has been especially useful as latent growth models (Oshri, Duprey, Kogan, Carlson, & Liu, 2018), and grouping qualitative data by population profile (e.g., high risk, low resilience vs. high risk, high resilience)(Ungar, Hadfield, & Ikeda, 2017) has helped to demonstrate the differential impact of environmental factors on individual change (Ungar, 2017).

Taken together, these approaches to research have helped show that from a social ecological standpoint, it is a naïve to employ pre-determined and rigid concepts related to what is, and is not, resilience. For example, Trzesniak, Liborio, and Koller (2013) highlight that it would be a mistake to consider risk factors as *always/only* a risk without a deeper consideration of the complexity of the social environment which can turn a risky pattern of behavior into a necessary adaptation for survival. To illustrate, child labor is considered a worldwide problem and a violation of human rights. However, some researchers have found that a more in-depth examination of the child's experience of work reveals some benefits such as positive sources of efficacy and cohesion, a strong identity, feelings of well-being, positive relationships, and access to material and social capital (Liborio & Ungar, 2010). Any conclusions about working children, then, must be seen contextually if we are to make suggestions for meaningful and culturally attuned interventions that support socially desirable outcomes. The same would be true for military personnel and their families, or for that matter, any other population.

Even if we are able to study resilience ecologically, it still remains challenging to account for aspects of the individual and his or her environment in the same model (Ungar, 2015b). In order to advance our understanding of complex social issues such as the phenomenon of resilience, we must employ methods that study them in their entirety, as a system, instead of separating the system into parts and assuming that the sum of the parts will give a coherent understanding of the whole. Complexity thinking means accepting unpredictability and uncertainty, and acknowledging that there are a multitude of perspectives that may lead to a particular culturally accepted assumption of resilience.

Finally, in order to support individuals in the dual processes of navigation and negotiation which are part of a social ecological understanding of resilience (Ungar, 2008), issues of power and voice must be considered as they "remind us that knowledge generation is a profoundly political act, concerning the power to define and to shape how resources are created and shared" (Sanders & Munford, 2009, p. 77). Researchers need to understand how actors within a particular system think and how their mental models influence decision-making and behavior. The use of action research, for example, is methodological congruent with the ecological study of resilience. Participatory action research is different from traditional research in that it engages the participants of the study throughout the entire research process as co-creators of knowledge through action. As such, it is well-suited to the study of resilience in different social ecologies (Coghlan & Brannick, 2010; Sanders & Munford, 2009). In particular, it ensures that factors and processes that are most relevant to a population under stress are included in the research. This has been especially true in work with Indigenous peoples globally where their voices have been marginalized and their own strategies for adaptation under stress misunderstood, pathologized, or ignored altogether (Bohensky & Maru, 2011). Developing local advisory committees, ensuring member checks with participants, hiring local stakeholders as co-researchers, and including in studies questions of local relevance can all help to reveal hidden patterns of resilience that are contextually specific. Collaborative forms of inquiry like this will allow us to develop research and practice that is culturally attuned and meaningful to those who we seek to support achieving resilient outcomes in the face of adverse conditions.

Recommendations and Conclusion

Understanding resilience, and the environments that potentiate it, is not an easy endeavor. Resilience requires methods of inquiry that examine the interface of person-in-environment. Resilience is necessarily contextual, as it requires elements of risk in order to manifest itself. It must, therefore, be studied in context. This is essential to the success of interventions seeking to support resilient outcomes and their capacity to be offered in culturally meaningful ways.

Understanding social ecologies and measuring developmental processes is difficult. Challenges remain in identifying which kinds of relational processes matter, and at what points in the developmental trajectory of an individual's life they matter most (Panter-Brick & Eggerman, 2013). If we are to continue to evolve the study of resilience in meaningful ways, an inversion of thinking is required so as not to miss the many pathways through which people experience resilience in the very diverse contexts where they are compelled to confront adversity.

References

Anderson, J. R., Amanor-Boadu, Y., Stith, S. M., & Foster, R. E. (2013). Resilience in military marriages experiencing deployment. In D. Becvar (Ed.), *Handbook of family resilience* (pp. 105–118). New York, NY: Springer.

American Psychiatric Association. (2013). In 5th ed. (Ed.), *Diagnostic and statistical manual of mental disorders*. Washington, DC: Author.

Berger, E. L., Diaz-granados, N., Herrman, H., Jackson, B., Stewart, D. E., & Yuen, T. (2011). What is resilience? *Canadian Journal of Psychiatry, 56*(5), 258–265.

Bohensky, E. L., & Maru, Y. (2011). Indigenous knowledge, science, and resilience: What have we learned from a decade of international Literature on "integration"? *Ecology and Society, 16*(4), 6.

Bonanno, G. A., & Mancini, A. D. (2012). Beyond resilience and PTSD: Mapping the heterogeneity of responses to potential trauma. *Psychological Trauma, 4*(1), 74–83.

Bottrell, D. (2009). Understanding 'marginal' perspectives: Towards a social theory of resilience. *Qualitative Social Work, 8*, 321–339.

Brown, K. (2016). *Resilience, development and global change*. New York, NY: Routledge.

CBC. (2015, July 16). PTSD diagnoses nearly triple amongst veterans in 8 years. *CBC News Nova Scotia*. Retrieved from http://www.cbc.ca/news/canada/nova-scotia/ptsd-diagnoses-nearly-triple-amongst-veterans-in-8-years-1.3154518

Coghlan, D., & Brannick, T. (2010). *Doing action research in your own organization* (3rd ed.). Thousand Oaks, CA: Sage Publications.

Crawford, P., Gilbert, P., Gilbert, J., Gale, C., & Harvey, K. (2013). The language of compassion in acute mental health care. *Qualitative Health Research, 23*(6), 719–727.

Crawford, P., Brown, B., Kvangarsnes, M., & Gilbert, P. (2014). The design of compassionate care. *Journal of Clinical Nursing, 23*(23–24), 3589–3599.

DiClemente, C. M., Rice, C. M., Quimby, D., Richards, M. H., Grimes, C. T., Morency, M. M., … Pica, J. A. (2018). Protective enhancing effects of neighborhood, family and school cohesion following violence exposure. *Journal of Early Adolescence, 38*(9), 1286–1321.

Folke, C. (2016). Resilience (Republished). *Ecology and Society, 21*(4), 44.

Galloway, G. (2016, Jan 22). One in 10 Canadian vets of Afghan war diagnosed with PTSD. *The Globe and Mail*. Retrieved from http://www.theglobeandmail.com/news/politics/one-in-10-canadian-vets-of-afghan-war-diagnosed-with-ptsd/article28360290/

Garmezy, N., & Rutter, M. (1983). *Stress, coping and development in children*. New York, NY: McGraw-Hill.

Hernandez-Wolfe, P., Killian, K., Engstrom, D., & Gangsei, D. (2015). Vicarious resilience, vicarious trauma, and awareness of equity in trauma work. *Journal of Humanistic Psychology, 55*(2), 153–172.

Hill, R. (1949). *Families under stress*. Westport, CT: Greenwood Press.

Killian, K. D. (2008). Helping till it hurts: A multi-method study of burnout, compassion fatigue and resilience in clinicians working with trauma survivors. *Traumatology, 14*(2), 32–44.

Lee, J. (2011). Higher-order model of resilience in the Canadian forces. *Canadian Journal of Behavioural Science, 43*(3), 222–234.

Liborio, R. M. C., & Ungar, M. (2010). Children's perspectives on their economic activity as a pathway to resilience. *Children and Society, 24*(4), 326–338.

Luthar, S. S. (2006). Resilience in development: A synthesis of research across five decades. In D. Cicchetti & D. J. Cohen (Eds.), *Developmental psychopathology: Vol.3. Risk, disorder and adaptation* (2nd ed., pp. 739–795). New York, NY: Wiley.

Masten, A. (2001). Ordinary magic. *American Psychologist, 56*(3), 227.

Masten, A. S. (2014). Global perspectives on resilience in children and youth. *Child Development, 85*(1), 6–20.

Masten, A. S., & Wright, M. O. (2010). Resilience over the lifespan: Developmental perspectives on resistance, recovery, and transformation. In J. W. Reich, A. J. Zautra, & J. S. Hall (Eds.), *Handbook of adult resilience* (pp. 213–237). New York, NY: Guilford.

McCubbin, L. D., & McCubbin, H. I. (2013). Resilience in ethnic family systems: A relational theory for research and practice. In D. Becvar (Ed.), *Handbook of family resilience* (pp. 175–195). New York, NY: Springer.

McCubbin, H. I., & Patterson, J. M. (1983). The family stress process: The Double ABCX model of adjustment and adaptation. *Marriage and Family Review, 6*, 7–37.

Murphy, L. B., & Moriarty, A. E. (1976). *Vulnerability, coping, and growth from infancy to adolescence*. New Haven, CT: Yale University Press.

Oshri, A., Duprey, E. B., Kogan, S. M., Carlson, M. W., & Liu, S. (2018). Growth patterns of future orientation among maltreated youth: A prospective examination of the emergence of resilience. *Developmental Psychology, 54*(8), 1456–1471.

Panter-Brick, C. (2015). Culture and resilience: Next steps for theory and practice. In L. Theron, L. Liebenberg, & M. Ungar (Eds.), *Youth resilience and culture: Commonalities and complexities* (pp. 233–244). London, UK: Springer.

Panter-Brick, C., & Eggerman, M. (2013). Understanding culture, resilience and mental health: The production of hope. In M. Ungar (Ed.), *The social ecology of resilience: A handbook of theory and practice* (pp. 369–386). New York, NY: Springer.

Prince-Embury, S., & Saklofske, D. H. (2013). *Resilience in children, adolescents, and adults: Translating research into practice*. New York, NY: Springer Science Business Media.

Rutter, M. (1987). Psychosocial resilience and protective mechanisms. *The American Journal of Orthopsychiatry, 57*(3), 316–331.

Rutter, M. (2013). Resilience: Causal pathways and social ecology. In M. Ungar (Ed.), *The social ecology of resilience: A handbook of theory and practice* (pp. 33–42). New York, NY: Springer.

Sanders, J., & Munford, R. (2009). Participatory action research. In M. Ungar (Ed.), *Researching resilience* (pp. 77–102). Toronto, ON: University of Toronto Press.

Sroufe, L. A., Egeland, B., Carlson, E. A., & Collins, W. A. (2005). The development of the person: The Minnesota study of risk and adaptation from birth to adulthood. New York, NY: Guilford.

Southwick, S., Bonanno, G., Masten, A., Panter-Brick, C., & Yehuda, R. (2014). Resilience definitions, theory, and challenges: Interdisciplinary perspectives. *European Journal of Psychotraumatology, 5*(1), 25338–25338.

Steeves, S. (2016, Aug 29). 22 Push-Ups Canada PTSD fundraiser exceeding expectations. *Global News*. Retrieved from http://globalnews.ca/news/2909538/22-push-ups-canada-challenge-ptsd-fundraiser-exceeding-expectations/

Supkoff, L. M., Puig, J., & Sroufe, L. A. (2013). Situation resilience in developmental context. In M. Ungar (Ed.), *The social ecology of resilience: A handbook of theory and practice* (pp. 127–142). New York, NY: Springer.

Theokas, C., & Lerner, R. M. (2006). Observed ecological assets in families, schools, and neighbourhoods: Conceptualisation, measurement and relations with positive and negative developmental outcomes. *Applied Developmental Science, 10*(2), 61–74.

Trzesniak, P., Liborio, R. M. C., & Koller, S. H. (2013). Resilience and children's work in Brazil: Lessons from physics for psychology. In M. Ungar (Ed.), *The social ecology of resilience: A handbook of theory and practice* (pp. 53–65). New York, NY: Springer.

Ungar, M. (2004). A constructionist discourse on resilience: Multiple contexts, multiple realities among at-risk children and youth. *Youth & Society, 35*(3), 341–365.

Ungar, M. (2008). Resilience across cultures. *British Journal of Social Work, 38*(2), 218–235.

Ungar, M. (2011). The social ecology of resilience: Addressing contextual and cultural ambiguity of a nascent construct. *American Journal of Orthopsychiatry, 81*(1), 1–17.

Ungar, M. (2013). Social ecologies and their contribution to resilience. In M. Ungar (Ed.), *The social ecology of resilience: A handbook of theory and practice* (pp. 13–31). New York, NY: Springer.

Ungar, M. (2015a). Patterns of family resilience. *Journal of Marital and Family Therapy, 42*(1), 19–31.

Ungar, M. (2018). Systemic resilience: Principles and processes for a science of positive change in contexts of adversity. *Ecology & Society, 23*(4), 34.

Ungar, M. (2015b). Practitioner review: Diagnosing childhood resilience: A systemic approach to the diagnosis of adaptation in adverse social ecologies. *Journal of Child Psychology and Psychiatry, 56*(1), 4–17.

Ungar, M. (2015c). Social ecological complexity and resilience processes. Commentary on 'A conceptual framework for the neurobiological study of resilience'. *Behavioral and Brain Sciences, 38,* 50–51.

Ungar, M. (2017). Which counts more? The differential impact of the environment or the differential susceptibility of the individual? *British Journal of Social Work, 47*(5), 1279–1289.

Ungar, M., Hadfield, K., & Ikeda, J. (2017). Young people's experiences of therapeutic relationships at high and low levels of risk and resilience. *Journal of Social Work Practice, 31,* 277–292.

Werner, E. E., & Smith, R. S. (2001). *Journeys from childhood to midlife: Risk, resilience, and recovery.* Ithaca, NY: Cornell University Press.

Werner, E. E. (2012). What can we learn about resilience from large-scale longitudinal studies? In S. Goldstein & R. Brooks (Eds.), *Handbook of resilience in children* (pp. 87–102). New York, NY: Springer.

World Health Organization. (2011). *World report on disability.* Geneva, Switzerland: World Health Organization.

Wright, M. O., Masten, A. S., & Narayan, A. J. (2013). Resilience processes in development: Four waves of research on positive adaptation in the context of adversity. In S. Goldstein & R. Brooks (Eds.), *Handbook of resilience in children* (2nd ed., pp. 15–37). New York, NY: Springer.

Zautra, A. J., Hall, J. S., & Murray, K. E. (2010). Resilience: A new definition of health for people and communities. In J. W. Reich, A. J. Zautra, & J. S. Hall (Eds.), *Handbook of adult resilience* (pp. 3–29). New York, NY: Guilford.

Part II
Methodological Considerations

Relational Research (Trans)forming Practices

Sheila McNamee

It might appear ethnocentric and self-interested to center this chapter on relational research with a story about American politics. However, I think this story offers an excellent entre into the most contested area of relational research. That most contested area takes the form of a critique that relational research is not rigorous, is relativist, and therefore does not contribute to our knowledge base. And, based on this critique, relational research is viewed as not helping us, as a global community, progress (Boghossian, 2006; Slife & Richardson, 2011). Hold on to that critique. We will return to it.

But before I launch into how contemporary American politics serves as a useful response to naïve critiques of relational research, it is important to note that I am using the terms relational, constructionist, and systemic as synonyms. I do so because of the cultural variation of these terms. In Europe, systemic theory and practice has long been identified within the legacy of Gregory Bateson (1972) and the innovative work of the Milan Team (Boscolo, Cecchin, Hoffman, & Penn, 1987; Palazzoli, Cecchin, Prata, & Boscolo, 1978) and Tom Andersen's reflecting processes (1990). How these systemic ideas have evolved is presented in McCarthy and Simon's (2016) volume, *Systemic Therapy as Transformative Practice.*

Yet, in North America, these same ideas – blended as well with the philosophical influences of Wittgenstein (1953), Bakhtin (1983), and Foucault (1979), to name a few – are more commonly referred to as constructionist (Gergen, 2015a, 2015b) or relational (McNamee & Hosking, 2012). It is beyond the scope of this chapter to detail the various trajectories and diversions of these terms and their implications for theory and practice. In an attempt to be as inclusive as possible, I am proposing

S. McNamee (✉)
University of New Hampshire, Durham, NH, USA

Taos Institute, Chagrin Falls, OH, USA
e-mail: Sheila.McNamee@unh.edu

© Springer Nature Switzerland AG 2020
M. Ochs et al. (eds.), *Systemic Research in Individual, Couple, and Family Therapy and Counseling*, European Family Therapy Association Series,
https://doi.org/10.1007/978-3-030-36560-8_7

that systemic, relational, and constructionist are terms that encompass common assumptions and forms of practice.

American Politics and Relational Research

In January of 2017, on national television, one of the American President's senior advisors, Kellyanne Conway, defended the President's Press Secretary, Sean Spicer's, claim that Trump's inaugural crowd surpassed any other. She said to her interviewer, "You're saying it's a falsehood. And… Sean Spicer, our press secretary… gave alternative facts."

In other words, the senior advisor to the president was basically claiming, "you have your facts and we have our (alternative) facts." This could be interpreted (and, in fact, was) as a challenge – to whom is unclear but purportedly, the American public – to determine whose facts were actually True; and this is why this story is relevant in our discussion of relational research.

The interviewer, Chuck Todd, responded, "Alternative facts aren't facts; they are falsehoods." Facts vs. Falsehoods? Facts vs. Lies? This is the critical ground upon which a systemic, constructionist, relational philosophy and a traditional, modernist, individualist philosophy is distinguished. And, this is why this American story is relevant to our understanding of relational research.

Traditional Versus Relational Research

The dominant research tradition has emerged within a modernist worldview.

Modernism assumes that, with the proper tools and techniques, we will be able to discover reality, as well as describe it, *as it really is*. Of course, part and parcel of this assumption is the belief that there is a reality to be discovered. Science and the scientific method serve as cornerstones of modernist thinking and thus the belief that research should follow accepted scientific methods remains the hallmark of modernism.

Systemic/constructionist/relational thinking, on the other hand, challenges the notion that there is one reality to be discovered. In fact, relational research challenges the very idea of discovery, itself (Gergen, 2015a, 2015b; McNamee & Hosking, 2012). Rather than discover reality, we create it in our interactions with each other and the environments in which we participate. Therefore, we propose that our ways of talking and relating with each other and the world should be the focus of study, and thus the idea of multiple truths, multiple realities, and multiple methods for exploring such realities is paramount. We are curious about what sorts of worlds can be made possible through particular forms of interaction. Focus is on relational processes that construct our worlds, and this is understood as something very different from a focus on discovering how the world (really) is.

The focus on relational processes is the hallmark of a constructionist/systemic orientation. This focus represents a shift from examining entities (whether they be individuals, groups, organizations or physical matter) to attending to what we refer to as language or language processes. To the constructionist, language is not simply a tool or vehicle used to transmit or exchange information about reality. Rather, language is seen as constructing reality. What we do together actually makes our social worlds. This distinction is significant because it invites a deconstruction of our accepted, dominant view of research. In other words, it suggests that we ask: *How else might we imagine research? How do we conceptualize what research is when we start from the position of seeing research – like any other interaction – as a relationally/systemically constructed process?*

Problems with the Modernist Critique of Relational Research

Let me return to our American story: Alternative Facts. Critics of systemic/constructionist ideas would be quick to claim that all who adopt a systemic/constructionist stance would completely agree with the notion of alternative facts. Why not? As constructionists, we acknowledge that meaning emerges in what people do together. In other words, meaning is *negotiated.* And, different communities, groups, and cultures can rightfully negotiate very different meanings and thus live in very different realities. To offer one example, in many cultures death is unequivocally the end of life. In other cultures (those perhaps more spiritually oriented), death is the beginning of life.

So, if the Trump administration negotiates "alternative facts," that is their constructed reality – they, too, are "facts." But, as a self-avowed constructionist, I cannot agree with the Press Secretary's comment that Trump's inauguration crowd was "the largest audience to ever witness an inauguration." Even if everyone in the White House, as well as everyone who supports Trump (both in the USA and elsewhere), has *negotiated* this *alternative fact*, as a constructionist, it cannot simply stand as the truth.

Critics of systemic/constructionist ideas would say that this last statement (the alternative fact is not the truth) illustrates an incoherence and inconsistency of the systemic/constructionist stance. More colloquially a critic might say, "You claim there is no Truth; there are multiple truths. But then you authoritatively claim that some of those multiple truths are false. Thus, you – the constructionist – are showing us that you really do believe in A TRUTH! And it's *your* truth!"

Both the inconsistency critique and the rampant relativist critique (anything goes) are hardline talking points for those who oppose systemic/constructionist ideas. They also unveil a lack of understanding about the philosophical premises of a systemic/constructionist orientation. Let me address this misunderstanding.

Philosophical Assumptions of a Systemic/Constructionist Stance

While we recognize that meaning – and therefore reality – are created in what people do together, that does not imply, nor even lightly suggest, that we can make up anything we want about the world. This is where critics make their biggest mistake.

We live within traditions that are culturally, relationally, and environmentally situated. Within those traditions – or interpretive communities, as Wittgenstein (1953) would call them – there are established forms of practice, established meanings, and established expectations. These established ways of being are the byproduct of coordinated actions among people who are operating within traditions and ways of talking and acting they have inherited. Because we all participate in many different, local traditions and communities, the possibility for negotiating diverse and multiple understandings of any given phenomenon are always present. This is the relativist position of systemic/constructionist thinking; it is not an "anything goes" position (see McNamee, 2017).

Let me explain how constructionist relativism is not rampant. The communities, traditions, and relations within which we live and act keep constructionists from slipping into an anything goes mentality. This is precisely what Garfinkel (1967) explained; we use words and actions to refer to the world and, in so doing, what we take for granted remains so precisely because we do not question these conventions. We draw upon negotiated ways of acting in order to achieve a sense of "rationality." In other words, we work very hard to maintain the social order.

Let's think about that. Every time a researcher designs an experiment with carefully controlled conditions, that researcher is participating in the world of traditional research. That is, the researcher is doing what is expected of a trained researcher. *In other words, it is what the researcher (and all others like him/her) is doing that "maintains the social order – or truth – about what counts as research."*

But consider this: What might happen if several researchers began to question (we would use the word, deconstruct) the assumptions that, for example, with the right method we can discover reality? What if a community of traditional, modernist laboratory scientists decided to explore how people who are HIV positive make meaning of an HIV prevention pill? What if they also explore how the popular press and religious groups make meaning of this pill (Koester, 2017; Koester & Grant, 2015)? Suppose these two groups view the pill in very different terms. Those who are HIV positive see the pill (much like the birth control pill) as allowing them to live a normal sexual life without fear of undesired consequences (e.g., infecting their partners or becoming gravely ill). Yet those in the popular press, some factions of oversight boards for pharmaceuticals, and religious groups see the pill as an invitation to promiscuous sexual behavior. In a modernist world, these would be competing (or alternative) facts/truths, and the logical next step would be to "prove" which is right and which is wrong.

But, as relational researchers, our focus is directed toward an exploration of these different communities and how such a focus might help us to understand the success or failure of this pill. What such an examination might yield is the *complexity* of the issue. If approached with curiosity (as opposed to certainty that the right method will produce the Truth), this relational research might find a way to bring these opposing communities together, and perhaps in so doing, those who are HIV positive have a chance to provide humanizing narratives about their lives, narratives that transform them (in the eyes of the press and religious groups) from sexual perverts to people valuing the health and safety of their partners and themselves. And similarly, perhaps in such a coming together, the oppositional press and religious factions are able to be viewed as also caring for people's safety. This research moves from two conflicting truths to two different approaches to making sure people are safe (Koester, 2017). The shared narrative is about safety. Now we have something to work with that embraces complexity rather than polarization.

This is transformation, not anything goes. The kinds of questions we ask focus our attention on the implications – or unintended consequences – of our communally constructed worlds. And, it is this attention to what our meanings make possible (or impossible) that is critical for systemic/constructionists. The attention is not on *proving* anything to be right or wrong but on exploring the implications of stepping into and embracing any particular truth. A researcher's curiosity about the very different worlds/realities/truths of those who live with HIV and who see the prevention pill as a good thing and those who oppose the pill makes it possible to see the "local coherence" for each group. From there, Any attempt to prove the truth or facticity of one view over another recedes when we attempt, instead, to understand difference. Attempting to understand difference opens possible ways to move forward together.

Let me return to the idea of maintaining the social order, because this is important. As systemic scholars and practitioners, we acknowledge that the social order emerges from what people do together. It is constructed. This means that all that we take for granted (e.g., that people will stop at a red light) is maintained by an often (but not always) unspoken social contract. It is amazing to think about this. Some people eat three meals a day – because that's what you're supposed to do in their world. Children go to school because that's what they are supposed to do. This *coordinated, negotiated* social order hinges entirely upon our participating in its maintenance. Thus, the social order that we take for granted is fragile.

Change, from this perspective, emerges in a couple of ways. Change occurs when a sub-community begins to question the taken-for-granted way of being. A good example is the women's movement. Yet, as we well know, one woman alone could not and did not alter the dominant patriarchal order. Change also occurs when diverse communities come together. We need only look historically to see the rampant transformation of the meaning of family (Coontz, 1992), organization (Kegan & Lahey, 2001; Morgan, 1997), healthcare (Charon, 2006; Kleinman, 1988), and more as associated with the increasing ability of cultures and communities to move and share resources. As one small illustration, many people, as well as medical practitioners, now see value in homeopathic treatments. For them, scientific medicine vs. homeopathic remedies is no longer a battle over competing truths.

What's Wrong with Alternative Facts?

Returning to alternative facts, why, you might wonder, am I claiming that Kellyanne Conway's alternative facts are questionable? In and of themselves, these alternative facts are not necessarily objectionable. What is objectionable is that those support- ing these alternative facts have demonstrated no interest in coordinating among competing views. Instead, the alternative facts have been proclaimed. End of conversation.

At this juncture, many in the media and general public turn to empiricism – the idea that all knowledge emerges from sense experience. In the case of Kellyanne's alternative facts, we were shown two side-by-side photographs of the National Mall – the stretch of land between the United States Capitol and the Lincoln Memorial. One photo was of Barak Obama's inaugural crowd and the other of Trump's. I'm sure many of you have seen these photos. Empirically, the Trump photo shows a good deal of empty space, whereas the Obama photo is packed with people.

Now, a traditional researcher would claim with certainty that, because we can see the substantial difference between the two crowds, we have empirical evidence that allows us to say that Obama's crowd was significantly larger than Trump's. Yet, the spokespeople for the White House (as well as the current president, himself) claim that empirical fact is false and that, alternatively, Trump's crowd was the largest in history.

But what if we introduced curiosity and asked about one's point of view? The comparative photographs we saw were both taken from the back of the crowd – looking toward the inaugural platform. But Trump and his advisors were positioned at the opposite end, looking out over the mall toward the back of the crowd. Had either the Press Secretary or Senior Advisor to the President or the media enter- tained the question of perspective, the hardline Fact/Alternative Fact (or Truth/Lie) could well have been softened. Also worthy of consideration is what the Administration meant by "crowd." Those physically present? Those watching online? Those watching on TV? And, additionally, is a crowd 100 people, 1000, 10,000, … 100,000?

Here, I am reminded of Gregory Bateson's (1972) metalogue, *What is an Instinct?*

> In this metalogue, his daughter asks him: Daughter: Daddy, what is an instinct?
> Father: An instinct, my dear, is an explanatory principle.
> D: But what does it explain?
> F: Anything – almost anything at all. Anything you want it to explain. (p. 38)

And like explanatory principles, empirical evidence is not immune to social coordination and negotiation. Bateson's daughter continues by claiming that instinct does not explain gravity, to which Bateson responds: "No. But that is because nobody wants 'instinct' to explain gravity. If they did, it would explain it." (p. 38)

His argument, as mine in this chapter, is that what counts as empirical evidence does so because we agree to certain parameters (this is what maintains the social order). In the present case, two contrasting photographs of people standing on the National Mall in Washington, DC serve to document that one president had a larger crowd than another. In order to challenge that empirical fact, one would need to create an explanatory principle that others agreed with or accepted, an explanatory principle that either granted the possibility of a perspectival shift of empirical evidence (i.e., photos from the opposing angle) or that deemed photographs of crowds as only a partial piece of the "crowd."

Most of the media, as well as most ordinary people, talked non-stop about the White House's alternative fact with great disbelief. How could they make such an obviously false claim? At this point, we must examine a common and dangerous misunderstanding about systemic/constructionist ideas.

Constructionists are not claiming that we can create reality at will. Constructionists are not claiming there is no physical/material reality. And yet, this is a common misunderstanding that many share. The dangerous effect of this misunderstanding is that there is no recognition that meaning emerges in social processes and is maintained only as people act in accordance with that meaning. Rather, this unintended effect of misunderstanding the acceptance of multiple worldviews claims that the social order can be altered at whim by those in powerful positions who wish to do so – what Foucault (1980) refers to as the "normalizing gaze."

But in a situation such as this one, the ability to normalize (declare) what is the case, despite competing views, invites us into the territory of rampant relativism – or, "you can have your fact and we will have ours, but we are in power so we all know ours will be deemed Truth." This is the rampant relativism so heavily critiqued by opponents to systemic/constructionist ideas. But again, let me repeat: This is not what a social construction or systemic stance proposes. Let me also say that I am simply pointing out that, when those with power make claims that disrupt the accepted social order, and when those claims are taken up with great enthusiasm by the media, the relational/systemic/constructionist stance of curiosity is ignored, thereby turning a possibility for coordinating a useful way forward into a debate about fact vs. falsity.

When we adopt a systemic/constructionist stance, we recognize that the material, physical world exists but how we come to name it, what it means to us, and how we interact with it are all a byproduct of social negotiation. Thus, you might say, "The White House negotiated their reality. Why can't that count?" Indeed, they have. And, most important, we must note that they declared that they had the right to claim what counts as a fact and what doesn't. There is no interest in the "other facts." Excuse the pun, but to the White House, their alternative facts trump any other facts.

The systemic/constructionist philosophical stance, on the other hand, presumes there will be multiple truths (facts) and – *a crucially important distinction* – is curious to attempt to understand how those facts were created and how they are viewed as coherent and rational. This small move toward curiosity is what divides the philosophical stance of systemic/constructionist work and the dangerous effects of misunderstanding its stance. I say the misunderstanding of the constructionist view of multiplicity is dangerous because such misunderstanding produces a world of universal right and wrong; a world of us and them. Such divisiveness invites conflict, violence, oppression, and war. Yet, when we adopt the philosophical orientation of systemic/relational work, we ask ourselves and others, "What stories are we developing?" "What are the unintended consequences of these stories on our own lives and on the lives of others?" "Are there more useful stories that could be told?"

But rather than ask these questions, those who presume nothing exists until we say so, stand firm in the belief that their facts are the only ones that matter with no curiosity to explore different beliefs, nor to understand how such beliefs could emerge in the first place as rational and coherent.

Relational Research

How does this argument help us think about research and, in particular, think about research as (trans)forming practices?

Systemic/relational/constructionist research is premised on the idea that what comes to be labeled as truth or fact – what appears to be empirical about the world – enjoys that status *only by virtue of communal engagement*. In other words, we return to people interacting (relating) in the world. It is not the world, itself, that is or is not factual or truthful; it is the negotiated agreements that people create and sustain (and also change) that are factual or truthful *within context* and this means that there will always be multiple truths. Yet living in a world of multiple truths does not mean anything goes. It means that our job – as researchers, consultants, therapists, teachers, managers – is to attempt to *coordinate* multiplicity, not eradicate it by speaking with authority in an attempt to dismiss multiplicity.

My point here is not so much about American politics as it is about moving from a position of "competing facts" (which, of course, implies some deliberation to determine which is right) to a position of competing beliefs that circulate within the parameters of a constructed social order. As systemic/constructionist researchers, we should occupy the latter. This shifts the focus and attention of our research from a proof-based rhetoric to a collaborative consideration of the implications and unintended consequences of what we study, how we study it, and what we ultimately do with our "results."

We must avoid perpetuating bi-polar, divisive conclusions (e.g., this was the largest inaugural crowd in history). Because we live in a complex and diverse world, the best our research can do it provide access to that diversity and complexity. We, as researchers, should not have the authorial and fateful last word.

And yet, the results of our inquiry must offer something. We are invited to explore what sorts of worlds we are generating, as well as what sorts of knowledge and understandings are being crafted, when we engage in any inquiry process. To that end, important questions to ask include:

- In what ways is this inquiry *useful*? And for whom?
- Does this inquiry generate new forms of understanding? For whom?

- Does this inquiry generate new forms of practice? For whom?

Returning to the common critique that relational research is not rigorous, is relativist and therefore not contributing to our knowledge base and thus not helping us, as a global community, progress, I would offer the following. Rigor is created in context; what counts as rigorous research in the lab will be very different from rigorous research in the field. Given the complexity of today's world, research must be relativist and, to that end, it adds to multiple knowledge bases. The ethics of relational research demand that, as researchers, we attempt to coordinate these multiple views – not for purposes of discerning which is true or right or factual but for purposes of initiating new forms of understanding. And, I would argue, it is this new form of understanding – understanding that embraces (rather than repels) the multiplicity of truths – that will humanize our world.

References

Andersen, T. (Ed.). (1990). *The reflecting team*. Kent, UK: Borgmann Publishing.

Bateson, G. (1972). *Steps to an ecology of mind*. New York, NY: Ballentine Books.

Boghossian, P. A. (2006). *Fear of knowledge: Against relativism and constructivism*. Oxford, UK: Clarendon Press.

Bakhtin, M. M. (1983). The dialogical imagination. M. Holquist (Ed.), C. Emerson & M. Holquist (Trans.). Texas: University of Texas Press.

Boscolo, L., Cecchin, G., Hoffman, L., & Penn, P. (1987). *Milan systemic family therapy*. New York, NY: Basic Books.

Charon, R. (2006). *Narrative medicine*. London, UK: Oxford University Press.

Coontz, S. (1992). *The way we never were: American families and the nostalgia trap*. New York, NY: Basic Books.

Foucault, M. (1979). Discipline and punish. New York: Vintage.

Foucault, M. (1980). *Power/knowledge: Selected interviews and other writings 1972–1977* (C. Gordon, et al., Trans.). New York, NY: Pantheon.

Garfinkel, H. (1967). *Studies in ethnomethodology*. Englewood Cliffs, NJ: Prentice- Hall.

Gergen, K. J. (2015a). *An invitation to social construction*. London, UK: Sage.

Gergen, K. J. (2015b). *Relational being: Beyond self and community*. Oxford, UK: Oxford University Press.

Kegan, R., & Lahey, L. L. (2001). *How the way we talk can change the way we work*. San Francisco, CA: Jossey-Bass.

Kleinman, A. (1988). *The illness narratives*. New York, NY: Basic Books.

Koester, K.A. (2017). *A pill to prevent HIV: Revising destructive narratives and re-writing our relationship to HIV disease* (Unpublished doctoral dissertation). Vrije Universiteit Brussels, Belgium.

Koester, K. A., & Grant, R. M. (2015). Keeping our eyes on the prize: No new HIV infections with increased use of HIV pre-exposure prophylaxis. *Clinical Infectious Disease, 61*(10), 1604–1605.

McCarthy, I., & Simon, G. (2016). *Systemic therapy as transformative practice*. Farnhill, UK: Everything Is Connected Press.

McNamee, S. (2017). Far from "anything goes": Ethics as communally constructed. *Journal of Constructivist Psychology, 31*, 361–368.

McNamee, S., & Hosking, D. M. (2012). *Research and social change: A relational constructionist approach*. New York, NY: Routledge.

Morgan, G. (1997). *Images of organization*. London, UK: Sage.

Palazzoli, M. S., Cecchin, G., Prata, G., & Boscolo, L. (1978). *Paradox and counterparadox*. New York, NY: Jason Aronson.

Slife, B., & Richardson, F. (2011). The relativism of social constructionism. *Journal of Constructivist Psychology, 24*, 333–339.

Wittgenstein, L. (1953). *Philosophical investigations*. Oxford, UK: Blackwell.

Discourse Analysis and Systemic Family Therapy Research: The Methodological Contribution of Discursive Psychology

Eleftheria Tseliou

My aim in this chapter is to discuss certain ways in which the theoretical and methodological approach of discursive psychology can contribute to systemic, couple and family therapy research. Discursive psychology is part of the wider trend of qualitative, hermeneutic research methodologies as well as theoretical proposals for the study of discourse, which are usually clustered under the over-inclusive, trans-disciplinary term, discourse analysis (Potter & Hepburn, 2005; Tseliou, 2013, 2018; Willig, 2013). Discourse analysis has incorporated epistemological and theoretical advances in humanities and social sciences, which have highlighted the constitutive role of language use for all phenomena, widely known as the discursive turn (Bozatzis, 2014; Tseliou, 2013, 2018; Tseliou & Borcsa, 2018). The field of systemic family therapy has also witnessed the effects of the discursive turn, as evident in the shift toward constructivist and social constructionist epistemological perspectives, which gave birth to post-modern therapeutic approaches, like collaborative, dialogic, and narrative approaches. More recently, it seems that the field has also welcomed the use of discourse analysis research methodologies mostly for the study of couple and family therapy process (Borcsa & Rober, 2016; Tseliou, 2017, 2018; Tseliou & Borcsa, 2018). Nevertheless, the deployment of discursive psychology in particular remains marginal. This is striking given the common episte-mological background and certain isomorphic tenets between systemic family therapy and discursive psychology. Like in the case of systemic family therapy, discursive psychology advances a re-thinking of psychological phenomena in discursive and interactional terms in that it prioritizes the context of language-use in interaction as *the context* per se for their constitution and study (Edwards & Potter, 1992; Wiggins, 2017). Most importantly, however, discursive psychology

E. Tseliou (✉)
Laboratory of Psychology, Department of Early Childhood Education,
University of Thessaly, Volos, Greece
e-mail: tseliou@uth.gr

© Springer Nature Switzerland AG 2020
M. Ochs et al. (eds.), *Systemic Research in Individual, Couple, and Family Therapy and Counseling*, European Family Therapy Association Series,
https://doi.org/10.1007/978-3-030-36560-8_8

can provide methodological input to systemic couple and family therapy process research suitable to address systemically informed inquiries concerning the therapeutic dialogue.

In this chapter, my aim is to introduce three specific theoretical and methodological proposals of discursive psychology which are indicative of its potential for systemic couple and family therapy research, due to their affinity with systemic family therapy tenets. These include the pragmatic orientation to theorizing and studying discourse, the intersubjective/interactional theoretical and methodological approach to the understanding and the study of psychological phenomena, and specific suggestions for studying the ways in which historical and socio-cultural and political contexts shape discourse use in therapy. Prior to discussing in detail these three proposals, I will first briefly introduce discursive psychology as well as its up-to-date deployment in the field of systemic couple and family therapy research.

Discursive Psychology and Systemic Family Therapy

In this section, I will start with a brief introduction concerning the place of discursive psychology in the broader spectrum of discourse analysis research. I will then present the history and some basic tenets of discursive psychology, which denote its affinity with systemic family therapy. Then I will conclude with a brief overview of its up-to-date use in systemic couple and family therapy research.

Discourse Analysis and Discursive Psychology: A Brief Introduction

Currently there is extensive use of the term discourse analysis across disciplines like education, psychology, linguistics, literary theory and criticism, etc. (Tseliou, 2013, 2017). Irrespective of differences in theoretical, epistemological, and methodological preferences, the term broadly refers to approaches which have incorporated main premises of constructivist, social constructionist, or post-structuralist frameworks. Such frameworks have introduced the idea that language is central for the constitution of every phenomenon. Knowledge, including scientific knowledge, is more a construction than a reflection of an independently existing reality, inseparable from the knowing subject or else the observer (Burr, 2015). Furthermore, they have forwarded the idea that language use is not neutral. Instead, history, culture, and ideology shape language use and delineate certain power relationships (Willig, 2013). Against this epistemological backcloth, discourse analysis approaches introduce certain methodological proposals for the study of talk and texts while sharing the premise that research is an interpretative process of knowledge construction, a process considered as historically and socio-culturally situated. These methodological proposals share the idea that the object of study is language per se. However, there is variability in the ways that different discourse analysis trends approach both the theorizing but also the study of discourse. This variability accounts for the treatment of discursive psychology as a distinct theoretical and methodological approach.

Discursive psychology is affiliated with discourse analysis approaches which focus on the study of how people use language to manage the course of their everyday interactions and how language use shapes interpersonal interaction. These approaches are rooted in the Anglo-Saxon tradition of the linguistic philosophy of Wittgenstein and Austin (Tseliou, 2013, 2017; Willig, 2013). They also utilize the intellectual heritage of conversation analysis (Sacks, Schegloff, & Jefferson, 1974), a tradition distinct from discourse analysis, which is rooted in ethnomethodology. Conversation analysis aims at the identification of the normative structure of talk-in-interaction or else at the investigation of conversational structures, which depict how the social world is performed via talk-in-interaction (Antaki, 2014). Analysis entails a micro-detailed scrutiny of both the content and the process of talk-in-interaction with an emphasis on the local context/setting of conversations. According to a frequently reiterated distinction in the field of psychology (Tseliou, 2013, 2015, 2017, 2018; Tseliou & Borcsa, 2018; Willig, 2013), these discourse analysis approaches differ from a second group of approaches, which focus on highlighting how the historical and socio-political contexts of language use restrict our choices when we use language over the course of our everyday interactions (Tseliou, 2013, 2017; Willig, 2013). In drawing from post-structuralist thinking like Foucault's theorizing (Foucault, 1972/1969) or post-Marxist contributions, like the ones by Laclau and Mouffe (Laclau & Mouffe, 1985) such approaches highlight issues interrelated with power and hegemonic conditions which shape language use. The main idea is that while people talk, they draw from historically available, ideologically laden, systematic ways to construct versions of the world, which they then negotiate and re-construct in the course of their everyday interactions. According to this approach, talk is not politically or ideologically neutral. Thus, post-structurally informed discourse analysis aims at the identification of systematic ways for speaking and for constructing objects/subjects, which are historically constituted and ideologically laden.

Despite what comes across as an "ontological quality" of such a distinction, discourse analytic practice often includes creative cross-loans between the different traditions. Furthermore, critical approaches to discursive psychology (see e.g., Bozatzis, 2009, 2016; Wetherell, 1998, 2007) mostly undertake a "both–and" perspective in that they combine the micro-detailed analysis of the "bottom–up" discursive approaches with the macro-orientation of the "top–down," post-structuralist approaches to discourse.

Discursive Psychology: A "Systemically" Informed Psychology?

Up-to-date, there are very engaging narratives of the historical origins of discursive psychology as well as of its evolution (Potter, 2012a, 2012b; Tileagă & Stokoe, 2016). Furthermore, there are many, very informative sketches of its basic tenets (e.g., Hepburn & Wiggins, 2005; Lester, 2014; O'Reilly, Lester, & Kiyimba, 2018; Potter, 2011, 2012a) including presentations of its main features, which I have reported elsewhere (Tseliou, 2015; Tseliou & Borcsa, 2018; Tseliou, Smoliak, LaMarre, & Quinn-Nilas, 2019). Thus, here, I will inevitably reiterate some key points concerning the history, the evolution, and the basic tenets of the discursive psychology approach to discourse analytic research.

Like in the case of discourse analysis, there is variety in the narratives concerning the history of discursive psychology and the elaboration of the term (e.g., Augoustinos & Tileagă, 2012; Billig, 2012; Edwards, 2012; Tileagă & Stokoe, 2016). Furthermore, there are different narratives, which attempt to delineate the various, existing trends of discursive psychology as well as its historical evolution (Hepburn & Wiggins, 2005; Potter, 2012a, 2012b; Wetherell, 2007). As concerns its origins, Edwards and Potter (1992) seem to have introduced the term, whereas most narratives (e.g., Billig, 2012; Hepburn & Potter, 2011; Potter, 2012b) relate the emergence of discursive psychology with a broader attempt to introduce a re-conceptualization of mainstream psychology and social psychology in particular. Such attempt included a critique of mainstream psychology for entailing an essentialist, ahistorical, and mostly cognitivist approach and is reflected in earlier writings of scholars like Jonathan Potter, Derek Edwards, Margaret Wetherell, and Michael Billig in the 1980s (see e.g., Billig, 1987; Potter & Wetherell, 1987).

Broadly speaking, discursive psychology is not simply a methodological proposal for the analysis of talk and texts. It further constitutes a theoretical proposal for a radical re-conceptualization of psychological phenomena, in ways similar to the re-conceptualization of psychopathology and psychotherapy introduced by systemic family therapy. For discursive psychology, psychological phenomena like cognition, memory, identity, etc. are treated as "matters of interested communication between speakers" (Antaki, 2014, p. 75) or else are "re-conceptualized as language-based activities" (Billig, 2014, p. 159). In that sense, discursive psychology is interested in how psychological phenomena are evoked in talk-in-interaction (Edwards, 1997, 2012; Potter, 1996). It thus shifts the locus of interest from the intra-psychic realm where psychology traditionally locates the understanding and the study of psychological phenomena to the realm of language use and interaction.

Like in the case of systemic approaches (Bateson, 1979), discursive psychology approaches discourse as interrelated with context and places particular emphasis on both the local context of discourse use, that is the specific occasion of language use, but also on the wider, social, historical and institutional context. This emphasis on the latter, although not identical, is reminiscent of post-structural developments in the field of systemic family therapy like the narrative approaches (White & Epston, 1990) which have been inspired by Foucault's thinking.

Furthermore, for discursive psychology the emphasis on theoretically and analytically approaching discourse is rather on its pragmatics as compared to its semantics, like in the case of pragmatic, systemic theoretical conceptualizations of communication (e.g., Watzlawick, Beavin-Bavelas, & Jackson, 1967). Discursive psychology also undertakes a rhetorical perspective in approaching discourse (Billig, 1987), according to which we constantly engage into an attempt of persuasion and argumentation concerning our views. Finally, discursive psychology subscribes to the ethnomethodological emphasis on how speakers themselves make sense of the conversations in which they participate (Tseliou, 2017, 2018), thus adhering to the interpretative and intersubjective quality of meaning-making processes.

As concerns analytic practice, discursive psychology shares the emphasis that conversation analysis places on the importance of disentangling what is constructed in talk utterance by utterance, while doing analysis. It also shares the ethnomethodological principle for analyzing naturally occurring talk, that is, talk as it naturally occurs, like in the case of transcribed, recorded counseling/psychotherapy sessions. Following a brief overview of the use of discursive psychology in family therapy research, I will explicate the above features in detail while elaborating on their potential for theoretical and methodological contributions in the field.

Discursive Psychology and Systemic Family Therapy Research

Despite the resonance between discursive psychology and systemic family therapy tenets, the deployment of discursive psychology in systemic family therapy research remains particularly marginal. Systemic family therapy research has grown out of polarized debates concerning the preference for either quantitative or qualitative research methodologies and currently undertakes a "both/and" perspective for the study of therapy process and outcome (Tseliou, 2018; Tseliou & Borcsa, 2018). Nevertheless, the use of qualitative research methodologies remains marginal, as they are mostly deployed for the study of therapy process (Tseliou, 2018; Tseliou & Borcsa, 2018). This is isomorphic to what seems to be the case in the broader spectrum of psychotherapy research, where qualitative research methodologies are minimally used.

In this context, there is growing use of discursive methodologies like conversation or discourse analysis (Borcsa & Rober, 2016; Tseliou & Borcsa, 2018), with few of the existing studies undertaking a systematic, discursive psychology methodological perspective (for an overview, see Tseliou, 2013). On the other hand, the literature of discursive psychology research of couple and family therapy seems to be growing rapidly (e.g., O'Reilly et al., 2018; Patrika & Tseliou, 2016a, 2016b; Sametband & Strong, 2018).

To date, discursive psychology has been utilized by small-scale studies which entail a limited number of sessions as data or which follow a case-study type of research design. The laborious nature of the detailed micro-analysis which discursive psychology necessitates coupled with the difficulty of acquiring access to the naturally occurring data of recorded or video-taped family therapy sessions possibly account for this scarcity. Such studies have investigated a range of topics, like family therapy problem talk in respect of attributions (O'Reilly, 2007; Patrika & Tseliou, 2016a, 2016b; Stancombe & White, 2005), the use of circular questioning in initial systemic family therapy sessions (Diorinou & Tseliou, 2014), or the negotiation and construction of cultural identities in the case of immigration (Sametband & Strong, 2018). However, this limited application of discursive psychology as a methodology for the study of couple and family therapy process does not pay justice to its potential for addressing questions concerning therapy process (and outcome) framed in systemic terms, that is, in ways which highlight an inter-subjectively oriented, discursive perspective.

In the remainder of this chapter, I will discuss three specific aspects of the methodological practice of discursive psychology which I think can add to systemic, family therapy process research, as they bear strong affinity with certain premises of systemic family therapy. These aspects relate to main adherences of discursive psychology which I will further elaborate in the following section by also engaging into a more specific demonstration of how they can be pursued in the context of analytic practice.

Discursive Psychology: Methodological Contributions to Systemic Family Therapy Research

Discursive psychology can facilitate the study of systemic family therapy process, by providing methodological tools for its study, which allow for the study of the therapeutic dialogue in tune with systemic/constructionist premises. Elsewhere (Tseliou, 2018) I have elaborated on the methodological potential of conversation analysis and discursive psychology for psychotherapy research. I have argued that they allow for the study of psychotherapy by highlighting interdependency in respect of therapist and client interaction while simultaneously allowing for an "insider's view," i.e., for investigating psychotherapy from therapist and clients' perspective. Here, I will focus on three specific, theoretical, and methodological aspects of discursive psychology. These include the pragmatic approach to the understanding (and study) of therapeutic dialogue, an intersubjective approach to the understanding (and study) of psychological phenomena, and also the potential for addressing the political and ideological aspects of therapeutic dialogue.

Argumentation and Rhetorics: The Pragmatics of Psychotherapeutic Discourse

Theorizing Discourse Early systemic theorizing (Bateson, 1979; Watzlawick et al., 1967) introduced a pragmatic approach to the understanding of communication, in that the emphasis was placed not so much on the content of discourse but on its function in the context of interaction as well as on its consequences for behavior and interaction. Similarly, discursive psychology adheres to the notion that talk is social, performative, and not neutral. This suggests that while in talk-in-interaction we are not simply transmitting content or information in an unproblematic way. Instead, discursive psychology places particular emphasis on what we perform by means of discourse use. For discursive psychology, discourse is action and has consequences for behavior. In that sense it has a functional aspect, we *do* things by words in the context of our discursive exchanges. Thus, discourse entails an *action orientation* in that we actively construct phenomena or versions of the world by means of discourse use and such constructions attend to interpersonal aims, like when we construct a complaint (Edwards & Potter, 1992; Potter & Wetherell, 1987). For discursive psychology, this performative aspect of talk-in-interaction is also rhetorically structured in the sense that we engage into a constant effort of persuasion as we argue for the "truth" and the "reality" of our views. However, for discursive psychology views are neither stable nor consistent. Instead, people express contradictory views even within the same course of interaction as each view is constructed in relation to its opposite. In that sense talk and thinking are approached as being dilemmatic, i.e., as always entailing two contrasting sides (Billig, 1987; Billig et al., 1988). Therefore, whenever we engage in talk, it is not so straightforward to adopt one view or another. For discursive psychology, co-conversants are always faced with dilemmas posed by the rhetorical context of their talk-in-interaction. The key dynamic for such "dilemmas of stake," in discursive psychology terminology, is how to talk so that our co-discussants cannot undermine our arguments as arising out of personal interest (Edwards & Potter, 1992, 1993). "Factual" discourse is a discourse structure, which facilitates the management of this dilemma. "Factual discourse" is any discourse where views are constructed as facts existing as a reality beyond speakers' personal views or preferences. This *fact and interest* perspective is interrelated with the notion of *accountability* (Edwards & Potter, 1992, 1993). For discursive psychology, discourse structure and content are revealing of the ways in which we attempt to manage accountability issues, that is, issues concerning the undertaking of responsibility for our choice to say (or not say) something as well as for what we choose to say (discourse content). These three aspects which constitute the pragmatic/rhetorical perspective of discursive psychology, namely, the *action orientation*, the *fact and interest*, and the *accountability* features, are depicted in the Discursive Action Model (DAM) (Edwards & Potter, 1993). DAM was originally introduced as an alternative to mainstream, social psychology theorizing for attributions and is extensively presented in the discursive psychology literature (e.g., Edwards & Potter, 1993; Potter, 2012a; Potter & Hepburn, 2005) as well as in family therapy research which deploys DAM for analysis (e.g., Diorinou & Tseliou, 2014; O'Reilly et al., 2018; Patrika & Tseliou, 2016a, 2016b).

Except of the rhetorical/argumentative perspective, there is a further important dimension concerning the discursive psychology approach to the theorizing and the study of discourse. This is the interactional perspective, a perspective very similar to systemic, family therapy theorizing concerning communication. Discursive psychology, in tune with ethnomethodology and conversation analysis, places emphasis on how we *intersubjectively* make sense of each other's discursive contributions and *jointly* construct phenomena in talk-in-interaction (Tseliou, 2018).

Analysis of Discourse The theoretical orientation that discursive psychology undertakes concerning discourse indicates a set of certain methodological principles for the analysis of any discourse, including psychotherapeutic discourse. Here, due to my particular focus, I will indicatively select the setting of initial systemic family therapy sessions, to briefly explicate these methodological principles. I will draw examples from studies, which have deployed discursive psychology for the analysis of initial systemic family therapy sessions.

A first methodological principle entails the *analysis of the rhetorical context*. From a discursive psychology perspective, when the therapist and the family members meet, they do not simply exchange their views concerning what seems to be troubling in an unproblematic way. Instead, they engage into argumentation concerning their perspectives, their epistemologies, and their worldviews about "the problem." Research (Ugazio, Fellin, Pennacchio, Negri, & Colciago, 2012) has indicated that in the case of systemic family therapy, these entail significant discrepancies. Family members usually share a linear epistemology according to which the identified patient has a problem for which they should not be held responsible. On the contrary, the systemic therapist espouses a perspective, which favors circular causality and relational responsibility. According to this, everyone contributes to the construction of the relational/discursive pattern within which the reported problem is embedded. This dynamic sets the ground for analyzing what is "at stake" for both sides. Patrika and Tseliou (2016b) present a detailed analysis of the "dilemma of stake" for family members and for the systemic therapist. For family members problem talk is challenging. On the one hand, the family therapy setting is a setting where problem talk is normatively expected as people enter therapy in order to ask for help about their problems. Problem talk, however, raises issues of attributions of responsibility and often denotes a search for a cause, i.e., for someone who is accountable or to be blamed for the reported difficulties. In a family therapy setting, family members are potential candidates. Consequently family members seem entangled within the dilemma of how to speak about problems but without facing risks concerning the attribution of responsibility (Patrika & Tseliou, 2016b). Correspondingly, the systemic family therapist seems equally caught in a difficult to handle dilemma: how to speak about problems without simultaneously blaming family members including the "identified patient," given that on the one hand, there is a normative expectation from an expert to diagnose problems and their cause(s) but on the other, the systemic perspective necessitates a neutrality perspective (Patrika & Tseliou, 2016b).

For discursive psychology analysis, this dynamic is critical as it provides the context for the interpretation of what is uttered by both sides. Such analysis, however, is not merely a descriptive analysis of the content of therapist and family members' discourse. Instead, a second methodological principle dictates a *shift from the level of content to the level of process*, in systemic terms. A discursive analyst needs to de-code what is performed by what the therapist and family members say: he/she needs to analyze the function of their words. Diorinou and Tseliou (2014) exemplify this feature in their analysis of a father's discourse in an initial systemic family therapy session. They show how father's factual discourse concerning his son's problem behavior, i.e., a discourse constructing the problem behavior as a fact existing independently of father's report about it, seems to attend to a multi-faceted function. It addresses the preceding invitation by the therapist to talk about the problem in a way, which delicately manages accountability issues. Father's factual discourse seems to eschew the risk of constructing his son as being responsible for the problem behavior while simultaneously eschews the risk of constructing himself as a father who accuses his son for the family's troubles (Diorinou & Tseliou, 2014). Diorinou and Tseliou (2014) analyze in detail the features which add factuality to father's discourse, like the use of direct quotation in the phrase, "there is no harmony in our house, no coordination, no consistency and all this may come up, let's say, through certain phrases like when my older son said "in my life I feel alone" (Diorinou & Tseliou, 2014, p. 110).

In order to reach an interpretation of what is performed in talk, analysis needs to follow a third methodological principle, which dictates a *sequential analysis of talk-in-interaction* in discursive psychology terms. This implies that the interpretation of the function of each utterance needs to take into account its conversational context. In other words, analysis of one utterance needs to take in into account both the preceding as well as the subsequent utterances. It further implies that the analyst needs to examine in detail, utterance by utterance, how therapist and family members de-code each other's discursive contributions. To accomplish this kind of analysis, discursive psychology makes use of contributions by ethnomethodology and conversation analysis. The first tradition has contributed the idea that talk entails reflexive markers, which indicate how speakers themselves interpret each other's contributions (Garfinkel, 1967). It thus acknowledges that talk has a reflexive quality, in that it is revealing of the constant process of interpretation and construction of meaning in which co-conversants engage. The second has provided an extensive body of empirical research concerning normative conversational structures (see, e.g., Sacks et al., 1974). Such normative expectations about what is anticipated or not in talk-in-interaction suggest a social accountability, intersubjective perspective to the study of therapeutic dialogue. For example, conversation analysis literature has identified normative structures which have the form of pairs and which are termed adjacency pairs (Sacks et al., 1974). In their case, when a first part of a pair is uttered, like an invitation, the second is normatively expected, like acceptance. However, breaches of such normative structures are often the case, e.g., denial of invitation, and these are of great analytic interest. In that sense, a detailed, sequential analysis of this kind can shed light to the function of a question in the place of a normatively expected answer by a family member, following a therapist's question. Patrika and Tseliou (2016a) present an example of this kind of sequential analysis, when they show how mother's question as a response to the therapist's circular question – "Who is happy with this?"– (Patrika & Tseliou, 2016a, p. 476) is part of a sequence which seems to contribute to the construction of a blaming pattern where both family members and the therapist seem to contribute.

An Interactional Perspective to Psychological Phenomena in Psychotherapeutic Discourse: The Case of Identity

The pragmatic/rhetorical perspective, which I have discussed in the previous section, is interrelated with the overall approach that discursive psychology undertakes concerning psychological phenomena. Discursive psychology suggests their re-considering in discursive and interactional terms, an orientation also undertaken by systemic family therapy. In order to further explicate this perspective, both on the level of theorizing but also in analytic terms; here I will indicatively select the notion of identity. Once more, I will draw examples from studies of initial systemic family therapy sessions, which have deployed discursive psychology as a method for analysis of therapy discourse.

Perhaps one of the most relevant identity categories as concerns the psychotherapeutic setting is the one of the patient. Systemic family therapy has deliberately selected the category of the identified patient aiming to denote a non-essentialist and non-pathologizing approach to the diagnosis of psychological problems. Similarly, when identity categories like "the hyperactive child," "the problematic child," "the depressed," or the "stressed mother" are deployed in family therapy talk, instead of ascribing to them a realist, ontological quality, the systemic therapist engages into an attempt to translate such categories in semantic or pragmatic sequences entangled in interactional patterns by means of circular questioning (for the latter see Penn, 1982; Tomm, 1985). For example, he/she may investigate both the meaning of such categories but also the pattern(s), which connects all family members' behaviors in relation to such a category. Circular questioning facilitates this investigation with questions like, "what does he/she do that makes him hyperactive?", "what does father do when he/she does that?", etc.

Discursive psychology undertakes a very similar perspective. Instead of approaching the deployment of identity categories in talk as pointing to an unmediated, one-by-one relationship between the category and the individual's identity, it attempts to decode their function in talk-in-interaction. In that sense, it approaches identity as a matter which speakers make relevant in their discourse and which they construct, often in various and contradictory ways, while they speak. There is extensive discursive psychology literature on identity (see, e.g., Antaki & Widdicombe, 1998) where an alternative approach to mainstream, social psychology theorizing about identity is discussed. There is also extensive debate within the discursive psychology literature, which reflects wider tensions concerning psychological theorizing about subjectivity correspondingly reflecting wider ontological and epistemological debates. For example, discursive psychology scholars are criticized for undertaking a "blank subjectivity" approach when they restrict notions like identity to the discursive deployment of relevant categories in talk-in-interaction and solely lean to the analysis of conversational exchanges (Parker, 2012). Some lean to psychoanalysis for handling this issue (e.g., Billig, 2014) whereas others, like Margaret Wetherell (1998, 2007), strive for theoretical articulations without resorting to a psychoanalytic perspective. Wetherell's proposal (Wetherell, 2007) suggests an approach, which combines an analysis of how identities are constructed in the micro context of discursive exchanges with an analysis which further seeks to identify regularities both in interpersonal relationships but also in the drawing of broader, culturally available and historically constituted ways of talking about certain categories, e.g., gender. This reflects an attempt to combine a conversation analytic perspective as depicted in membership categorization theory (Sacks, 1989) with post-structural theorizing which uses the notion of subject positioning to refer to the ways that speakers position themselves and their co-conversants in identity terms (see, e.g., Guilfoyle, 2018). A full discussion of such debates definitely extends the scope of this text. Once more, what seems striking here is the resonance of such debates with debates concerning the place of the individual in systemic theorizing and therapy (e.g., Flaskas & Pocock, 2009).

As exemplified in the previous section, analytic practice in the case of identity categories deployment follows the main methodological principle of interpreting its *function in the particular rhetorical and sequential context* of its deployment. O'Reilly's (2007) analysis of the deployment of the category of the "naughty" child by parents in initial systemic family therapy sessions is a good example of such an orientation. O'Reilly (2007) has shown how the deployment of this category facilitates the management of accountability issues concerning the family's troubles or the construction of the identity of a "good parent." Similarly, Patrika and Tseliou (2016a) in their analysis highlight how the category of the "stressed mother," deployed by mother, seems interwoven with the construction of her child as "problematic" and seems to facilitate the management of accountability issues concerning the family's reported difficulties. For an example, see the following lines from the analyzed extract (Patrika & Tseliou, 2016a, p. 476): "I was an anxious mother... Because since he started walking, I was following him all the time, because I didn't know what he was going to do."

Ideological Aspects of Psychotherapeutic Discourse: History and Socio-Political Context

Critical discursive psychology scholars (e.g., Bozatzis, 2009, 2016; Wetherell, 1998, 2007; Wetherell & Edley, 2014) argue for the necessity of contextualizing the pragmatic/rhetorical perspective with an analysis of the historical and ideological conditions of discourse use. This indicates that interpretation should extend the micro-rhetorical and sequential context of the local setting where talk-in-interaction takes place. Instead, it should include an analysis of the historical and the political genealogy of patterns of language use. In discursive psychology literature, this perspective is elaborated by means of notions like "interpretative repertoires" (Potter & Wetherell, 1987) and "ideological dilemmas" (Billig et al., 1988). Interpretative repertoires indicate that there are historically and culturally available, systematic sets of constructions of phenomena from which speakers draw when in talk-in-interaction.

These can be traced by means of analyzing the content of discourse, including its grammar and structure (Potter & Wetherell, 1987). Here I choose to focus on the notion of ideological dilemmas, which is less popular in the discursive psychology research literature.

Billig et al. (1988) discuss ideology as "lived ideology," meaning that ideology is constantly constructed and re-constructed in the context of peoples' everyday interactions. Thus, dilemmas of stake, like the ones explicated in the previous section, are not ideologically neutral. Instead, they are interwoven with wider, historically constituted ideological dilemmas. Addressing the ideological aspect as well as the interrelated aspect of power relations can also grant access to interpreting what is not said, what speakers refrain from uttering (Billig, 2014). This perspective is potentially attentive to arguments concerning the necessity of addressing the political and ideological aspects of family therapy discourse in the context of criticisms levelled against initial systemic family therapy models of the first cybernetic era (e.g., Hare-Mustin, 1994). It further resonates with therapeutic approaches, which have undertaken a more political, activist stance to therapy in light of Foucault's theorizing (White & Epston, 1990).

Undertaking such an orientation in analysis necessitates linking discourse tensions of the local context with wider ideological tensions. Analysis should further trace the ideological conditions of the historical constitution of what is talked about. Up-to-date it seems that no discursive psychology study of family therapy discourse undertakes this perspective in analysis, although there are such examples in the critical discursive psychology literature (Bozatzis, 2009, 2016) as well as examples of critical perspectives in discourse analysis of family therapy (e.g., Guilfoyle, 2018; Kogan, 1998). Here I will attempt to provide an example by discussing the phenomenon of psychologization (see, e.g., Sapountzis & Vikka, 2015) in family therapy discourse, under the light of Billig et al. (1988) notion of ideological dilemmas. Such phenomenon entails the use of terminology of expertise in respect of psychological matters, like diagnostic discourse as indicated by the use of terms like "depression," "hyperactivity," etc. by lay speakers like family members. This may be coupled with appeals to the therapist for providing a diagnosis for the problem. For example, family members may pose questions to the systemic family therapist like, "Will you now tell us what the problem is?" In order to highlight the broader, ideological dynamic of this kind of discourse, I will draw from Billig et al.'s (1988) discussion of a specific ideological dilemma. This is the "expertize vs. equality" ideological dilemma, which I think that is of critical relevance for systemic family therapy discourse.

For Billig et al. (1988) an expert's position in a democratic society is not that straightforward in the sense that the power exercised by an expert may be in conflict with the democratic ideal of equality: the more expertise the more that equality is at stake. On the other hand, democracy does not necessarily go together with equality, given that power has not entirely vanished in democratic societies. For Billig et al. (1988) this creates a context of ambivalence as concerns the relationships between experts and non-experts. In this context, there seems to be a constant process of negotiation between the expert and the non-expert concerning the limits of the expert's power. Furthermore, and paradoxically so, the more that experts try to establish equality the more inequality may be established, for it is not that easy to eliminate the tension between equality and inequality. For example, non-experts may respond to such efforts with further pleas on experts to practice expertise, like in the case of the question addressed to therapists reported above. As Billig et al. (1988) put it, especially concerning professions like the one of the psychotherapist, the more one tries to become friendly and equalitarian the more there is the danger that he or she may be accused for doing something that anyone could do and thus the more he/she seems in danger of losing his/her professional identity. On the other hand, the more he/she stays with (professional) distance the more he/she is in danger of being accused that he/she adheres to non-democratic ideals by attempting to establish the non-symmetrical position of an expert.

In Patrika and Tseliou (2016b, p. 11) there is analysis of an excerpt of an initial family therapy session where mother repeatedly poses the following question to the therapist: "Is this normal?" She does so in respect of her son's behavior which she has previously referred to as hyperactive. The therapist refrains from giving an answer to this question and instead reciprocates the question by asking mother whether she considers the child's behavior as being normal: "I am wondering, do you consider it as being normal or don't you consider it as being normal?" (Patrika & Tseliou, 2016b, p. 11). In their analysis, Patrika and Tseliou (2016b) address the local, rhetorical context of mother's appeal and highlight the related tension, concerning both the therapist and mother. Mother is there for getting an expert's view concerning her troubles, and her question can be seen as an attempt to evoke the therapist's expertise. On the other hand, the systemic therapist tries to eschew the risk of adopting a straightforward expert's role by providing an answer, given his/her commitment to an equalitarian, non-expert, non-interventive role, as a systemic, post-modern, collaborative therapist (Patrika & Tseliou, 2016b). If interpreted under the light of the ideological dilemmas perspective, such tension can be seen as also reflecting wider ideological tensions concerning expertise as juxtaposed to equality. Expert's effort – in this case the therapist's – to collaboratively share expertise with non-experts by assigning them power seems to intensify their efforts to evoke his expertise. Simultaneously, though, he/she remains the one "in control" of their dialogue and the one assigning power, for "nobody wants to take democracy that far" (Billig et al., 1988, p. 70). As Billig et al. (1988) put it, this tension is not so easy to handle, as power differentials do not simply vanish out of our wish to act collaboratively, given the institutional assignment of the role of an expert.

Conclusions

In this chapter, I have argued that discursive psychology can fruitfully contribute to systemic family therapy process research. I have discussed how undertaking a discursive psychology methodological approach can facilitate the investigation of therapeutic dialogue in ways, which resonate with systemic adherences. I have discussed three specific ways, which include a pragmatic approach to discourse, an interactional perspective to the understanding and study of psychological phenomena, as well as a historical and ideological approach to discourse use. Discursive psychology analysis can shed light to the subtle ways in which the therapist and family members co-construct the therapeutic dialogue, while they argue for their views and struggle with certain dilemmas. Further, it can allow for approaching both the therapist and family members as competent, social actors, whose discourse seems entangled with wider, ideological tensions.

My proposal, however, should not be considered as an appeal to replace other qualitative or quantitative methodologies for the study of therapeutic discourse, which have and still prove particularly illuminating (Tseliou & Borcsa, 2018). Discursive psychology has potential but also bears certain limitations as it can address specific research questions framed in the context of certain epistemological adherences. Further to that, analysis is a laborious endeavor, which necessitates a rather sophisticated expertise and this may discourage researchers from giving it a chance. There are also unresolved tensions, which further complicate the venture of doing discursive psychology type of analysis, like debates over what constitutes proper analysis (Bozatzis, 2014). The latter coupled with the lack of specific guidelines of how to go about an analysis and with the so far limited deployment of discursive psychology for the study of systemic couple and family therapy further complicate the picture. My prejudiced view, given my "close relationship" both with systemic family therapy and with discursive psychology, is that their meeting can contribute to both fields. My wish is that this chapter will contribute to this aim.

References

Antaki, C. (2014). Conversation analysis and the discursive turn in social psychology. In N. Bozatzis & Th. Dragonas (Eds.), *The discursive turn in social psychology* (pp. 74–86). Chagrin Falls, OH: Taos Institute Worldshare Books.

Antaki, C., & Widdicombe, S. (1998). *Identities in talk*. London, UK: Sage.

Augoustinos, M., & Tileagă, C. (2012). Twenty five years of discursive psychology. *British Journal of Social Psychology, 51*(3), 405–412. https://doi.org/10.1111/j.2044-8309.2012.02096.x

Bateson, G. (1979). *Mind and nature: A necessary unity*. Glascow, Scotland: Fontana/Collins.

Billig, M. (1987). *Arguing and thinking: A rhetorical approach to social psychology*. Cambridge, UK: Cambridge University Press.

Billig, M., Condor, S., Edwards, D., Gane, M., Middleton, D., & Radley, A. (1988). *Ideological dilemmas: A social psychology of everyday thinking*. London, UK: Sage.

Billig, M. (2012). Undisciplined beginnings, academic success, and discursive psychology. *British Journal of Social Psychology, 51*(3), 413–424. https://doi.org/10.1111/j.2044-8309.2011.02086.x

Billig, M. (2014). Towards a psychoanalytic discursive psychology: Moving from consciousness to unconsciousness. In N. Bozatzis & T. Dragonas (Eds.), *The discursive turn in social psychology* (pp. 159–170). Chagrin Falls, OH: Taos Institute Worldshare Books.

Borcsa, M., & Rober, P. (2016). *Research perspectives in couple therapy: Discursive qualitative methods*. Switzerland: Springer.

Bozatzis, N. (2009). Occidentalism and accountability: Constructing culture and cultural difference in majority Greek talk about the minority in Western Thrace. *Discourse & Society, 20*(4), 431–453. https://doi.org/10.1177/0957926509104022

Bozatzis, N. (2014). The discursive turn in social psychology: Four nodal debates. In N. Bozatzis & T. Dragonas (Eds.), *The discursive turn in social psychology* (pp. 25–50). Chagrin Falls, OH: Taos Institute Worldshare Books.

Bozatzis, N. (2016). Cultural othering, banal occidentalism and the discursive construction of the 'Greek crisis' in global media: A case study. *Suomen Antropologi: Journal of the Finnish Anthropological Society, 41*(2), 47–71. Retrieved from https://journal.fi/suomenantropologi/article/view/59642

Burr, V. (2015). *Social constructionism* (3rd ed.). London, UK: Routledge.

Diorinou, M., & Tseliou, E. (2014). Studying circular questioning 'in situ': Discourse analysis of a first systemic family therapy session. *Journal of Marital and Family Therapy, 40*(1), 106–121. https://doi.org/10.1111/jmft.12005

Edwards, D. (1997). *Discourse and cognition*. London, UK: Sage.

Edwards, D. (2012). Discursive and scientific psychology. *British Journal of Social Psychology, 51*, 425–435. https://doi.org/10.1111/j.2044-8309.2012.02103.x

Edwards, D., & Potter, J. (1992). *Discursive psychology*. London, UK: Sage.

Edwards, D., & Potter, J. (1993). Language and causation: A discursive action model of description and attribution. *Psychological Review, 100*(1), 23–41. https://doi.org/10.1037/0033-295X.100.1.23

Flaskas, C., & Pocock, D. (2009). *Systems and psychoanalysis: Contemporary integrations in family therapy*. London, UK: Karnac.

Foucault, M. (1972). *The archaeology of knowledge* (A. M. Sheridan, Trans.). London: Tavistock. (Original work published 1969).

Garfinkel, H. (1967). *Studies in ethnomethodology*. Englewood Cliffs: NJ: Prentice Hall.

Guilfoyle, M. (2018). Constructing unfinalizability: A subject positioning analysis of a couple's therapy session hosted by Tom Andersen. *Journal of Marital and Family Therapy, 44*, 426. https://doi.org/10.1111/jmft.12305

Hare-Mustin, R. T. (1994). Discourses in the mirrored room: A postmodern analysis of therapy. *Family Process, 33*(1), 19–35. https://doi.org/10.1111/j.15455300.1994.00019.x

Hepburn, A., & Potter, J. (2011). Threats: Power, family mealtimes, and social influence. *British Journal of Social Psychology, 50*(1), 99–120. https://doi.org/10.1348/014466610X500791

Hepburn, A., & Wiggins, S. (Eds.). (2005). Developments in discursive psychology. *Discourse & Society, 16*(5), 595–601. https://doi.org/10.1177/0957926505054937

Kogan, S. (1998). The politics of making meaning: Discourse analysis of a 'postmodern' interview. *Journal of Family Therapy, 20*, 229–251. https://doi.org/10.1111/1467-6427.00085

Laclau, E., & Mouffe, C. (1985). *Hegemony and socialist strategy: Towards a radical democratic politics*. London, UK: Verso.

Lester, J. N. (2014). Discursive psychology: Methodology and applications. *Qualitative Psychology, 1*(2), 141–143. https://doi.org/10.1037//qup0000015

O'Reilly, M. (2007). Who's a naughty boy then? Accountability, family therapy, and the "naughty" child. *The Family Journal: Counseling and Therapy for Couples and Families, 15*(3), 234–243. https://doi.org/10.1177/1066480707301316

O'Reilly, M., Lester, M., & Kiyimba, N. (2018). Discursive psychology as a method of analysis for the study of couple and family therapy. *Journal of Marital and Family Therapy, 44*, 409. https://doi.org/10.1111/jmft.12288

Parker, I. (2012). Discursive social psychology now. *British Journal of Social Psychology, 51*(3), 471–477. https://doi.org/10.1111/j.2044-8309.2011.02046.x

Patrika, P., & Tseliou, E. (2016a). Blame, responsibility and systemic neutrality: A discourse analysis methodology to the study of family therapy problem talk. *Journal of Family Therapy, 38*(4), 467–490. https://doi.org/10.1111/1467-6427.12076

Patrika, P., & Tseliou, E. (2016b). The 'blame game': Discourse analysis of family members and therapist negotiation of problem definition in systemic family therapy. *European Journal of Counseling Psychology, 4*(1), 101–122. https://doi.org/10.5964/ejcop.v4i1.80. Retrieved from: http://ejcop.psychopen.eu/article/view/80

Penn, P. (1982). Circular questioning. *Family Process, 21*(3), 267–280. https://doi. org/10.1111/j.1545-5300.1982.00267.x

Potter, J. (1996). *Representing reality: Discourse, rhetoric and social construction*. London, UK: Sage.

Potter, J. (2011). Discursive psychology and discourse analysis. In J. P. Gee & M. Handford (Eds.), *Routledge handbook of discourse analysis* (pp. 104–119). London, UK: Routledge.

Potter, J. (2012a). Discourse analysis and discursive psychology. In H. Cooper (Ed.), *APA handbook of research methods in psychology* (Quantitative, qualitative, neuropsychological, and biological) (Vol. 2, pp. 119–138). Washington, DC: American Psychological Association.

Potter, J. (2012b). Re-reading discourse and social psychology: Transforming social psychology. *British Journal of Social Psychology, 51*(3), 436–455. https://doi. org/10.1111/j.2044-8309.2011.02085.x

Potter, J., & Hepburn, A. (2005). Discursive psychology as a qualitative approach for analysing interaction in medical settings. *Medical Education, 39*, 338–344. https://doi. org/10.1111/j.1365-2929.2005.02099.x

Potter, J., & Wetherell, M. (1987). *Discourse and social psychology: Beyond attitudes and behaviour*. London, UK: Sage.

Sacks, H. (1989). Lecture six. The M.I.R. membership categorization device. *Human Studies, 22*, 271–281. Retrieved from: http://www.jstor.org/stable/

Sacks, H., Schegloff, E. A., & Jefferson, G. (1974). A simplest systematics for the organization of turn-taking for conversation. *Language, 50*, 696–735. https://doi.org/10.2307/412243

Sametband, I., & Strong, T. (2018). Immigrant family members negotiating preferred cultural identities in family therapy conversations: A discursive analysis. *Journal of Family Therapy, 40*(2), 201–223. https://doi.org/10.1111/1467-6427.1216

Sapountzis, A., & Vikka, K. (2015). Psychologization in talk and the perpetuation of racism in the context of the Greek school. *Social Psychology of Education, 18*(2), 373–391. https://doi. org/10.1007/s11218-014-9258-6

Stancombe, J., & White, S. (2005). Cause and responsibility: Towards an interactional understanding of blaming and 'neutrality' in family therapy. *Journal of Family Therapy, 27*, 330–351. https://doi.org/10.1111/j.1467-6427.2005.00326.x

Tileagă, C., & Stokoe, E. (2016). Contemporary discursive psychology. In C. Tileagă & E. Stokoe (Eds.), *Discursive psychology: Classic and contemporary issues*. London, UK: Routledge.

Tomm, K. (1985). Circular interviewing: A multifaceted clinical tool. In D. Campbell & R. Draper (Eds.), *Applications of systemic family therapy* (pp. 33–45). New York, NY: Grune and Stratton.

Tseliou, E. (2013). A critical methodological review of discourse and conversation analysis studies of family therapy. *Family Process, 52*(4), 653–672. https://doi.org/10.1111/famp.12043

Tseliou, E. (2015). Discourse analysis and educational research: Challenge and promise. In T. Dragonas, K. Gergen, S. McNamee, & E. Tseliou (Eds.), *Education as social construction: Contributions in theory, research and practice* (pp. 263–282). Chagrin Falls, OH: Taos Institute Worldshare Books Publications. http://www.taosinstitute.net/ education-as-social-construction

Tseliou, E. (2017). Conversation and discourse analysis for couple and family therapy. In J. Lebow, A. Champers, & D. C. Breunlin (Eds.), *Encyclopedia of couple and family therapy*. Springer. https://doi.org/10.1007/978-3-319-15877-8_941-1

Tseliou, E. (2018). Conversation analysis, discourse analysis and psychotherapy research: Overview and methodological potential. In O. Smoliak & T. Strong (Eds.), *Therapy as discourse: Practice and research* (pp. 163–186). London, UK: Palgrave.

Tseliou, E., & Borcsa, M. (2018). Discursive methodologies for couple and family therapy research: Editorial to special section. *Journal of Marital and Family Therapy, 44*(3), 375–385. https://doi.org/10.1111/jmft.12308

Tseliou, E., Smoliak, O., LaMarre, A., & Quinn-Nilas, C. (2019). Discursive psychology as applied science. In K. O'Doherty & D. Hodgetts (Eds.), *The Sage handbook of applied social psychology* (pp. 400–419). London, UK: Sage.

Ugazio, V., Fellin, L., Pennacchio, R., Negri, A., & Colciago, F. (2012). Is systemic thinking really extraneous to common sense? *Journal of Family Therapy, 34*, 513–1791. https://doi.org/10.1111/j.1467-6427.2011.00538.x

Watzlawick, P., Beavin-Bavelas, J., & Jackson, D. D. (1967). *Pragmatics of human communication: A study of interactional patterns, pathologies and paradoxes*. New York, NY: Norton.

Wetherell, M. (1998). Positioning and interpretative repertoires: Conversation analysis and post-structuralism in dialogue. *Discourse & Society, 9*, 387–412. https://doi.org/10.1177/0957926598009003005

Wetherell, M. (2007). A step too far: Discursive psychology, linguistic ethnography and questions of identity. *Journal of SocioLinguistics, 11*(5), 661–681. https://doi.org/10.1111/j.1467-9841.2007.00345.x

Wetherell, M., & Edley, N. (2014). A discursive psychological framework for analyzing men and masculinities. *Psychology of Men and Masculinities, 15*(4), 355–364. https://doi.org/10.1037/a0037148

White, M., & Epston, D. (1990). *Narrative means to therapeutic ends*. New York, NY: Norton.

Wiggins, S. (2017). *Discursive psychology: Theory, method and applications*. London, UK: Sage.

Willig, C. (2013). *Introducing qualitative research in psychology* (3rd ed.). Berkshire, UK: McGraw Hill.

From Research on Dialogical Practice to Dialogical Research: Open Dialogue Is Based on a Continuous Scientific Analysis

Jaakko Seikkula

The Psychiatric Approach

Open dialogue was originally initiated in Western Lapland in Finland. The approach has developed through specific decisive steps, which were based on the Finnish need-adapted approach tradition integrating psychodynamic individual psychotherapy with systemic family therapy (Alanen, 1997). After taking the first step in 1984 – and the most decisive one on the whole – by reorganizing the planning of the treatment in open meetings with the hospitalized patient and the family, it took 11 years before the entire comprehensive system of care was named as open dialogue. This happened in a research project led by professor Jukka Aaltonen (Aaltonen, Seikkula, & Lehtinen, 2011).

Research has played an essential role in the development from family-centered psychiatric care to a comprehensive description of a system of care. Actually open dialogue is totally based on systematic research and seems to be the most scientifically analyzed system of care on the whole. In every new phase of the development and reorganization of the psychiatric organization, research was needed for both understanding the phenomenon of the therapeutic processes and detecting the outcome of the new approach. Being involved since its inception in 1987, these processes have also contributed to a new understanding of research. This includes understanding the study design, data collection methods, data analysis methods, and data interpretation methods for observations done in the research. In summary, following are the three elements of research:

J. Seikkula (✉)
Department of Psychology, University of Jyväskylä, Jyväskylä, Finland
e-mail: jaakko.a.t.seikkula@jyu.fi

© Springer Nature Switzerland AG 2020
M. Ochs et al. (eds.), *Systemic Research in Individual, Couple, and Family Therapy and Counseling*, European Family Therapy Association Series,
https://doi.org/10.1007/978-3-030-36560-8_9

1. The research is "naturalistic" in the way that it takes place within the everyday – natural – clinical practice following what happens there. Research designs do not change the clinical practice for the research, as so often done in empiristic clinical trials.
2. The research includes "mixed method research" with the intention to identify all the possible elements of the object of the research. Statistical information is needed to analyze the treatment effects of the entire group of patients in the research. However, qualitative methods are needed to study the information in detail to understand the meaning of outcome statistics in the real-life clinical practice.
3. The research has a strong dialogical emphasis both in concerning how to be in dialogue with the observations of the research to make them available in the everyday clinical practice and in the way that the observations are done about the dialogical processes of therapeutic meetings.

Studies on Western Lapland Psychiatric System

Studies can be classified into two categories. The first part of the studies was concretely related to the Western Lapland psychiatric system. The second part of the studies has been developed to see dialogues in different contexts and no longer connected only to the Western Lapland, but actually opening a new dialogical research tradition.

Admission to the Hospital: The System of Boundary

The first large research project took place in 1988–1992. It was initiated to change the practice of admission of the patients into the hospital in the way that a specific admission team was founded to organize the first meeting with the referred patient and hopefully with the family before the final decision of admission was made. The aim was to find out what happened in the first meeting and which were the elements affecting the admission and the possible decision not to admit the patient. At that time including the family into the inpatient treatment was already an everyday practice, and inviting families into open meetings created a specific way of interactions that we started to name as the system of boundary. Jaakko Seikkula (1991, 1994) and the chief psychiatrist Jyrki Keränen (1992) both conducted their Ph.D. theses about this data.

The design and methods Including all the patients referred to the Keropudas hospital within 2-month period. The aim was to follow up the treatment process and outcomes for 1–4 years in the everyday clinical practice. Research methods included statistical information regarding the psychological status – GAF, psychological tests such as WAIS intelligence test and Rorschach personality test, and psychiatrist anamnestic interview – followed by evaluation of the coevolution of the team and the family by applied use of Olson Circumplex Model. The Clinical Rating Scale was used to analyze the family interactional style. The scale was adjusted to analyze the team interaction to compare how much interaction within the team resembled the one of the family system. In addition to these specific methods that were statistical analyses, qualitative analysis was conducted by giving case descriptions about the coevolution process.

Results The decision of the admission differed significantly according to the previous experiences about psychiatric hospitalizations. *First-time patients* were admitted in only 2 cases out of 14, and families participated in every case. Among *recurrent patients*,14 out of 26 were hospitalized, and among *long-term* patients,26 out of 32 patients. Out of total 70 patients referred to the psychiatric hospital, 28 decided to be treated by home visits without the hospitalization. In the 1-year follow-up, the decision was seen as a correct one in all cases in the way that those patients did not need hospitalization during the 1-year period (Seikkula, 1991). The admission interview of a single doctor focused on symptoms and finding a solution for the treatment rapidly. By having a team in charge of the first interview, it was possible to focus on the social network of the patients and consequently on the resources available (Keränen, 1992).

Conclusions It is possible to find alternatives for hospitalization if there is a team in charge of the admission interview and in case this team takes the responsibility of the outpatient treatment afterwards. The need for hospitalization can be reduced to 40%. Teams learned to consider how both the previous history of the families and the form of dialogue with the families are used. This study encouraged to change the organization of the psychiatric system in the way that hospital beds were reduced from 330 to 60 and instead a network of mobile crisis intervention teams were organized for the province.

Qualitative Content Analysis: Defining Open Dialogues

Professor Jukka Aaltonen initiated a research project for the comprehensive community-based care in 1993 to 1995 (Aaltonen et al., 1997; Aaltonen et al., 2011).The aim was twofold: to understand the elements of the new system of care that had been going on some 5 years after the change of the organization and to see if change occurred in the incidence of schizophrenia in the province to prevent chronification.

Design and methods The patient records of all the patients taking the first contact to psychiatry during the years 1985 to 1994 were analyzed ($N = 1918$) to find out the nonaffective psychotic patients or prodromal cases ($N = 250$). The patient records of these 250 patients were analyzed to find out the optimal elements of the new treatment during 1990 to 1994 in comparison to the traditional hospital base treatment from 1985 to 1989. In the qualitative content analysis, the main elements were found and summarized. In addition to this, a statistical test was conducted to see if the diagnosis of nonaffective psychosis had changed in proportion between those two periods of time.

Results

1. The optimal treatment of psychotic patients within the new system of care includes main elements as follows:
2. Immediate help is guaranteed by having the first meeting within 24 hours after the contact was taken to the psychiatric system.
3. Social network perspective is included by always inviting the family and in some cases other members of the social network as early as possible to participate throughout the treatment process.
4. Flexibility is realized by adapting to the unique needs of every patient and family by using a reliable therapy method. Different methods of treatment are integrated with each other. Often this also means mobility by going to the homes of the patients.
5. Responsibility is guaranteed if whichever staff member was contacted takes the responsibility of organizing the first meeting, in which the case-specific treatment team was formed.
6. Psychological continuity was realized in the way that the case-specific team can include staff members from different units in and outside psychiatry, as from social care. This team takes charge of the entire treatment process as long as needed.
7. Tolerating uncertainty is a decisive element of the team's action in the way that it aims at increasing the safety, which is enough for the family to tolerate the situation, in which there are no ready-made solutions or any ready-made manuals of treatment to be followed.
8. Generating dialogue is the focus of the team to increase understanding about what happened to the patients and to the family and what would be the best ways to go on in the treatment.

After summing up these main elements of the optimal treatment in the new era of care, it was thought how to name the system. In this discussion, the decision emerged to name the system of care as open dialogue approach (Seikkula et al., 1995).It was also found that the incidence of schizophrenia was significantly lower in the 1990s compared to the one in the 1980s. In 1985, there emerged 33 new schizophrenia patients per 100,000 inhabitants, and in 1994, there were 7 new schizophrenia patients.

Conclusions: This research meant a step into a more general description of the family-centered, crises intervention services. A hypothesis was formed that the decline of the incidence of schizophrenia was related to the change of treatment system of family involvement in the open dialogical processes.

Voices of the Treatment Meeting: Dialogical Approach

Dialogues and dialogism had become the main ideas of the therapeutic practices, first initiated in the dissertation (Seikkula, 1991) and thereafter in the research project conducted by Aaltonen et al., 2011. As a continuation of the question, in which ways the treatment team become connected with the family on the boundary, psychologist Kauko Haarakangas (1997) studied what happened in dialogues in the treatment meetings.

Design and methods   Following the live supervision taking place in three systemic family therapy training groups. Out of the patients followed, one case in each group was selected. In 10 therapy meeting sessions with the trainees and the supervisor, a specific dialogical analysis was conducted.

Results   If the meaning system of the family and the team co-evolved with each other a possibility emerged to shift from a symptom focused discourse to a more resource-orientated discourse. A specific model about the interaction between the inner and outer voices of the team members, and of the family members, was formed. As a part of this, the specific functions of the horizontal and vertical polyphony were described. It was also found that an advanced therapist tolerated more uncertainty in dialogues, thus emphasizing the importance of psychotherapy training.

Conclusions   The research contributed with increased knowledge regarding the importance of listening in the way that everyone is heard by respecting everyone's opinion and perspective as equal and important as all others. This research was also important to realize that within the open therapy meetings, a new way of family therapy work is initiated, that is, different in respect to other language-orientated approaches, as narrative therapy for instance.

Integrated Treatment of Acute Psychosis: Three Open Dialogue Data Sets

Western Lapland was one of the six psychiatric treatment centers that were research sites in the Finnish National API (Integrated Treatment of Acute Psychosis) project organized by the National Research and Development Centre for Welfare and Health (STAKES), the Department of Psychology at the University of Jyväskylä, and the Department of Pharmacology at the University of Turku. The total catchment area included 600,000 inhabitants (Lehtinen, Aaltonen, Koffert, Räkkölöinen, & Syvälahti, 2000).

In this project, the specific focus was on improving community treatment and increasing the knowledge of the role of medication in the treatment of psychosis. Every new first-episode psychotic patient was asked to give permission for the project. In three of the six districts, treatment was arranged as usual, and in the other three, the treatment was community and family centered. In these three, it was decided to organize the treatment according to theneed adaptive approach and to try to postpone hospitalization and neuroleptic treatment in the beginning of the treatment. Neuroleptics were advised to be used only in case intensive help in the crises is not helpful enough for decreasing the symptoms and other problems.

The API project took place from April 1992 to the end of 1993. In Western Lapland, we continued our research of first-episode psychotic patients locally named as the Open Dialogue in Acute Psychosis (ODAP) project (1994–1997) (Seikkula, Aaltonen, Alakare, Haarakangas, & Keränen, 2006; Seikkula et al., 2003). After this a new study was conducted referred to as ODAPII 2003–2005 with the aim to determine the stability of the results from the earlier research projects.

Designs and methods The study included all first-episode patients between 16 and 50 years of age with nonaffective psychosis (using DSM-III-R and DSM-IV for the third period, ODAP2003–2005). The diagnostic consistency of the schizophrenia diagnosis was 78% (Kappa = 0.453; $p = 0.002$). The main sources of information were (1) premorbid variables such as psychiatric and employment status at the outset, and duration of untreated psychosis (DUP) (defined as the time between first psychotic symptoms and the start of psychosocial intervention); (2) process variables, i.e., the number of hospital days, number of family meetings, and the use of neuroleptic medication and individual psychotherapy; and (3) outcome variables, i.e., number of relapses (defined as making a new contact for treatment after terminating the original treatment, or as an intensification of existing treatment because of new psychotic or other severe symptoms), employment status, and the mental state of the patients on the Brief Psychiatric Rating Scale (BPRS), the Global Assessment of Function Scale (GAF), and a five-category subscale of the Strauss–Carpenter Rating Scale (Opjordsmoen, 1991; Strauss & Carpenter, 1972). During the API and ODAP periods, ratings were conducted jointly by Jaakko Seikkula and chief psychiatrist Birgitta Alakare. These authors worked as researchers and were not involved as therapists in the treatment process. During the third study period, ODAPII2003–2005, all registrations and ratings were performed by an experienced nurse together with Birgitta Alakare.

Ratings were performed at the baseline and at the 2-year follow-up. During the first treatment meetings, the family was interviewed to determine DUP. Birgitta Alakare verified this during an individual interview with the patient. The follow-up interviews took place in the presence of both the case-specific treatment team and the family. The statistical analysis was conducted using the Pearson Chi-square in cross-tables, and a one-way analysis of variance (ANOVA) for comparison of the means of independent groups. With the two first sets of data during the API and ODAP1, a 5-year follow-up was also conducted.

Results In one of the studies, *schizophrenia patients were compared in a quasi-experimental design* with the patients from another API project research site (Seikkula et al., 2003).The comparison groups used neuroleptic medication in all cases compared to 35% use in the ODAP 1 group (Table 1). Significantly more

Table 1 Frequencies in treatment process variables in the three groups at the 2-year follow-up, a pair comparison

	API group N = 22	ODAP group N = 23	Comparison group N = 14	Chi-square	P	
Use of neuroleptics						
Started	8	8	14	14.58	<0.001[a]	
Ongoing	5	4	10	8.35	< 0.05[a]	
Individual psychotherapy						
Yes	12	11	8			
No	10	12	6	0.49	NS	

[a]API and Comparison groups

Table 2 Means of treatment process and outcome variables in the three groups at the 2-year follow-up, t-test pair comparison

	API group N = 22	ODAP group N = 23	Comparison group N = 14	t-value	P	η^2
Hospitalization days						
Mean	35.9	14.3	116.9	3.29	< 0.01[a]	0.242
SD	44.0	25.0	102.2			
Number of family meetings						
Mean	26.1	20.1	8.9	−4.291	< 0.001[a]	0.351
SD	14.1	20.6	6.2			
BPRS score						
Mean	32.3	24.9	26.5	2.532	< 0.05[b]	0.144
SD	13.7	5.2	7.1			

Note: BPRS is a 19-item scale, each item rated 1–9
[a]t-Test for independent samples between API and comparison groups
[b]t-test for independent samples between API and ODAP groups

family meetings emerged in the API and ODAP groups compared to comparison groups. Comparison group patients were hospitalized ten times more compared to ODAP1 group (Table 2).

Respectively, the outcomes of the treatment after 2 years were significantly different between open dialogue and comparison group (Tables 2 and 3).

Relapses occurred in 71% of comparison groups compared to 34% in API and 27% in ODAP group. A total of 50% of comparison group patients had remaining moderate psychotic symptoms left compared to 17% in ODAP group. Out of the ODAP patients, 91% had returned to full employment or were actively job seeking compared to 43% in comparison group.

In another study, a historical comparison was conducted to find out differences in processes and outcomes between the three inclusions periods in Western Lapland (Seikkula, Alakare, & Aaltonen, 2011). In this analysis, all the nonaffective psychotic patients were included. In the first two periods of API and ODAP1, only few of the patients intended to treat did not participate, whereas in the ODAP2 period 10 years

Table 3 Frequencies of outcome variables in the three groups at the 2-year follow-up

	API group	ODAP group	Comparison group	Chi-square	P
	N = 22	N = 23	N = 14		
Number of relapsed patients	8	6	10	4	< 0.05[a]
Employment status					
Studying or working	13	15	3		
Unemployed	1	6	3		
Disability allowance	8	2	8	10.36	< 0.001[b]
Residual psychotic symptoms					
0–1	14	19	7	4.43	< 0.05[b]
2–4	6	4	7		

Note: Unemployed means to have been working during the last 2 years, but now unemployed and job-seeking
[a]API and comparison groups
[b]ODAP and comparison groups

Table 4 Historical comparison of API, ODAP 1, and ODAP 2 (Seikkula et al., 2011)

	API 1992–1993	ODAP1 1994–1997	ODAP2 2003–2005
	N = 33	N = 43	N = 18
Patient's age (mean years)	26.6	26.8	20.6***
Duration of symptoms (months)	19.6	10.2	11.4 **
DUP (months)	4.3	3.3	0.9
Therapy meetings with social network	21,8	16,3	26,3
Inpatient days	26	18	14

after the attrition was much higher. This was probably partly due to the fact that psychotic problems were not as clear as in the 1990s, which may illustrate the change in the treatment system in Western Lapland during the 15 years of the new practice. DUP had declined to less than 1 month before the treatment start, which means problems do not have time to develop as such a severe psychotic reaction. Also, the mean age of the patients was significantly lower at 2000. In addition to differences in age and DUP, the only difference occurred in the remaining psychotic symptoms at the 2-year follow-up in the way that ODAP2 patients had significantly less symptoms (Table 4).

Poor Outcomes Situations

One of the aims is to find problems in the treatment to be taken care of in the clinical practice. Seikkula et al. (2003) conducted a research comparing the good and poor outcome cases in the API and ODAP1 cohorts. Out of 78 (22%) patients, 17 were living in retirement or had more than moderate psychotic symptoms. The group of poor outcomes had poorer social networks, and they were more probably unemployed or were not actively searching for a job. They also had more probably the diagnosis of schizophrenia and longer DUP. When comparing the treatment process variables, it was noted that poor outcome patients had more hospital days, and they were using more often neuroleptic medication.

In another study, differences in dialogues during the first meetings were analyzed (Seikkula, 2002). In poor outcome situations, the topical episodes of dialogues were mainly monological, i.e., the team failed in generating dialogical, reflective way of being in dialogues. In poor outcome situations, the clients seldom had semantic or interactive dominance; i.e., they did not have access to take the initiative to a new topic of discussion or to the way it was discussed. In addition to these notions in poor outcome, the language area was mostly indicative without access to symbolic meaning making, while dialogues handled concrete issues of life and treatment. In the crisis, families may have poorer linguistic capabilities for symbolic reflections. This forms a challenge to the team, and in some of the poor outcome situations, the team did not succeed to construct the way to more open dialogue. In one case, it became evident that the team disregarded the patient's first reflections about his violent acts towards his mother and his first reflections about his psychotic thoughts. They were more present in the story that the patient was telling about incidents that had happened at home and not present in the dialogue in the meeting when all of a sudden he started to speak of his hallucination. When the team did not answer this reflection, it never after became possible during the entire therapeutic process.

Long-Term Outcome in Open Dialogue

The long-term outcome was first clarified in a 5-year follow-up study of the first two inclusion periods API and ODAP (Seikkula et al., 2006). However, it was found that the 2-year outcomes had stayed. Nineteen percent were living on a disability allowance, and 33% of the patients used psychosis medication.

In the contemporary research project (Bergström et al., 2018), all the first-episode psychotic patients included in the three inclusions periods between 1992 and 2005 ($N = 108$) were followed mostly over 20 years' time. The Finnish national health register information was used to make a comparison to the entire Finnish national cohort of first-episode psychotic patient ($N = 1763$).

In Table 5, the main variables are described, in which significant differences were noted. In addition, a significant difference was noted in the mortality (OD = 2.8; TAU = 9.2) when suicides and accidents were excluded.

Conclusions In this consistent long-term follow-up, outcomes and differences to treatment as usual have stayed on the same line throughout the process of years. This as such is already surprising, because usually it is noted that over a longer time the outcome differences decline or disappear because of the multiplicity of mediating

Table 5 Psychiatric treatment and disability pensions in year 2015 approximately 20 years after the start of treatment

	OD (N = 108) (%)	TAU (N = 1763) (%)	Chi-square test x^2	p
Thirty or more hospital days at onset	18.5	94	32.4	0.000
Neuroleptics started at onset	16.7	75.5	389.7	0.000
Neuroleptics in 2015	36.1	81.1	110.4	0.000
Treatment contact in 2015	27.8	49.2	16.7	0.000
Disability pension in 2015	33	61	28	0.000

variables in life. From the research point of view, these observations also verify the importance of naturalistic designs, since the outcomes seemed to be stable during the course of treatment and life processes even if the treatment has been terminated.

These outcomes also pose a question of the psychiatric treatment system that strongly emphasizes using medication as the basis of treatment in psychosis. Open dialogue focuses entirely on the other part of the story, working intensively with the family in open dialogical meetings for searching new meanings in life. But as was seen in the poor outcome analyses, the team can also fail in generating a dialogue that is helpful enough. By combining the information of the statistical outcome analysis with the investigation of the dialogues, it is possible to find precise points of challenging practice.

Studies on Dialogism

The second part of the studies developed based on the experiences of the studies on Western Lapland psychiatric system and open dialogues, but they go beyond the concern of the actual context of care. They can be seen to be forming a basis for the overall dialogical research tradition.

Dialogical and Narrative Processes in Depression: Multicentre Randomized Study

Western Lapland was part of the national Dialogical and Narrative Process in Couple Therapy for Depression (DINADEP) research project. In this randomized trial project, the data consisted of comparing couple therapy added to treatment as usual in three health districts in Finland. When comparing the differences between the three districts, it was noted that in Western Lapland, the recovery from depression was significantly better than in the other two districts. These results support the use of the dialogical approach also in other severe mental health problems than psychosis.

Experiences of Both the Patients and the Psychiatrists

Psychiatrist Pekka Borchers (2014) and nurse Jukka Piippo (2008) have evaluated our treatment as a part of their doctoral thesis. They interviewed some of our patients, families, and case-specific teams. Pekka Borschers's research described the inner dialogues of psychiatrists in the context of the need-adapted treatment of psychosis. Jukka Piippo found in his study that shared discussions created the feeling of safety for all sides.

The Way to Dialogical Research on Dialogical Practices: Making Sense of the Dialogues by DIHC Method

Kauko Haarakangas (1997) research project was the first one to examine the dialogical processes in open dialogue practice. Later, more needs emerged to see the qualities of dialogues in relation to the treatment outcomes. In the first attempt of this (Seikkula, 2002) good and poor outcome, psychotic patients were compared during the API and ODAP1 research projects. In comparison of the very first open dialogue therapy meetings at the outset, some significant differences seem to appear in the dialogue. In poor outcome cases, the language used was often indicative instead of symbolic meaning making. The difference also occurred in the way that in a good outcome situation, most of the episode of dialogues were dialogical instead of monological ones.

When starting the DINADEP project including couples in the therapy of depressed clients, the dialogical inquiry was systematized by creating a specific method dialogical investigations of happening of change (DIHC).

Designing the Studies

Before the analysis can be started, the multiactor session must be video-recorded and transcribed. Depending on the focus of the study, a specific part of the session can be transcribed or the entire session. To make a multiactor perspective possible, the transcript of the therapy conversation is printed in columns, one column for each speaker. Utterances are written in columns in temporal order. For a successful exploration, it is good to read the text simultaneously while watching the video recording of the session. In what follows the description of the methods is taken from the first paper, where this method was described (Seikkula et al., 2012).

The research process proceeds in steps, as follows:

STEP I: Exploring Topical Episodes in the Dialogue

Defining topical episodes means taking them as the main object for analysis (Linell, 1998). Topical episodes are defined in retrospect, after the entire dialogue of one session has been divided into sequences. Episodes are defined by the topic under discussion and are regarded as a new episode if the topic is changed. The researcher can choose, out of all themes, some specific important topics for further analysis. After dividing the session into topical episodes, within each episode certain variables are identified, as specified below.

STEP II: Exploring the Series of Responses to the Utterances

In each sequence, the way of responding is explored. Responses are often constructed within a series of utterances made by each participant in the actual dialogue. Within each topical episode, the responses to each utterance are registered, to gain a picture of how each interlocutor participates in the creation of the joint experience in the conversation. A three-step process is followed. The meaning of the response becomes visible in the next utterance to the answering words. It can start with whatever utterance is regarded as the initiating utterance (IU). The *answer* given to this IU is categorized according to the following aspects:

A. The participant takes the initiative (i.e. who is dominant) in each of the following respects:

- *Quantitative dominance*: this simply refers to who does most of the speaking within a sequence.
- *Semantic or topical dominance*: this refers to who is introducing new themes or new words at a certain moment in the conversation. This individual shapes most of the content of the discourse.
- *Interactional dominance:* this refers to the influence of one participant over the communicative actions, initiatives, and responses within the sequence. It is possible that this individual will have more influence on other parties than that exerted by the actual interlocutors (Linell, Gustavsson, & Juvonen, 1998; Linell, 1998). For instance, when a family therapist is inviting a new speaker to comment on what was previously said, he/she is having the interactional dominance. Also, someone who is very silent can have interactional dominance, by evoking solicitous responses from others.

- Rather than identifying the person who is dominant in the family session, the main focus of the investigation is on the *shifting patterns* of these three kinds of dominance.

B. *What* is responded to. The speakers may respond to:

- Their experience or emotion while speaking of the thing at this very moment (implicit knowing)
- What is said at this very moment
- Some previously mentioned topics in the session
- *What* or *how* it was spoken

- • External things, outside this session
- • Other issues. If so, what are these issues?

- • These are not mutually exclusive categories, since in a single utterance many aspects can be presented. The special form of answers in a situation in which the speaker introduces several topics is considered to form one utterance. The interest is on looking at how the answer helps to open up a space for dialogues in the response to that answer.

C. What is *not* responded to:
What voices in the utterance – bearing in mind that a single utterance by a single participant can include many voices – are *not* included in the response of the next speaker?

D. *How* the utterance is responded to:
Monological dialogue refers to utterances that convey the speaker's own thoughts and ideas without being adapted to the interlocutors. One utterance rejects another one. Questions are presented in a form that presupposes a choice of one alternative. The next speaker answers the question, and in this sense, his/her utterance can be regarded as forming a dialogue, but it is a closed dialogue. In *dialogical dialogue*, utterances are constructed to answer previous utterances, and also to wait for an answer from utterances that follow. A new understanding is constructed between the interlocutors (Bakhtin, 1984; Luckman, 1990; Seikkula, 1995). This means that in his/her utterance, the speaker includes what was previously said, and ends up with an *open* form of utterance, making it possible for the next speaker to join in what was said.

E. How the present moment, the implicit knowing of the dialogue, is taken into account. When one looks at videos of dialogues in which there are sequences of responses, one observes body gestures, gazes, and intonation. Often this includes, for example, observing tears or anxiety – aspects not seen when one merely reads the transcript. The present moment becomes visible also in comments on the present situation, for example, comments on the emotions felt concerning the issue under scrutiny.

STEP III: Exploring the Processes of Narration and the Language Area
This step can be conducted in two alternative ways:

(III a) Indicative Versus Symbolic Meaning
This distinction refers to whether the words used in the dialogue are always being used to refer to some factually existing thing or matter (indicative language), or whether the words are being used in a symbolic sense; in other words, whether they are referring to other *words*, rather than to an existing thing or matter (Haarakangas, 1997; Seikkula, 1991, 2002; Wertsch, 1985; Vygotsky, 1981). Each utterance is categorized as belonging to one of these two alternatives.

(III b) Narrative Process Coding System
The preliminary development of this coding system was undertaken by Angus, Levitt, and Hardtke (1999) within individual psychotherapy. Laitila, Aaltonen,

Wahlström, and Agnus (2001) further developed the system for the family therapy setting. Three types of narrative processes are distinguished. The speaker uses either (1) *external language*, giving a description of things that happened; (2) *internal language*, describing his/her own experiences in the things he/she describes; or (3) *reflective language*, exploring the multiple meanings of things, the emotions involved, and his/her own position in the matter.

After the investigation of the responses in the chosen topical episodes, a conclusion is reached concerning how the chosen topic is handled in this specific therapy process.

The Way to Dialogical Research on Dialogical Practices: Relational Mind and Embodiment in Dialogue

In dialogism, it is looked in more detail what happens in human communication. All human life is based on a dialogical interchange with other human minds, and we as humans become humans only within a dialogical responsive relationship with each other. The Russian philosopher Mikhail Bakhtin put the matter thus: "To live means to participate in dialogue: to ask questions, to heed, to respond, to agree, and so forth. In this dialogue a person participates wholly and throughout his whole life: with his eyes, lips, hands, soul, spirit, with his whole body and deeds" (Bakhtin, 1984). According to Bakhtin, we participate in this active dialogical relationship throughout our entire lives with our entire body and with all our actions. Thus, dialogue is not only spoken words and responding in words. Dialogue is an ongoing process of responding in the stream of sensing similarities or dissimilarities in our bodies. Responses are created in milliseconds, not primarily in mediated actions through meanings formed in words. Life is participation in the ongoing dance with whoever is present at the moment.

Humans are connected to each other in such a way as to generate the human mind. In order to manage this, human beings constantly attune themselves to each other on many domains:

1. In dialogues between participants, participants give utterances that wait for an answer, and thus jointly coauthor stories that are generated in the present moment. The dialogue in action incudes both the spoken content, but perhaps even more importantly, the prosodial part of the utterances, i.e., the rhythm of speech, the timbre, the pitch, pauses, and silent moments.
2. There is attunement in central nervous system (CNS) and autonomic nervous system (ANS) activity. The involuntary ANS operates between becoming alert and prepared for action (the sympathetic nervous system), and relaxing, becoming soothed, and recovering (the parasympathetic nervous system).
3. Participants attune in their bodily movements and gestures.
4. Participants attune in facial expressions. Smiling is particularly important, as both a regulator of one's affective arousal and as a form of communication and

connectedness with the listener. Another essential element is the connection through gaze.

5. There is attunement in experiences that every participant feels in given situations. These experiences are stored both in the memory of the body (as sensations) without explicit formulation in words, and in the words, which can be recalled if desired. Experiences are the orientation basis for the next interactional setting, either in general or specifically with certain individuals.

Design and methods In a research project funded by the Academy of Finland, Seikkula, Karvonen, Kykyri, Kaartinen, and Penttonen (2015) operationalized the relational mind within couple therapy. For the first time, the entire interactional system was described and analyzed from the point of view of the embodied action of both clients and two therapists, working together. In addition to precise facial and corporeal video filming of the couple therapy session, the ANS of both the couple and the therapists was measured. We looked at how therapists and clients attuned to each other in their breathing, in their heart rate, in their bodily movements (including facial expression), and in their speech. In addition, the electrodermal activity ("skin conductance") was measured from each of the four participants simultaneously to see how therapists and clients attuned to each other with their sympathetic nervous system. In an individual interview (Stimulated Recall Interview, or SRI) conducted within one day of the session, each participant saw four brief meaningful episodes from the session, selected by the researcher. They were asked to give information on their inner feelings and thoughts during those episodes (i.e., aspects that had not been said aloud).

Results In general, it was found that therapists' and clients' sympathetic nervous system activity became synchronized during therapy (Karvonen, Kykyri, Kaartinen, Penttonen, & Seikkula, 2016). Often, the attunement seems to be a complex, dyadic, or triadic phenomenon which changes over time (Seikkula et al., 2015). For instance, in one case, strong synchrony emerged between one therapist and one client in terms of their ANS arousal level throughout the therapy session. That high stress – estimated from heart rate variability (HRV) – could occur when others (e.g., the therapists in their reflective comments with each other) were discussing issues relating to the index person. In the sympathetic nervous system (SNS) arousal in cases where intimate partner violence had occurred, it was noted that criticism towards each other did not in itself increase the arousal. Nevertheless, at the moment when criticism included criticism of the identity of the other, a significant increase in SNS arousal took place. The fight-or-flight mechanism was activated. This may be related to the use of violence in emotionally loaded situations between the couples (Päivinen et al., 2016). Change in the prosody of speech has an important role in speaking about the most relevant emotional experiences of the client. This applies to showing affiliation with the client's expressed sorrow, and also to instances in which a notable change in meaning-making takes place (Kykyri et al., 2016). The therapist's softer and lower volume of voice, and use of silences, was related to assisting the client to continue expressing and processing her emotions concerning previously unspoken experiences. SNS arousal and dialogical change seldom happened at the same time. Most often the SNS arousal emerged first in relation to some specific, emotionally important topic for the couple. In the new dialogical understanding, high SNS arousal seldom occurred; instead the arousal was observed as taking place after the emotion-arousal experience (Haapanen & Niemi, 2016).

Conclusions In the Relational Mind projects, the origins of the synchronization of the human communication in multirelational setting were operationalized. Observations for the first time included both the therapist and clients. In relation to the expectations, the synchronization proved to be a much more complicated phenomenon. In dialogue with several participants, there seem to be several different positions to become attuned as a part of the communication. Two speakers may be involved in the dialogue through their simultaneous ANS arousal, thus all the time responding to each other by feeling and sensing the same type of bodily experiences. At the same time, the other in listening position may have more distance from the actual dialogue, thus participating on a more linguistic and rational level. They may become involved into the embodied arousal by changing the intonation or having silent moments in the dialogue. All these observations are only preliminary ideas of the multiplicity of the process of creating an embodied relational mind.

What Can We Learn About the Studies Presented?

I have described only some of the studies that have been conducted about Western Lapland psychiatry or about open dialogue system. The focus has been on studies, in which I have either been the principal investigator or participated in other ways by data gathering or acting as scientific supervisor, e.g., in doctoral dissertations. All studies have played an important role at least in three respects. (1) They are relevant to describe the outcomes of the treatment and consequently the problems in the outcomes in Western Lapland psychiatric system. This was especially important in the early years of development, when no systematic description existed about the comprehensive system of care of open dialogues. But it was important also during the last years to see the long-term outcomes of psychotic and depressed patients in the era of evidence-based medicine – EBM – where everything done should be based on guidelines of excellence, which strongly emphasize the use of medication, whereas open dialogue studies have reported outcomes improve when medication is decreased.

(2) They have been relevant to build up the foundations of open dialogue approach overall. Open dialogue would not exist without these studies. Open dialogue as a concept was described in the study where the patient records were analyzed to find out the optimal elements of the new family-centered approach that emphasizes crises services. As the summary of the observation, the main elements were defined and thereafter it was thought how to name the new system. Thereafter, several stud-

ies have been conducted within the frame of open dialogues showing positive outcomes of the treatment of psychotic and other most severe mental health problems. If these studies would not exist, most probably the idea of open dialogue could not be alive within the EBM era, since many of the basic elements are so different compared with the emphasis in treatment of excellence guidelines. The main question is that of using psychosis medication in the treatment of acute psychosis. In open dialogue studies, it has been shown that the treatment outcome improves by selective use of medication.

The second part of the information received in the outcome studies is the notion of poor outcome patients. In these studies, there is important knowledge to be taken to develop the practice in the way that failures could be minimized by the actions of the therapeutic team. For instance, in one of the studies (Seikkula, 2002), based on the statistical information about good outcome and poor outcome patients, a comparison was conducted concerning the quality of dialogues in the very first meeting at the outset of the crises. In this study, it was noted that the quality of dialogical practice seemed to be different in the poor outcome patients, for instance, in the ways that the team seemed to focus more on indicative language by asking for concrete happening in treatment and life, instead of being able to generate dialogical exchange. In a case example presented in the chapter, it was seen that the team was interested about what happened in the home of the patient, where he had been violent towards his mother. At the same time, however, in the dialogue the young man started to reflect on his own behavior and about his strange (psychotic) thoughts, but the team members never answered to these reflections. After this first meeting, it never became possible to discuss about the psychotic ideations in the way that the patient himself would have been scrutinizing the possibilities that his thoughts could be related to his stressful life situation. The inquiry of the basic elements of dialogues was a starting point to realize the importance of being present in the moment and responding to the utterances of the clients more than focusing on stories that clients are telling about their life happening before the meeting. These types of observations probably never would have been done without the systematic registration of the therapy sessions and analyzing of them. And thus, the development of dialogical practice would not have been possible in the way that we have seen afterwards.

(3) They have been relevant for me personally in my own way to develop my understanding about the meaning of treatment systems, family inclusion into the treatment processes, psychotic problems in the life of the patient and the families, and the dialogical practice. I suppose that making the observations in psychotherapy training and clinical supervision would not have been enough for opening up a new frame – or could we say new paradigm – about the human mind, about the mental health problems as a part of human mind, and especially about the dialogism as the core of human existence and consequently becoming the core of the new productive clinical practice.

Making research is a process of multiple ingredients to be considered all the time. Starting to plan the research, we must make several decisive decisions and choices. If we plan an empiricistic trial, we need to control the given treatment by manualizing it; by restricting the patients' possibilities for other needed treatment during the process of the research, we need to guarantee that the entire group of patients receives the same treatment that is not too much adopted to their unique individual needs; we need to select the methods for data gathering in the way that guarantees the neutrality in relation to the patients and so on. All these decisions cultivate a specific kind of psychological understanding through which our thinking is in risk of coming to focus on pathologies, symptoms, and causes of the outcomes. In these trials, the statistics of the group means become the most relevant source of information in defining the differences between study and control/comparison groups.

In the outcome studies that I have been involved, the point of origin is in many respects quite different. The big aim is not to have explanatory models of cause and effect but having a description about the entire system of care with some specific defined elements in it. In the studies, we do not want to control too much other elements of treatment but want to make possible for integrating different therapeutic methods according to the unique needs of clients. The design is often planned in the way that the therapeutic team participates in the outcome interviews, thus having immediate feedback of their work in the specific therapeutic processes. We also want to guarantee that the data gathering methods are not too pathologizing, but instead guarantee the possibility to see the crises as a part of life along with resources that the patients and families are having. By all this we can guarantee that the external validity of the research is much higher compared to empiricistic trials.

This is something that we have verified in our studies. It is a well-known fact that the outcomes received in empiricistic controlled trials lose 20% of their efficacy when applied in real life, everyday clinical practice. This has been noted in the psychotherapy studies but also in the medication trials. In concrete, this means that if it is observed in a research that some medication can cause 50% improvement of the patients in the trial and 30% improvement in the real life. But still the treatment of excellence guidelines is written based on the empiricistic trials by knowing the loss of effect of the study method. In the three ODAP studies conducted, we have observed the opposite. After the first two periods of research in 1992 to 1993 and 1994 to 1997, the same procedure of research was replicated 10 years after 2003–2005, and the outcomes of the psychotic patients were the same, registering, e.g., that 84% of the first episode psychotic patients could return to full employment after 2 years, as it had been in the first two study periods. No loss of the efficacy of the treatment was noticed, which is quite extraordinary. Actually, I do not know any other research projects within our field, where this would had been tested. This is what is meant by having higher external validity of the research. The topic of the research is really the one that we meet in everyday clinical practice and not an artificial laboratory kind of practice that is constructed to make the empiricistic trail possible.

Criticism to the Research

Within science and within the clinical practice, critical points of view should be considered all the time to develop best possible practice and best possible research about the practice. Concerning the research on open dialogues and dialogical methods, there are several types of criticism presented. Mostly criticism has been focused on outcome studies, but there is criticism also towards the dialogical methods and towards the research of embodiment on the dialogical processes.

In the outcome studies of first episode psychosis, the main criticism has been pointed towards the study design. The critical voices are saying that these studies do not contribute with evidence-based knowledge, because they are not randomized or do not even follow a quasi-experimental design. Some other have quite heavily accused about a fraud by saying that in some of the papers, there is not enough information about the intention to treat group of patients and thus giving possibility to exclude the most severe psychotic patients (Friis, Larsen, & Melle, 2003). Some have also criticized that in the studies the reliability of the use of research methods such as rating scales are not enough reported. Part of this type of criticism is justified because of what I said in the previous paragraph. When having emphasis on guaranteeing the external validity of the research, randomization of the patients into a study group and control group within Western Lapland is impossible. This is because the core idea of open dialogue approach is having the entire system of care following the basic principles to make the dialogical processes optimal. Thus, all staff had training in open dialogue, which makes it impossible to conduct other type of treatment in a reliable way in the same sample of patients. Comparison however is needed to make it possible to conclude if the outcomes of the treatment are coming from the reported approach. Thus, historical comparison is used (Seikkula et al., 2006), which is many times seen as the most vulnerable comparison design. In this study, the historical comparison was done to the phase of development of open dialogue having already the key element of it, but not in the defined form. The criticism is not justified in the sense that it dis-acknowledges the fact that there is a quasi-experimental study (Seikkula et al., 2003), in which it was shown that schizophrenia patients had significantly better outcome in open dialogue treatment compared to treatment as usual. In the ongoing research with 20-year follow-up, this challenge is overcome by having a comparison to the entire Finland first-episode psychotic patients. This comparison shows significant differences in the outcomes in mortality, use of treatment services, use of medication, and the amount of early retirement – all in favor of Western Lapland open dialogue approach.

A very relevant part of the criticism is that, so far, the open dialogue studies have only been conducted in Western Lapland, which may be strongly biased. In the future, really a lot more studies of the outcomes in open dialogues are needed in other countries and in other contexts.

Another line of criticism has been shown from the systemic family and social constructionism supporters. According to them, it is ethically questionable to conduct research, in which the patient groups are categorized by diagnosis and in which statistical methods for evaluating the symptoms by rating scales information are used.

According to some of the criticisms, this will objectify the patients, and only their symptoms or pathological parts are seen instead of looking at the entire human being. According to this criticism, only qualitative methods of inquiries could be justified. From my point of view, this criticism often makes all too simple conclusions by seeing any kind of outcome research as an empiricistic laboratory-type trial. I would recommend these people to be more aware of the possibilities of the naturalistic design, where the practice itself is followed taking place in real life and the methods used are adapted to the unique contexts. Other way round, using rating scales as such does not objectify the patients, when we are precise as to what purposes we use the rating scales about the experiences of the informants. For me the information received in the rating scales is more information about the experiences of the informant concerning his/her own life at the moment. In the outcome studies about Western Lapland, we can realize that the use of these evaluation methods and diagnosis for grouping the patients in the studies has not impacted negatively on the treatment outcomes. I suppose that it has affected the opposite by improving the outcomes of the treatment by having all the time systematic information about the recipients of the interventions.

A very interesting and illustrative criticism has been directed to the relational mind research project, in which the embodied participation in the dialogues is measured. From the social constructionism point of view, this research has been condemned as unnecessary, saying that having information about the embodied reactions is an effort to have an objective knowledge about the reactions of the clients in therapy. Some even more critical voices have said this being contra to dialogism overall. These critics have not exactly followed the basic idea of looking at the dialogical process by including all the different domains of communications simultaneously and having the information about how do we humans synchronize to each other in multirelational situations. The basic idea of the research is the contrary: to across the reductionist idea of human behavior being able to reduce into brain functions and instead to open the possibilities for looking at the entire human communication in the way that there is no hierarchy between the different domains of communication. Actually, relational mind research may be seen as criticism to the overemphasis on spoken language that I sense being the case within social constructionism. As far as we exclude the information of our bodies in the research and in the description of human life, we continue the dualistic division of mind and body.

References

Aaltonen, J., Seikkula, J., Alakare, B., Haarakangas, K., Keränen, J., & Sutela, M. (1997). Western Lapland project: A comprehensive family-and network centered community psychiatric project. *ISPS. Abstracts and Lectures, 12*, 124.

Aaltonen, J., Seikkula, J., & Lehtinen, K. (2011). Comprehensive open-dialogue approach I: Developing a comprehensive culture of need-adapted approach in a psychiatric public health catchment area the Western Lapland Project. *Psychosis, 3*, 179–191.

Angus, L., Levitt, H., & Hardtke, K. (1999). The narrative process coding system: Research applications and applications for therapy. *Journal of Clinical Psychology, 50*, 1244–1270.

Alanen, Y. (1997). *Schizophrenia.Its origins and need-adapted-treatment*. London: Karnac Books.

Bakhtin, M. (1984). *Problems of Dostojevskij's poetics: Theory and history of literature, Vol.* Manchester, UK: Manchester University Press.

Borchers, P. (2014). "Issues like this have an impact" the need-adapted treatment of psychosis and the Psychiatrist's inner dialogue. Jyväskylä studies in education, psychology and Social Research 507.

Bergström, T., Seikkula, J., Alakare,B., Mäki, P., Köngäs-Saviaro, P., Taskila, J., ... Aaltonen, J. (2018). The family-oriented open dialogue approach in the treatment of first-episode psychosis: Nineteen–year outcomes. Psychiatry Research 270 (2018) 168–17.

Friis, S., Larsen, T. K., & Melle, I. (2003). Terapivedpsykoser. *TidsskrNorLægeforen, 123*, 9.

Haapanen, K. & Niemi, P. (2016). *Moments of change in multiactor therapy dialogues: The embodied and linguistic attunement of four cases*. Master Thesis. University of Jyväskylä. Department of Psychology. June 2016

Haarakangas, K. (1997). Hoitokokouksen äänet: Dialoginen analyysi perhekeskeisen psykiatrisen hoitoprosessin hoitokokouskeskusteluista työryhmän toiminnan näkökulmasta [The voices in treatment meeting. A dialogical analysis of the treatment meeting conversation in family-centered process in regard to the team activity.] In Finnish with English abstract. Jyväskylä: Jyväskylän yliopisto.

Karvonen, A., Kykyri, V.-L., Kaartinen, J., Penttonen, M., & Seikkula, J. (2016). Sympathetic nervous system synchrony in couple therapy. *Journal of Marital and Family Therapy, 42*(3), 383–395.

Keränen, J. (1992). Avohoitoon ja sairaalahoitoon valikoituminen perhekeskeisessä psykiatrisessa hoitojärjestelmässä. [The Choice between Outpatient and Inpatient Treatment in a Family Centered Psychiatric Treatment System.] In Finnish with English abstract. Jyväskylä: Jyväskylän yliopisto.

Kykyri, V.-L., Karvonen, A., Wahlström, J., Kaartinen, J., Penttonen, M., & Seikkula, J. (2016). Soft prosody and embodied attunement in therapeutic interaction: A multi-method case study of a moment of change. *Journal of Constructivist Psychology, 30*, 211–234. https://doi.org/10.1080/10720537.2016.1183538

Laitila, A., Aaltonen, J., Wahlström, J., & Agnus, L. (2001). Narrative process coding system in marital and family therapy: An intensive case analysis of the formation of a therapeutic system. *Contemporary Family Therapy, 23*, 309–322.

Lehtinen, V., Aaltonen, J., Koffert, T., Räkkölöinen, V., & Syvälahti, E. (2000). Two year outcome in first-episode psychosis treated according to an integrated model. Is immediate neuroleptisation always needed? *European Psychiatry, 15*, 312–320.

Linell, P. (1998). Approaching dialogue: Talk, interaction and context in dialogical perspectives. Amsterdam: John Benjamin.

Linell, P., Gustavsson, L., & Juvonen, P. (1998). Interactional dominance in dyadic communication: A presentation of initiative-response analysis. *Linguistics, 26*, 415–442.

Luckman, T. (1990). Social communication, dialogue and conversation. In I. Markova & K. Foppa (Eds.), *The dynamics of dialogue* (pp. 45–61). London: Harvester.

Opjordsmoen, S. (1991). Long-term clinical outcome of schizophrenia with special reference to gender difference. *Acta Psychiatr Scand, 83*, 307–313.

Päivinen, H., Holma, J., Karvonen, A., Kykyri, V.-L., Tsatsishvili, V., Kaartinern, J., ... Seikkula, J. (2016). Affective arousal during blaming in couple therapy: Combining Analyses of Verbal Discourse and Physiological Responses in Two Case Studies. *Contemporary Family Therapy, 38*, 373–384.

Piippo, J. (2008). Trust, autonomy and safety at integrated network- and family-oriented model for co-operation: A qualitative study. Jyväskylä studies in education, psychology and social research 347.

Seikkula, J. (1991). Perheen ja sairaalan rajasysteemi potilaan sosiaalisessa verkostossa. [The Family-Hospital Boundary System in Social Network.) In Finnish with English summary. Jyväskylä: Jyväskylän yliopisto.

Seikkula, J. (1994). When the boundary opens: Family and hospital in co-evolution. *Journal of Family Therapy., 16*, 401–414.

Seikkula, J. (1995). From monologue to dialogue in consultation with larger systems. *Human Systems, 6*, 21–42.

Seikkula, J. (2002). Open dialogues of good and poor outcome in psychotic crisis. Example on family violence. *Journal of Marital and Family Therapy, 28*, 263–274.

Seikkula, J., Aaltonen, J., Alakare, B., Haarakangas, K., & Keränen, J. (2006). Five year follow-up of nonaffective psychosis in open-dialogue approach: Treatment principles, follow-up outcomes, and two case studies. *Psychotherapy Research, 16*(2), 214–228.

Seikkula, J., Aaltonen, J., Alakare, B., Haarakangas, K., Sutela, M., & Keränen, J. (1995). Treating psychosis by means of open dialogue. In S. Friedman (Ed.), *The reflecting team in action: Collaborative practice in family therapy*. New York: Guilford Press.

Seikkula, J., Alakare, B., & Aaltonen, J. (2011). The comprehensive open-dialogue approach in western Lapland: II. Long-term stability of acute psychosis outcomes in advanced community care. *Psychosis, 3*(3), 192–204.

Seikkula, J., Alakare, B., Aaltonen, J., Holma, J., Rasinkangas, A., & Lehtinen, V. (2003). Open dialogue approach:Treatment principles and preliminary results of a two-year follow-up on first episode schizophrenia. *Ethical Human Sciences and Services., 5*(3), 163–182.

Seikkula, J., Karvonen, A., Kykyri, V.-L., Kaartinen, J., & Penttonen, M. (2015). The embodied attunement of therapists and a couple within dialogical psychotherapy: An introduction to the Relational Mind Research Project. *Family Process, 54*(4), 703–715.

Seikkula, J., Laitila, A., & Rober, P. (2012). Making sense of multifactor dialogues. *Journal of Marital and Family Therapy, 38*(4), 667–687. https://doi.org/10.1111/j.1752-0606.2011.00238.x

Strauss, J., & Carpenter, W. (1972). The prediction of outcome in schizophrenia. *Archives of General Psychiatry, 27*, 739–746.

Seikkula, J., Alakare, B & Aaltonen, J. (2001) Open Dialogue in psychosis II: A comparison of good and poor outcome. *Journal of Constructivist Psychology* 14, 267–284.

Seikkula, J., Aaltonen, J., Alakare, B., Haarakangas, K., Sutela, M. & Keränen,J. (1995) Treating psychosis by means of open dialogue. In S. Friedman (Ed.) The Reflecting team in action: Collaborative practice in family therapy. New York: Guilford Press.

Vygotsky, L. (1981). The development of higher forms of attention in childhood. In J. Wertsch (Ed.), *The concept of activity in Soviet psychology* (pp. 189–240). New York: M. E. Sharpe.

Wertsch, J. (1985). Vygotsky and social formation of mind. Cambridge: Harvard University Press.

Systemic Practitioner Research – Some (Epistemological) Considerations and Examples

Matthias Ochs, Lucie Hornová, and Andrea Goll-Kopka

Research

The OECD (2015, p. 44) defines research as "a creative and systematic work undertaken to increase the stock of knowledge, including knowledge of humans, culture and society, and the use of this stock of knowledge to devise new applications." This definition seems in line with our own metaphorical formulation made to stimulate students and practitioners to dare to try research (Ochs, 2012b), that research should consist of two ingredients: "adventure" (creative work) and "bookkeeping" (systematic work). "Adventure" means that research should be driven by a yearning, an interest, a love for gaining specific knowledge, that it should be even "libido-loaded"; "bookkeeping" has to be gained in a systematic, methodological-driven, transparent, comprehensible, and documented way.

This rather broad definition of research is a good starting point and umbrella for our perspective on systemic research, that there exists a variety of different research discourses with their specific logics, premises, methodologies, and scopes, that relate to each other in a heterarchical way, e.g., high frequent time series designs, randomized controlled studies, qualitative phenomenological studies – and practitioner

M. Ochs (✉)
Department of Social Work, Fulda University of Applied Sciences, Fulda, Germany
e-mail: matthias.ochs@sw.hs-fulda.de

L. Hornová
Psychologická ambulance, Rychnov nad Kněžnou, Czech Republic

A. Goll-Kopka
School of Social Science and Law, SRH University Heidelberg, Heidelberg, Germany

© Springer Nature Switzerland AG 2020   165
M. Ochs et al. (eds.), *Systemic Research in Individual, Couple, and Family Therapy and Counseling*, European Family Therapy Association Series,
https://doi.org/10.1007/978-3-030-36560-8_10

research.[1] A good example for that perspective is, e.g., "Research Methods in Family Therapy" (Sprenkle & Piercy, 2005), where you can find ethnography alongside multilevel growth models and program evaluation methodology.[2]

Systemic Research – Or What Makes Research Systemic?

Systemic research is a notation used for a very wide range of research approaches (Ochs, 2013; Ochs & Schweitzer, 2012). This wide range refers to the many fields of application of systemic practice (e.g., social work, psychotherapy, various formats of counseling, supervision, coaching, pedagogy and organizational development), to different research methodologies (e.g., qualitative, quantitative, mixed-methods),[3] and to various epistemological perspectives (e.g., social/relational constructionism, discourse theory, dynamical systems theory, hermeneutics, critical rationalism). This diversity of approaches to "systemic research" invites experts from a variety of disciplines with a plurality of views of investigations. It makes it difficult to define systemic research in a more rigorous way and to differentiate systemic from non-systemic research. Some authors suggest the term "systemic inquiry" (e.g., Simon & Chard, 2014) instead of "systemic research," because "research" seems too strongly associated with (academic) investigation endeavors, that could produce intended or unintended hegemonic, "outvoting" effects to the disadvantage of alternative inquiry/research perspectives.[4] Also defining systemic research by the "object of research" seems problematic: Why should systemic research be limited to the investigation of social systems, such as organizational units, teams, families, or couples? What about researching interaction between biological, psychological, and social systems, as in relational neurobiology (e.g., Ditzen & Heinrichs, 2014; Fishbane, chapter "From Reactivity to Relational Empowerment in Couple Therapy: Insights from Interpersonal Neurobiology" this

---

[1] It is worth mentioning that evidence-based medicine (EBM) pioneer David Sackett also emphasizes, that despite the fact, that the EBM hierarchies reflect the relative authority of various types of research, "it's about integrating individual clinical expertise and the best external evidence" (Sackett, Rosenberg, Gray, Haynes, & Richardson, 1996, p. 71; see also Satterfield et al. (2009) for a transdisciplinary model of evidence-based practice, that also respects e. g. patients' preferences).

[2] For our own (German language) textbook of systemic research (Ochs & Schweitzer, 2012), we chose a similar approach.

[3] Stock (2015, p. 25) underlines that systemic thinking "values qualitative and quantitative data."

[4] Reynolds (2014, p. 129) cites Maori researcher Linda Tuhiwai Smith: "'research' is probably one of the dirtiest words in the indigenous world's vocabulary… It stirs up silence, it conjures up bad memories, it raises a smile that is knowing and distrustful… The ways in which scientific research is implicated in the worst excesses of colonialism remains a powerful remembered history for many of the world's colonized peoples. It is a history that still offends the deepest sense of our humanity."

volume; see also Nyman et al., chapter "Significant Moments in a Couple Therapy Session: Towards the Integration of Different Modalities of Analysis" this volume),[5] or neurophysiological pattern forming using systems theory model (e.g. Tass & Haken, 1996)?

Are There Existing Systemic Research Methods?

There is an ongoing debate whether there exist research methods specific for systemic research. Schiepek and Strunk (1994) explicate that for the empirical description of complex systems, one has to collect hundreds to thousands of measurement time points so that one can, e.g., differentiate white noise from a deterministic chaotic attractor (e.g., by using the Kolmogorov-Sinai-entropy, a hint for the "chaoticity" of a signal, or the spectrum of the Lyapunov-exponent for characterization of chaoticity). On the other hand, researchers with a relational constructionist perspective favor, e.g., rhizomic, messy, fluid, expansive inquiry (Reynolds, 2014) by referring to French philosopher Gilles Deleuze or to Norwegian qualitative researcher Steinar Kvale's "hermeneutics of suspicion" (and analyzing and describing data, e.g., by handmade drawings). Hildenbrand (1998, p. 114) argues that, "quantitative studies follow linear-causal patterns of thought and because of that, they are not first choice in systemic research, while qualitative approaches often come from a reconstructive perspective of the analysis of social reality" – and that fits better with a systemic constructivist epistemology. Schiepek (2010) explains (measuring as an important part of systemic research means the transformation of an empirical into a numeric relative) that qualitative data (e.g., phenomenological descriptions, casuistic) are useful only for the formulation of hypothesis, which can be empirically tested in "real" quantitative systemic research in the next step. Ochs (2012a) considers that the entanglement of multiple research perspectives (e.g., EEG measures, questionnaires, observational data, interviews, available documents, artefacts), as practiced in mixed-methods designs (Creswell & Plano Clark, 2017), is a good "systemic" way of approaching an "object" of research. Our position is that there are no "systemic research methods," but a lot of very diverse qualitative, quantitative, and mixed research methods, that all could be useful for systemic investigations (see Ochs, 2013). But, of course: We must systematically, comprehensively and thoroughly explicate in which way a specific research endeavor is viewed as "systemic."

---

[5] In the context of a Heidelberg university hospital research program, we investigated, e.g., associations and feedback-loops between different systems-levels: visual evoked potentials (VEPs), emotional and family problems in migraine children (Just et al., 2003; Ochs et al., 2005; Oelkers et al., 1999).

The Research of the Practice or the Practice of Research?

Is systemic research the investigation and evaluation of systemic practice? In that sense, an RCT study, such as Knekt et al. (chapter "The Effectiveness of Three Psychotherapies of Different Type and Length in the Treatment of Patients Suffering from Anxiety Disorders" this volume), which evaluates solution focused therapy, could be labeled systemic research? But what about undertaking a study in a psychoanalytical setting, which investigates the complex interactions between therapist and patient (e.g., Shapiro, 2015), or a study researching resource and solution orientation in CBT (e.g., Willutzki, Teismann, & Schulte, 2012)? Or is systemic research simply, when systemic practitioners doing inquiry of their own practice – doing practitioner research?

These considerations demonstrate the plurality of systemic research. But what about systemic practice?

Systemic Practice – As "Applied/Practiced Epistemology"

In our perspective, systemic practice is "applied/practiced epistemology" (Schlippe & Schweitzer, 2019) build upon two complementary epistemological columns (see Fig. 1)[6]: (1) Column: systems theory (dynamical systems theory, sociological systems theory); (2) Column: constructivism (biological/radical constructivism, social/relational constructionism, psychological/moderate constructivism (rooted in critical rationalism)) (see also Ochs, 2020).[7]

Similarly, SPR needs to reflect both epistemological perspectives. For example, second-order cybernetics (as an important aspect of systems theory) recognizes the therapist as a part of the therapeutic system. In a research context, the observer needs to include self-observation as a key element in "operationalized" ways, e.g., by writing a research diary with personal process notes. Autoethnographic research approaches conceptualize the researcher as part of the "object" of investigation (see Ellis and Ellingson (2007) for an autoethnographic perspective in a constructionist research context). Systemic researchers, such as Günter Schiepek (chapter "Contributions of Systemic Research to the Development of Psychotherapy" this

---

[6] Of course, there are "overlappings" of these two epistemological columns: Gloy (2006, S. 221) formulates in a philosophy textbook: "If someone is talking about system or systems theory, constructivism is not far away." Moser (2011, p. 10) uses the term "systems theoretical constructivism" to describe the "observation of construction processes in the context of theories of self-organization." On the other hand, Lock and Strong (2010) retrace the manifold philosophical and theoretical influences on social constructionism, such as Phenomenology, Hermeneutics, Marxism, or Dialogism, that have nothing to do with systems theory.

[7] It is well known that there are many other concepts forming the broad stream of systemic practice like "solution-focused" therapy, dialogical-systemic approaches or narrative therapy – but they all could be tracked down systematically to these two epistemologies of a systemic way of thinking.

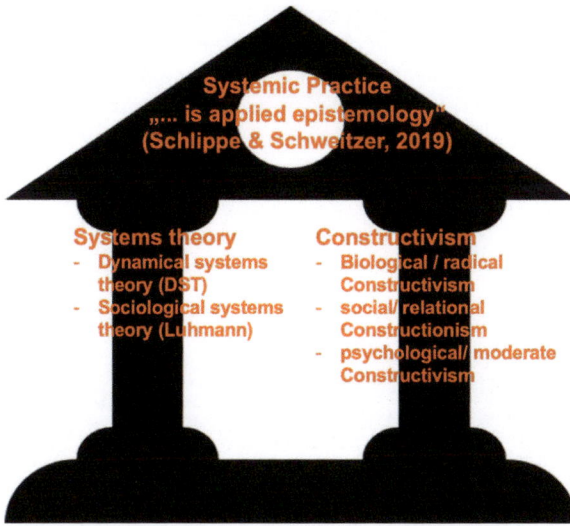

Fig. 1 The two epistemological columns of systemic practice. (Ochs, 2020)

volume), Wolfgang Tschacher (chapter "The Social Present in Psychotherapy: Duration of Nowness in Therapeutic Interaction" this volume), or Jürgen Kriz (e.g. 2001), do quantitative time series analysis with questionnaires, physiological or videographed data. These methods are well-grounded in dynamic systems theory (DST), such as Synergetics (Haken, 1983).[8] Baecker (2012), a scholar of Germany's most famous systems theory sociologist Niklas Luhmann (1984), states as the main contribution of systems theory to empirical research is the sorting, reflection, and interpretation of qualitative or quantitative primary data by concepts such as "information," "communication," "control," "system," "environment," "function," "observation," "form," "self-reference," or "complexity" – but not first of all collecting that primary data.

Another prominent understanding of "systemic" practice (now referring to the second column), especially in an Anglo-American context, is formed by social/relational constructionist epistemology, and the key concept that all of our understandings are socially constructed. McNamee (chapter "Relational Research (Trans) forming Practices" this volume) summarizes relational constructionist research as a co-created, generative process introducing locally useful change, new understandings, and new possibilities (SPR example 1 below leans on such a perspective). Another epistemological perspective is moderate constructivism (Sydow, 2015, p. 44–45; Stierlin, 1997), which values and differentiates between "hard data" (e.g., blood pressure, income, genetic parenthood) and "soft data" (e.g., description of feelings, personal narrations, subjective health) in a biopsychosocial model context, e.g., systemic family medicine practice (McDaniel, Hepworth, & Doherty, 1992).

---

[8] It's worth mentioning that in 2019 the Springer Book Series in Synergetics has 125 titles.

The biopsychosocial model potentially also has the capacity to integrate the vast amount of empirical evidence from a lot of psychological disciplines, such as social psychology, psychology of perception and memory, cognitive psychology, and neuropsychology (Myers, 2014), which demonstrate that human knowledge forming is a highly constructed matter on many process levels. Moderate constructivism can also be understood as psychological constructivism[9] – so if a practitioner is investigating his own systemic practice by undertaking (family) diagnostic questionnaires constructed in terms of psychological/psychometric test theory (such as Example 2 below), this can also be considered as systemic (practitioner) research.

(Systemic) Practitioner Research

Practitioner research refers to workplace research performed by individuals who work in the respective professional field as opposed to being full-time academic researchers (e.g., Fox, Martin, & Green, 2007). Coghlan (2003) names this "insider research," "because it draws on the experience of practitioners as members of their organizations and so makes a distinctive contribution to the development of insider knowledge about organizations and organizational change" (p. 451). Helps (2017) refers to the distinction of Shotter (1993) between "aboutness" and "withness" positions and assigns practitioner research to the latter. Shaw (2005) understands practitioner research "as a phenomenon that manifests a pervasive cluster of concerns about good professional practice in contemporary society" and not "a fringe operation—a 'street market' version of mainstream research" (p. 1231).

Some important developments took place in education (e.g., Schön, 1983), nursing (e.g., Molde & Diers, 1985), and social work (e.g., Flynn & McDermott, 2016; Fuller & Petch, 1995; Lunt & Shaw, 2017; Powell & Orme, 2011; Shaw, 2005; Wade & Neuman, 2007).[10] Harvey et al. (2013) investigate practitioner research capacities of social workers. They find that although "very few social workers had high levels of experience in complex research tasks that include conducting, reporting, presenting, and publishing research" and identified "research anxiety and research avoidance as significant challenges," social workers were "generally enthusiastic about research" (p. 551).

---

[9] The term "psychological constructivism" is not very well defined: sometimes it is used, when referring to individual conditions of perception, attention and cognition in the context of construction of knowledge; sometimes this term is associated with the Personal Construct Psychology of George A. Kelly or the Genetic Epistemology of Jean Piaget (Sutter, 2009).

[10] Especially the last-mentioned profession is of great interest in the systemic context, because social workers represent, e.g., in Germany, but also UK, the major profession of systemic practitioners (roundabout half of the members of the systemic associations in Germany are social workers/social pedagogues).

The practitioner research scenario seems attractive for some reasons:

- *Potential of professional systemic practitioners*
  The systemic approach evolved mainly in practice and private training (and not in university) contexts (Schweitzer & Ochs, chapter "The Heidelberg Systemic Research Conferences: It´s History, Goals, and Outcomes" this volume). Until recently, systemic conferences (such as the EFTA conferences or the annual conferences of the German systemic associations DGSF and SG) were mainly practitioner driven in terms of presenters and participants. There exists a bigger potential of systemic professionals that could do research in professional practice, than in universities or research institutes. As Helps (2017) complements: "Many systemic researchers have conducted research using actual clinical material" (p. 351), such as video recordings and transcripts of clinical sessions.

- *In line with (social) constructionist epistemology*
  The social/relational constructionist stance seems in line with a research perspective that strengthens and underlines the role of the researcher as a participant and co-constructivist of the context and the "object" of research. Ever since the "second-order cybernetics" position of the observer/therapist has been recognized as part of the system (von Foerster, 1981), the observer is no longer seen as "neutral and detached" but rather as a part of the observing system. The observer cannot stand in an "objective" or "object defining position," without stepping into "self-transforming" and "object-transforming" processes. That epistemological point of view served as an inspiration for a lot of systemic practice concepts, such as the "non-expert position" (Anderson & Goolishian, 1992), the "co-creation" of practice discourses (Shotter, 1993), or the "dialogue of different perspectives" (Andersen, 1987). A researcher that approaches practice from the outside (e.g., a university or research institute context) is always in danger of doing this intended or unintendedly with a problematic power discourse in the sense of Foucault (1984). This danger may be avoided by researching one's own practice on an "eye to eye level" with the subjects of research (Anderson, 1997). Allwright (2005) underlines in the context of language teacher practitioner research that "the ethical and epistemological dimensions are the most critical, with the emphasis on understanding rather than problem-solving" (p. 353). In addition, as van der Donk and van Lanen (2018) remind us, constructivism has become one of the major approaches in professional teaching and learning: Learners construct their own knowledge from interpreting their experiences and exploring naturally occurring practice.

- *Systemic practice sometimes even looks like (qualitative) research already*
  The counseling/therapy discourses of systemic practices are characterized by "a vast and extraordinary library of questions," as Simon (2014, S. 8) puts it; some authors even talk about systemic "interviewing" (e.g., Hanot, 2006; Sheinberg & Brewster, 2014; Tomm, 1987) instead of therapy or counseling – which comes even closer to (qualitative) research. Burck (2005) states that "many of the qualitative research methods developed in the social sciences are well suited to explore research questions pertinent for the systemic field, and make a good fit with

systemic thinking"(S. 237). So, if (re-)framing systemic practice with a research perspective, a SPR scenario may appear anyway.

- *A possibility of bridging research and practice*
  Not only, but also in the systemic field, there is often a call for "bridging research and practice" (e.g., Borcsa & Rober, 2016; Burns, 2007; Wulff & St. George, 2016) – the practitioner research scenario seems to be one possible appropriate answer to that demand.

On the other hand, practitioner research is accompanied by some non-trivial theoretical challenges – not only, but especially with a systemic stance. Of course, as suggested above, this depends very much on the epistemological base of the particular systemic stance (e.g., dynamic systems theory, sociological systems theory, social constructionism, moderate constructivism):

- *A lot of terms and approaches, that mean more or less (not) the same*
  There are a lot of ((systemic) practitioner) research approaches in the context of a broader social constructionist framework that emphasize as an essential part of the research endeavor the subjectivity and involvement of both researcher and researched ones just as the interaction between them, e.g., systemic action research (Burns, 2007), constructivist research (Holstein & Gubrium, 2007), participatory (action) research (Bargold & Thomas, 2010), postmodern qualitative inquiry (Cooper & White, 2012), and performative inquiry (Fels & McGiven, 2002) – a term that Gergen and Gergen (2012) favor – collaborative research (Fraenkel, chapter "Collaborative Family Program Development: Research Methods that Investigate and Foster Resilience and Engagement in Marginalized Communities" this volume), community-based research (Strand et al. 2003), relational constructionist research approach (McNamee & Hosking, 2012, McNamee, chapter "Relational Research (Trans)forming Practices" this volume) – to name only a few. This situation is not only confusing for researchers[11] but even more for practitioners, that are planning to investigate their own practice: Harvey et al. (2013) found in a survey about practitioner research capacity in social workers that anyway a lack of confidence, limited knowledge and skills, and practical constraints are impeding research activity – this situation is for practitioners aggravated by this potentially dizzying designation of research approaches.
- *Research and practice belongs to different social functional systems*
  From a sociological systems theory perspective (e.g., Luhmann, 1977, 1984), which merges Talcott Parsons structural functional theory with the autopoiesis theory of Humberto Maturana and Francesco Varela, research and practice could be considered as associated with respective different social functional systems,[12]

---

[11] An article exploring and describing in a systematic way the differences and similarities of all these approaches could be a good and useful service.

[12] In his original theory of social systems, Luhmann (1977, 1984) discriminates three types of social systems (interactions, organizations and functional social systems); later he and his followers add groups, families and networks to that typology. Furthermore Luhmann discriminates social systems (that are made out of communication – not out of humans, as someone could think streetwise) from biological (with living as core process) and psychological (with consciousness as core process) systems.

which are in a heterarchical way environments for each other, and that provide for each other "only" intransparency, non-instructive and non-directive stimulation, complexity, paradoxes, and contingency. Each social functional system follows a specific binary code as communicative core process: research is part of the social functional system "science" (with the specific binary code: true/untrue) and, e.g., psychosocial counseling practice is part of the social functional system "social work" (with the binary code help/not help), psychotherapy part of the social functional system "medicine" (illness/health). While it is a commonplace that humans operate in the context of a lot of social systems, it could be helpful to reflect the possible benefits and pitfalls of the operation of communicative core processes of the respective systems (see Ochs & Thom, 2014).

- *Research and practice acts are not interchangeable or simply the same*
  In an earlier publication, Wright (1990) reminds us that research is also a family therapy intervention technique and sensitizes, and in this way there are "therapeutical" effects of undertaking research in the practice. Of course, this is "grist to the mill" for a social constructionist's research perspective (e.g., McNamee & Hosking, 2012; Simon & Chard, 2014), which has at its core, that a researcher co-constructs social reality and so the "object" of research with their (embodied) concepts, mediated by interaction and communication acts in the research process. On the other hand, treating research and practice acts, just as synonyms for social reality transforming endeavors (an impression, that one could receive from ideas such as "From Mirroring To World-Making: Research As Future Forming" (Gergen, 2015)) with no connotative or substantial differences, could be associated with the risk of somewhat "theoretical decompensation."

- *SPR is not equivalent to a social constructionist perspective*
  One distinction, that is often made, is that between conventional/(post-)positivistic and reflexive/constructivist research (e.g., Guba & Lincoln, 1989; McNamee & Hosking, 2012). A lot of systemic advocates state that systemic research, and so systemic practitioner research, has to be placed on the reflexive/constructivist side. One of these advocates is Gail Simon (e.g., 2013), who did some pioneering work to elaborate a systemic practitioner research approach (Burck & Simon, 2017).[13] As mentioned above, our understanding of the systemic approach – and also of SPR – is that it is founded on two epistemological columns, constructivism and systems theory (Ochs, 2020). The practitioners in the SNS network (an informal association, that are working with the dynamical systems theory based Synergetic Navigation System) call themselves systemic practitioner researchers – for instance, addiction therapist Judith Patzig investigates regulation of emotions of in-patient patients of her own practice with the SNS (Patzig &

---

[13] The "Journal of Family Therapy" special issue "Developments in systemic practitioner research", edited by Burck and Simon (2017), presents practitioner research endeavors in that line: Brown (2017) analyzes the intersubjective process between the researcher (herself) and the client based on the conceptualization of five poetic images that recur in Martin Buber's work on dialogism; Salter (2017) introduce a narrative inquiry design for systemic group work with women who have experienced abuse and oppression, that she co-facilitated.

Schiepek, 2015; Schiepek, chapter "Contributions of Systemic Research to the Development of Psychotherapy" this volume).

- *Improving practice by SPR is something different from reflexive formats (e.g., supervision), training, self-learning or by documentation (e.g., for quality control purposes)*
  We have argued above, that there has to be "a difference, that makes a difference," between practice and research; the same accounts for practitioner research and other reflexive and quality control formats for practice, such as professional self-reflection (supervision or colleague exchanges, like intervision), documentation (e.g., by a certificated quality control system), training, and self-learning by, e.g., reading professional journals. Wulff and St George (2014) define research as daily practice as "continuously examining data/information from our own clinical work reflexively in order to better understand what we do and what we could do" (p. 296). But to investigate in a systematically, theoretical, and methodological driven as well as transparent way one's own practice (that's practitioner research) has to lead to other insights as, e.g., documentation by a certificated quality control system or a supervision session. Differences between practitioner research and other reflexive formats are, e.g., that in practitioner research exploring the potential of subjects is of greater quality and consistency as well as being more literature linked and driven; the self-practice/−observation/−reflection is also more oriented at the elementary research questions. Practitioners normally don't have time for complex, rigid, consistent ways of self-observation/−reflection (e.g., writing a research journal after every session).

- *"Maps" of each other*
  Besides the mentioned "theoretical" challenges, there are some attitudes or preconceptions by practitioners and academics of each other, which challenge the "bridging" of practice and research.
  In the academic field, one can experience a lot of "opinions" (preconceptions) concerning practitioner research:

- It is classified as a "street market" version of "real" research, as "dirty research" (not proper research); actually a lot of university colleagues don't know anything about the concept of practitioner research and tend to wrinkle their noses at it, because they suppose the crashing of all quality criteria in the so called empirical research endeavor.

- Practitioners are too long out of academic/research contexts and so lost a lot of their skills and competencies for undertaking proper research and writing about it.

- Practitioners are not interested in research; actually Padberg (2012) investigates the question, why practitioners don't read ((research) literature); he comes to the conclusion that for practitioners this kind of literature isn't instructive, informative, and inspiring.

- They are not capable of stepping back from their (emotional) involvement into their practice and because of that the distorting and confounding effects they are producing while doing research are gigantic.

- On the other side, in the practice field, one can also experience a lot of "opinions" (preconceptions) concerning academic research:
- Research by university people is not of interest for the practice field, because academics investigate topics that don't really matter to practitioners.
- The language of the academic "ivory tower" is not compatible with the practice field.
- Academics want to dominate practitioners with some kind of hegemonial stance and tell them how to do practice, out of their academic research results.
- Systemic practitioners are doing very well without academics; as mentioned above systemic practice flourished and is flourishing perfectly outside the academic world (only when it comes to issues of funding systemic practice, e.g., by health insurances, there is a call from the practice for empirical evidence).
- Healing and helping are something completely different, than producing knowledge and truth (see the sketches of Luhmann's social functional systems above).

Two Examples of SPR Projects

We want to sketch now two SPR projects, their benefits, pitfalls and challenges, and the practitioner and researcher perspective. We try to give a hint how SPR could broaden options of research. In both examples researching one's own practice plays a key role in developing both practice and theory. These two examples were strongly stimulated by the participation of the second (LH) and third author (AGK) in the Heidelberg systemic research conference; the first author (MO) did PhD consultation/supervision.

"Co-therapy as a Team Transforming Experience" (LH)

This practitioner research example builds on the relational constructionist perspective. It invites all the research participants to become co-researches of the project. The goal is to develop a shared understanding and generate new practice. Research is viewed as a process of learning, and the main method is shared and reflected self-reflexivity.

Context

This project was undertaken by a team of a psychology/psychotherapy out-patient service placed in a general hospital in a rural area of Czech Republic. The team is multidisciplinary (psychologists, psychotherapists, art therapist, social worker), consisting of four men and four women. All come from different therapeutic backgrounds, i.e., systemic, Gestalt, and analytical; most of the team members are double or triple trained. The team is also well "weaved into" the network of other services (e.g., social services, psychiatric community services, juvenile courts and hospital environment). The ambulance also serves as a teaching/training place for students in psychotherapy trainings, so there was a curiosity in the team of its own processes of learning and transformation in order to improve teaching training abilities.

Challenge

We learnt about the research results of the need adapted treatment/open dialogue approach with psychotic patients (Seikkula, chapter "From Research on Dialogical Practice to Dialogical Research: Open Dialogue is Based on A Continuous Scientific Analysis" this volume, Ochs et al., 2020). These results seemed convincing for us. The principles of the "open dialogue" seemed very familiar to what we already did, so it was hard to believe that something that "we almost do" could bring such drastic change in results when applied with greater radicalness. The results seemed to be putting into question the whole system of established treatment of psychotic patients that is known in Czech Republic – so we felt both inspired and challenged.

At the same time, we could see how applying "more radicalness" and "dialogical principles" could be useful and potentially transforming in all areas of our work, not just in treating psychotic patients. We could also see that "converting into dialogism" could bring a potential danger of division into the team and into the network collaborating with us as, e.g., "open dialogue" introduces some controversial use of medication and can create a space for misunderstandings and misinterpretations. We needed to "re-discover" the dialogical approach for ourselves, within our local professional and socio-cultural context. We felt we needed to develop our own language for "dialogical changes." We somewhat "hoped" that, through our own gradual transformation, the whole network connected to our practice could somehow absorb the change. We were interested in how a team of well-established and well-experienced practitioners can be transformed, and how can dialogism be re-discovered in the environment of extremely busy day-to-day practice.

Why (Systemic Practitioner) Research? Why Not a Training, Supervision or Improved Regular Documentation?

The first logical option would have been to send some team members on training courses on dialogical practices. First of all, there were no courses on dialogical practices available at that time. But also, dialogism seemed to be addressing the way we are with the clients and each other rather than what we do. As a team, we very much value the diversity of our perspectives. With dialogism, it seemed that each one of us was seeing something slightly different as "what makes it work," would use their own theoretical background to describe it and examples of their own work for how they use it. We were as much interested in "what is already dialogical" in our own practice as much as in what "could be more dialogical." The research gave us time and legitimization to experiment with new ways of working. Regarding our professional network, the fact that the changes in our behavior and language are part of a "research project" offered a safer framework. It made us to constantly switch between the experiment and the meta-position of reflecting about it.

We were looking for a research design compatible with our work ethics, influenced by the broader Postmodern Turn; all the different therapeutic orientations that we are using, turning our attention to language, making us attentive to the position of the observer, viewing self-reflexivity as one of the main sources of information and valuing difference as one of the main sources of change together with the basic systemic principles, the "non-expert position" and collaborative approach. We were looking for a research, which would honor this work ethics; we have found a good theoretical background in the research perspective of relational constructionism (e.g., McNamee & Hosking, 2012, McNamee, chapter "Relational Research (Trans) forming Practices" this volume). So, we turned to the TAOS institute[14] to supervise the way we co-construct/research/establish our change.

Goals

We used SPR to explore the dialogical aspects already present in our team context and to develop knowledge of what new dialogical perspectives could be within our team context. We also wanted to map our own transformation process to gain more knowledge about the transformation process itself. We have decided that it is a co-therapy setting where we feel that we learn most, and feel safe and ready to experiment. We felt that during our co-therapy sessions, we tend to use the behavior which we see from different perspectives as the most dialogical. We reflect on our own ability to use the dialogical qualities with the co-therapist right after the session.

Design

Through a series of questions answered in writing and discussions, we co-created the design of our research to gain the maximum involvement. We created a so-called "dialogical loop" to slowly build up our understanding together with the practice transformation. We reflected our co-therapy session in the co-therapy couple using set up questions (see below), and then brought the answers to a focus group. The focus group[15] was taped, transcribed, and analyzed, and the results were presented

---

[14]TAOS institute is an American non-profit organization founded 1991 by Ken Gergen, Mary Gergen, Sheila McNamee, Harlene Anderson, David Cooperrider, Suresh Srivastva, and Diana Whitney to promote the ideas of social/relational constructionism in academic and practical aspects of life.

[15]By "focus group"we understand a set time, where all the team-members were meeting and discussing a given topic. We all were familiar and have followed the general rules of a focus group coducting as given by, for example, Krueger & Casey (2000).

for discussion in the beginning of the next focus group. The process was repeated till everyone was happy with the amount of our understanding and the transformation of our practice.

"Dialogical Loop"

- *Questions answering*

  Throughout a 1.5-year time period, we kept meeting regularly for minimum two co-therapy sessions a week. As we prefer male-female co-therapy couples, and we are four male and four female therapists, each one of us had worked with four different partners, creating 16 co-therapy couples. After each co-therapy session, we had the time slot of 45 minutes to discuss in-between the two therapists and answer in writing the two main questions: (1) what have I learned today about the co-therapy process and (2) what have I learned today about myself. These questions were developed by the team to increase our self-reflexivity.[16]

- *Focus groups*

  Every 2–3 months a focus group was organized, where the results were shared. The focus groups were taped, transcribed, and analyzed, and the results of the analysis were fed back in the beginning of the next focus group and then discussed in an ongoing circle. Additionally, we have decided to do some common readings and tape observations. Reflections of these readings and observations were part of the focus groups.

- *Data analysis*

  For the data analysis, we have used the Charmaz (2006) version of grounded analysis to analyze the transcript. We have also paid attention to "high and low energy moments" in the discussion to the appearance of metaphors and re-appearances of phrases used in the previous focus groups later on in the process. The basic analysis was done by the author herself as impulses for possible interpretations and repeatedly re-done according to the reactions and possible interpretations of the rest of the team.

Results

There are several areas, where we see effects/results of our research. There is of course a greater sum of knowledge about dialogism, but there is also the increase of the emotional ability to transform it into new skills:

- We have created an understanding of what dialogism is for us and found ways to build it into our practice as described in literature.

---

[16] Even though it seems that these two questions have nothing to do with dialogism, we recognized them as helpful. Our understanding of dialogism was to increase our ability to of shared self-reflexivity and through empathic listening to each other develop our own ability to express our thoughts and feelings. Through answering these questions in this context, we stepped straight into "practice of dialogism"with each other while reflecting our feelings and thoughts during the session.

- We have defined and adopted into our practice the dialogical way of co-working.
- Adopting this new practice has enabled us to address new client groups which we have found until then "frustrating" or "scary" in a manner which we actually find energizing.
- We are now teaching dialogical co-working at a university-based course using many examples from our own learning process and practice.
- We have formulated the concept of "dialogical ethics" – not as a concept we "own" but a direction toward which we want to develop. We now use the concept in our teaching sessions in different contexts. We also use it to introduce new team members, who did not participate in the research with us into our work ethics.
- We reflected on the series of practical changes which we see as a part of our transformation. Not just changes in, for example, furniture settings but also, for example, the diagnosing/report writing, which we still have to do for medical/legal purposes, we increasingly see as a tool with a therapeutic potential.

Example Two "Systemic Practitioner Research of Out-Patient Social-Pediatric Multifamily Groups" (AGK)

The second example demonstrates the use of quantitative and qualitative methods while doing systemic practitioner research. The researcher included both herself and the clients in gaining deeper mutual understanding and deeper understanding of the issue involved. Participating in the research (as reflected in the results) gave the clients sense of importance and opened new learning/therapeutic potential for both – clients and the therapist.

Context

Our Multifamily Groups (MFG) were developed and have been implemented since 1995 for over 20 years at a large out-patient pediatric center in a Children's Hospital Medical Center in Frankfurt/Main, Germany (Goll-Kopka, 2009, 2012). This center provides comprehensive diagnostic evaluation and therapy for complex or serious childhood illness, developmental delays and disabilities. The MFG project originated when families at the pediatric center, for whom the disabilities caused great distress, had difficulties decoding the language of the medical and rehabilitation system, and who felt a deep sense of isolation and a lack of understanding coming from others in their social context. It is headed by a multidisciplinary team consisting of two group facilitators – one social worker and one psychologist (AGK), both experienced family-therapists – and four trainees in special education. Experimenting with different settings, it finally led us to a structure for the MFG as a two-day workshop, running Friday afternoon until Sunday afternoon, and held in a service-oriented facility in a tranquil outdoor region near Frankfurt. This format best accommodated the needs of these exhausted families, taking into account the work/school schedules of family members. There are three 90-minute sessions for entire families and all facilitators together; six 90-minute sessions for several parallel subgroups (the parents, older siblings, and the children themselves), time slots for informal socialization opportunities: seven shared meals and two evening activities that are attended by the group leaders as well. Different media, like art collages, and specific drawing and moving exercises, bring family members of all ages together and allow the families to represent their experiences and feelings in different modalities.

During my clinical work as a family therapist, consultant, and clinical psychologist in that Children's Hospital Medical Center, I undertook different practitioner research projects – two research projects (Goll-Kopka, 2009; Retzlaff, Brazil, & Goll-Kopka, 2008) without a bridge to the academic field and one big research project still working as a family therapist, consultant and clinical psychologist, but also being a PhD candidate within a doctorate program at the University of Oldenburg.[17]

Challenges

The challenges which we faced are common in current pediatric family research in real-life settings: small sample sizes, recruitment, and adherence concerns. Working as a family therapist and clinician you relate to the burden of the families you work with and as a researcher you would like those families to "work" for the research requirements – for example, take some more extra time for interviews and filling out questionnaires. These ambivalences arise sharply when being in both roles – a practitioner and a researcher in the same field. We solved it by trying to reduce the burden of the research requirements, for example, by doing the interviews with the families at their houses. Research needs time, money and a network with other people, who do research. The Systemic Research Conferences and being a PhD candidate at the university of Oldenburg – especially presenting the project and discussing it at both places – was very productive for the research process.

Goals

One purpose and goal of the research project was to examine, how the participating family members describe specific intervention components of MFG and how the therapeutic process and the outcome of a multifamily group are assessed by participants, and to detect whether there is evidence that participation in an MFG changes parental coping behavior and parental competence. Or, in other words, How can our systemic interventions help and support families, who face-life-long challenges in better, effective ways? Families are experts of their everyday life situation and in

---

[17] This difference whether you have a bridge to the academic field like a university setting, academic network, and its resources or not, makes a big difference by being a practitioner researcher and looking at practitioner research projects.

bringing the empowerment attitude also into research, we were curious about the subjective perspectives of the members of our multifamily groups in a more profound way than just an evaluation. "Understanding the participants' perspectives and experiences of therapy is particularly important for treatment approaches which emphasize empowerment (and this is true of most multifamily treatments)"(Lemmens, Eisler, Dierick, Lietaer, & Demyttenaere, 2009, p. 251).

My own practitioner research motifs or reasons originate from the same attitude as a family therapist or clinical psychologist – one is curiosity or my longing for understanding thoroughly and deeper – I want to understand better, more differentiated and discriminated the social world of the people I work with or the complex phenomena I encounter in my (clinical) work, and find better and more useful ways of helping the people. The aims for the research are to understand, evaluate, and improve the practice and also to disseminate the findings more widely. Research meant investigating my clinical work and the themes connected to it – it raised my own awareness or my own self-reflexivity; it evolved an evaluating reflexive process. These two fields affected each other recursively in a broadening and developmental sense.

Design

The study examined the perspectives of all participating family members regarding specific intervention components and the therapeutic process and its outcomes of a heterogeneous, closed MFG. We must attempt to hear the "'family conversational voice' as a whole. This cannot be done if we talk to only one family member" (Dahl & Boss, 2005, S. 66). A mixed – method design was administered:

- A problem-centered interview with all eight families and their members of one multifamily group was undertaken by a qualified psychologist, who did not belong to the institutional context. The interviews were transcribed and analyzed by a group of three raters using qualitative content analysis.
- In addition, a single-group pre-post-design was administered by using three common questionnaires concerning the therapeutic process and outcome, parental coping behavior, and parental competence. They were assessed at three measuring points before the MFG Intervention, 3 weeks and 12 weeks after the intervention.

Results

Through the results and the study, we could connect and integrate the multifamily group intervention into a broader theoretical systemic understanding and conceptualize a systemic model (Goll-Kopka & Born, 2018). Specific intervention components such as the provided therapeutic environment and the mutual support that was facilitated by offering different opportunities for contact with families in similar situations are highlighted as particularly helpful:

- The distance from everyday life and its demands and restrictions was considered to be a therapeutic aspect of this MFG setting. The regenerating effect through a service-oriented facility in a tranquil outdoor region was seen as a beneficial prerequisite, allowing for the focused reflection on family and personal issues. Group cohesion builds faster through being together as an entire group for two days in one facility. It is this aspect of closeness that is effective for processing for example stress and grief. Attendance of and satisfaction with the group were high.
- The activation of and work on intense emotions and the space given to one's own and other families' concerns during the MFG were considered essential for a favorable therapeutic process. The participation with one's partner deepened the mutual understanding among parental partners. Participation in an MFG can be associated with an increased level of togetherness of parental partners, and a higher level of perceived parental competence. Increased feelings of parental togetherness and competence were reported.
- For most of the families, this was the first time they spoke in depth about their stories with other families affected by the same issues. Telling stories in a group of knowledgeable others provides a meaningful context that has a dramatically restorative effect on group members. Further, the comparison with their own stories helps the families to put their experiences into different perspectives.
- Results suggest that this MFG for families of children with chronic diseases or disabilities is highly feasible for these families so they come to terms with the life-long challenges and develop better ways in coping with their situation (Goll-Kopka & Born, 2018).

Discussion

We will discuss some benefits and challenges of doing SPR that emerge among others out of the two examples above. Much of the published research in the systemic context is/was outcome research for legitimization reasons, trying to validate the field (IQWIG, 2017). SPR seems to be very interesting and appealing to generate knowledge about what is happening in daily systemic practice (Simon & Chard, 2014; Burck & Simon, 2017).

Benefits of Doing (Systemic) Practitioner Research

The research benefits of both examples could be seen in a more general way as benefits common in systemic practitioner research.

Benefits for the Researchers, Co-researchers, and the Participants

In both examples, the co-researchers (exp. 1) and the researcher and the participants (exp. 2) mention as a result of the research increased self-reflexivity and creation of a learning/therapeutic environment which help to see difficulties within the practice as "experiences" which are carefully "listened to" by the others. This attitude helps to create a common vocabulary open to all the parties involved-scientific community, practitioners, clients, etc. with new therapeutic perspectives and potentials.

Benefits for the Practice

In both examples, the researchers see the experience as "self-transformative" not just in terms of new skills but also in terms of creating a space to think about "who am I" as a therapist, colleague, and human being. The space for this type of reflection was experienced as having a burn-out prevention potential. The practice also benefits from the researchers /co-researchers developing other related skills like writing or doing analysis. By gaining a more specific understanding of the effective factors of the therapeutic work, its setting and framework – the research results helped implementing the MFG project better in the organization and its funding for example through the City of Frankfurt.

Benefits for the Scientific Community

In both cases the research has helped to increase theoretical awareness of the issue involved in the professional community, has helped with funding and created a potential inspiration for new colleagues. The well-discussed gap between practice and academia grew smaller (LH and AGK both got positions at universities in the aftermath of their practitioner research PhDs).

Pitfalls, Downfalls, and Challenges of Doing (Systemic) Practitioner Research

Doing Systemic Practitioner Research Inside or Outside an Academic Context?

It is extremely helpful to have some kind of access and connection to the academic context while doing practitioner research,[18] e.g., for securing empirical quality criteria, such as validity, reliability and objectivity – all mainstream quality criteria,

---

[18] One possibility to do so is to participate in a PhD program specific for systemic (practitioner) research: e.g., "Professional Doctorate in Systemic Practice"-Programme at the University of Bedfordshire/UK (https://www.beds.ac.uk/research-ref/rgs/programmes/profdoc/pdsp/) or Taos Institute Ph.D. Program (https://www.taosinstitute.net/taos-phd-program)

which could turn over for and translate to every kind of practitioner research (see also Simon, 2018), e.g., for ensuring inter-rater-reliability of interview-data-analysis (better access to co-raters), for face validity of interview-manuals (by colleagues), or for improving its own theoretical and empirical considerations by presenting and discussing them with colleagues. For practitioners, there is a tendency to be closed up in their "own little practitioner world," with, e.g., language or vocabulary. Also the academic context is helpful for approaching up to date, relevant literature (via access to literature date bases); practitioners sometimes are too narrow in the literature and not so sure what is important and what unimportant literature.

"Conflict of Interests" Between the Practitioner and Researcher

"Caution must be used to protect families from our potential conflict of interest. While we are doing therapy, we cannot put the gathering of research data first; while we are doing research, we need to recognize that we are not doing therapy …" (Dahl & Boss, 2005, S. 68). The conflict between doing practice and research and the ambivalence and complications being in both roles was in the two examples always present and had to be considered. The main difference between "practitioner research" and academic research is the position and the role of the researcher in the research process. But in both you have to keep in mind "This is research 'with' people, not 'on' people, and participants` lives are affected in … ways through the research and its consequent changes …" (Mendenhall & Doherty, 2005, p. 105). Generally, the issue of ethics is discussed very thoroughly and broadly in the context of (systemic) practitioner research (see e.g. Chan, Teram, & Shaw, 2017; Helps, 2017). In example 2 it an attempt was made to follow the movement of "Service-User-Led-Research" (Faulkner & Thomas, 2002). This means, always to reflect on and keep in mind the "side effects" or consequences of the research for the field and the "service users." "This dearth of supportive research has been due, as outlined earlier, to the mismatch between the requirements of research protocols and the needs of overextended caregiving families ... a third difficulty for conducting research of the medical multifamily groups is recruitment of participant families. Variation in illness course often puts family support needs in direct opposition to research requirements!" (Gonzalez & Steinglass, 2002, p. 318 and p. 338).

"A Touch Too Much" Emotional Work Involvement

Doing practitioner research and learning on such a personal and emotional level (such as example 1) can also stir up some deep personal processes, and group dynamics within the team involved can be both emotionally exhausting and exciting at other times. It is questionable if participants want to be emotionally involved with their work on such a deep level.

Lack of Resources

One main problem in doing SPR is lack of resources (e.g., time, money, and staff); these (contextual) factors limit the research and its possibilities, for example, in gathering and evaluating data or writing a research article. In both examples the whole research was considered a quite time-consuming process. Of course, it was seen as time invested into the team education in example 1 – but still, it was time taken away from the client sessions and of the private life. The time invested is usually done "for free" in the practitioner contexts, which raises the question of cost-effectiveness of the time invested into the research.

The Perspective of Academics Involving in Practitioner Research

Also for academics there are benefits and challenges of being engaged in practitioner research. Benefits are, e.g., to have access to the fields of application; this is especially of interest for systemic academics since, as mentioned above, important systemic approach developments are happening more in practice than in academic contexts. A very important aspect of having contact with the fields of systemic application is to learn about perspectives and experiences "out there" so research does proceed with important aspects of systemic real life practice and is not happening "in the Ivory tower." For the cooperation with practitioners, challenges for academics are, e.g., their lack of time for doing research, what is problematic for the whole research process, from planning, data collection, analysis, and interpretation to process of writing; also practitioners are no longer well skilled and familiar in doing research and its processes.

Conclusion

In our perspective, SPR includes broad options of research building on system theory and the constructionist perspective while researching one's own practice. It is also a very useful approach in the context of bachelor, master, and PhD thesis: social work and psychotherapy students at Universities of Applied Sciences, for example, are often already employed and use their professional contexts for empirical endeavors. We see SPR furthermore as a good opportunity to connect the world of practice, where systemic ideas are put to a good use, challenged, and developed on a day-to-day basis, with the world of academia and it's theoretical and research challenges and possibilities. In our experience, even though challenging, SPR plays a key role in developing both practice and academic perspectives toward deeper self-reflexivity and broader awareness of the context of our work – which is key for professional competencies development (Orlinsky et al., 1999).

References

Allwright, D. (2005). Developing principles for practitioner research: The case of exploratory practice. *The Modern Language Journal, 89*, 353–366.

Andersen, T. (1987). The reflecting team: Dialogue and meta-dialogue in clinical work. *Family Process, 26*, 415–428.

Anderson, H. (1997). *Conversation, Language and Possibilities: A Postmodern Approach to Therapy*. New York: Basic Books.

Anderson, H., & Goolishian, H. (1992). The client is the expert: A not-knowing approach to therapy. In S. McNamee & K. J. Gergen (Eds.), *Inquiries in social construction. Therapy as social construction* (pp. 25–39). Thousand Oaks, CA: Sage.

Baecker, D. (2012). Die Texte der Systemtheorie. In M. Ochs & J. Schweitzer (Eds.), *Handbuch Forschung für Systemiker* (pp. 153–186). Göttingen: V&R.

Bargold, J., & Thomas, S. (2010). Partizipative Forschung. In G. Mey & K. Mruck (Eds.), *Handbuch Qualitative Forschung in der Psychologie* (pp. 333–344). Wiesbaden: VS/Springer.

Borcsa, M., & Rober, M. (2016). *Research Perspectives in Couple Therapy. Discursive Qualitative Methods*. Cham, CH: Springer International.

Brown, J. M. (2017). A dialogical research methodology based on Buber: Intersubjectivity in the research interview. *Journal of Family Therapy, 39*, 415–436.

Burck, C. (2005). Comparing qualitative research methodologies for systemic research: The use of grounded theory, discourse analysis and narrative analysis. *Journal of Family Therapy, 27*, 237–262.

Burck, C., & Simon, G. (2017). Editorial. Developments in systemic practitioner research. *Journal of Family Therapy, 39*, 285–287.

Burns, D. (2007). *Systemic action research: A strategy for whole system change*. Bristol: Policy Press.

Chan, T. M. S., Teram, E., & Shaw, I. (2017). Balancing methodological rigor and the needs of research participants: A debate on alternative approaches to sensitive research. *Qualitative Health Research, 27*, 260–270.

Charmaz, K. (2006). *Constructing grounded theory*. London: Sage.

Coghlan, D. (2003). Practitioner research for organizational knowledge. Mechanistic- and organistic-oriented approaches to insider action research. *Management Learning, 34*, 451–463.

Cooper, K., & White, R. E. (2012). *Qualitative research in the post-modern era contexts of qualitative research*. Amsterdam: Springer Netherlands.

Creswell, J. W., & Plano Clark, V. L. (2017). *Designing and conducting mixed methods research* (3rd ed.). Thousand Oaks, CA: Sage.

Dahl, C. M., & Boss, P. (2005). The use of phenomenology for family therapy research: The search for meaning. In F. Piercy & D. Sprenkle (Eds.), *Research methods in family therapy* (2nd ed., pp. 63–84). New York: Guilford Press.

Ditzen, B., & Heinrichs, M. (2014). Psychobiology of social support: The social dimension of stress buffering. *Restorative Neurology and Neuroscience, 32*, 149–162.

Ellis, C., & Ellingson, L. L. (2007). Autoethnography as constructionist project. In J. A. Holstein & J. F. Gubrium (Eds.), *Handbook of constructionist research* (pp. 445–466). New York: Guilford.

Faulkner, A., & Thomas, P. (2002). User-led research and evidence-based medicine. *The British Journal of Psychiatry, 180*, 1–3.

Fels, L. & McGivern, L. (2002). Intertextual Play through Performative Inquiry: Intercultural Recognitions. In G. Brauer (Ed.). Body and Language: Intercultural Learning Through Drama (pp. 19–35). Greenwood Academic.

Flynn, C., & McDermott, F. (2016). *Doing research in social work and social care. The journey from student to practitioner researcher*. London: Sage.

Foucault, M. (1984). In P. Rabinow (Ed.), *The Foucault reader*. New York: Pantheon.

Fox, M., Martin, P., & Green, G. (2007). *Doing practitioner research*. New Delhi: Sage.

Fuller, R., & Petch, A. (1995). *Practitioner-research: The reflective social worker.* Buckingham: Open University Press.

Gergen, K. J. (2015). From mirroring to world-making: Research as future forming. *Journal for the Theory of Social Behaviour, 45*, 287–310.

Gergen, M. M., & Gergen, K. J. (2012). *Playing with purpose. Adventures in performative social science.* London: Routledge.

Gloy, K. (2006). *Grundlagen der Gegenwartsphilosophie: Eine Einführung.* Stuttgart: UTB.

Goll-Kopka, A. (2009). Multi-family therapy with families of children with developmental delays, chronic illness and disabilities: "the Frankfurt multi-family therapy model". *Praxis der Kinderpsychologie und Kinderpsychiatrie, 58*, 716–732.

Goll-Kopka, A. (2012). *Multifamiliengruppen als therapeutisches Angebot bei somatischer Erkrankung und Behinderung (PhD thesis).* Oldenburg: Carl von Ossietzky Universität Oldenburg.

Goll-Kopka, A., & Born, A. (2018). Multifamilygroups as a psychosocial and Contextoriented intervention for somatic illness and disability. *Praxis der Kinderpsychologie und Kinderpsychiatrie, 67*, 568–586.

Gonzalez, S., & Steinglass, P. (2002). Application of multifamily groups in chronic medical disorders. In W. R. McFarlane (Ed.), *Multifamily groups in the treatment of severe psychiatric disorders.* New York: Guilford.

Guba, E. G., & Lincoln, Y. S. (1989). *Fourth generation evaluation.* Thousand Oaks, CA: Sage.

Haken, H. (1983). *Synergetics. An introduction.* Heidelberg: Springer.

Hanot, M. (2006). Systemic interviewing techniques for the social worker. *Thérapie Familiale, 27*, 75–89.

Harvey, D., Plummer, D., Pighills, A., & Tilley, P. (2013). Practitioner Research Capacity: A Survey of Social Workers in Northern Queensland. *Australian Social Work, 66*(4), 540–554.

Helps, S. (2017). The ethics of researching one's own practice. *Journal of Family Therapy, 39*, 348–365.

Hildenbrand, B. (1998). Qualitative Forschung in der systemischen Therapie. *System Familie, 11*, 112–119.

Holstein, J. A., & Gubrium, J. F. (2007). *Handbook of constructionist research.* New York: Guilford.

IQWIG Institut für Qualität und Wirtschaftlichkeit im Gesundheitswesen (2017). Systemische Therapie bei Erwachsenen als Psychotherapieverfahren. IQWiGBerichte – Nr. 513. Köln: IQWIG.

Just, U., Oelkers, R., Bender, S., Parzer, P., Ebinger, F., Weisbrod, M., & Resch, F. (2003). Emotional and behavioural problems in children and adolescents with primary headache. *Cephalalgia, 23*, 206–213.

Kriz, J. (2001). Self-Organization of Cognitive and Interactional Processes. In M. Matthies, H. Malchow, & J. Kriz (Eds.), *Integrative systems approaches to natural and social dynamics* (pp. 517–537). Heidelberg: Springer.

Krueger, R. A., & Casey, M. A. (2000). *Focus groups: A practical guide for applied research* (3rd ed.). Thousand Oaks, CA: Sage.

Lemmens, G. M. D., Eisler, I., Dierick, P., Lietaer, G., & Demyttenaere, K. (2009). Therapeutic factors in a systemic multi-family group treatment for major depression: patients' and partners' perspectives. *Journal of Family Therapy, 31*, 250–269.

Lock, A., & Strong, T. (2010). *Social constructionism: Sources and stirrings in theory and practice.* New York: Cambridge University Press.

Luhmann, N. (1977). Differentiation of society. *The Canadian Journal of Sociology, 2*, 29–53.

Luhmann, N. (1984). *Soziale Systeme.* Frankfurt am Main: Suhrkamp.

Lunt, N., & Shaw, I. (2017). Good practice in the conduct and reporting of practitioner research: Reflections from social work and social care. *Practice, 29*, 201–218.

McDaniel, M., Hepworth, J., & Doherty, W. J. (1992). *Medical family therapy: A biopsychosocial approach families with health problems.* New York: Basic.

McNamee, S., & Hosking, D. M. (2012). *Research and social change: A relational constructionist approach.* London: Routledge.

Mendenhall, T. J., & Doherty, W. J. (2005). Action research methods in family therapy. In F. Piercy & D. Sprenkle (Eds.), *Research methods in family therapy* (2nd ed., pp. 100–118). New York: Guilford.

Molde, S., & Diers, D. (1985). Nurse practitioner research: Selected literature review and research agenda. *Nursing Research, 34*, 362–367.

Moser, S. (Ed.). (2011). *Konstruktivistisch forschen. Methodologie, Methoden, Beispiele.* Wiesbaden: Springer VS.

Myers, D. G. (2014). *Psychologie.* Heidelberg: Springer.

Ochs, M. (2012a). Systemisch forschen per Methodenvielfalt – konzeptuelle Überlegungen und Anwendungsbeispiele. In M. Ochs & J. Schweitzer (Eds.), *Handbuch Forschung für Systemiker* (pp. 395–422). Göttingen: V&R.

Ochs, M. (2012b). Ein kleiner "Leitfaden" für die Durchführung systemischer Forschungsvorhaben (nicht nur) für Praktiker. In M. Ochs & J. Schweitzer (Eds.), *Handbuch Forschung für Systemiker* (pp. 423–448). Göttingen: V&R.

Ochs, M. (2013). Pluralität und Diversi(vi)tät systemischer Forschung. *Familiendynamik, 38*(1), 4–11.

Ochs, M. (2020). Die erkenntnistheoretischen Säulen und praxeologischen Grundorientierungen systemischen Arbeitens. In P. Bauer & M. Weinhardt (Eds.), *Systemische Kompetenzen entwickeln. Grundlagen, Lernprozesse und Didaktik.* Göttingen: Vandenhoeck & Ruprecht.

Ochs, M., Pfautsch, B., Schweitzer, J., Aderhold, V., Borst, U., & Cubellis, L. (2020). Systemic family work in the context of severe mental illnesses: Three evidence-based approaches. In K. Wampler (Ed.), *The handbook of systemic family therapy.* New York: Wiley.

Ochs, M., & Schweitzer, J. (Eds.). (2012). *Handbuch Forschung für Systemiker.* Göttingen: Vandenhoeck & Ruprecht.

Ochs, M., Seemann, H., Franck, G., Wredenhagen, N., Verres, R., & Schweitzer, J. (2005). Primary headache in children and adolescents: Therapy outcome and changes in family interaction patterns. *Families, Systems & Health, 23*, 30–53.

Ochs, M., & Thom, J. (2014). Psychotherapie(–forschung) in postpolitischen Zeiten. In I. J. Zwack & E. Nicolai (Eds.), *Systemische Streifzüge. Herausforderungen in systemischer Therapie und Beratung* (pp. 212–245). Göttingen: Vandenhoeck & Ruprecht.

OECD. (2015). *Frascati manual. The measurement of scientific, technological and innovation activities.* Paris: OECD Publishing.

Oelkers, R., Grosser, K., Lang, E., Geisslinger, G., Kobal, G., Brune, K., & Lötsch, J. (1999). Visual evoked potentials in migraine patients: Alterations depend on pattern spatial frequency. *Brain, 1122*, 1147–1155.

Orlinsky, D. E., Ambühl, H., Ronnestad, M. H., Davis, J., Gerin, P., Davis, M., … Cierpka, M. (1999). Development of psychotherapists: Concepts, questions, and methods of a collaborative international study. *Psychotherapy Research, 9*, 127–153.

Padberg, T. (2012). Warum lesen Psychotherapeuten keine Forschungsliteratur? *Psychotherapeut, 11*, 10–17.

Patzig, J., & Schiepek, G. (2015). Emotionsregulation und emotionsfokussiertes Prozessmonitoring in der Suchttherapie. In I. Sammet, G. Dammann, & G. Schiepek (Eds.), *Der psychotherapeutische Prozess. Forschung für die Praxis* (pp. 124–135). Stuttgart: Kohlhammer.

Powell, J., & Orme, J. (2011). Increasing the confidence and competence of social work researchers: What works? *British Journal of Social Work, 41*, 1566–1585.

Retzlaff, R., Brazil, S., & Goll-Kopka, A. (2008). Multifamily therapy in children with learning disabilities. *Praxis der Kinderpsychologie und Kinderpsychiatrie, 57*, 346–361.

Reynolds, V. (2014). A solidarity approach: The rhizone & messy inquiry. In G. Simon & A. Chard (Eds.), *Systemic inquiry. Innovations in reflexive practice research* (pp. 127–154). Farnhill: Everything is Connected Press.

Sackett, D. L., Rosenberg, W. M. C., Gray, J. A. M., Haynes, R. B., & Richardson, W. S. (1996). *Evidence based medicine: what it is and what it isn't. BMJ, 312*, 71–73.

Salter, L. (2017). Research as resistance and solidarity: 'Spinning transformative yarns'- a narrative inquiry with women going on from abuse and oppression. *Journal of Family Therapy, 39*, 366–385.

Satterfield, J. M., Spring, B., Brownson, R. C., Mullen, E. J., Newhouse, R. P., Walker, B. B., & Whitlock, E. P. (2009). Toward a transdisciplinary model of evidence-based practice. *The Millbank Quarterly, 87*, 368–390.

Schiepek, G. (2010). *Systemische Forschung. Eine Positionsbestimmung. Familiendynamik, 35*, 60–70.

Schiepek, G., & Strunk, G. (1994). *Dynamische Systeme. Grundlagen und Analysemethoden für Psychologen und Psychiater*. Heidelberg: Asanger.

Schön, D. A. (1983). *The reflective practitioner: How professionals think in action*. New York: Basic Books.

Shapiro, Y. (2015). Dynamical systems therapy (DST): Theory and practical applications. *Psychoanalytic Dialogues, 25*, 83–107.

Shaw, I. (2005). Practitioner research: Evidence or critique? *British Journal of Social Work, 35*, 1231–1248.

Sheinberg, M., & Brewster, M. K. (2014). Thinking and working relationally: Interviewing and constructing hypotheses to create compassionate understanding. *Family Process, 53*, 618–639.

Shotter, J. (1993). *Conversational realities: Constructing life through language*. London: Sage.

Simon, G. (2013). Relational ethnography: Writing and Reading in and about research relationships. *Forum Qualitative Forschung, 14*(1), Art. 4.

Simon, G. (2018). Eight criteria for quality in systemic practitioner research. *Murmurations: Journal of Transformative Systemic Practice, 1*, 42–60.

Simon, G., & Chard, A. (Eds.). (2014). *Systemic inquiry. Innovations in reflexive practice research*. Farnhill: Everything is Connected Press.

Simon, G. (2014). Systemic Inquiry as a form of Qualitative Research. In G. Simon, G., & A. Chard, (Eds.), Systemic inquiry. Innovations in reflexive practice research (pp. . Farnhill: Everything is Connected Press.

Sprenkle, D. H., & Piercy, F. P. (2005). *Research methods in family therapy*. New York: Guilford.

Stierlin, H. (1997). Zum aktuellen Stand der systemischen Therapie. *Familiendynamik, 22*, 348–362.

Stock, D. P. (2015). *Systems thinking for social change*. White River Junction, VT: Chelsea Green.

Strand, K., Cutforth, N., Stoecker, R., Marullo,S., & Donohue, P. (2003). Community-Based Research in Higher Education: Principles and Practices. San Francisco: Jossey-Bass/John Wiley Periodicals.

Sutter, T. (2009). *Interaktionistischer Konstruktivismus*. Wiesbaden: Springer VS.

Tass, P., & Haken, H. (1996). Synchronized oscillations in the visual cortex—a synergetic model. *Biological Cybernetics, 74*, 31–39.

Tomm, K. (1987). Interventive interviewing: Part I. strategizing as a fourth guideline for the therapist. *Family Process, 26*, 3–13.

Van der Donk, C., & van Lanen, B. (2018). Practitioner research in the practice and education of healthcare professionals in the Netherlands. *Texto & Contexto – Enfermagem, 27*, https://doi.org/10.1590/0104-070720180000650017.

von Foerster, H. (1981). *Observing Systems*. Seaside, Cal: Intersystems Publications.

von Schlippe, A., & Schweitzer, J. (2019). *Gewusst wie, gewusst warum: Die Logik systemischer Interventionen*. Göttingen: Vandenhoeck & Ruprecht.

von Sydow, K. (2015). *Systemische Therapie*. München: Reinhardt.

Wade, K., & Neuman, K. (2007). Practice-based research. *Social Work in Health Care, 44*, 49–64.

Willutzki, U., Teismann, T., & Schulte, D. (2012). Psychotherapy for social anxiety disorder: Long-term effectiveness of resource-oriented cognitive-behavioral therapy and cognitive therapy in social anxiety disorder. *Journal of Clinical Psychology, 68*, 581–591.

Wright, L. M. (1990). Research as a family therapy intervention technique. *Contemporary Family Therapy, 12*, 477–483.

Wulff, D., & St George, S. (2014). Research as daily practice. In G. Simon & A. Chard (Eds.), *Systemic inquiry: Innovations in reflexive practitioner research* (pp. 292–308). Farnhill: Everything is Connected Press.

Wulff, D., & St. George, S. (2016). Researcher as practitioner: Practitioner as researcher. In S. S. George & D. Wulff (Eds.), *Family therapy as socially transformative practice: Practical strategies (AFTA SpringerBriefs in Family Therapy)* (pp. 25–40). New York: Springer International.

Family Secrecy – A Challenge for Researchers

Eva Deslypere and Peter Rober

Introduction

A family secret has been defined as the intentional concealment of information by one or more family members who are impacted by it (Berger & Paul, 2008; Bok, 1982; Vangelisti & Caughlin, 1997). In dealing with family secrets, according to Imber-Black (1993), the questions "who knows the secret?" and "who does not know the secret?" are central. Several authors have emphasized that in family secrets the information that is withheld is critical to the one who the information is concealed from because it has impact on his/her life (Berger & Paul, 2008; Bok, 1982; Vangelisti & Caughlin, 1997). Interestingly, Imber-Black (1998) suggests secrecy is unhealthy (p. 19). Secrets can be "toxic" (p. 21) and "dangerous" (p.21) as they can seriously affect family relationships (Imber-Black, 1998). They create barriers and coalitions and affect family communication (Imber-Black, 1998; Karpel, 1980; Vangelisti & Caughlin, 1997). Family members may experience tension, anxiety, loneliness, and stress-related symptoms like sleeplessness, headaches, etc. (Imber-Black, 1998; Karpel, 1980).

Viewed from that perspective, the concept *family secret* fits well with some of the implicit truths of our Western culture. We live in a culture where open communication is promoted and openness is considered a sign of a healthy relationship (Merrill & Afifi, 2015). Some talk about the ideology of openness (Afifi, Shahnazi, Coveleski, Davis, & Merrill, 2016), as there seems to be a bias against secrecy (Caughlin, Afifi,

E. Deslypere (✉) · P. Rober
Institute for Family and Sexuality Studies (IFSS), Department of Neurosciences in the School of Medicine KU Leuven, Leuven, Belgium
e-mail: eva.deslypere@upckuleuven.be

© Springer Nature Switzerland AG 2020
M. Ochs et al. (eds.), *Systemic Research in Individual, Couple, and Family Therapy and Counseling*, European Family Therapy Association Series,
https://doi.org/10.1007/978-3-030-36560-8_11

Carpenter-Theune, & Miller, 2005): open communication is valued, and revealing secrets is considered to be healing and morally superior to keeping them (Ellis, 2008).

Notwithstanding the cultural bias against secrets, some authors have described also positive *aspects* of concealing information. Afifi, Olson, and Armstrong (2005), for instance, describe how a person can protect him/herself by concealing information from close others who are powerful and potentially violent. Ellis (2008) states that secrets can help establish bonds between people and might permit social order to continue uninterrupted. Other authors have highlighted the good intentions of people who hold secrets, highlighting how secret holders want to protect others by withholding information (e.g., Afifi et al., 2005; Papp, 1998).

Clinical Case Studies

Research into family secrecy is not an easy task. Particularly data collection poses a challenge. Because of the covert and sensitive nature of secrets, family members' loyalty and fear for negative reactions when the secret is disclosed, enquiry into secrecy is extremely difficult. This can help us understand why a great deal of research on family secrecy is based on anecdotal data like *clinical case studies*. Imber-Black (1993, 1998) and Selvini (1997), for instance, wrote about family secrets as they surfaced in the therapy room. They recount their struggles with what seems to be a dichotomous choice: Should I disclose the secrets or not? Imber-Black's case studies led her to conclude that a one-size fits-all approach does not apply to secrecy, as no two families with secrets are the same. Instead she argues for an "it all depends" position toward secrecy.

The case study research on family secrecy has led to interesting findings. Authors like Imber-Black and others have succeeded in mapping a lot of the territory (Imber-Black, 1998). They defined family secrets as an intentional concealment of information by one or more family members who are impacted by it. They distinguished family secrets from privacy, stating that in family secrets information that is withheld is critical to the one who the information is concealed from because it has impact on his/her life. Furthermore, they categorized the main topics of family secrets (suicide, adoption, etc.), and they identified the different types of family secrets. Importantly, they also mapped some of the destructive effects family secrets can have on family members. Implicitly or explicitly these family therapeutic approaches advised family therapists to carefully and expertly aim at disclosure of the family secret, as it would free the family members from the burden of the secret (Imber-Black, 1998).

Autoethnography

Besides clinical case studies, also autoethnography has been used to study family secrecy. Autoethnography is an approach to qualitative inquiry in which narrative writing about personal experiences is seen as a road to shared understanding

(Holman Jones, 2005; Lapadat, 2009). In the field of family therapy, autoethnography as a method is very rare. The first autoethnographic study in a family therapy journal was published in 2015 (Olson, 2015). In other fields like sociology and cultural anthropology, autoethnography is much more used. And as it happens, in the field of sociology, there have been a lot of interesting publications around the issue of family secrecy based on autoethnographic methods. In these publications, more than in the case study research, the complexity of family secrecy is highlighted (e.g. Goodall Jr., 2006, 2008; Kuhn, 1995; Pelias, 2008; Poulos, 2008).

Probably the best known and influential autoethnographic study of secrecy is Goodall's study (Goodall Jr., 2005). In his book *A Need to Know* (Goodall Jr., 2006), he tells the story of growing up in a "nuclear family with toxic secrets." He wrote about his father who was a CIA spy during the Cold War and the secrecy this entailed. In Goodall's family, the secrecy regarding his father's job was covered up with the story of his father being an ordinary government worker. It is not until inheriting his father's diary that Goodall discovered the true story and became the inheritor of his father's toxic secret. Even though his father was already dead, the discovery of the secret poisoned Goodall's relationship with his father. Goodall spent 2 years researching his father's life only to conclude, "in the end the story I have constructed remains incomplete" (Goodall Jr., 2005, p. 498). Following Goodall, other researchers wrote about their family secrets (e.g., Ellis, 2008; Pelias, 2008). In comparison with the traditional family therapy literature based on clinical case studies, autoethnographic research offers a fresh, humane perspective on family secrecy. It has an open-minded view on family secrecy as all families have secrets. The constructive as well as destructive powers of secrets led some of these researchers to the question *do we need to know?* or *do we, as a part of growing up, have to accept our families as they were and the secrets that they lived?* (Ellis, 2008). Maybe we don't have to know everything, and maybe some secrets help us lead a more satisfying life. Maybe we don't need to know the whole truth; maybe we just need a story to live with. For example, the story Goodall constructed allowed him to come to a better appreciation and understanding of his parents' need to keep secrets, and to move on (Goodall Jr., 2005).

Methodologically autoethnography is very inspiring, and in recent years, it has led to research on family secrecy along less obvious lines, also in the field of family therapy. In this chapter, we will refer to the study of family secrecy using an autoethnographical film, an autobiographical novel, and finally to an autoethnographical study of a family therapist's own family.

Study of an Autoethnographical Documentary Film

While most case studies used to research family secrecy are clinical case studies, Rober, Walravens, and Versteynen (2012) studied a nonclinical case of a family with a secret. The documentary film *Familiegeheim (trans. "family secret")* by Jaap van

Hoewijk tells the story of van Hoewijk's investigation into the death of his father and portrays a family in which the suicide of the father is kept secret from the three children. The film begins with van Hoewijk telling the viewers *"I wanted to find out what I was not allowed to discover."* During his quest to discover the truth, it became clear that everybody knew about his father's suicide except Jaap and his two younger sisters. They had been told their father died in a motorcycle accident. After the funeral, his father's existence was erased from the house: all his belongings, including photographs of him, were removed. This gave the children the impression that their father was a forbidden topic and that questions about him would not be appreciated by their mother. Remarkably, mother did not destroy the pictures of father. Instead she put them in three envelopes, one for each child.

The film shows that in trying to discover the untold story of his father's death, van Hoewijk bombards his mother with questions. However, she is reluctant to answer them and keeps concealing and hiding information. It seems as if she is constantly making a selection about what she can reveal and what not. For example, in talking with neighbors and family members, van Hoewijk learns that his parents did not have a happy marriage and his father even embezzled money from his employer. However, his mother insists everything was fine in her marriage. This leads van Hoewijk to call into question what his mother tells him. More than answers to his questions, what van Hoewijk is searching for is a dialogical space in which questions can be asked and truthful answers can be given.

The film portrays the gradual discovery of the untold story of the father's death. Knowing the truth about his father's death only raised more questions for van Hoewijk. Why did his father commit suicide? How did he die exactly? This shows that a new discovery does not necessarily lead to closure, but it may raise more questions. The suggestion in the film is clear: Probably there will always be things left untold (Goodall Jr., 2005).

The analysis of the film shows that the concept of family secrets does not fully grasp the complexity of family secrecy. The concept implies that the truth is hidden and that the real story is concealed. Also, the concept indicates that some family members know what is concealed while others do not. Furthermore, the concept suggests that because of the detrimental effects of the concealment, it would be better to disclose the hidden information. Finally, the concept indicates that the disclosure of what really happened would resolve the uncertainty of those who did not know. van Hoewijk's movie points out that what happens in a family when a traumatic experience is concealed is more complex than the concept of family secrets suggests. For example, although van Hoewijk's mother did not tell her children about the father's suicide, she did tell them he died in an accident. It seems that while some stories were left untold, other stories were told instead. Also, while the children did not know about the suicide, other people, for instance, mother's sister, knew. This indicates that mother made a selection in the disclosure of the information. Some information was said to all, some information was said to some, and some information was said to none.

Although the concept of family secrets implies that there is a truth that is hidden which may be revealed when the whole story is told, van Hoewijk's film demonstrates this is not the case. The disclosure of the father's suicide did not resolve van Hoewijk's uncertainty, instead it raised more questions and a deeper distrust.

These findings led the researchers (Rober et al., 2012) to propose the use of the concept *selective disclosure* as this concept seemed to better comprehend the complexities of family communication when sensitive information is not revealed. The concept refers to a process of selection as to whom to tell what, how much, and when. It is a continuing process in time filled with tensions, small decisions, and good intentions. The concept also implies that the disclosure of information will not resolve everything as there will always be things left untold. Thus, rather than more information what is needed is a dialogical space where some things can be said, while admitting that not everything will be said and respecting that there are good reasons for not revealing.

Interview Studies in the Field of Medically Assisted Procreation

While the study of a film, however interesting it might be, may not be enough grounds to question the usefulness of the concept of *family secret*, the importance of the alternative concept *selective disclosure* was further illustrated in interview studies in the field of assisted reproductive technologies (e.g., Indekeu, D'Hooghe, Daniels, Dierickx, & Rober, 2014; Van Parys et al., 2016; Wyverkens et al., 2017). In the beginning (second half of the twenty-first century) in the domain of medically assisted procreation secrecy was the preferred course of action. When undergoing medically assisted infertility treatments, couples were advised not to disclose their use of donor insemination and egg donation to their child (Golombok et al., 1996). The ethics committee of the *American Society for Reproductive Medicine* recommended to encourage couples to have intercourse immediately following insemination, to create ambiguity about the child's genetic identity which, in turn contributed further to secrecy (Paul & Berger, 2007). Policy changes in recent decades led to the removal of donor anonymity in several countries (e.g., New Zealand, The Netherlands, Sweden, Norway, etc.) (Wyverkens, Van Parys, & Buysse, 2015). Despite these changes, many parents of donor-conceived children remain silent about their child's biological origin (Murray, MacCallum, & Golombok, 2006; Wyverkens et al., 2017). Parents believe it would be more harmful than beneficial for their child and the family to reveal the truth. For instance, they feel disclosure would endanger the relationship between the child and nongenetic parent. In addition, parents want to protect the partner unable to conceive (Ilioi, Blake, Jadva, Roman, & Golombok, 2017).

Some research has focused on the process of disclosure. These researchers have noticed that disclosure is not a dichotomous issue (secret vs. disclosure); it is more complex than that. For instance, parents who decide to disclose the conception story do so gradually (Readings, Blake, Casey, Jadva, & Golombok, 2011; Van Parys et al., 2016). This means that the information given by parents to their child is tailored to the child's age, maturity, and questions. As such it can be viewed as a bidirectional process of building an acceptable *story they can live with* (Rober et al., 2012), with the best interest of the child in mind (Van Parys et al., 2016). Furthermore, it is a process of *selective disclosure* (Rober et al., 2012; Rober & Rosenblatt, 2013; Van Parys et al., 2016).

The Study of an Autobiographical Novel

Rober and Rosenblatt (2013) studied a chapter from James Agees novel *A death in the family*. This novel was published in 1957. *A Death in the Family* is considered a masterpiece of American literature. It is an autobiographical novel that tells the story of the way a family deals with the sudden death of the father Jay, who was killed in a car accident. Rober and Rosenblatt focused on the fourth chapter, in which the mother (Mary) is informed of the death of the father by her brother Andrew. Since the disclosure of the death of a loved one involves a choice process as what to tell and what not to tell, the focus of the study is on the process of selective disclosure.

More than traditional research methods, the analysis of detailed descriptions of the thoughts and concerns of the characters and their interactions gives insight in the inner process of family members' communication. It shows that before and during the bringing of the horrible news of the accident, a comprehensive thought process takes place. The family agrees without much discussion that Andrew, Mary's brother, should disclose what happened to Jay. The setting and time of the disclosure are carefully chosen. The sharing of the news is postponed until Mary's parents are present and the children are asleep. The spacious living room is chosen as location of disclosure. Mary's mother urges Mary to sit next to her, allowing Mary to hold her mother's hand for support. Also, in the telling of the story, a well thought-out selection takes place. The main elements Andrew wants Mary to hear are: Jay was alone in the car, and thus he did not have an affair; Jay died instantly, he did not suffer; and although Jay used to have a drinking problem, at the time of the accident he was not drunk. Andrew does not share the information that a witness suspected that Jay was drunk driving. This suggests that full disclosure is not the objective but creating a shared story they can all live with is.

At some point during the telling of the story, Mary starts to cry. Andrew stops talking instantaneously, and the family focuses on comforting Mary. When she is calmed down Andrew resumes his story. However, his fear of making Mary cry again affects his storytelling. This suggests that the storytelling is regulated by the emotions of the person considered the most emotionally vulnerable and by the discomfort of the other family members with the display of emotions. Silences are inserted when emotions are running high. Only when control is regained does the storytelling continue.

The study of Rober and Rosenblatt highlights that the process of selective disclosure is regulated by what they call *systemic emotion management*. To prevent emotionally vulnerable family members from being deluged by emotions, family members avoid certain topics and certainly would not want to put the deceased in a bad light. Silences are preferred when one is unsure as to what is acceptable to say and when the risk of overwhelming emotions is high. Systemic emotion management is not only directed at managing the emotions of the most vulnerable family member but also the emotions of the other family members. Self-reproach and feelings of guilt of the speaker for causing emotional outbursts may mediate the process of systemic emotion management. Furthermore, the analysis shows that although selective disclosure of the death of a loved one is often described as an interpersonal process, sometimes the negotiation on what to say and what not to say surfaces. For instance, after Mary's emotional outburst she insists *"I want to know - all of it .... Everything there is to tell."* (p. 181). The interpersonal and intrapersonal process of selective disclosure leads to an emotionally acceptable and shared story, a story to live by.

Interview Studies in the Field of Grief

This process of *systemic emotion management* can also be found in the communication process of grieving parents. Hooghe, Rosenblatt, and Rober (2018) explored the experiences of grieving parents related to the process of talking and not talking. They found that a process of emotional attunement, on an intrapersonal and interpersonal level, takes place when bereaved parents communicate about their child. On an intrapersonal level parents search for a balance between staying close to the child and not being overwhelmed by the pain of the loss. To be able to keep this balance, this sometimes meant withdrawing from the outside world. Not talking can be seen as a form of respect for one's own and each other's need to withdraw and not burden or be burdened by the emotions of the partner. On a relational level emotional regulation took place by observing the other when talking about the loss. A conversation is stopped, and words may be left unspoken as a way to spare each other.

An Autoethnographic Study of a Family Therapist's Own Family

An example of an autoethnographic study in the field of family therapy is Rober's study of the secrecy surrounding his grandfather's war experiences (Rober & Rosenblatt, 2015). His grandfather had been a prisoner of war during World War II. He was imprisoned in Stalag XVIIB were prisoners had to face poor living conditions, freezing temperatures, food scarcity, and death. Throughout his captivity, Rober's grandfather wrote letters to his family, the main message always being "I'm ok."

In his letters Rober's grandfather speaks about the good times they had in the past or he refers to the future when they will all be reunited. He never mentions the present and his life in the camp. After he was liberated, the silence about his war experiences remained.

Silence can be conceptualized as being the result of psychological or political processes. In a psychological conceptualization silence is viewed as a symptom of posttraumatic stress. Silence can also be regarded as a result of political suppression. Both conceptualizations of silence are considered to be problematic. The solution lies in giving words so the repressed stories and experiences can be voiced. However, Rober points out that silence can also be life-giving. The "it's ok" messages in his grandfather's letters can be viewed as a way to reassure himself. The messages allowed him to keep traumatic experiences at a distance, not to dwell on his dreary living conditions and survive the camp. Research on prisoners of war (Makepeace, 2017) and studies in the field of trauma acknowledge the life-giving power of silence. Especially in cases of prolonged or chronic stress or trauma, emotionally ventilating and working through traumatic events and painful experiences from the past may cause overwhelming re-experiencing of painful events, impeding the healing process. (Dalgaard & Montgomery, 2015; Raphael, Meldrum, & McFarlane, 1995; Summerfield, 1999).

The "it's ok" messages not only protected his own sanity and survival, they were probably also meant to reassure his family. Knowing their husband and father was safe allowed his family to focus on their own survival. After the war, the camp and what Rober's grandfather went through were never mentioned. The continued silences about his experiences after the war can be understood as his grandfather's way of protecting himself and his loved ones from the pain of his past.

Rober and Rosenblatt's research on Rober's grandfather led them to conclude that not all family secrets are toxic. This may be very important for systemic practice. Rober and Rosenblatt urge therapists not only to consider the destructive aspects of silence but the life-giving aspects as well. Furthermore, it is important for therapists to listen, not only to what a client says but also to the client's silences and hesitations to speak. Working with the dialectical tension between those family members who want to speak and those who are hesitant often leads to the creation of a space to talk safely about things that had been left unsaid.

Family Secrecy and Selective Disclosure

The research on family secrecy – using different methodological approaches – has led to a general model of *selective disclosure as a relational attunement process* (see Fig. 1). When a parent is confronted with a shocking experience (e.g., a death in the family, an unexpected pregnancy, an unspeakable trauma, etc.), the parent will sense his/her own vulnerability as well as the vulnerability of one's loved ones. In order to protect oneself and one's loved ones, the parent will selectively disclose what happened in the form of a narrative. Some things are said, other things remain

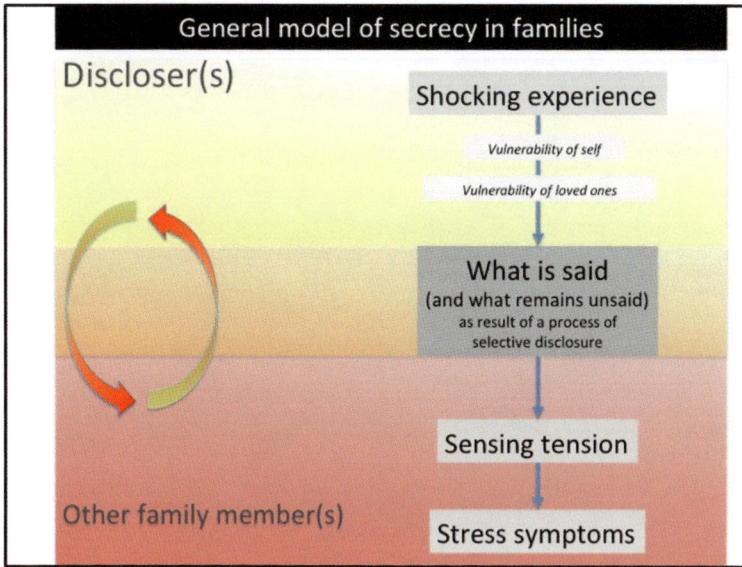

Fig. 1 General model of selective disclosure

unspoken. While this narrative may partly fill in a gap, the other family members (partner, son, daughter, etc.) may sense tensions, and this may result in stress symptoms for some of them (probably the most vulnerable ones).

The research on family secrecy highlights the complexity of family dynamics when important information is not shared and has led to reflection on the concept of family secret itself. It strongly suggests that the question should be posed if a concept like *selective disclosure* is not better fitted to capture the complexity of secrecy than the concept of *family secret*. Disclosure is not viewed as dichotomous (secrecy or disclosure) and is not defined as a "moment in time" act but rather as an ongoing process through time (Indekeu et al., 2013; Rober et al., 2012). The concept highlights that what we are dealing with is a multifaceted, bidirectional attunement process; a process filled with tensions, small decisions, and good intentions (Van Parys et al., 2016). It refers to a process of selection of what to tell, to whom, how to tell, when to tell, and so on (Rober & Rosenblatt, 2013). It seems to essentially be an intrapersonal and interpersonal process of responsive emotional attunement (Hooghe et al., 2018; Rober, 2017), in which the discloser has the vulnerability of his/her loved ones at heart, as well as one's own vulnerability (see Fig. 2).

While disclosing, the discloser monitors the reactions of the family members to which he/she tells his/her story. The selection of what is said and what remains unsaid seems to be moderated by the family member that is considered most vulnerable emotionally, very often, but not always, one of the children (Rober & Rosenblatt, 2013) (see Fig. 3).

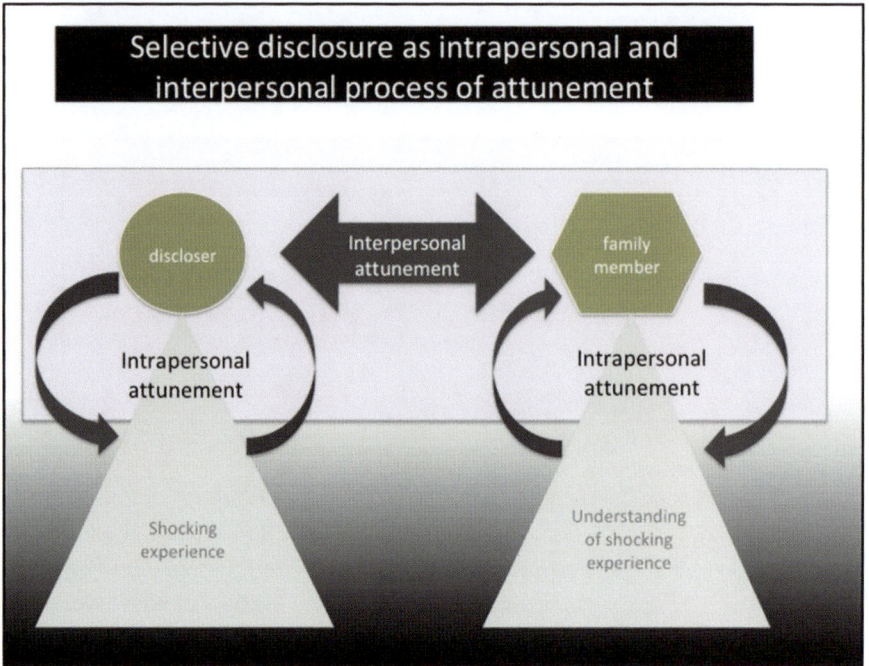

Fig. 2 Summarizes the main characteristics of the process of selective disclosure when there is one discloser and one family member to which the information is disclosed

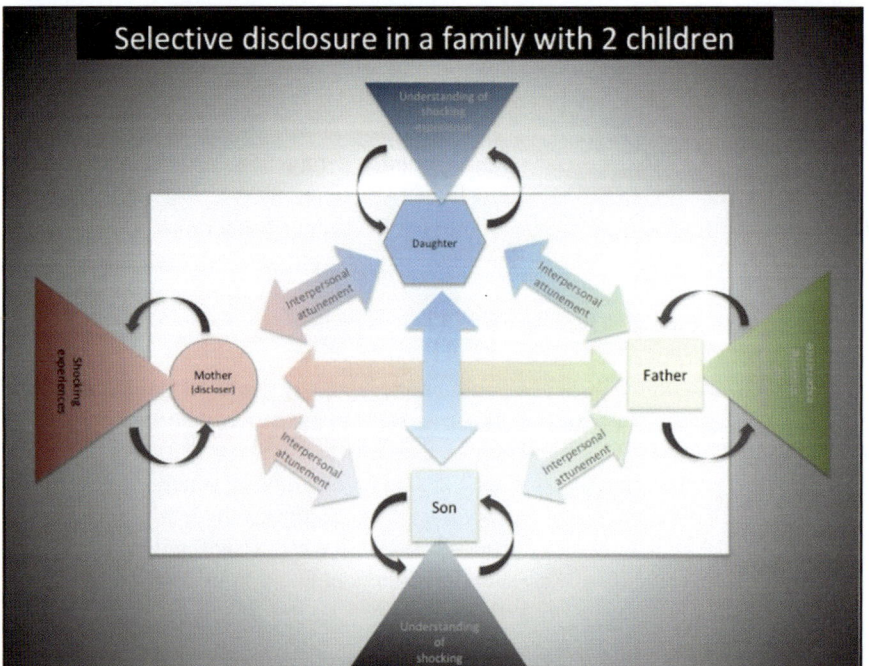

Fig. 3 Summarizes these characteristics in a family with one discloser (by way of example, the mother), and three other family members (father, son, daughter)

Implied in the concept of *selective disclosure* is the idea that whatever is said, other things remain unsaid as the main aim of family members is to tell stories that don't harm loved ones (Pelias, 2008). In addition, the concept suggests that what is needed, rather than more information, is the creation of a dialogical space in which questions can be asked and some things can be said; knowing and accepting that not everything will be revealed (Rober et al., 2012).

The Family Therapist

While it is clear that the research of family secrecy has led to interesting findings, it is remarkable that the focus of the research is almost exclusively on the family and on the harmful consequences of secrets (e.g., Imber-Black, 1998). As far as we know there is only one study that focuses on the perspective of the professional helper: a focus group study of experienced family therapists. In this study of Deslypere and Rober (2018), the researchers want to try to understand the experiences of family therapists when they are confronted with secrets. The data indicate that family secrets evoke strong experiences, like powerlessness and anger, in therapy sessions. Managing these emotions poses a challenge for therapists. The findings highlight that therapists employ several strategies for dealing with these challenges. One of the strategies therapists use is to try to avoid being cornered by the secret. However, they not always succeed in this difficult task. So, when this avoiding strategy does not work, and they are confronted with family secrets, therapists seem to make a choice between trying to bear the secret with the secret keeper and – what they call – "taking action." For most of the participants taking action entails trying to create space to talk about what was kept unsaid in the family. This strategy is meant as an invitation to disclose and as such corresponds with the traditional view on secrecy where the objective is disclosure. For a minority of participants in our study however taking action consisted not only of moving toward disclosure but also of exploring the secret without actual disclosing it. Therapists who use this strategy explored the silences, hesitations, and the good reasons clients have for keeping secrets. This strategy builds on the concept of selective disclosure.

Toward the Future

Based on the findings of this focus group research, we are preparing further research, using a methodology that has hardly been used in the context of the study of family secrecy: *tape-assisted recall (TAR) interviewing* (Elliott, 1986). This method of data collection has been used mainly in psychotherapy process research on the experiences of clients in therapy (e.g., Rennie, 1990, 1992, 1994). We used this method to study the therapist's inner conversation during psychotherapy sessions (Rober, Elliott, Buysse, Loots, & De Corte, 2008a, 2008b). Recently we also used it in our research of selective disclosure of traumatic experiences in refugee families (e.g., Kevers, Rober, & De Haene, 2018; Kevers, Rober, Rousseau & De Haene, submitted). We are confident that the use of the TAR methodology will lead to a deeper understanding of the ways family therapists deal with family secrecy in their practices.

References

Afifi, T. A., Olson, L., & Armstrong, C. (2005). The chilling effect and family secrets. Examining the role of self-protection, other-protection, and communication efficacy. *Human Communication Research, 31*(4), 564–598.

Afifi, T. A., Shahnazi, A. F., Coveleski, C., Davis, S., & Merrill, A. (2016). Testing the ideology of openness: The comparative effects of talking, writing, and avoiding a stressor on rumination and health. *Human Communication Research, 43*(4), 76–101.

Berger, R., & Paul, M. (2008). Family secrets and the family functioning: The case of donor assistance. *Family Process, 47*(4), 553–566.

Bok, S. (1982). *Secrets: On the ethics of concealment and revelations.* New York: Pantheon Books.

Caughlin, J. P., Afifi, T. D., Carpenter-Theune, K. E., & Miller, L. E. (2005). Reasons for, and consequences of, revealing personal secrets in close relationships: A longitudinal study. *Personal Relationships, 12,* 43–59. https://doi.org/10.1111/j.1350-4126.2005.00101.x

Dalgaard, N. T., & Montgomery, E. (2015). Disclosure and silencing: A systematic review of the literature on patterns of trauma communication in refugee families. *Transcultural Psychiatry, 52*(5), 579–593. https://doi.org/10.1177/1363461514568442

Deslypere, E. & Rober, P. (2018). Family Secrecy in Family Therapy Practice: An Explorative Focus Group Study. *Family Process* (published online), doi.org/10.1111/famp.12409

Elliott, R. (1986). Interpersonal process recall (IPR) as a psychotherapy process research method. In L. S. Greenberg & W. M. Pinsof (Eds.), *The psychotherapeutic process: A research handbook* (pp. 503–527). New York: Guilford.

Ellis, C. (2008). Do we need to know? *Qualitative Inquiry, 14*(7), 11314–11320. https://doi.org/10.1177/1077800408322681

Golombok, S., Brewaeys, A., Cook, R., Giavazzi, M. T., Guerra, D., Mantovani, A., … Dexeus, S. (1996). The European study of assisted reproduction families: Family functioning and child development. *Human Reproduction, 11*(10), 2324–2331.

Goodall, H. L., Jr. (2008). My family secret. *Qualitative Inquiry, 14*(7), 1305–1308.

Goodall, H. L., Jr. (2005). Narrative inheritance: A nuclear family with toxic secrets. *Qualitative Inquiry, 11,* 492–513.

Goodall, H. L., Jr. (2006). *A need to know: The clandestine history of a CIA family.* Walnut Creek, CA: Left Coast Press.

Holman Jones, S. (2005). Autoethnography: Making the personal political. In N. K. Denzin & Y. S. Lincoln (Eds.), *Handbook of qualitative research* (3rd ed., pp. 763–792). London: Sage.

Hooghe, A., Rosenblatt, P., & Rober, P. (2018). "We hardly ever talk about it": Emotional responsive attunement in couples after a child's death. *Family Process, 57,* 226–240. https://doi.org/10.1111/famp.12274

Ilioi, E., Blake, L., Jadva, V., Roman, G., & Golombok, S. (2017). The role of age of disclosure of biological origins in the psychological wellbeing of adolescents conceived by reproductive donation: A longitudinal study from age 1 to age 14. *Journal of Child Psychology and Psychiatry, 58*(3), 315–324.

Imber-Black, E. (1993). Secrets in families and family therapy: An overview. In E. Imber-Black (Ed.), *Secrets in families and family therapy* (pp. 3–28). New York: Norton.

Imber-Black, E. (1998). *The secret life of families.* New York: Bantam Books.

Indekeu, A., D'Hooghe, T., Daniels, K. R., Dierickx, K., & Rober, P. (2014). 'Of course he's our child': Transitions in social parenthood in donor sperm recipient families. *Reproductive Biomedicine Online, 28*, 106–115.

Indekeu, A., Dierickx, K., Schotsmans, P., Daniels, K. R., Rober, P., & D'Hooghe, T. (2013). Factors contributing to parental decision-making in disclosing donor conception: A systematic review. *Human Reproduction Update, 19*(6), 714–733. https://doi.org/10.1093/humupd/dmt018

Karpel, M. (1980). Family secrets. *Family Process, 19*, 295–306.

Kevers, R., Rober, P., & De Haene, L. (2018). Unraveling the mobilization of memory in research with refugees. *Qualitative Health, 28*(3), 456–465. https://doi.org/10.1177/1049732317746963

Kevers, R., Rober, P., Rousseau, C. & De Haene, L. (submitted). Silencing or Silent Transmission? An Exploratory Study on Trauma Communication in Kurdish Refugee Families.

Kuhn, A. (1995). *Family secrets: Acts of memory and imagination*. London: Verso.

Lapadat, J. C. (2009). Writing our way into shared understanding: Collaborative autobiographical writing in the qualitative methods class. *Qualitative Inquiry, 15*, 955–979.

Makepeace, C. (2017). *Captives of war: British prisoners of war in Europe in the second world war*. Cambridge (UK): Cambridge University Press.

Merrill, A. F., & Afifi, T. D. (2015). Attachment-related differences in secrecy and rumination in romantic relationships. *Personal Relationships, 22*, 259–274. https://doi.org/10.1111/pere.12078

Murray, C., MacCallum, F., & Golombok, S. (2006). Egg donation parents and their children: Follow-up at age 12 years. *Fertility and Sterility, 85*(3), 610–618. https://doi.org/10.1016/j.fertnstert.2005.08.051

Olson, M. (2015). An auto-ethnographic study of "open dialogue": The illumination of snow. *Family Process, 54*, 716–129.

Papp, P. (1998). The worm in the bud: Secrets between parents and children. In E. Imber-Black (Ed.), *Secrets in families and family therapy* (pp. 66–85). New York: Norton.

Paul, M. S., & Berger, R. (2007). Topic avoidance and family functioning in families conceived with donor insemination. *Human Reproduction, 22*(9), 2566–2571.

Pelias, R. J. (2008). H.L. Goodall's a need to know and the stories we tell ourselves. *Qualitative Inquiry, 14*(7), 1309–1313. https://doi.org/10.1177/1077800408322680

Poulos, C. N. (2008). *Accidental ethnography: An inquiry into family secrecy*. Walnut Creek, CA: Left Coast Press.

Raphael, B., Meldrum, L., & McFarlane, A. (1995). Does debriefing after psychological trauma work? *British Medical Journal, 310*, 1479–1480. https://doi.org/10.1136/bmj.310.6993.1479

Readings, J., Blake, L., Casey, P., Jadva, V., & Golombok, S. (2011). Secrecy, disclosure and everything in-between: Decisions of parents of children conceived by donor insemination. *egg donation and surrogacy. Reproductive BioMedicine Online, 22*, 485–495. https://doi.org/10.1016/j.rbmo.2011.01.014

Rennie, D. L. (1990). Toward a representation of the client's experience of the psychotherapy hour. In G. Lietaer, J. Rombauts, & R. Van Balen (Eds.), *Client-centered and experiential therapy in the nineties* (pp. 155–172). Leuven: Leuven University Press.

Rennie, D. L. (1992). Qualitative analysis of the client's experience of psychotherapy: The unfolding of reflexivity. In S. G. Toukmanian & D. L. Rennie (Eds.), *Psychotherapy process research: Paradigmatic and narrative approaches* (pp. 211–233). London: Sage.

Rennie, D. L. (1994). Storytelling psychotherapy: The client's subjective experience. *Psychotherapy, 31*, 234–243.

Rober, P. (2017). *Therapy together: Family therapy as a dialogue*. London: Palgrave Macmillan.

Rober, P., Elliott, R., Buysse, A., Loots, G., & De Corte, K. (2008a). What's on the therapist's mind? A grounded theory analysis of family therapist reflections during individual therapy sessions. *Psychotherapy Research, 18*(1), 48–57.

Rober, P., Elliott, R., Buysse, A., Loots, G., & De Corte, K. (2008b). Positioning in the therapist's inner conversation: A dialogical model based on a grounded theory analysis of therapist reflections. *Journal of Marital and Family Therapy, 34*, 406–421.

Rober, P., & Rosenblatt, P. C. (2013). Selective disclosure in a first conversation about a family death in James Agee's novel "a death in the family". *Death Studies, 37*, 172–194.

Rober, P., & Rosenblatt, P. C. (2015). Silence and memories of war: An autoethnographic exploration of family secrecy. *Family Process, 56*(1), 250–261. https://doi.org/10.1111/famp.12174

Rober, P., Walravens, G., & Versteynen, L. (2012). "In search of a tale they can live with": About loss, family secrets, and selective disclosure. *Journal of Marital and Family Therapy, 38*(3), 1–13. https://doi.org/10.1111/j.1752-0606.2011.00237.x

Selvini, M. (1997). Family secrets: The case of the patient kept in the dark. *Contemporary Family Therapy, 19*(3), 315–335. https://doi.org/10.1023/A:1026131609210

Summerfield, D. (1999). A critique of seven assumptions behind psychological trauma programmes in war-affected areas. *Social Science and Medicine, 48*(10), 1449–1462.

Van Parys, H., Wyverkens, E., Provoost, V., De Sutter, P., Pennings, G., & Buysse, A. (2016). Family communication about donor conception: A qualitative study with lesbian parents. *Family Process, 55*(1), 139–154. https://doi.org/10.1177/1049732315606684

Vangelisti, A. L., & Caughlin, J. P. (1997). Revealing family secrets: The influence of topic, function, and relationships. *Journal of Social and Personal Relationships, 14*(5), 679–705.

Wyverkens, E., Provoost, V., Ravelingen, A., Pennings, G., De Sutter, P., & Buysse, A. (2017). The meaning of the sperm donor for heterosexual couples: Confirming the position of the father. *Family Process, 56*(1), 203–216. https://doi.org/10.1111/famp.12156

Wyverkens, E., Van Parys, H., & Buysse, A. (2015). Experiences of family relationships among donor-conceived families: A meta-ethnography. *Qualitative Health Research, 25*(9), 1223–1240. https://doi.org/10.1177/1049732314554096

Part III
Answering Clinical Issues Using Scientific Knowledge and Methods

Mentalization in Systemic Therapy and Its Empirical Evidence

Eia Asen and Peter Fonagy

The Emergence of Mentalizing Approaches

Mentalizing (Fonagy, Steele, Steele, Moran, & Higgitt, 1991) refers to the attitude and skills involved in understanding mental states, both one's own as well as those of others, and their connections with feelings and behaviour. The terms 'mentalization' and 'mentalizing' are often used interchangeably; the latter is derived from a verb and therefore perhaps more accurately captures that this is a continuous activity rather than a fixed state of mind or the specific characteristic of an individual. Mentalizing mostly occurs without effort or specific consciousness; it is a process of perceiving and interpreting human behaviour in terms of intentional mental states such as feelings, needs, reasons or purposes. Mentalizing enables us to create a picture of the thoughts, feelings and intentions of those around us and to help us make sense of their actions in the same terms that we organize our own subjective experiences. It is important for representing, communicating and regulating feelings and belief states linked to one's wishes and desires. Some of the characteristics of effective mentalizing are listed in Table 1.

'Effective mentalizing' does not mean that one has to be reflective and to mentalize explicitly at all times, but to find a balance between intuition and reflection, reasons and feelings, between being self-reflective and considering external situations, between thinking about one's own reactions and the experiences of others.

Mentalizing is a fundamentally bidirectional or transactional social process which develops in the context of interactions with others, and in the first instance in the context of early attachment relationships. Its quality in relation to understanding others is influenced by how well those around us mentalize. The experience of how other people mentalize is internalized, enabling us to enhance our own capacity for

E. Asen (✉) · P. Fonagy
Anna Freud National Centre for Children and Families, University College London,
London, UK

© Springer Nature Switzerland AG 2020
M. Ochs et al. (eds.), *Systemic Research in Individual, Couple, and Family Therapy and Counseling*, European Family Therapy Association Series,
https://doi.org/10.1007/978-3-030-36560-8_12

Table 1 Some characteristics of effective mentalizing

Openness to discovery: a stance of curiosity towards mental states
Impact awareness: understanding how one is affected by the mental states of other people and that one may affect their states of mind
Safe uncertainty: the knowledge that one can never be really sure about what goes on in other people's mind
Perspective-taking: the ability to see oneself through the eyes of others and appreciation that others can see the world in ways different from us
Ability to show empathy
Ability to 'give and take': the skill of turn-taking
Autobiographical continuity: the capacity to connect past and present experiences
Belief in changeability
Taking responsibility and assuming accountability for one's feelings, thoughts and actions
Ability to trust and to assume a non-paranoid stance
Playfulness and self-mocking humour
Humility; knowing the limits of one's abilities and knowledge

empathizing and better engaging in interactive social processes (Fonagy, Gergely, Jurist, & Target, 2002). In situations of stress, difficulties in mentalizing almost inevitably arise. If mentalizing cannot be restored, a rapidly emerging vicious cycle can emerge, with intense emotions erupting, leading to a temporary loss of the capacity to think about the thoughts and feelings of others and the self in a balanced way (Bateman & Fonagy, 2016). For example, when stressed, a parent's mind might become temporarily closed to seeing his child from a perspective other than his own. So when she is calling out for her father to play with her, whilst he is working on his computer, he might see this as her just 'being difficult', and call out to her to "*be quiet and wait*" and to entertain herself. If the child feels that she is not being appropriately responded to, she may escalate her demands and accompanying behaviours to 'get through' to the father in the hope that he will respond. However, the intensification of the child's behaviour is likely to further derail the father's capacity to mentalize (his child and, recursively so, himself), and the two are quite likely to end up in a vicious cycle of non-mentalizing. In other words, the child's emotional arousal compromises the parent's capacity to provide the psychological recognition that the child craves. This happens intermittently a lot in ordinary family life, but when this non-mentalizing cycle becomes chronic, it can lead to more serious difficulties.

A major objective of mentalization-informed family work is to enhance and maintain mentalizing during emotionally highly charged family discourses which so often trigger and sustain family conflicts, including intra-family violence. The focus of this type of work is on the contexts that generate the specific feelings, needs, desires, beliefs and thoughts that may contribute to the collapse of mentalizing, with the aim of disrupting the feedback cycle of non-mentalizing that generates confusing and destructive interactions between family members. The ability to see oneself through the eyes of others and appreciate that others can see the world in ways different from us is at the heart of effective mentalizing. Perspective-taking is often impaired, and at times completely lacking, in families where acrimony, violence and mutual blame are common currency.

Over the past 10–20 years many systemic practitioners have attempted to 'remember' and integrate psychodynamic concepts. Bridges were re-built between the psychoanalytic and systemic worlds (Akister & Reibstein, 2004; Dallos, 2006; Diamond & Siqueland, 1998; Flaskas, 2002; Fraenkel & Pinsof, 2001) and the arrival of mentalization-based therapy (MBT), developed initially for adults presenting with borderline personality disorder (Bateman & Fonagy, 2016), further inspired systemic practitioners. A family-focused form of MBT emerged, MBT-F, leading to various attempts to manualize this approach (Asen & Fonagy, 2012b; Fearon et al., 2006; Keaveny et al., 2012). However, questions were raised soon whether MBT-F could really be regarded as yet another new 'brand' of family therapy, or whether one was dealing merely with a new emphasis when working with families, with some innovative and plenty of rather familiar techniques. Our own view is that mentalizing is an important ingredient of *all* psychotherapies (Fonagy & Allison, 2014) and that it can enrich systemic practice; it brings forth a set of strategies and techniques that can be grafted on to well-established systemic approaches.

The Basic Clinical Model

As in systemic therapy, the key proposition of the mentalizing approach is that emotional and behavioural problems are essentially relational in nature. However, MBT specifically holds that it is the breakdown in mentalizing which gives rise to relational problems that undermine family coping, creativity and resilience. Families and individuals vary in their capacity to mentalize for a multitude of reasons (e.g. genetics, early experience, trauma, current stressors). Chronic problems with mentalizing can contribute to distressing and stressful family interactions which further undermine mentalization. Given that the consideration, interpretation and appraisal of mental states (in self and others) are all essential for healthy relationships, the primary goal of therapy is to terminate non-mentalizing interactions and communications and to restore effective mentalizing. To that effect the primary therapeutic focus is on the mental states – the thoughts, feelings, wishes, needs, desires and beliefs – of each member of the family, and the relationships between them (Asen & Fonagy, 2012a).

To achieve this, the therapist shows a genuine interest in wanting to understand family members' different perspectives – even those of family members not present. He pays careful attention to levels of arousal and comments when family mentalizing appears to go 'off line'. He notices and names family patterns of interaction and works with them directly in the 'here and now'. He explores thoughts, needs and emotions in a relational context; and he remembers to mentalize himself – in other words, he pays attention to his own mental states and is prepared to explore openly the impact these may have on the family. The therapist acknowledges and positively connotes different perspectives put forward by family members, checking repeatedly and explicitly that he has properly understood what somebody has said or means (*"let me just check that I've got this right"*). The therapist also continuously demonstrates that he can simply not know what anyone feels, without asking questions to find out. He may assist family members to communicate and express what they feel by, for example, stopping the conversation to ask what it is that the person feels she cannot say or explain. When a family member engages in blaming statements, such as "*he's always trying to wind me up!*" the therapist may inquire: "*and does this feel to you that he is being deliberately annoying? Or could there be other reasons?*" The therapist can follow this up with 'triadic mentalization-eliciting' questions, such as for one of the family members to comment on the relationship between two other people: "*what do you think it was like for your Mum that time that you had a tantrum in the car?*" or "*how do you think your parents felt towards each other when you were screaming so much?*" Invoking hypothetical scenarios and using 'what if' questions explicitly encourages people to temporarily slip into the shoes of another family member: "*what would you think she would have felt if he had just walked out of the room at that point? And do you think your father might have felt the same or something quite different? What if your mother had just left the room*" and to the mother: "*what did you think he would think and feel if you did stop?*"

These questions are reminiscent of the 'circular questions' put forward by the Milan team many decades ago (Selvini Palazzoli, Boscolo, Cecchin, & Prata, 1980). However, their aims were both similar and yet somewhat different from those in the use of questioning in MBT. The Milan team's questioning process aimed to create and highlight differences, to draw connections and distinctions between family members in order to provide information that framed problems in new ways and released new information about the problem into the system. This, they argued, would encourage new ways of viewing family interactions and communications. The Milan team invented specific questions to achieve this by, for example, investigating a dyadic relationship by asking a third person for their perceptions on that relationship. The focus was primarily on behavioural sequences and each person's interpretation of behaviour by, for example, asking family members to rank each other on specific behaviours so that discrepancies in the views of various family members became more noticeable as a way of establishing circularity and new meaning. One of the aims of these techniques was to "*fix the point in the history of the system when important coalitions underwent a shift and the subsequent adaptation of that shift became problematic for the family*" (Penn, 1982, p. 272) so that the differences in family relationships before and after the problem emerged became more evident.

Whilst mentalization-focused techniques also aim to encourage family members to adopt new and different perspectives, the main goal is to focus on the states of mind of each family member and, via a recursive process, on each individual's own state of mind in relation to everyone else. The aim is *not* to ask circular questions in order to devise elaborate hypotheses on problem emergence and family dynamics, but to strengthen attachments and other aspects of family relationships by promoting effective mentalizing. Mentalization-focused interventions often move from initial orienting questions to creating an agreed language about affect. The interpersonal and emotional context of important events will always be explored by reference to

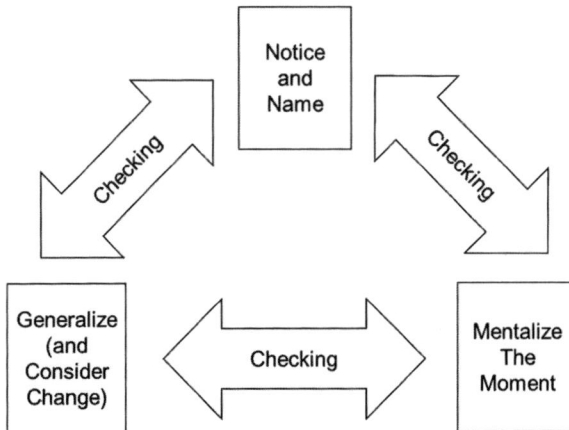

Fig. 1 The mentalizing loop

accompanying mental states. This can be quite a taxing demand, as family members often want to restate the sequence of concrete events and what they see as 'facts'.

Therapists themselves may serve as appropriate role models for mentalizing when they ask for clarification and reflection, using the sequence of 'stop, replay, explore and reflect'. This is particularly useful when faced with crass examples of non-mentalizing. The reviewing process by which mentalizing was impaired or lost is a key effective component of the approach. Unless the therapists determinedly 'stop' or 'pause' non-mentalizing narratives, so that the feelings and thoughts at the moment before the loss of mentalization can be re-captured, they may inadvertently feed into the proliferation of a non-mentalizing stance. The 'pause and review' technique, part of the mentalizing loop (see Fig. 1), has the effect of slowing down interactions, thereby gradually permitting each family member to resume effective mentalizing, in which emotion is integrated with cognition, and the focus on self and others gets equal weight. The sequence of (1) action, (2) pause and (3) reflection aims to restore balance to mentalizing. The rebalancing will be reflected in relevant commentary that implies (1) curiosity, (2) respect for the opacity of other minds, (3) awareness of the impact of affect on self and others, (4) perspective-taking, (5) narrative continuity and (6) a sense of agency and trust.

The Mentalizing Loop

In order to facilitate the emergence of productive mental states, the therapist constantly tracks the family members' ability to mentalize. When the capacity to mentalize is undermined, the therapist helps the family member to recover from this disruption and to reinstate mentalizing processes. The mentalizing loop (Asen & Fonagy, 2012b) is a tool as well as a 'route map' which defines the therapist's stance, allowing him to support both his own and the family members' effective mentalizing. The mentalizing loop can describe and draw attention to specific interactions and communications between family members. Focusing explicitly on these states of mind – by *'noticing and naming'* them – has the effect of putting family interactions temporarily on hold. Here the therapist might notice a meaningful family interaction and decide to punctuate it: *"I noticed that when you father talked about the fight you had with your son James, you mother, looked away. Has anybody noticed this or is this my own imagination?"* The therapist's emphasis on a certain event is followed by an act of checking whether this observation has also any validity for the family members: *"has anybody else noticed this?"* The act of checking is of great importance and repeats itself throughout all phases of the loop because it models the mentalizing process. Furthermore, it creates a respectful and inquisitive setting and protects the therapist's own position from becoming a non-mentalizing one. After all, the therapist's mentalizing capacity – like anyone's – inevitably falters at times and the mentalizing approach encourages honesty about this. It may, for example, be sometimes appropriate for the therapist to talk about how mentalizing fluctuates and, if temporarily lost, how it comes back 'online'.

Once the therapist has received acknowledgement and permission from the family members to further explore the subject, the main part of the intervention can begin: *'mentalizing the moment'*. The therapist facilitates this by encouraging everyone to contemplate other family members' feelings and thoughts, for example by asking: *"what are your thoughts about what just happened? What do you imagine mother is feeling that makes her behave like this? And how does this affect others? What do you make of it, father? Can I ask you, Mary, what it feels like for you when this happens between your parents? And what do you think, mother, it feels like for Mary or your husband? If one could see thought bubbles coming out of your wife's head, what might be 'written' in them?"* In this way, the therapist animates family members to bring in their perspectives, to brainstorm about states of mind ('mindstorming'), and to always check with others whether they see matters similarly or differently. This process of continuous checking – which includes the therapist – creates a loop: what has been noticed is named and what has been named is questioned, and perceptions are checked all round. When family members are encouraged to rewind and review a specific sequence, a meta-perspective is generated, which can reignite an effective mentalizing stance. At some point, the therapist may ask a family member to connect the here and now mental states to other similar situations that may arise in the course of ordinary family life, in an attempt to link the specifics of the acute interactions to the general and habitual patterns unfolding at home. This can be facilitated by a simple open question: *"Have you noticed that things like this are also happening at home?"* This, in turn, puts family members into a position that allows them to contemplate how similar situations could be managed in less problematic ways in the future, perhaps in response to the therapist asking: *"and how might you manage this differently next time something like this happens?"* It is this move to *'generalizing and considering change'* which appeals to family members' creativity and self-help potential and, if it leads to suggestions by one family member, then this is *'noticed and named'* by the therapist: *"I can see that Dad thinks if this happens, Mum should take him calmly aside and not talk in front of the child – have I got that right?"* and the *'checking'* loop starts again.

Innovative Techniques to Stimulate Mentalizing

Various playful techniques, described in more detail elsewhere (Asen & Fonagy, 2017), have been developed with the aim to stimulate mentalizing in a family context. Winnicott (Winnicott, 1971) has written extensively about the therapeutic use of play and stated that playing happens in the interface between our inner world and external reality, in that space where our imagination is able to shape the external world without the experience of compliance or too much anxiety. This offers the experience of a 'non-purposive state' in which 'creative reaching-out' can take place (Winnicott, 1971); it opens up a space of trust and relaxation in which the need to make sense is – at least temporarily – absent. Playful games and exercises encourage implicit mentalizing and provide a balance to primarily language-oriented methods which generally tend to be based on question-and-answer formats. Play can also counterbalance the intellectualizing tendencies for hyper-reflectiveness of some adult family members. The invitation to 'play' creates a different therapeutic context, one which is seemingly less 'serious', overtly experimental, prompting creativity and surprise – and being fun! What playful exercises achieve is the simultaneous experience of intense emotion and the contextualizing and containing effect of thoughts, building the capacity to regulate affect during episodes of emotion escalation (Fishbane, 2007). Below we describe a few playful games and exercises that stimulate mentalizing.

In the exercise *'reading the mind behind the face'* all family members are asked to name any feelings they know, with the therapist writing each of these down on separate cards. Once 15–20 feelings have been chosen, each person draws a card and displays the feeling state without using words, with the other family members having to speculate what is being conveyed. Usually, there is much guessing and laughter, followed by discussions about how feelings can be correctly identified or how facial expressions can be misleading. If these expressions are captured photographically (via a camera, iPad or mobile phone) there may be, after several rounds of this, a collection of 20 or more photographs, which can be printed and placed on the wall of the consulting room, like exhibits in an art gallery, and be viewed and discussed in turn by the family members. This may trigger memories, particularly if they are asked about times when they felt the way they are depicted in the photographs and whether anyone else in the family had spotted their 'state' – and if they had not, whether this would have been 'ok' or not. Some or all of the photos can be taken home and specific photos may be prominently displayed, serving as a reminder of how 'mental state snapshots' can lead to useful conversations and how they can continue to stimulate inter-session curiosity about mental states. Affect state snapshots can thus enable cognition to bring about improvements in the regulation of affect within the family.

Another version of *'reading the mind behind the face'* involves the *'therapeutic use of selfies'*, with the aim to address the brittle nature of self-representations, particularly when working with teenagers and their families. Taking pictures of oneself in a range of different individual as well as social situations with a mobile phone is very much in fashion these days. The therapist can ask the young person to prepare 10 'selfies' for the subsequent session when they are jointly viewed with family members who are encouraged to speculate about the thoughts and feelings depicted in each photo and comment on them from their perspective. This can also be done when the parents bring 'selfies' and get their children to respond to questions such as "*what is Mum thinking and feeling*", "*what went on in his mind when he took this photo*" and "*what might your parents wish or fear when they see this photo?*" The work can be extended by getting each family member to bring three photos of themselves to the next session. In the session, they are asked to fill in 'mental state thought bubbles', first on their perception of the feelings and thoughts of the other, followed by the way they think the others might fill in the thought bubbles belonging to their own photos. At the core of taking and mentalizing 'selfies' is the encouragement of mental movement from 'within' to 'without'. The essence of effective mentalizing is recognizing the tension between accepting the opaqueness of minds and yet desiring transparency which the interpretation of actions in terms of mental states offers. This requires a continuous awareness of the limitations of one's capacity to 'know for sure' what others feel and think, as well as playful imagination in guessing what is motivating others around us.

Work with masks is another playful activity as people tend to behave differently when wearing a mask; they are more willing to explore and expose parts of their private thoughts and feelings which they tend not to make public in their everyday life. The use of masks in therapy aims to create a playful frame to overcome barriers imposed by fears of social condemnation, ridicule or blame and generate curiosity through revealing the mind, or more about the mind, behind the mask. The activity '*Masked Ball*' specifically utilizes one of the freedoms masks can afford to their wearers, namely to encourage story telling. If this is focused on oneself, or one's self, then 'prospective life stories' or 'prospective CVs' can be constructed, enabling each family member to examine their (imagined) life 'story' from a future perspective. This allows otherwise unthinkable – or indeed non-mentalizable – possibilities to emerge. Each family member is asked to choose a theatrical mask, depicting a dramatic looking person. All put on the mask at the same time and look at each other, having formed a circle – with the therapist sitting outside the circle. He explains that the year is 2070, everyone is alive but that, for whatever reason, family members have lost touch with each other and that this is the first time they all are meeting in decades. Each family member is asked to role-play themselves as at the suggested age, meeting up in 2070 for a family dinner party and exchanging their lifetime experiences. The therapist starts by asking each family member as to where they are 'now' (the year 2070), what they do and how they got there. He slants the narratives by sharpening focus on mental states – probing their 2070 needs, disappointments, beliefs, hopes and fears. He gradually encourages mutual exploration and discussion, keeping up the playful and 'fantasy' character of the 'masked ball'. Having created a distant future, the imaginary clock is gradually rewound by one or two decades each time, and the family members imagine themselves meeting up in ever more recent periods eventually finding themselves one year from now. Conversation at each of these times centres around: "*when you look back on your life, what were the turning points? What made a difference? What might other family members think and feel if that really came true?*" The focus can then be on the concrete steps family members can undertake to achieve particular 'scenarios'. In this way the family may be helped to create a mentalized continuity of its functioning and a potential change that can be achieved which is (a) rooted in current experience and (b) entails the changes in thoughts in relation to others, feelings about oneself and beliefs about each family members' contribution, which may be necessary to get there. Quite a number of different applications of the therapeutic use of masks to stimulate mentalizing have been developed and these can be found elsewhere (see Asen & Fonagy, 2017).

Playful exercises and activities involving the body can be employed to stimulate mentalizing, and non-mentalizing affective and somatic states can thus be made accessible to mentalization. Maps, or other types of visual representation, encourage a collaborative approach. A large piece of paper on a table with family members and therapist sitting around it allows participants to look at their representations from an external or meta-perspective. The cognitive perspective on bodily states if shared with family members allows a distancing from physical experience and places the individual in the position of an onlooker permitting alternative perspectives. In the presence of other members of the family this becomes a collaborative venture and can give rise to and shape a new narrative. These exercises start from involving the body, literally placing the mind in the physical body and the brain, then moving to create physical representations of family fights via 'conflict maps' and ultimately translating relational constructs from physical into psychological language. For example, putting affective states on a body map, 'externalizing' these so to speak, permits family members to view and examine mental states. In the presence of other members of the family, this becomes a collaborative venture and can give rise to, and shape, a new shared narrative. In the exercise 'body-feeling scan', each family member is asked, in turn, to lie on a large piece of paper or paper roll. The outlines of each person are drawn with a pen, and each family member is then asked to draw or paint their feelings into their body shape, using different colours, shapes and forms, and label them. In the 'mind–brain scan', each family member is provided with a paper diagram of a cross section of the human brain, but adapted so that instead of the usual four ventricles, there are altogether 10 larger and smaller spaces depicted in the diagram. Everyone is asked to speculate about "*what goes on in the head*" of one other family member and then to fill in the spaces with the feelings, wishes, beliefs or thoughts they imagine that person harbours.

Family conflicts can also be made 'visible' via sculptures, made out of clay or similar materials. This can either be a joint exercise, with all family members working together on a family sculpture, or alternatively, each family member can be given the materials to do their very own sculpture of how they see their family at this moment. Once the sculptures are completed, each family member is asked to speculate about the mental states of the various sculpted figures, an exercise in both mentalizing self and others. The 'sculptor' then explains what had been on his mind. At some stage, family members can be asked how the sculpture would be different if it had been made before a major event in the family (illness, death, social welfare intervention) and some re-sculpting or re-positioning of figures can take place. Similarly, future scenarios can be explored by asking how family members might want the family to look like in months or years – and how this might affect each person's state of mind.

Building Epistemic Trust

The formation of a good therapeutic alliance counts as one of the main factors for positive outcomes in any form of psychotherapy (Falkenstrom, Granstrom, & Holmqvist, 2013; Tasca & Lampard, 2012). Above all it is essential to establish a relationship where the client(s) can trust the therapist and the therapeutic process; this will hugely assist them to take onboard new ideas and perspectives. Mentalization-focused practitioners have introduced the notion of *epistemic trust* in order to conceptualize the process of how the 'learning' of effective mentalizing takes place; it refers to a person's trust in the authenticity and personal relevance of interpersonally transmitted information (Fonagy, Luyten, & Allison, 2015). We acquire this early in our lives: securely attached children treat their parents as an authentic source for processing important new information. Feeling recognized in terms of their needs and thoughts makes children trust that source as they believe that their subjectivity is important to the parent. What the trusted person tells us we can accept as part of our culture. In a therapeutic context, being recognized and validated as a person in one's own right and having agency, is a precondition for the opening up of epistemic trust.

The qualities required for a person to earn epistemic trust are, above all, benevolence and reliability. They trigger epistemic trust and open up channels that allow us to receive knowledge about a personally relevant social world – knowledge that transcends specific experiences and becomes relevant in, and generalizable to, many different settings (Fonagy et al., 2015). However, we also need to learn to discern not just who is to be trusted and who is benevolent and reliable as a source of information, but also who is uninformed, unreliable or downright bad-intentioned. Being excessively and uncritically open to receiving any new information is as maladaptive as is being excessively closed to the possibility of receiving new information (Sperber et al., 2010; Wilson & Sperber, 2012). If an attachment figure is a source of both fear and trust, the child – and later on the adult – will seek assurance from elsewhere but feel doubtful at the same time. This position of 'epistemic mistrust' is often associated with 'epistemic hyper-vigilance': a seemingly restless, if not obsessive, preoccupation with reading contextual cues (Fonagy et al., 2015; Fonagy & Allison, 2014). Children, for example, who continuously watch their parents' facial expressions, anxiously anticipating any possible sudden 'changes of mind' in their parents, often have considerable difficulties tuning into their own states of mind. Being mentalized in the context of attachment relationships in the family generates epistemic trust within that family unit. Mentalization-focused work aims to enhance effective mentalizing and build attachments all round and thereby build epistemic trust so that even if a parent is, for example, temporarily not able to stop their own work and immediately attend to their child, that very parent nevertheless recognizes that the child's wish to have the parent nearby may come from anxiety or excitement, or a worry that the parent has 'forgotten' them.

The Evidence Base of Mentalizing Work with Families

Mentalization-based therapy (MBT) for adults presenting with borderline personality disorder has a strong evidence base, as indicated in recent reviews of psychological interventions for Borderline Personality Disorder (BPD) (e.g. Budge et al., 2013; Nelson et al., 2014; Stoffers et al., 2012). An early Randomized Controlled Trial (RCT) of MBT in a partial hospital setting found that an 18-month programme resulted in lasting and significant changes in mood states and interpersonal functioning (Bateman & Fonagy, 1999, 2001). In comparison to treatment as usual (TAU), benefits were large and they continued to grow during the 18-month follow-up. A follow-up, 8 years on from initial entry into treatment found that the MBT group continued to do better than TAU, with better outcomes in levels of suicidality (23% in the MBT group vs. 74% in TAU group), diagnostic status (13% vs. 87%), service use (2 years vs. 3.5 years) and other measurements such as use of medication, global functioning and vocational status (Bateman & Fonagy, 2008).

A trial of MBT in an adult outpatient setting has also found better results to TAU (Bateman & Fonagy, 2009), particularly in the long term (Bateman & Fonagy, 2013). Significantly in this trial, control treatment was a manualized, highly efficacious treatment, structured clinical management (Bateman & Fonagy, 2009). A study of the treatment of adolescents who self-harm with outpatient MBT found that the MBT group showed a recovery rate of 44%, compared to 17% of those who received TAU (Rossouw & Fonagy, 2012). A study in Denmark investigated the efficacy of MBT versus a less intensive, manualized supportive group therapy in patients diagnosed with BPD (Jørgensen et al., 2013). The combined MBT was superior to the less intensive supportive group therapy on clinician-rated Global Assessment of Functioning. An 18-month naturalistic follow-up found that treatment effects at termination were sustained at 18 months (Jørgensen et al., 2014). Half of the patients in the MBT group met criteria for functional remission at follow-up, compared with less than one-fifth in the supportive therapy group, but three-quarters of both groups achieved diagnostic remission, and almost half of the patients had attained symptomatic remission. In a second study from Denmark (Petersen et al., 2010), a cohort of patients treated with partial hospitalization followed by group MBT showed significant improvements after treatment (average length 2 years) on a range of measures including Global Assessment of Functioning, hospitalizations and vocational status, with further improvement at 2-year follow-up.

A naturalistic study by Bales et al. (2012) in the Netherlands investigated the effectiveness of an 18-month manualized program of MBT in 45 patients diagnosed with severe BPD. There was a high prevalence of comorbidity of DSM-IV Axis I and Axis II disorders. Results showed significant positive change in symptom distress, social and interpersonal functioning and personality pathology and functioning; effect sizes were moderate to large ($d = 0.7–1.7$). This study however is limited by the absence of a control group. Another study (Bales et al., 2015) applied propensity score matching to determine the best matches for 29 MBT patients from within a larger ($n = 175$) group who received other specialized psychotherapeutic treatments. These other specialized treatments yielded improvement across domains, which was generally only moderate; in contrast, pre–post effect sizes were consistently large for MBT, with Cohen's d for reduction in psychiatric symptoms of -1.06 and -1.42 at 18 and 36 months, respectively, and ds ranging from 0.81 to 2.08 for improvement in domains of personality functioning. Given the non-randomized study design and the variation in treatment dose received by participants, the between-condition difference in effects should be interpreted cautiously. A multi-site randomized trial by the same group comparing intensive outpatient and partial hospitalization-based MBT for patients with BPD is currently under way (Laurenssen et al., 2014).

Mentalization-based work with families has not yet been reliably evaluated. At least one clinical trial is currently under way (Midgley et al., 2017), but there are no data available at this stage. Some small-scale evaluation studies have been carried out, mostly in the UK. For example, in a naturalistic evaluation of the effectiveness of short-term MBT work with families (up to 10 sessions), findings from the parent-report Strengths and Difficulties Questionnaire (SDQ) (Goodman, 1997) showed a statistically significant reduction in behavioural and emotional difficulties in children and young people. Over the course of therapy, parents reported an overall reduction in the impact that their child's difficulties were having on both individual and family functioning (Keaveny et al., 2012). In a small-scale qualitative study (Etelaapa, 2011), most parents spoke about their sense of 'stuckness' prior to starting therapy, and went on to describe the ways they felt the therapy had helped them. When asked to reflect on the impact of the therapy, most of the young people (aged 8 to 15) commented on the importance of feeling listened to and understood, and some described the way in which the sessions had positively affected the relationships within their family. Although small-scale, the evaluation studies described above provide some initial indication that families can be helped by a mentalization-informed family approach, and that this way of work is acceptable to families themselves. Further research is urgently needed, however, to explore whether a mentalization-informed family approach is effective, either as a 'stand-alone' model of therapy or as a supplement to existing systemic approaches to working with families.

References

Akister, J., & Reibstein, J. (2004). Links between attachment theory and systemic practice. *Journal of Family Therapy, 26*, 2–16.

Asen, E., & Fonagy, P. (2012a). Mentalization-based family therapy. In A. Bateman & P. Fonagy (Eds.), *Handbook of mentalizing in mental health practice* (pp. 107–128). Arlington, VA: American Psychiatric Publishing.

Asen, E., & Fonagy, P. (2012b). Mentalization-based therapeutic interventions for families. *Journal of Family Therapy, 34*(4), 347–370. https://doi.org/10.1111/j.1467-6427.2011.00552.x

Asen, E., & Fonagy, P. (2017). Mentalizing family violence part 2: Techniques and interventions. *Family Process, 56*(1), 22–44. https://doi.org/10.1111/famp.12276

Bales, D., Timman, R., Andrea, H., Busschbach, J. J., Verheul, R., & Kamphuis, J. H. (2015). Effectiveness of day hospital mentalization-based treatment for patients with severe borderline personality disorder: A matched control study. *Clinical Psychology & Psychotherapy, 22*(5), 409–417. https://doi.org/10.1002/cpp.1914

Bales, D., van Beek, N., Smits, M., Willemsen, S., Busschbach, J. J., Verheul, R., & Andrea, H. (2012). Treatment outcome of 18-month, day hospital mentalization-based treatment (MBT) in patients with severe borderline personality disorder in the Netherlands. *Journal of Personality Disorders, 26*(4), 568–582. https://doi.org/10.1521/pedi.2012.26.4.568

Bateman, A., & Fonagy, P. (1999). Effectiveness of partial hospitalization in the treatment of borderline personality disorder: A randomized controlled trial. *American Journal of Psychiatry, 156*(10), 1563–1569. https://doi.org/10.1176/ajp.156.10.1563

Bateman, A., & Fonagy, P. (2001). Treatment of borderline personality disorder with psychoanalytically oriented partial hospitalization: An 18-month follow-up. *American Journal of Psychiatry, 158*(1), 36–42. https://doi.org/10.1176/appi.ajp.158.1.36

Bateman, A., & Fonagy, P. (2008). 8-year follow-up of patients treated for borderline personality disorder: Mentalization-based treatment versus treatment as usual. *American Journal of Psychiatry, 165*(5), 631–638. https://doi.org/10.1176/appi.ajp.2007.07040636

Bateman, A., & Fonagy, P. (2009). Randomized controlled trial of outpatient mentalization-based treatment versus structured clinical management for borderline personality disorder. *American Journal of Psychiatry, 166*(12), 1355–1364. https://doi.org/10.1176/appi.ajp.2009.09040539

Bateman, A., & Fonagy, P. (2013). Impact of clinical severity on outcomes of mentalisation-based treatment for borderline personality disorder. *British Journal of Psychiatry, 203*, 221–227. https://doi.org/10.1192/bjp.bp.112.121129

Bateman, A., & Fonagy, P. (2016). *Mentalization-based treatment for personality disorders: A practical guide*. Oxford, UK: Oxford University Press.

Budge, S. L., Moore, J. T., Del Re, A. C., Wampold, B. E., Baardseth, T. P., & Nienhuis, J. B. (2013). The effectiveness of evidence-based treatments for personality disorders when comparing treatment-as-usual and bona fide treatments. *Clinical Psychology Review, 33*(8), 1057–1066. https://doi.org/10.1016/j.cpr.2013.08.003

Dallos, R. (2006). *Attachment Narrative Therapy*. Maidenhead & New York: Open University Press.

Diamond, G. S., & Siqueland, L. (1998). Emotions, attachments and relational reframe. *Journal of Structural and Strategic Therapy, 17*, 36–50.

Etelaapa, K. (2011). *Families' experiences of Mentalization Based Treatment for Families (MBT-F)*. (MSc),. London: University College London.

Falkenstrom, F., Granstrom, F., & Holmqvist, R. (2013). Therapeutic alliance predicts symptomatic improvement session by session. *Journal of Counseling Psychology, 60*(3), 317–328. https://doi.org/10.1037/a0032258

Fearon, P., Target, M., Fonagy, P., Williams, L., McGregor, J., Sargent, J., & Bleiberg, E. (2006). Short-Term Mentalization and Relational Therapy (SMART): An integrative family therapy for children and adolescents. In J. G. Allen & P. Fonagy (Eds.), *Handbook of mentalization-based treatment*. Chichester, UK: John Wiley & Sons.

Fishbane, M. (2007). Wired to connect: Neuroscience, relationships, and therapy. *Family Process, 46*(3), 395–412. https://doi.org/10.1111/j.1545-5300.2007.00219.x

Flaskas, C. (2002). *Family Therapy Beyond Postmodernism*. Hove, UK: Brunner-Routledge.

Fonagy, P., & Allison, E. (2014). The role of mentalizing and epistemic trust in the therapeutic relationship. *Psychotherapy (Chicago, Ill.), 51*(3), 372–380. https://doi.org/10.1037/a0036505

Fonagy, P., Gergely, G., Jurist, E., & Target, M. (2002). *Affect regulation, mentalization, and the development of the self*. New York: Other Press.

Fonagy, P., Luyten, P., & Allison, E. (2015). Epistemic petrification and the restoration of epistemic trust: A new conceptualization of borderline personality disorder and its psychosocial treatment. *Journal of Personality Disorders, 29*(5), 575–609. https://doi.org/10.1521/pedi.2015.29.5.575

Fonagy, P., Steele, M., Steele, H., Moran, G. S., & Higgitt, A. C. (1991). The capacity for understanding mental states: The reflective self in parent and child and its significance for security of attachment. *Infant Mental Health Journal, 12*(3), 201–218. https://doi.org/10.1002/1097-0355(199123)12:3<201::Aid-Imhj2280120307>3.0.Co;2-7

Fraenkel, P., & Pinsof, W. (2001). Teaching family therapy-centred integration: Assimilation and beyond. *Journal of Psychotherapy Integration, 11*, 59–86.

Goodman, R. (1997). The strengths and difficulties questionnaire: A research note. *Journal of Child Psychology and Psychiatry, 38*(5), 581–586.

Jørgensen, C. R., Bøye, R., Andersen, D., Døssing Blaabjerg, A. H., Freund, C., Jordet, H., & Kjølbye, M. (2014). Eighteen months post-treatment naturalistic follow-up study of mentalization-based therapy and supportive group treatment of borderline personality disorder: Clinical outcomes and functioning. *Nordic Psychology, 66*(4), 254–273. https://doi.org/10.1080/19012276.2014.963649

Jørgensen, C. R., Freund, C., Boye, R., Jordet, H., Andersen, D., & Kjolbye, M. (2013). Outcome of mentalization-based and supportive psychotherapy in patients with borderline personality disorder: A randomized trial. *Acta Psychiatrica Scandinavica, 127*(4), 305–317. https://doi.org/10.1111/j.1600-0447.2012.01923.x

Keaveny, E., Midgley, N., Asen, E., Bevington, D., Fearon, P., Fonagy, P., . . . Wood, S. D. (2012). Minding the family mind: The development and initial evaluation of mentalization-based treatment for families. In N. Midgley & I. Vrouva (Eds.), *Minding the child* (pp. 98–112). Hove, UK: Routledge.

Laurenssen, E. M., Westra, D., Kikkert, M. J., Noom, M. J., Eeren, H. V., van Broekhuyzen, A. J., . . . Dekker, J. J. (2014). Day hospital mentalization-based treatment (MBT-DH) versus treatment as usual in the treatment of severe borderline personality disorder: Protocol of a randomized controlled trial. BMC Psychiatry, 14, 149. doi:https://doi.org/10.1186/1471-244X-14-149

Midgley, N., Besser, S., Dye, H., Fearon, P., Gale, T., Jefferies-Sewell, K., . . . Wood, S. (2017). The Herts and minds study: Evaluating the effectiveness of mentalization-based treatment (MBT) as an intervention for children in foster care with emotional and/or behavioural problems: A phase II, feasibility, randomised controlled trial. Pilot and Feasibility Studies, 3, 12. doi:https://doi.org/10.1186/s40814-017-0127-x

Nelson, K. J., Zagoloff, A., Quinn, S., Swanson, H. E., Garber, C., & Schulz, S. C. (2014). Borderline personality disorder: Treatment approaches and perspectives. *Clinical Practice, 11*(3), 341–349. https://doi.org/10.2217/CPR.14.24

Penn, P. (1982). Circular questioning. *Family Process, 21*(3), 267–280. https://doi.org/10.1111/j.1545-5300.1982.00267.x

Petersen, B., Toft, J., Christensen, N. B., Foldager, L., Munk-Jorgensen, P., Windfeld, M., . . . Valbak, K. (2010). A 2-year follow-up of mentalization-oriented group therapy following day hospital treatment for patients with personality disorders. Personality and Mental Health, 4(4), 294–301. doi:https://doi.org/10.1002/Pmh.140

Rossouw, T. I., & Fonagy, P. (2012). Mentalization-based treatment for self-harm in adolescents: A randomized controlled trial. *Journal of the American Academy of Child and Adolescent Psychiatry, 51*(12), 1304–1313. https://doi.org/10.1016/j.jaac.2012.09.018

Selvini Palazzoli, M., Boscolo, L., Cecchin, G., & Prata, G. (1980). Hypothesizing—circularity—Neutrality: Three guidelines for the conductor of the session. *Family Process, 19*(1), 3–12. https://doi.org/10.1111/j.1545-5300.1980.00003.x

Sperber, D., Clement, F., Heintz, C., Mascaro, O., Mercier, H., Origgi, G., & Wilson, D. (2010). Epistemic vigilance. *Mind & Language, 25*(4), 359–393. https://doi.org/10.1111/j.1468-0017.2010.01394.x

Stoffers, J. M., Vollm, B. A., Rucker, G., Timmer, A., Huband, N., & Lieb, K. (2012). Psychological therapies for people with borderline personality disorder. *Cochrane Database of Systematic Reviews, 8*(8), CD005652. https://doi.org/10.1002/14651858.CD005652.pub2

Tasca, G. A., & Lampard, A. M. (2012). Reciprocal influence of alliance to the group and out-come in day treatment for eating disorders. *Journal of Counseling Psychology, 59*(4), 507–517. https://doi.org/10.1037/a0029947

Wilson, D., & Sperber, D. (2012). *Meaning and relevance*. Cambridge, UK: Cambridge University Press.

Winnicott, D. W. (1971). *Playing and reality*. London: Routledge.

Mindfulness- and Compassion-Based Interventions in Relational Contexts

Corina Aguilar-Raab

> *There is a strong current in contemporary culture advocating holistic views as some sort of cure-all... Reductionism implies attention to a lower level while holistic implies attention to higher level. These are intertwined in any satisfactory description: and each entails some loss relative to our cognitive preferences, as well as some gain... there is no whole system without an interconnection of its parts and there is no whole system without an environment.*
> *Varela (1977)*

Introduction

In this chapter, the constructs of mindfulness and compassion are introduced and the evidence base on mindfulness- and compassion-based interventions in relational contexts is reviewed. Whereas in the last decades a growing body of empirical evidence suggests the multiple benefits of such secular approaches for physiological and psychological health for individuals, still less is known for couples, children, and families. Rooted in traditionally individual contemplative practices, applying mindfulness and compassion in relational contexts requires unique adaptations. Several programs were adapted for a variety of contexts and settings, which will be illustrated based on a few examples.

To explain, why and how such programs support not only the reduction of individual distress but also the enhancement of relationship quality underlying mechanisms such as co-regulation processes will be addressed. Finally I will conclude by discussing communalities and divergences between Buddhist-rooted and systemic approaches and outline possible perspectives for research and application.

C. Aguilar-Raab (✉)
Institute of Medical Psychology, Center of Psychosocial Medicine, Heidelberg University Hospital, Heidelberg, Germany
e-mail: Corina.Aguilar-Raab@med.uni-heidelberg.de

© Springer Nature Switzerland AG 2020
M. Ochs et al. (eds.), *Systemic Research in Individual, Couple, and Family Therapy and Counseling*, European Family Therapy Association Series,
https://doi.org/10.1007/978-3-030-36560-8_13

223

Mindfulness and Compassion

Mindfulness

Normally, in order to make the most of my time at the train station, I make appointments, short phone calls, and have breakfast on the side. My mind is full of overlapping thoughts, feelings, and automatic actions without being aware of this "fullness." This seems to be the usual way of living for millions of people to cope with the challenges of an achievement-based world. To meet the demands of this fast-moving world, we respond with multitasking and self-optimization. Contra intuitively, however, this usually only contributes to a perceived increase in demands and stress.

Instead, devoting myself to one single thing in this present moment at the same time using my accepting self-awareness to observe a possible wandering mind or how my mind gets impressed by distractions is a moment of "mind-*fulness*": *Intentionally focusing a certain object, wandering, re-focusing by means of mindfulness, trying not to lose the chosen object of attention* (Bishop et al., 2004; Kabat-Zinn, 1990, 1994).

While trying to establish necessary measurements and scales, mindfulness can be regarded as either a state of mind or a trait (Baer, Smith, Hopkins, Krietemeyer, & Toney, 2006; Brown & Ryan, 2003), with one or multiple sub-dimensions (Bergomi, Tschacher, & Kupper, 2013; but see also for a critical comment on the assessment of mindfulness: Grossman, 2011). Basically, it involves the intention to focus my attention towards a certain object, and at the same time using a mental faculty on a meta-level, a kind of self-awareness, interoceptive awareness, or meta-cognition (Vago & Silbersweig, 2012), which is able to recognize any mind wandering, being able to re-direct in case of losing stability, or clarity of the intentionally focused object (Shapiro, Carlson, Astin, & Freedman, 2006).

Practicing this contemplative technique continuously, formally and informally in daily life, leads to an attitude, which turns us from a *doing* to a *being* mode, helping us to answer challenging and stressful events more adaptively and healthily (Santorelli, Meleo-Meyer, Koerbel, & Kabat-Zinn, 2017).

Since Jon Kabat-Zinn introduced the secular Mindfulness-Based Stress Reduction (MBSR) program, an 8-week-long group-training in the 1970s, mindfulness has gained an amazing popularity in research and society (Kabat-Zinn, 1990, 1994, 2003).

In the last decades, a growing body of research has shown the efficacy of Mindfulness-Based Interventions (MBIs) in preventative and clinical settings (Baer, 2003; Gotink et al., 2015; Khoury, Sharma, Rush, & Fournier, 2015; Vøllestad, Nielsen, & Nielsen, 2012).

Such interventions contribute to well-being and quality of life (Godfrin & van Heeringen, 2010), life satisfaction, psychological functioning such as decrease in anxiety, depression, distress and burnout (e.g., Chiesa & Serretti, 2009; Gotink et al., 2015; Khoury et al., 2015). At the same time, they lead to an increase in resilience and distress tolerance in healthy adults (Feldman, Dunn, Stemke, Bell, &

Greeson, 2014). In the clinical field, MBIs have been tested in physical disorders such as chronic pain, cancer, cardiovascular disorders, and others (e.g., Grossman, Tiefenthaler-Gilmer, Raysz, & Kesper, 2007) as well as mental disorders such as depression (Kuyken et al., 2008, 2016; Strauss, Cavanagh, Oliver, & Pettman, 2014; Teasdale et al., 2000), anxiety (Hofmann, Sawyer, Witt, & Oh, 2010), addiction (Bowen et al., 2014), trauma (Kearney, McDermott, Malte, Martinez, & Simpson, 2011; King et al., 2013), and many more (e.g., Green & Bieling, 2012; Hempel et al., 2014). Among others, results indicate a reduction in depressive and anxiety symptoms (Hofmann et al., 2010; Strauss et al., 2014) with moderate effect sizes (e.g., in pre-post comparison with $n = 72$, Hedge's $g = 0.55$, or in comparison with a wait-list-control group with $n = 67$ and Hedge's $g = 0.53$; Khoury et al., 2013) comparable to other therapeutic interventions or a significant decrease in risk of relapse in depression (Teasdale et al., 2000) and addiction (see also Goldberg et al., 2018).

One of the essential mechanisms behind this, which is mostly investigated experimentally, is attentional processing, not least due to a possible operationalization (see also Jha, Krompinger, & Baime, 2007): For example, in visual attention processing, participants of the mindfulness meditation group showed more precise, effective, and flexible visual attentional processing in different tasks such as multiple perspectives images compared to participants of the non-meditation group (Hodgins & Adair, 2010).

Other psychological mechanisms underlying the preventative effects of such interventions are mindfulness and its different factors – as we could show, for example, that especially the sub-dimensions of mindfulness – *acceptance*, *decentering*, and *relativity* – are important mediators for resilience and distress tolerance (Nila, Holt, Ditzen, & Aguilar-Raab, 2016), but also rumination and worry have been stated to be relevant (Gu, Strauss, Bond, & Cavanagh, 2015; for a content based synopsis on mechanisms see: Shapiro et al., 2006).

From a neuroscience perspective, the effects of mindfulness meditation are related to the interacting components that are involved in basic self-regulation processes, which are (1) attention control, (2) emotion regulation, and (3) self-awareness (Tang, Hölzel, & Posner, 2015), differing depending on the stage of practice. Taylor et al. (2011) were able to demonstrate that mindfulness in long-term meditators compared to beginners deactivated the default mode networks during processing of different emotional stimuli, whereas beginners revealed a downregulation of the amygdala.

Overall, the neurophysiological findings indicate both functional (anterior cingulate cortex (ACC) and posterior cingulate cortex (PFC) – attentional and emotional control; Amygdala – emotional regulation; prefrontal cortex (PCC) – self-awareness, etc.) and structural (cortical thickness, grey matter volume or density) change effects, such as a decrease in the density of grey matter in the amygdala correlated with a decrease in perceived stress (Hölzel et al., 2010).

Compassion

Pity is not compassion but empathic distress: As I walk through the forest, I hear calls for help until I discover that someone has slipped into a hole in the ground and can't get out by herself. While I perceive the suffering and the pain and finally feel it myself, I am completely taken by the hopelessness of the situation. From my identification with the suffering and in my numbness I lose my stability and fall into the hole myself. Since I've lost my ability to act, I get desperate myself (Fig. 1).

Compassion can also be understood as empathic concern (Singer & Klimecki, 2014): In this same story, while resonating with the suffering and recognizing the need for relief of the person being stuck in the hole, feeling connected and close, I feel the urge to help. As I am able to keep the ability to take into account different and widened perspectives, I self-efficaciously make use of my scope of actions, throw a rope down so she can climb out (Fig. 2).

Compassion is a complex construct containing cognitive, affective, motivational, and behavioral components (Feldman & Kuyken, 2011). Instead of being totally overwhelmed by the suffering and being identified with it, it activates a motivation to help and if possible also a prosocial and helping behavior (Goetz, Keltner, & Simon-Thomas, 2010; Strauss et al., 2016).

This is rooted in the understanding of a basic common ground between others and myself, wanting happiness and avoiding suffering (Lama & Ekman, 2008). The closeness and connectedness contribute to resiliently tolerating this distress, understanding that suffering realistically pervades all our lives. Staying grounded, it is guided by the possibilities of dealing with the changing nature of suffering or alleviating it while mindfully applying any actions – including changing perspectives and attitudes – needed (Singer & Boltz, 2013).

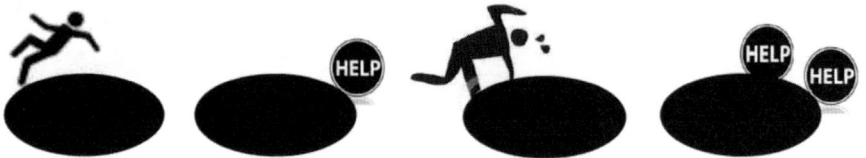

Fig. 1 Simplified representation of pity or empathic distress

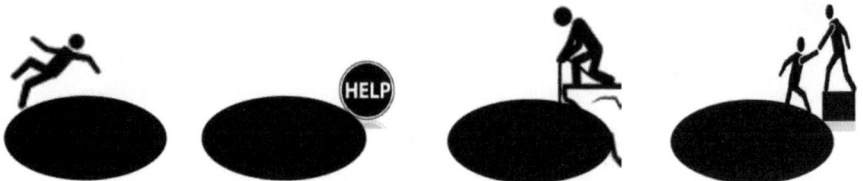

Fig. 2 Simplified representation of compassion or empathic concern

Similar to mindfulness, compassion can be deepened and expanded by training (Brito, 2014; see also Germer & Barnhofer, 2017). Several secular trainings exist to enhance the compassionate response to suffering in ourselves and others. Currently around eight secular training protocols are published and tested (for an overview see Kirby, Tellegen, & Steindl, 2017; and see also for *Compassion Focused Therapy*: Gilbert, 2009, 2010, 2013; Shonin, Gordon, & Griffiths, 2014). The Cognitively-Based Compassion Training (CBCT®), a secular group-based 6-, 8-, or 10-week long training, was established by Prof. Dr. Lobsang Negi in 2004–2005 at the Emory University, GA, USA, taking into account scientific findings on psychological and neurophysiological functioning of mind, experience, and behavior (Ozawa-de Silva & Negi, 2013).

In a successive process, the psychological and cognitive preconditions are taught and practiced in six modules via different stabilizing and analytic meditative practices in order to cultivate and strengthen empathic concern and compassionate resonating. The modules and key components are: (1) developing attentional stability and clarity, (2) cultivating insight into the changing nature of the moment-to-moment mental experience combined with non-reactivity, (3) cultivating self-compassion – recognizing and understanding biased cognitions and reactions and enhancing self-efficacy, (4) increasing impartiality by reflecting basic similarities with others, (5) developing appreciation and affection for others by acknowledging our interdependent nature, and finally (6) developing empathy and realizing engaged compassion – as a motivation and readiness to unselfishly act if possible and needed (Aguilar-Raab, Jarczok, Warth, et al., 2018; Dodds et al., 2015; Ozawa-de Silva & Negi, 2013).

CBCT® is one of the most scientifically researched compassion trainings so far (Shonin, Van Gordon, Compare, Zangeneh, & Griffiths, 2015). In college students it helped to increase self-rated compassion and quality of sleep and reduced the feeling of loneliness and depression (Mascaro et al., 2018). Those who practiced more often showed less stress responses and better immune responses after a social stress test in the laboratory post training (Pace et al., 2009; Pace et al., 2010). Desbordes et al. (2012) provided evidence for post CBCT® effects in non-meditative states with regard to higher amygdala response to negative-valanced stimuli, which was significantly associated with a reduction of depressive symptoms. Mascaro, Rilling, Negi, and Raison (2013) found significant increases in empathic arousal and neural activity in the inferior frontal gyrus and dorsomedial prefrontal cortex for CBCT® participants compared to an active control group.

Overall, significant changes with average medium effect sizes in self-reported (self-)compassion (compassion: $d = 0.55$, $k = 4$, 95% CI [0.33–0.78]; self-compassion: $d = 0.70$, $k = 13$, 95% CI [0.59–0.87]), mindfulness ($d = 0.54$, $k = 6$, 95% CI [0.38–0.71]), well-being ($d = 0.51$, $k = 8$, 95% CI [0.30–0.63]), psychological distress ($d = 0.47$, $k = 14$, 95% CI [0.19–0.56]), depression ($d = 0.64$, $k = 9$, 95% CI [0.45–0.82]), and anxiety ($d = 0.49$, $k = 9$, 95% CI [0.30–0.68]) compared to (active) control groups could be found (Kirby et al., 2017; but see also: Hofmann, Grossman, & Hinton, 2011).

Some authors propose that the key mechanism of compassion is the activation of the parasympathetic system, which helps to provide feelings of safeness and via experiencing affiliative behavior from others calming down (Gilbert, 2014; Gilbert et al., 2008; Kirby, 2017).

Reviewing the Evidence Base on Mindfulness and Compassion in Social Contexts

Humans are social beings and therefore their well-being is essentially associated with positive social relationships (Kok & Fredrickson, 2014). Social integration, social support, bonding, and the feeling of closeness even affect the likelihood of survival (Holt-Lunstad, 2018; Holt-Lunstad, Smith, & Layton, 2010). In particular, a high relationship quality improves various health outcomes (Robles, Slatcher, Trombello, & McGinn, 2014). This seems to be related to the functional dimension of positive relationships: They help to buffer against stress, and constitute a social-emotional resource (Ditzen, Hoppmann, & Klumb, 2008). Nurturing social environments are proposed to consist of several factors: the reduction and minimization of negative interpersonal emotions, motives, cognitions and behaviors such as aggression, devaluation, conflict, etc., and at the same time the encouragement and strengthening of a shared sense of ethical/non-harming values, and based on that empathic, supportive, positive, and compassionate resonance and interactions (Biglan, 2015; Biglan, Flay, Embry, & Sandler, 2012; Kirby, 2016).

The long-standing tradition of research on attachment and psychosexual development of children and adolescents has shown how important the family environment is for coping with ever new developmental challenges (Fonagy, 2018). The probability to develop a secure attachment system is associated with better family relationships, which in turn is linked to a broad variety of mental and physical advantages: Responsive, warm-hearted, and caring parents that are able to find the right balance between providing clear circumscribed limits and autonomy reduce the chance for antisocial problem behavior, substance abuse, and other health risk behaviors (Allen, Moore, Kuperminc, & Bell, 1998; O'Brien et al., 2006; Smetana, Campione-Barr, & Metzger, 2006). At the same time, it is undoubtedly verified that those healthy environments promote good psychological functioning in terms of the development of social, emotional, and ethical intelligence (Bethell et al., 2017; Di Fabio & Kenny, 2016). In prediction of future abilities, children who grew up in such contexts are more prone to build and maintain healthy – personal and professional – relationships in later life. They are more capable of responding flexibly and adaptively to changing internal and external needs and requirements, to make use of their resources, to understand problems as challenges, and to find effective solutions (Grevenstein, Bluemke, Schweitzer-Rothers, & Aguilar-Raab, 2019; Guajardo, Snyder, & Petersen, 2009; Gutman & Feinstein, 2010; Moffitt et al., 2011; Stack, Serbin, Enns, Ruttle, & Barrieau, 2010).

The question is, therefore, what effects do mindfulness and (self-)compassion have in social contexts, such as couples and families, and how do relevant relational and interpersonal characteristics improve?

First studies in couples and families suggest that both mindfulness and compassion indirectly contribute to a more positive relationship through better self- and emotion-regulation (Brown, Creswell, & Ryan, 2015; Coatsworth, Duncan, Greenberg, & Nix, 2010; Duncan, Coatsworth, & Greenberg, 2009; Shonin et al., 2014).

A variety of published studies point to the fact, that higher mindfulness is linked to marital satisfaction and relationship quality (Barnes, Brown, Krusemark, Campbell, & Rogge, 2007; Burpee & Langer, 2005; Jones, Welton, Oliver, & Thoburn, 2011; Kozlowski, 2012; Wachs & Cordova, 2007). Enhanced mindfulness also leads to increased empathetic concern and an improved ability to take into account the perspective of the other (Atkinson, 2013; Burpee & Langer, 2005; Wachs & Cordova, 2007). Following meditation training, interpersonal problems diminish. In stressful interactions, mindfulness helps to apply more adaptive response skills, which also accompany more effective communication (Barnes et al., 2007). In association with higher meditation experience, interpersonal cooperative skills seem to increase in terms of acceptance, tolerance, empathy, helpfulness, compassion, etc. (Atkinson, 2013; Haimerl & Valentine, 2001). Furthermore, experienced meditators showed that in relationships the tendency to react automatically decreases connected to the feeling of safety and freedom with regard to the relationship (Pruitt & McCollum, 2010).

In a mindfulness-based relationship enhancement program for non-distressed couples, Carson, Carson, Gil, and Baucom (2004) showed that besides improved mindfulness also relationship satisfaction increased; similar findings were reported for expecting parents (Gambrel & Piercy, 2015a, 2015b).

Mindfulness parenting refers to techniques and attitudes in which (self/other)-awareness, listening, recognition, and self- as well as co-regulation is pervaded by non-judgmental, accepting warm-heartedness of the here-and-now experiences of all members in the family (Duncan et al., 2009). In a randomized-controlled trial with 65 families, Coatsworth et al. (2010) showed that the implementation of mindfulness in an existing intervention program (Mindful Strengthening Family Program, MSFP) resulted in positive effects through indirect enhancement of the quality of parent–youth relationships: The intervention led to an enhanced use of mindfulness as a technique and of management practices especially by the mothers' parenting their children and increased the emotional qualities between parents and children.

Current research suggests that self-compassion contributes to a more positive, compromising and caring behavior in relationships (Neff & Beretvas, 2013) and a stronger sense of social connectedness and relatedness (Bloch, 2018; Neff, 2003). In addition to better relationship quality and satisfaction (Jacobson, Wilson, Kurz, & Kellum, 2018), the willingness to provide emotional support is also positively influenced (Bloch, 2018).

In a study by Hutcherson, Seppala, and Gross (2008), a single loving kindness meditation compared to a neutral imaginative control condition led to an increase in perceived social connectedness and a more positive attitude towards a stranger.

In a study on compassionate actions in couple relationships it could be shown that, both, the recipient but particularly the benefactor benefit in terms of emotional well-being (Reis, Maniaci, & Rogge, 2014). Furthermore, a recent study demonstrated the importance of the partners helping behavior not only for relationship quality but also for the recipients' personal growth and self-improvement (Overall, Fletcher, & Simpson, 2010).

Furthermore, in groups, compassion leads to higher cohesiveness and cooperation (Gilbert, 2014), which is associated with less hostile and revengeful behavior.

From a psychobiological perspective, the neuropeptide oxytocin is related to compassionate feelings in combination with a stronger orientation towards others and a caring attitude for others (Goetz et al., 2010; Klimecki, Leiberg, Ricard, & Singer, 2013). At the same time, as oxytocin seems to buffer stress-responsiveness in our stress system, it may be connected to the stress-protective effects of positive relationships (Ditzen et al., 2009).

In a recent study, heterosexual couples, who engaged in a couple-discussion in the laboratory during which saliva cortisol samples were drawn, rated their levels of mindfulness. The results indicate that mindfulness in terms of curiosity moderated the effects of negative partner engagement in the conflict, whereas mindfulness in terms of decentering moderated the effect of partner withdrawal behavior or disengagement. At the same time, higher levels of mindfulness during the conflict were related to a better stress-response recovery in the occurrence of more negative interactions of the partner (Laurent, Hertz, Nelson, & Laurent, 2016).

Figure 3 summarizes the interconnection between contemplative practices, including mindfulness and compassion, and the improvement of interpersonal functioning, up to the positive outcomes for physical and mental health:

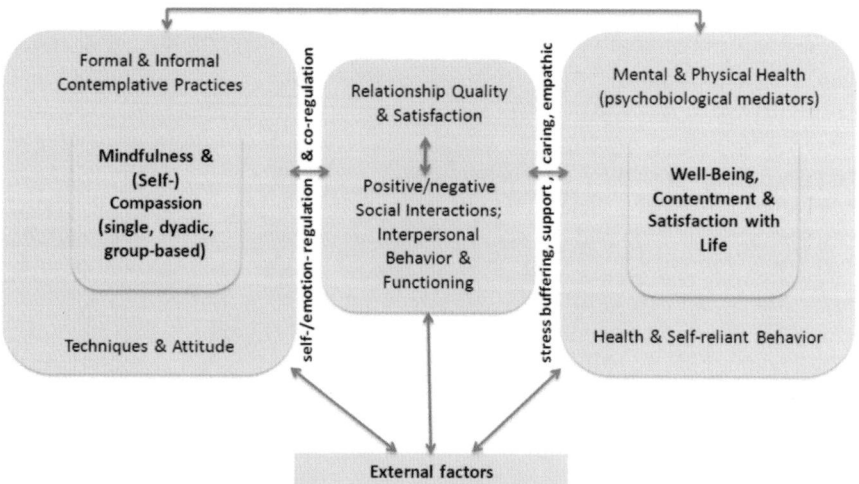

Fig. 3 Interconnection between contemplative practices, interpersonal functioning, and health

Specific Considerations When Applying Mindfulness and Compassion in Social Contexts

Rooted in traditionally individual meditation practices, applying mindfulness and compassion in relational contexts requires unique adaptations. There exist currently a variety of adapted mindfulness-based programs for different social contexts such as couples and families and their specific challenges, but less formalized compassion programs (Jones et al., 2011).

As stated above, the overall aim is to positively influence the relationship quality, relationship satisfaction, and the concrete social interaction behavior.

On the one hand, this succeeds based on an improved stress management, that is, the beneficial influence of coping mechanisms and self- or emotion-regulation strategies in the face of adverse, stress-related circumstances. On the other hand, adapted programs for couples and families address non-judgmental and accepting interaction behavior with each other. The idea is to cultivate an appreciative communication that is characterized by being present and open (see also the concept and practice of "Insight Dialogue": Kramer, Meleo-Meyer, & Turner, 2008).

The feedback processes in direct interactions should be characterized less by reactive impulses than by self-regulated and aware reactions. With an increasing ability to perceive attentively and to recognize what drives me in higher-order and underlying motives, for example, to say or do certain things, it is possible in the medium- and long-term to direct my own interaction behavior more self-regulated/controlled and, for example, to think along with potential consequences of action. Mindfulness supports the awareness of own emotional states and increases the chance for more flexible behavior instead of being mindlessly driven by strong (negative) thoughts and feelings (Brown, Whittingham, Boyd, McKinlay, & Sofronoff, 2014; Hayes, Strosahl, & Wilson, 2011). This makes it possible that more or less strong inner emotional reactions don't necessarily have to be verbally expressed to my partner unfiltered. The ability to pause mindfully helps me to reflect on how I can possibly express my own needs, desires, perspectives differently or more purposefully – and being and acting more in alignment with my own values (Duncan et al., 2009; Kabat-Zinn & Kabat-Zinn, 2009; Siegel & Hartzell, 2003). Furthermore, it increases the chance to extend my relationship and parenting repertoire – based on a developing mindful attitude (Bögels & Restifo, 2014).

Since verbal communication plays an important role in social contexts, especially alongside non-verbal communication, mindful communication is formally practiced, for example, in dyads (see also Kok & Singer, 2017).

Couple and Family Contexts

In specialized programs such as *Mindfulness-Based Relationship Enhancement* (Carson et al., 2004) or *Mindful Parenting* (Altmaier & Maloney, 2007; Bögels, Lehtonen, & Restifo, 2010; Sawyer Cohen & Semple, 2010), mindfulness is specifically practiced in order to increase the quality of relationships by means of fluent, flexible, and more appropriate interactions based on a more attuned and caring attitude between romantic partners or between parents and their children. In these adapted trainings, the specific and social context characteristics are given special consideration (see also the literature to co-regulation: Efklides, 2008; Horn & Maercker, 2016; Schoebi & Randall, 2015).

In couples, for example, the aspect of (physical) intimacy is addressed, which is practiced dyadically as a couple through mindful touch or massage (Carson et al., 2004).

Mindfulness exercises in the family take into account the children's developmental process and status and the changing role of the parents and their respective challenges to accompany the child in an age-appropriate and educational way. Practicing mindfulness exercises together can strengthen family cohesion. Additionally, it can contribute to the awareness of the interconnectedness and recursive interactions similar to systemic family interventions.

Introducing children to mindfulness requires the use of creative and playful techniques. Depending on their age, children find it much easier than adults to relate to the present and to discover themselves and the world curiously. Since many experiences actually have novelty value, younger children are more firmly anchored in the moment-to-moment experience.

If children become familiar with mindful awareness and understanding from an early stage onward, this can strengthen their (self-)regulatory abilities (Geisler & Muttenhammer, 2016).

Children usually discover the moment-to-moment experience and aspects of our own psychological functioning in a playful way – with greater involvement of the body. Additionally, they learn about mindfulness and compassion through tangible and actually comprehensible representations such as the use of visual materials, for example, working and playing with a glass of water, filling it with different ingredients symbolizing different mental states – often called the "mind jar" (Williard & Saltzman, 2015). Being whirled up by stirring or moving these ingredients, children can experience what it needs to establish a clear water glass: The same is true for the mind – they can notice how their thoughts wander and what it feels like to calm down inside – when the various substances (or mental states) in the *mind jar* have settled at the bottom.

Parents usually find themselves in a very exhausting and sometimes overwhelming everyday life, in which the behavior of the children themselves is often interpreted and understood as the trigger for experiencing stress (Dumas, 2005). Through a mindful attitude towards oneself and the children, it can be possible to engage in a more favorable and supportive way. If the bond and closeness to the child is reestablished in this way, negative interaction cycles can be interrupted, redirected, and shaped differently.

Social Contexts and Psychopathology

If individual members of the family suffer from psychopathological symptoms, these are usually tailored even more specifically to the conditions caused by the disorder (Bögels, Hellemans, van Deursen, Römer, & van der Meulen, 2014; Gehart, 2012). The use of mindfulness exercises in children with externalizing problem behavior such as ADHD is achieved, for example, through shorter exercise units with a higher degree of variation, which in turn are linked to repetitive movement sequences (Bögels, Hoogstad, van Dun, de Schutter, & Restifo, 2008). Most of such interventions contain sitting, movement-based, and body scan meditations (Burke, 2010).

Parental involvement is particularly important in childhood and adolescent psychopathologies. The therapy process can be supported by the parents' practice of mindfulness, not only in the sense of treating the affected child, but also to relieve the parents and help change their attitude towards themselves, their parenting style, and the child. Thus, in accordance with family therapeutic interventions, parents and their children are trained in mindfulness together but at the same time separately, parallel to the child (Bögels et al., 2008), or in a sequential order – first the parents, then the child (Singh et al., 2010).

Recent research has demonstrated that mindfulness trainings adapted in such contexts are not only feasible, acceptable, and efficacious for the child in terms of reduction of distress and increase of well-being, awareness, and executive functioning (Zylowska et al., 2007), but also from the perspective of the parents in their evaluation of the child's and their own goals; even more interestingly, the child's enhanced awareness also predicted the long-term ratings of child symptoms from the parents' perspective (Bögels et al., 2008). Overall, current research indicates that contemplative practices with children and their parents are effective in treating different child disorders, but due to methodological issues, further research is needed to shed more light on the actual effects differentially and without literature bias (Evans et al., 2018).

Compassion Programs in Social Contexts: CBCT-fC

An example for an adaptation of a formalized Compassion Training program is the CBCT-fC – the above-mentioned Cognitively-Based Compassion Training (CBCT®) – for Couples, where couples are treated in a multi-couple training (see also Asen & Scholz, 2010). In the SIDE-Study – the Social Interaction in Depression Study – the original CBCT® protocol was complemented by evidence-based couple therapeutic techniques and approaches (Aguilar-Raab, Jarczok, Warth, et al., 2018). As the association of depression and impaired social functioning is well known (Hirschfeld et al., 2000; Rehman, Gollan, & Mortimer, 2008), we focused on couples where one partner suffers from depression, hypothesizing that the enhancement of mindfulness and compassion led not only to a decrease in depressive symptoms, but may especially support improvements in social interactional skills such as perspective taking and empathically concerned communication. Additions to the protocol were made with regard to the following:

1. We added psychoeducational parts, emphasizing the connection of depression and social functioning on the one hand, and the linkage of social functioning, relationship skills, and physical and mental health parameters on the other hand.
2. We included several dyadic meditations, such as mindful listening and speaking – non-reactively/decentered, empathic listening and speaking, and dyadic compassionate resonancing without speaking but being aware of exchanging compassionate concern for each other (see Goldin & Jazaieri, 2017; Langri & Weiss, 2013).
3. Additionally, we adopted cognitive-behavioral exercises from partner communication programs (see Kröger, Heinrichs, & Hahlweg, 2009), appreciation in action and gratefulness in action verbally and non-verbally ("noticing, how the partner is doing something good for me").

Besides group-treatment-based advantages such as cohesion (Yalom, 1995), the additional approach is rooted in systemic practice and thinking (Aguilar-Raab, Grevenstein, & Schweitzer, 2015; Schlippe & Schweitzer, 2013): Taking into account that members of social systems such as partners in a romantic relationship are recursively and self-organized linked to each other, the major goal was to positively initiate a process of reframing, perspective taking and expansion through interpersonal meta-awareness. Moreover, while being connected to one's own needs and values, the training aimed to support partners to engage in partner-related issues with a more resource-oriented and active actor-based understanding (seeing oneself as a co-creator), comprehending the complexity of relational processes on the one hand, and the constructivistic nature of (relational) perceptions on the other (Cecchin, 1987; Schlippe & Schweitzer, 2013). Finally, we tried to emphasize the development of a warm-hearted and caring attitude towards oneself and the other, resulting in a more tendered and emotional self-disclosing way of interacting – as there is a long tradition of emotion-focused couple therapy (Greenberg & Goldman, 2008). The first results of the SIDE study suggest improvement in ways as hypothesized and that are in line with the above-mentioned evidence: The depression scores in female partners decreased, whereas self-compassion and mindfulness increased. Furthermore, saliva cortisol in the female partners decreased on average in a positive social interaction task in the laboratory post training; in qualitative feedbacks, overall couples reported, for example, a stronger sense of understanding for each other. Compassion as a capacity to approach another's suffering with its foundation in an attentive and self-caring attitude enriched by appreciation, affection, and empathic concern seems to be a helpful tool for improving relationship quality, satisfaction, and social functioning.

With regard to families and/or children, adapted compassion training is in its infancy: There are few published articles focusing on CBCT® in foster care (Pace et al., 2013) or for at-risk adolescents (Reddy et al., 2013), with first promising results in better regulation of emotions and stress or even an assessed positive impact on inflammatory reactions via saliva CRP concentrations.

Compassion programs could also have positive effects on families and educational contexts, but these have so far not been scientifically tested, if at all (see Kirby, 2016). A highly innovative approach is the so-called Social, Emotional, and Ethical Learning Program (SEE Learning), which was developed at the Center for Contemplative Science and Compassion-Based Ethics at the Emory University (GA, USA) and is comparable to the CBCT® in terms of theoretical concepts (Center for Contemplative Science and Compassion-Based Ethics, 2019). However, it differs in its differentiation and implementation of pedagogical and didactic teaching methods and has been developed to be integrated into teaching in different school contexts in all age groups (for an overview, see: http://compassion.emory.edu/index.html or http://compassion.emory.edu/see-learning/index.html).

"Please Read the Package Brochure or Contact...?": Unwanted Side Effects

Of course, the difficult aspects of mindfulness and compassion practice should not be missing from this synopsis: Research on the side on negative effects of interventions that focus on mindfulness or compassion is still in its infancy. This is certainly due not least to the hype of contemplative techniques as a whole, but above all to the limited empirical data available on this topic – only one in five published studies report these particular effects at all (Wong, Chan, Zhang, Lee, & Tsoi, 2018; with regard to compassion alone no study at all could be detected). The difficulties initially pointed out with the lack of uniform definitions of these constructs, but also with measuring difficulties, certainly contribute significantly to this situation. In addition, it is crucial to narrow down exactly what is meant by (negative) side effects, for example – at least a perceived or measurable damage or harm to the participant of a corresponding intervention. According to psychotherapy research, in which the factors responsible for the success of therapy can be identified and named after the explanation of variance, it can be said in summary that these are certainly factors which concern the client, the therapist/instructor and their relationship and the intervention applied therein. Harmful effects can also be presumed in this field – and, as shown in the same way, can also be empirically proven in rudiments – and depend to a large extent on inadequate pre-assessments according to the initial situation of an individual participant, but also to a large extent on psychologically inadequately qualified, poorly trained trainer/therapists. The lack of competence of a trainer/therapist is then also responsible for a poor selection of precisely fitting, didactically skillful – also in terms of time and space – applied mindfulness/compassion-based methods and techniques that can enable a change process in the "right" direction for a specific person (Dobkin, Irving, & Amar, 2012).

Now to the facts: In about 20 case study reports, the affected meditators or the supervising trainers reported the following serious or highly stressful effects caused by the meditation itself or in connection to it: psychosis, mania, depersonalization, anxiety, and panic episodes and other psychological dysfunctions (Van Dam et al., 2018). In a recent systematic review of RCTs, 3 out of 25 MBSR and 1 out of 11 MBCT trials reported negative effects such as anger or anxiety (Wong et al., 2018). With regard to the difficulties of contemplative interventions in the social context, a study of the effectiveness of an online mindfulness program for families living with mental illness could show that the negative effects relate to, for example, feelings of guilt not to practice, practicing as a perceived additional stress factor, stirring up emotions, or realizing that one has made "wrong" decisions in the past. It becomes clear that these have basically nothing to do visibly with the social dimension (Stjernswärd & Hansson, 2017). It can therefore be deduced that the usual criteria – comparable to those generally discussed in the systemic world – could also be used here: For example, if one of the participants in the social system does not have any (inner) access to the contemplative method used, or if it is necessary to give the individual members of the system separate therapeutic space at a certain point in time, and others.

In summary, persons with a history of trauma or a current severe psychiatric diagnosis, including acute suicidal tendencies, should not be treated, or should not be treated exclusively and primarily with a purely contemplative intervention. Mindfulness and compassion are no substitute for proper diagnosis and treatment by trained professionals.

Commonalities and Divergences between Buddhist-Rooted Approaches and Systemic Thinking

Systemic theory and thinking can be linked to Buddhist-rooted contemplative approaches (see also Prosky, 2016; Schmidt, 2016). As systemic therapists are mostly concerned with a constructivist way of thinking, it is very important to take into account first-person-perspectives understanding the variety of perceptions, which is true for Buddhist-oriented approaches in terms of experience-oriented techniques that support developmental processes of deepening perception and sophisticating valid reasoning (see also Varela & Shear, 1999). In both, techniques are employed to promote perspective taking, shifting and extending perspectives and understanding one's own feelings and thoughts not as given, rigid truths but as conditioned possibilities (see also Vogd, 2016). From a cognition point of view, meta-cognition and awareness are tools in both respects (see also Varela, Thompson, & Rosch, 1991): Systemically, cybernetics is being understood in the sense of governance as part of a whole that is more than its parts, however still part of the whole (as a therapist being part of the social system, co-creating and co-directing the social interrelational process) (Simon, 2009), while in a Buddhist approach, meta-cognition enables a practitioner to make use of an inner mental faculty that observes inner processes of mind wandering, being attentive, re-focusing, etc., helping to regulate attention and building upon it also to regulate impulses and reactions (see also Lutz, Jha, Dunne, & Saron, 2015).

Mindfulness- and compassion-based practices utilize a non-judgmental, non-reactive, and decentered way of dealing with inner impulses, which might be a helpful tool to establish intrinsic neutrality, which is regarded as an ideal goal of systemic professional competence (e.g., Cecchin, 1987).

Although mindfulness- and compassion-based programs do not primarily focus on the enhancement of positive thinking and feelings per se, still they can be regarded as resource-oriented approaches which on the one hand make use of the basic potential of psychological abilities (attention processes; bonding and affiliation, etc.), but on the other hand also consider the social situation of the human being, that its survival is rooted in cooperation and pro-sociality (Hare, 2017). This is comparable to systemic thinking in its resource orientation, but also in its theoretical understanding of complexity and circularity. At the same time, the interdependence theory is analogous to the understanding of the dependent arising nature of phenomena, which is the heart of Buddhist teachings (see also Prosky, 2016; Vogd, 2016).

Furthermore, the attitude of being curious and not-knowing towards individuals, the social system, its members' views and ideas seems to be in line with attitudes proposed in Buddhist-rooted approaches of non-judgment and "beginners mind" (Rosch, 2007).

In both, the systemic and in the Buddhist world, self-responsibility is conceived as a freedom and necessary self-care. Everyone has the chance to turn difficulties, problems and dysfunctions into a different (self-)understanding ("reframing") or to overcome stagnation, or to change what can be changed without resigning (Panichelli, 2013).

In addition, in both traditions, the reference to the present is considered a reliable means of avoiding unnecessary and useless references to the past or the future – in the sense of ruminative thinking about things one might regret or in terms of worries or excessive fears of the future.

Instead, it is a matter of looking at what is useful for one's personal (systemic) goals in a functional and purposeful way in accordance with one's own (systemic) values. Paradoxically, it is about a goal orientation in which the goal may define a way, but without losing the reference to the here-and-now experience, neither clinging to the past nor to the future.

After all, both are to a certain extent concerned with dealing with uncertainties, unpredictability, tolerance with ambiguities (see also Vogd, 2016), and last but not least with making use of a realm of possibilities that is shaped less by prejudices than by the connectedness and fundamental commonalities of individuals.

Although the psychological and Buddhist-rooted construct "compassion," as described above, has largely not explicitly been addressed in systemic circles so far, systemic practitioners deal also "unspokenly" with an intimate, related interaction based on understanding, tolerance, and respect. Even if less normatively a "good human" behavior such as prosociality and altruism is to be addressed, the warm-heartedness and closeness that every human being needs basically in order to at least feel safe and be able to flourish also applies here.

A good practical example of the implicit application of "compassion" in the systemic field is the so-called "Open Dialogue," as described by Seikkula and Trimble (2005): This is mainly used in social contexts, in which the participants are exposed to extreme stress having to tolerate ambiguities. All participants are present during this intervention, while special emphasis is placed on the respectful handling of the (heavy) emotional states of others and one's own. The social network structure creates a kind of language of its own and thus a kind of new meaning – dialogue as a collaborative construction of meaning. This is particularly supported in the sense of reflective dialogues of the professionals. The factors of healing specified by the authors, such as creation of community and others, "(…) are supported by powerful mutual emotional attunement, an experience that most people would recognize as feelings of love" (p. 465), (…) as referred to non- "(…) romantic, but rather another kind of loving feeling found in families, absorbing mutual feelings of affection, empathy, concern, nurturance, safety, security, and deep emotional connection." (p. 469). The authors further explain that only with the complete presence of the whole person, in the sense of an embodied being, with the direct here-and-now reference of the professionals the possibility of a dialogue can arise. Special emphasis is placed on compassionate listening.

Outlook and Upcoming Research

What remains to be said at the end?

Contemplative practices such as mindfulness and compassion will be continuously adapted in different social contexts, as current results are promising in its positive effects enhancing social connectedness, co-regulation, and positive relationship quality and thereby achieving preventative and clinical treatment goals.

Further research is needed to identify the differential effects, mediators, and mechanisms that are of particular significance in the social context. Some current endeavors point in the direction of further and deeper comparison of the systemic and Buddhist theoretical approaches and of really enabling an advanced understanding in order to obtain further insights into the mind, its functioning, and the complexity of social structures from this kind of synergies.

Finally, systemic practitioners can benefit from a practice of mindfulness and compassion by continuously and openly questioning their own attitudes; sensitizing themselves to their own inner automatisms, thereby positively shaping their relationship with themselves and their clients; and to improve self- and other-oriented regulation.

A compassionate resonance with oneself and others is embedded in being connected with own needs, wishes, perspectives, and limitations, which only really makes it possible to get in touch with others fundamentally.

To close the circle, start where you are, and shift your perspective(s)!

References

Aguilar-Raab, C., Grevenstein, D., & Schweitzer, J. (2015). Measuring social relationships in different social systems: The construction and validation of the Evaluation of Social Systems (EVOS) Scale. *PLoS One, 10*(7), e0133442–e0133442. https://doi.org/10.1371/journal.pone.0133442

Aguilar-Raab, C., Jarczok, M. N., Warth, M., Stoffel, M., Winter, F., Tieck, M., … Ditzen, B. (2018). Enhancing Social Interaction in Depression (SIDE study): Protocol of a randomised controlled trial on the effects of a Cognitively Based Compassion Training (CBCT) for couples. *BMJ Open, 8*(9), e020448. https://doi.org/10.1136/bmjopen-2017-020448

Allen, J. P., Moore, C., Kuperminc, G., & Bell, K. (1998). Attachment and adolescent psychosocial functioning. *Child Development, 69*(5), 1406–1419.

Altmaier, E., & Maloney, R. (2007). An initial evaluation of a mindful parenting program. *Journal of Clinical Psychology, 63*(12), 1231–1238. https://doi.org/10.1002/jclp.20395

Asen, E., & Scholz, M. (2010). *Multi-family therapy: Concepts and techniques.* New York, NY: Routledge.

Atkinson, B. J. (2013). Mindfulness training and the cultivation of secure, satisfying couple relationships. *Couple and Family Psychology: Research and Practice, 2*(2), 73.

Baer, R. A. (2003). Mindfulness training as a clinical intervention: A conceptual and empirical review. *Clinical Psychology: Science and Practice, 10*, 125–143.

Baer, R. A., Smith, G. T., Hopkins, J., Krietemeyer, J., & Toney, L. (2006). Using self-report assessment methods to explore facets of mindfulness. *Assessment, 13*, 27–45.

Barnes, S., Brown, K. W., Krusemark, E., Campbell, W. K., & Rogge, R. D. (2007). The role of mindfulness in romantic relationship satisfaction and responses to relationship stress. *Journal of Marital and Family Therapy, 33*(4), 482–500. https://doi.org/10.1111/j.1752-0606.2007.00033.x

Bergomi, C., Tschacher, W., & Kupper, Z. (2013). The assessment of mindfulness with self-report measures: Existing scales and open issues. *Mindfulness, 4*(3), 191–202.

Bethell, C. D., Solloway, M. R., Guinosso, S., Hassink, S., Srivastav, A., Ford, D., & Simpson, L. A. (2017). Prioritizing possibilities for child and family health: An agenda to address adverse childhood experiences and foster the social and emotional roots of well-being in pediatrics. *Academic Pediatrics, 17*(7S), S36–S50. https://doi.org/10.1016/j.acap.2017.06.002

Biglan, A. (2015). *The nurture effect: How the science of human behavior can improve our lives and our world.* Oakland, CA: New Harbinger Publications.

Biglan, A., Flay, B. R., Embry, D. D., & Sandler, I. N. (2012). The critical role of nurturing environments for promoting human well-being. *American Psychologist, 67*(4), 257.

Bishop, S. R., Lau, M., Shapiro, S., Carlson, L., Anderson, N. D., Carmody, J., … Devins, G. (2004). Mindfulness: A proposed operational definition. *Clinical Psychology: Science and Practice, 11*, 230–241.

Bloch, J. H. (2018). Self-compassion, social connectedness, and interpersonal competence. Graduate student theses, dissertations, & professional papers. 11224. Montana, Missoula: University of Montana. https://scholarworks.umt.edu/etd/11224

Bögels, S., & Restifo, K. (2014). *Mindful parenting: A guide for mental health practitioners.* New York, NY: Springer.

Bögels, S. M., Hellemans, J., van Deursen, S., Römer, M., & van der Meulen, R. (2014). Mindful parenting in mental health care: Effects on parental and child psychopathology, parental stress, parenting, coparenting, and marital functioning. *Mindfulness, 5*(5), 536–551. https://doi.org/10.1007/s12671-013-0209-7

Bögels, S. M., Hoogstad, B., van Dun, L., de Schutter, S., & Restifo, K. (2008). Mindfulness training for adolescents with externalizing disorders and their parents. *Behavioural and Cognitive Psychotherapy, 36*(2), 193–209.

Bögels, S. M., Lehtonen, A., & Restifo, K. (2010). Mindful parenting in mental health care. *Mindfulness, 1*(2), 107–120. https://doi.org/10.1007/s12671-010-0014-5

Bowen, S., Witkiewitz, K., Clifasefi, S. L., Grow, J., Chawla, N., Hsu, S. H., … Larimer, M. E. (2014). Relative efficacy of mindfulness-based relapse prevention, standard relapse prevention, and treatment as usual for substance use disorders: A randomized clinical trial. *JAMA Psychiatry, 71*, 547–556.

Brito, G. (2014). Secular compassion training: An empirical review. *Journal of Transpersonal Research, 6*(2), 61–71.

Brown, F. L., Whittingham, K., Boyd, R. N., McKinlay, L., & Sofronoff, K. (2014). Improving child and parenting outcomes following paediatric acquired brain injury: A randomised controlled trial of Stepping Stones Triple P plus Acceptance and Commitment Therapy. *Journal of Child Psychology and Psychiatry, 55*(10), 1172–1183.

Brown, K. W., Creswell, J. D., & Ryan, R. M. (2015). *Handbook of mindfulness: Theory, research, and practice*. New York, NY: Guilford Publications.

Brown, K. W., & Ryan, R. M. (2003). The benefits of being present: Mindfulness and its role in psychological well-being. *Journal of Personality and Social Psychology, 84*, 822–848.

Burke, C. A. (2010). Mindfulness-based approaches with children and adolescents: A preliminary review of current research in an emergent field. *Journal of Child and Family Studies, 19*(2), 133–144.

Burpee, L. C., & Langer, E. J. (2005). Mindfulness and marital satisfaction. *Journal of Adult Development, 12*(1), 43–51.

Carson, J. W., Carson, K. M., Gil, K. M., & Baucom, D. H. (2004). Mindfulness-based relationship enhancement. *Behavior Therapy, 35*(3), 471–494. https://doi.org/10.1016/S0005-7894(04)80028-5

Cecchin, G. (1987). Hypothesizing, circularity, and neutrality revisited: An invitation to curiosity. *Family Process, 26*(4), 405–413. https://doi.org/10.1111/j.1545-5300.1987.00405.x

Center for Contemplative Science and Compassion-Based Ethics. (2019). *SEE Learning - social, emotional and ethical learning. An initiative for educating heart and mind - framework*. Atlanta, GA, USA: Emory University.

Chiesa, A., & Serretti, A. (2009). Mindfulness-based stress reduction for stress management in healthy people: A review and meta-analysis. *Journal of Alternative and Complementary Medicine, 15*, 593–600.

Coatsworth, J. D., Duncan, L. G., Greenberg, M. T., & Nix, R. L. (2010). Changing parent's mindfulness, child management skills and relationship quality with their youth: Results from a randomized pilot intervention trial. *Journal of Child and Family Studies, 19*(2), 203–217.

Desbordes, G., Negi, L. T., Pace, T. W. W., Wallace, B. A., Raison, C. L., & Schwartz, E. L. (2012). Effects of mindful-attention and compassion meditation training on amygdala response to emotional stimuli in an ordinary, non-meditative state. *Frontiers in Human Neuroscience, 6*, 292.

Di Fabio, A., & Kenny, M. E. (2016). Promoting well-being: The contribution of emotional intelligence. *Frontiers in Psychology, 7*, 1182. https://doi.org/10.3389/fpsyg.2016.01182

Ditzen, B., Hoppmann, C., & Klumb, P. (2008). Positive couple interactions and daily cortisol: On the stress-protecting role of intimacy. *Psychosomatic Medicine, 70*(8), 883–889. https://doi.org/10.1097/PSY.0b013e318185c4fc

Ditzen, B., Schaer, M., Gabriel, B., Bodenmann, G., Ehlert, U., & Heinrichs, M. (2009). Intranasal oxytocin increases positive communication and reduces cortisol levels during couple conflict. *Biological Psychiatry, 65*(9), 728–731. https://doi.org/10.1016/j.biopsych.2008.10.011

Dobkin, P., Irving, J. A., & Amar, S. (2012). For whom may participation in a mindfulness-based stress reduction program be contraindicated? *Mindfulness, 3*, 44–50. https://doi.org/10.1007/s12671-011-0079-9

Dodds, S. E., Pace, T. W. W., Bell, M. L., Fiero, M., Negi, L. T., Raison, C. L., & Weihs, K. L. (2015). Feasibility of Cognitively-Based Compassion Training (CBCT) for breast cancer survivors: A randomized, wait list controlled pilot study. *Supportive Care in Cancer, 23*(12), 3599–3608. https://doi.org/10.1007/s00520-015-2888-1

Dumas, J. E. (2005). Mindfulness-based parent training: Strategies to lessen the grip of automaticity in families with disruptive children. *Journal of Clinical Child and Adolescent Psychology, 34*(4), 779–791.

Duncan, L. G., Coatsworth, J. D., & Greenberg, M. T. (2009). A model of mindful parenting: Implications for parent–child relationships and prevention research. *Clinical Child and Family Psychology Review, 12*(3), 255–270. https://doi.org/10.1007/s10567-009-0046-3

Efklides, A. (2008). Metacognition: Defining its facets and levels of functioning in relation to self-regulation and co-regulation. *European Psychologist, 13*(4), 277–287. https://doi.org/10.1027/1016-9040.13.4.277

Evans, S., Ling, M., Hill, B., Rinehart, N., Austin, D., & Sciberras, E. (2018). Systematic review of meditation-based interventions for children with ADHD. *European Child & Adolescent Psychiatry, 27*(1), 9–27.

Feldman, C., & Kuyken, W. (2011). Compassion in the landscape of suffering. *Contemporary Buddhism, 12*(1), 143–155. https://doi.org/10.1080/14639947.2011.564831

Feldman, G., Dunn, E., Stemke, C., Bell, J., & Greeson, J. (2014). Mindfulness and rumination as predictors of persisntece with a distress tolerance task. *Personality and Individual Differences, 56*, 154–158. https://doi.org/10.1016/j.paid.2013.08.040

Fonagy, P. (2018). What makes a difference? Supporting families in caring for children. In P. Leach (Ed.), *Transforming infant wellbeing: Research, policy and practice for the first 1001 critical days*. New York, NY: Routledge.

Gambrel, L. E., & Piercy, F. P. (2015a). Mindfulness-based relationship education for couples expecting their first child-part 1: A randomized mixed-methods program evaluation. *Journal of Marital and Family Therapy, 41*(1), 5–24.

Gambrel, L. E., & Piercy, F. P. (2015b). Mindfulness-based relationship education for couples expecting their first child-part 2: Phenomenological findings. *Journal of Marital and Family Therapy, 41*(1), 25–41.

Gehart, D. R. (2012). *Mindfulness and acceptance in couple and family therapy*. New York, NY: Springer Science & Business Media.

Geisler, U., & Muttenhammer, J. (2016). *Achtsamkeitsübungen mit kindern und jugendlichen in der psychotherapie*. Paderborn, Germany: Junfermann Verlag.

Germer, C., & Barnhofer, T. (2017). Mindfulness and compassion: Similarities and differences. In P. Gilbert (Ed.), *Compassion: Concepts, research and applications* (1st ed., pp. 69–86). London, UK: Routledge.

Gilbert, P. (2009). Introducing compassion-focused therapy. *Advances in Psychiatric Treatment, 15*(3), 199–208. https://doi.org/10.1192/apt.bp.107.005264

Gilbert, P. (2010). *The compassionate mind: A new approach to life's challenges*. London: Constable.

Gilbert, P. (2013). *Compassion focused therapy*. Paderborn, Germany: Junfermann.

Gilbert, P. (2014). The origins and nature of compassion focused therapy. *British Journal of Clinical Psychology, 53*(1), 6–41. https://doi.org/10.1111/bjc.12043

Gilbert, P., McEwan, K., Mitra, R., Franks, L., Richter, A., & Rockliff, H. (2008). Feeling safe and content: A specific affect regulation system? Relationship to depression, anxiety, stress, and self-criticism. *The Journal of Positive Psychology, 3*(3), 182–191. https://doi.org/10.1080/17439760801999461

Godfrin, K. A., & van Heeringen, C. (2010). The effects of mindfulness-based cognitive therapy on recurrence of depressive episodes, mental health and quality of life: A randomized controlled study. *Behavior Reserach and Therapy, 48*, 738–746.

Goetz, J. L., Keltner, D., & Simon-Thomas, E. (2010). Compassion: An evolutionary analysis and empirical review. *Psychological Bulletin, 136*(3), 351.

Goldberg, S.B., Tuckerd, R.P., Greene, P.A., Davidson, R.J., Wampold, B.E., Kearney, D.J., Simpson, T.L. (2018). Mindfulness-based interventions for psychiatric disorders: A systematic review and meta-analysis. Clinical Psychology Review, 59, 52–60. https://doi.org/10.1016/j.cpr.2017.10.011

Goldin, P., & Jazaieri, H. (2017). The compassion cultivation training (CCT) program. In *The Oxford handbook of compassion science*. Oxford, UK: Oxford University Press.

Gotink, R. A., Chu, P., Busschbach, J. J. V., Benson, H., Fricchione, G. L., & Hunink, M. G. M. (2015). Standardised mindfulness-based interventions in healthcare: An overview of systematic reviews and meta-analyses of RCTs. *PLoS One, 10*, e0124344.

Green, S. M., & Bieling, P. J. (2012). Expanding the scope of mindfulness-based cognitive therapy: Evidence for effectiveness in a heterogeneous psychiatric sample. *Cognitive and Behavioral Practice, 19*, 174–180.

Greenberg, L. S., & Goldman, R. N. (2008). *Emotion-focused couples therapy: The dynamics of emotion, love, and power.* Washington, D.C.: American Psychological Association.

Grevenstein, D., Bluemke, M., Schweitzer-Rothers, J., & Aguilar-Raab, C. (2019). Better family relationships – higher well-being: The connection between relationship quality and health related resources. *Mental Health and Prevention, 14*, 200160. https://doi.org/10.1016/j.mph.2019.200160

Grossman, P. (2011). Defining mindfulness by how poorly I think I pay attention during everyday awareness and other intractable problems for psychology's (re)invention of mindfulness: Comment on Brown et al (2011). *Psychological Assessment, 23*, 1034–1040.

Grossman, P., Tiefenthaler-Gilmer, U., Raysz, A., & Kesper, U. (2007). Mindfulness training as an intervention for fibromyalgia: Evidence of postintervention and 3-year follow-up benefits in weil-being. *Psychotherapy and Psychosomatics, 76*, 226–233.

Gu, J., Strauss, C., Bond, R., & Cavanagh, K. (2015). How do mindfulness-based cognitive therapy and mindfulness-based stress reduction improve mental health and wellbeing? A systematic review and meta-analysis of mediation studies. *Clinical Psychology Review, 37*, 1–12.

Guajardo, N. R., Snyder, G., & Petersen, R. (2009). Relationships among parenting practices, parental stress, child behaviour, and children's social-cognitive development. *Infant and Child Development: An International Journal of Research and Practice, 18*(1), 37–60.

Gutman, L. M., & Feinstein, L. (2010). Parenting behaviours and children's development from infancy to early childhood: Changes, continuities and contributions. *Early Child Development and Care, 180*(4), 535–556.

Haimerl, C. J., & Valentine, E. R. (2001). The effect of contemplative practice on intrapersonal, interpersonal, and transpersonal dimensions of the self-concept. *Journal of Transpersonal Psychology, 33*(1), 37–52.

Hare, B. (2017). Survival of the friendliest: Homo sapiens evolved via selection for prosociality. *Annual Review of Psychology, 68*, 155–186. https://doi.org/10.1146/annurev-psych-010416-044201

Hayes, S. C., Strosahl, K. D., & Wilson, K. G. (2011). *Acceptance and commitment therapy: The process and practice of mindful change.* New York, NY: Guilford Press.

Hempel, S., Taylor, S. L., Marshall, N. J., Miake-Lye, I. M., Beroes, J. M., Shanman, R., … Shekelle, P. G. (2014). *Evidence map of mindfulness.* In *VA Evidence-based Synthesis Program Reports.* Washington, D.C.: Department of Veterans Affairs (US).

Hirschfeld, R. M., Montgomery, S. A., Keller, M. B., Kasper, S., Schatzberg, A. F., Moller, H. J., … Bourgeois, M. (2000). Social functioning in depression: A review. *Journal of Clinical Psychiatry, 61*(4), 268–275.

Hodgins, H. S., & Adair, K. C. (2010). Attentional processes and meditation. *Consciousness and Cognition, 19*(4), 872–878.

Hofmann, S. G., Grossman, P., & Hinton, D. E. (2011). Loving-kindness and compassion meditation: Potential for psychological interventions. *Clinical Psychology Review, 31*(7), 1126–1132. https://doi.org/10.1016/j.cpr.2011.07.003

Hofmann, S. G., Sawyer, A. T., Witt, A. A., & Oh, D. (2010). The effect of mindfulness-based therapy on anxiety and depression: A meta-analytic review. *Journal of Consulting and Clinical Psychology, 78*, 169–183.

Holt-Lunstad, J. (2018). Why social relationships are important for physical health: A systems approach to understanding and modifying risk and protection. *Annual Review of Psychology, 69*, 437–458. https://doi.org/10.1146/annurev-psych-122216-011902

Holt-Lunstad, J., Smith, T. B., & Layton, J. B. (2010). Social relationships and mortality risk: A meta-analytic review. *PLoS Medicine, 7*(7), e1000316. https://doi.org/10.1371/journal.pmed.1000316

Hölzel, B. K., Carmody, J., Evans, K. C., Hoge, E. A., Dusek, J. A., Morgan, L., … Lazar, S. W. (2010). Stress reduction correlates with structural changes in the amygdala. *Social Cognitive and Affective Neuroscience, 5*(1), 11–17. https://doi.org/10.1093/scan/nsp034

Horn, A. B., & Maercker, A. (2016). Intra- and interpersonal emotion regulation and adjustment symptoms in couples: The role of co-brooding and co-reappraisal. *BMC Psychology, 4*(1), 51. https://doi.org/10.1186/s40359-016-0159-7

Hutcherson, C. A., Seppala, E. M., & Gross, J. J. (2008). Loving-kindness meditation increases social connectedness. *Emotion (Washington, DC), 8*(5), 720–724. https://doi.org/10.1037/a0013237

Jacobson, E. H. K., Wilson, K. G., Kurz, A. S., & Kellum, K. K. (2018). Examining self-compassion in romantic relationships. *Journal of Contextual Behavioral Science, 8*, 69–73.

Jha, A. P., Krompinger, J., & Baime, M. J. (2007). Mindfulness training modifies subsystems of attention. *Cognitive, Affective, & Behavioral Neuroscience, 7*(2), 109–119.

Jones, K. C., Welton, S. R., Oliver, T. C., & Thoburn, J. W. (2011). Mindfulness, spousal attachment, and marital satisfaction: A mediated model. *The Family Journal, 19*(4), 357–361.

Kabat-Zinn, J. (1990). *Full catastrophe living. Using the wisdom of your body and mind to face stress, pain and illness.* New York, NY: Delacorte.

Kabat-Zinn, J. (1994). *Wherever you go, there you are: Mindfulness meditation in everyday life.* New York, NY: Hyperion.

Kabat-Zinn, J. (2003). Mindfulness-based interventions in context: Past, present, and future. *Clinical Psychology: Science and Practice, 10*, 144–156.

Kabat-Zinn, M., & Kabat-Zinn, J. (2009). *Everyday blessings: The inner work of mindful parenting.* New York, NY: Hachette.

Kearney, D. J., McDermott, K., Malte, C., Martinez, M., & Simpson, T. L. (2011). Association of participation in a mindfulness program with measures of PTSD, depression and quality of life in a veteran sample. *Journal of Clinical Psychology, 68*(1), 101–116. https://doi.org/10.1002/jclp.20853

Khoury, B., Lecomte, T., Fortin, G., Masse, M., Therien, P., Bouchard, V., … Hofmann, S. G. (2013). Mindfulness-based therapy: A comprehensive meta-analysis. *Clinical Psychology Review, 33*(6), 763–771. https://doi.org/10.1016/j.cpr.2013.05.005

Khoury, B., Sharma, M., Rush, S. E., & Fournier, C. (2015). Mindfulness-based stress reduction for healthy individuals: A meta-analysis. *Journal of Psychosomatic Research, 78*, 519–528.

King, A. P., Erickson, T. M., Giardino, N. D., Favorite, T., Rauch, S. A. M., Robinson, E., … Liberzon, I. (2013). A pilot study of group mindfulness-based cognitive therapy (MBCT) for combat verterans with postraumatic stress disorder (PTSD). *Depression and Anxiety, 30*(7), 638–645. https://doi.org/10.1002/da.22104

Kirby, J. N. (2016). The role of mindfulness and compassion in enhancing nurturing family environments. *Clinical Psychology: Science and Practice, 23*(2), 142–157. https://doi.org/10.1111/cpsp.12149

Kirby, J. N. (2017). Compassion interventions: The programmes, the evidence, and implications for research and practice. *Psychology and Psychotherapy: Theory, Research and Practice, 90*(3), 432–455. https://doi.org/10.1111/papt.12104

Kirby, J. N., Tellegen, C. L., & Steindl, S. R. (2017). A meta-analysis of compassion-based interventions: Current state of knowledge and future directions. *Behavior Therapy, 48*(6), 778–792. https://doi.org/10.1016/j.beth.2017.06.003

Klimecki, O. M., Leiberg, S., Ricard, M., & Singer, T. (2013). Differential pattern of functional brain plasticity after compassion and empathy training. *Social Cognitive and Affective Neuroscience, 9*(6), 873–879.

Kok, B. E., & Fredrickson, B. L. (2014). Wellbeing begins with "we": The physical and mental health benefits of interventions that increase social closeness. In F. A. Huppert & C. L. Cooper (Eds.), *Interventions and policies to enhance well-being: A complete reference guide* (Vol. 6, pp. 1–29). https://doi.org/10.1002/9781118539415.wbwell042

Kok, B. E., & Singer, T. (2017). Effects of contemplative dyads on engagement and percieved social connectedness over 9 months of mental training: A randomized clinical trial. *JAMA Psychiatry, 74*(2), 126–134. https://doi.org/10.1001/jamapsychiatry.2016.3360

Kozlowski, A. (2012). Mindful mating: Exploring the connection between mindfulness and relationship satisfaction. *Sexual and Relationship Therapy, 28*(1–2), 92–104.

Kramer, G., Meleo-Meyer, F., & Turner, M. L. (2008). Cultivating mindfulness in relationship: Insight dialogue and the interpersonal mindfulness program. In S. F. Hick & T. Bien (Eds.), *Mindfulness and the therapeutic relationship* (pp. 195–214). Guilford Press, New York, NY.

Kröger, C., Heinrichs, N., & Hahlweg, K. (2009). In M. Hautzinger & P. Pauli (Eds.), *Kompetenz-, Kommunikations- und Problemlösetraining [Competence training, communication training, and problem-solving training]*. Göttingen, Germany: Hofgrefe.

Kuyken, W., Byford, S., Taylor, R. S., Watkins, E., Holden, E., White, K., … Teasdale, J. D. (2008). Mindfulness-based cognitive therapy to prevent relapse in recurrent depression. *Journal of Consulting and Clinical Psychology, 76*, 966–978.

Kuyken, W., Warren, F. C., Taylor, R. S., Whalley, B., Crane, C., Bondolfi, G., … Dalgleish, T. (2016). Efficacy of Mindfulness-Based Cognitive Therapy in prevention of depressive relapse: An individual patient data meta-analysis from randomized trials. *JAMA Psychiatry, 73*, 565–574.

Lama, D., & Ekman, P. (2008). *Emotional awareness: Overcoming the obstacles to psychological balance and compassion*. New York, NY: Holt Paperbacks.

Langri, T. J., & Weiss, L. (2013). Compassion cultivation training (CCT). In T. Singer & M. Bolz (Eds.), *Compassion: Bridging theory and practice* (pp. 441–451). Leipzig, Germany: Max Planck Institute for Human Cognitive and Brain Sciences.

Laurent, H. K., Hertz, R., Nelson, B., & Laurent, S. M. (2016). Mindfulness during romantic conflict moderates the impact of negative partner behaviors on cortisol responses. *Hormones and Behavior, 79*, 45–51. https://doi.org/10.1016/j.yhbeh.2016.01.005

Lutz, A., Jha, A. P., Dunne, J. D., & Saron, C. D. (2015). Investigating the phenomenological matrix of mindfulness-related practices from a neurocognitive perspective. *American Psychologist, 70*(7), 632–658. https://doi.org/10.1037/a0039585

Mascaro, J. S., Kelley, S., Darcher, A., Negi, L. T., Worthman, C., Miller, A., & Raison, C. (2018). Meditation buffers medical student compassion from the deleterious effects of depression. *The Journal of Positive Psychology, 13*(2), 133–142. https://doi.org/10.1080/17439760.2016.1233348

Mascaro, J. S., Rilling, J. K., Negi, L. T., & Raison, C. L. (2013). Pre-existing brain function predicts subsequent practice of mindfulness and compassion meditation. *NeuroImage, 69*, 35–42.

Moffitt, T. E., Arseneault, L., Belsky, D., Dickson, N., Hancox, R. J., Harrington, H., … Ross, S. (2011). A gradient of childhood self-control predicts health, wealth, and public safety. *Proceedings of the National Academy of Sciences, 108*(7), 2693–2698.

Neff, K. D. (2003). The development and validation of a scale to measure self-compassion. *Self and Identity, 2*(3), 223–250. https://doi.org/10.1080/15298860390209035

Neff, K. D., & Beretvas, S. N. (2013). The role of self-compassion in romantic relationships. *Self and Identity, 12*(1), 78–98.

Nila, K., Holt, D. V., Ditzen, B., & Aguilar-Raab, C. (2016). Mindfulness-based stress reduction (MBSR) enhances distress tolerance and resilience through changes in mindfulness. *Mental Health & Prevention, 4*(1), 36–41. https://doi.org/10.1016/j.mhp.2016.01.001

O'Brien, M. P., Gordon, J. L., Bearden, C. E., Lopez, S. R., Kopelowicz, A., & Cannon, T. D. (2006). Positive family environment predicts improvement in symptoms and social functioning among adolescents at imminent risk for onset of psychosis. *Schizophrenia Research, 81*(2–3), 269–275.

Overall, N. C., Fletcher, G. J., & Simpson, J. A. (2010). Helping each other grow: Romantic partner support, self-improvement, and relationship quality. *Personality and Social Psychology Bulletin, 36*(11), 1496–1513.

Ozawa-de Silva, B., & Negi, L. T. (2013). Cognitively-Based Compassion Training: Protocol and key concepts. In T. Singer & M. Bolz (Eds.), *Compassion: Bridging theory and practice* (pp. 416–438). Leipzig, Germany: Max Planck Institute for Human Cognitive and Brain Sciences.

Pace, T. W. W., Negi, L. T., Adame, D. D., Cole, S. P., Sivilli, T. I., Brown, T. D., … Raison, C. L. (2009). Effect of compassion meditation on neuroendocrine, innate immune and behavioral responses to psychosocial stress. *Psychoneuroendocrinology, 34*(1), 87–98. https://doi.org/10.1016/j.psyneuen.2008.08.011

Pace, T. W. W., Negi, L. T., Dodson-Lavelle, B., Ozawa-de Silva, B., Reddy, S. D., Cole, S. P., ... Raison, C. L. (2013). Engagement with cognitively-based compassion training is associated with reduced salivary C-reactive protein from before to after training in foster care program adolescents. *Psychoneuroendocrinology, 38*(2), 294–299.

Pace, T. W. W., Negi, L. T., Sivilli, T. I., Issa, M. J., Cole, S. P., Adame, D. D., & Raison, C. L. (2010). Innate immune, neuroendocrine and behavioral responses to psychosocial stress do not predict subsequent compassion meditation practice time. *Psychoneuroendocrinology, 35*(2), 310–315.

Panichelli, C. (2013). Humor, joining, and reframing in psychotherapy: Resolving the Auto-Double-Bind. *The American Journal of Family Therapy, 41*(5), 437–451. https://doi.org/10.1080/01926187.2012.755393

Prosky, P. (2016). From systems theory to compassion: Further steps to an ecology of mind. *Human Systems: The Journal of Therapy, Consultation and Training, 27*(2), 169–178.

Pruitt, I. T., & McCollum, E. E. (2010). Voices of experienced meditators: The impact of meditation practice on intimate relationships. *Contemporary Family Therapy, 32*(2), 135–154. https://doi.org/10.1007/s10591-009-9112-8

Reddy, S. D., Negi, L. T., Dodson-Lavelle, B., Ozawa-de Silva, B., Pace, T. W. W., Cole, S. P., ... Craighead, L. W. (2013). Cognitive-based compassion training: A promising prevention strategy for at-risk adolescents. *Journal of Child and Family Studies, 22*(2), 219–230.

Rehman, U. S., Gollan, J., & Mortimer, A. R. (2008). The marital context of depression: Research, limitations, and new directions. *Clinical Psychology Review, 28*(2), 179–198. https://doi.org/10.1016/j.cpr.2007.04.007

Reis, H. T., Maniaci, M. R., & Rogge, R. D. (2014). The expression of compassionate love in everyday compassionate acts. *Journal of Social and Personal Relationships, 31*(5), 651–676.

Robles, T. F., Slatcher, R. B., Trombello, J. M., & McGinn, M. M. (2014). Marital quality and health: A meta-analytic review. *Psychological Bulletin, 140*(1), 140.

Rosch, E. (2007). More than mindfulness: When you have a tiger by the tail, let it eat you. *Psychological Inquiry - An International Journal for the Advancement of Psychological Theory, 18*(4), 258–264. https://doi.org/10.1080/10478400701598371

Santorelli, S. F., Meleo-Meyer, F., Koerbel, L., & Kabat-Zinn, J. (2017). *Mindfulness-based stress reduction (MBSR) authorized curriculum guide*. Retrieved from https://www.umassmed.edu/cfm/training/mbsr-curriculum/

Sawyer Cohen, J. A., & Semple, R. J. (2010). Mindful parenting: A call for research. *Journal of Child and Family Studies, 19*(2), 145–151. https://doi.org/10.1007/s10826-009-9285-7

Schlippe, A. v., & Schweitzer, J. (2013). *Lehrbuch der systemischen therapie und beratung I: Das grundlagenwissen*. Göttingen, Germany: Vandenhoeck & Ruprecht.

Schmidt, S. (2016). Eine systemische perspektive auf die praxis der achtsamkeit. *Kontext, 47*(4), 335–353.

Schoebi, D., & Randall, A. K. (2015). Emotional dynamics in intimate relationships. *Emotion Review, 7*(4), 342–348. https://doi.org/10.1177/1754073915590620

Seikkula, J., & Trimble, D. (2005). Healing elements of therapeutic conversation: Dialogue as an embodiment of love. *Family Process, 44*, 461–475. https://doi.org/10.1111/j.1545-5300.2005.00072.x

Shapiro, S. L., Carlson, L. E., Astin, J. A., & Freedman, B. (2006). Mechanisms of mindfulness. *Journal of Clinical Psychology, 62*(3), 373–386.

Shonin, E., Gordon, W. V., & Griffiths, M. D. (2014). Loving-kindness and compassion meditation in psychotherapy. *Psychology of Religion and Spirituality, 6*, 123–127.

Shonin, E., Van Gordon, W., Compare, A., Zangeneh, M., & Griffiths, M. D. (2015). Buddhist-derived loving-kindness and compassion meditation for the treatment of psychopathology: A systematic review. *Mindfulness, 6*(5), 1161–1180.

Siegel, D. J., & Hartzell, M. (2003). *Parenting from the inside out*. New York, NY: Jeremy P. Tarcher - Penguin.

Simon, F. (2009). *Einführung in systemtheorie und konstruktivismus*. Heidelberg, Germany: Carl-Auer Verlag.

Singer, T., & Boltz, M. (2013). *Mitgefühl: In alltag und forschung.* Deutschland: Max-Planck-Gesellschaft.

Singer, T., & Klimecki, O. M. (2014). Empathy and compassion. *Current Biology, 24,* R875–R878. https://doi.org/10.1016/j.cub.2014.06.054

Singh, N. N., Singh, A. N., Lancioni, G. E., Singh, J., Winton, A. S., & Adkins, A. D. (2010). Mindfulness training for parents and their children with ADHD increases the children's compliance. *Journal of Child and Family Studies, 19*(2), 157–166.

Smetana, J. G., Campione-Barr, N., & Metzger, A. (2006). Adolescent development in interpersonal and societal contexts. *Annual Review of Psychology, 57,* 255–284.

Stack, D. M., Serbin, L. A., Enns, L. N., Ruttle, P. L., & Barrieau, L. (2010). Parental effects on children's emotional development over time and across generations. *Infants & Young Children, 23*(1), 52–69. https://doi.org/10.1097/IYC.0b013e3181c97606

Stjernswärd, S., & Hansson, L. (2017). Effectiveness and usability of a web-based mindfulness interventions for families living with mental illness. *Mindfulness, 8,* 751–764. https://doi.org/10.1007/s12671-016-0653-2

Strauss, C., Cavanagh, K., Oliver, A., & Pettman, D. (2014). Mindfulness-based interventions for people diagnosed with a current episode of an anxiety or depressive disorder: A meta-analysis of randomised controlled trials. *PLoS One, 9,* 1–13.

Strauss, C., Taylor, B. L., Gu, J., Kuyken, W., Baer, R., Jones, F., & Cavanagh, K. (2016). What is compassion and how can we measure it? A review of definitions and measures. *Clinical Psychology Review, 47,* 15–27.

Tang, Y.-Y., Hölzel, B. K., & Posner, M. I. (2015). The neuroscience of mindfulness meditation. *Nature Reviews Neuroscience, 16*(4), 213.

Taylor, V. A., Grant, J., Daneault, V., Scavone, G., Breton, E., Roffe-Vidal, S., … Beauregard, M. (2011). Impact of mindfulness on the neural responses to emotional pictures in experienced and beginner meditators. *NeuroImage, 57*(4), 1524–1533.

Teasdale, J. D., Segal, Z. V., Williams, J. M., Ridgeway, V. A., Soulsby, J. M., & Lau, M. A. (2000). Prevention of relapse/recurrence in major depression by mindfulness-based cognitive therapy. *Journal of Consulting and Clinical Psychology, 68,* 615–623.

Vago, D. R., & Silbersweig, D. A. (2012). Self-awareness, self-regulation, and self-transcendence (S-ART): A framework for understanding the neurobiological mechanisms of mindfulness. *Frontiers in Human Neuroscience, 6,* 296. https://doi.org/10.3389/fnhum.2012.00296

Van Dam, N. T., van Vugt, M. K., Vago, D. R., Schmalzl, L., Saron, C. D., Olendzki, A., … Meyer, D. E. (2018). Mind the hype: A critical evaluation and prescriptive agenda for research on mindfulness and meditation. *Perspectives on Psychological Science, 13*(1), 36–61. https://doi.org/10.1177/1745691617709589

Varela, F.J. (1977). On being autonomous: The lessons of natural history for systems theory. In: G. Klir (Ed.), *Applied systems research.* New York, NY: Plenum Press. p. 77–85 as cited in: Rudrauf, D. (2003). From autopoiesis to neurophenomenology: Francisco Varela's exploration of the biophysics of being. *Biology Research, 36,* 27–65.

Varela, F. J., & Shear, J. (1999). First-person methododologies: What, why, how? *Journal of Conciousness Studies, 6*(2–3), 1–14.

Varela, F. J., Thompson, E., & Rosch, E. (1991). *The embodied mind: Cognitive science and human experience.* Cambridge, MA: MIT Press.

Vogd, W. (2016). Wozu achtsam sein und worauf die Achtsamkeit lenken? Welten ohne Grund bauen und darin heimisch werden! *Kontext, 47*(4), 374–384.

Vøllestad, J., Nielsen, M. B., & Nielsen, G. H. (2012). Mindfulness- and acceptance-based interventions for anxiety disorders: A systematic review and meta-analysis. *British Journal of Clinical Psychology, 51,* 239–260.

Wachs, K., & Cordova, J. V. (2007). Mindful relating: Exploring mindfulness and emotion repertoires in intimate relationships. *Journal of Marital and Family Therapy, 33*(4), 464–481. https://doi.org/10.1111/j.1752-0606.2007.00032.x

Williard, C., & Saltzman, A. (2015). *Teaching mindfulness skills to kids and teens.* New York, NY: Guilford Press.

Wong, S. Y. S., Chan, J. Y. C., Zhang, D., Lee, E. K. P., & Tsoi, K. K. F. (2018). The safety of mindfulness-based interventions: A systematic review of randomized controlled trials. *Mindfulness, 9*, 1344–1357. https://doi.org/10.1007/s12671-018-0897-0

Yalom, I. D. (1995). *The theory and practice of group psychotherapy*. New York, NY: Basic Books.

Zylowska, L., Ackerman, D. L., Yang, M. H., Futrell, J. L., Horton, N. L., Hale, T. S., … Smalley, S. L. (2007). Mindfulness meditation training in adults and adolescents with ADHD: A feasibility study. *Journal of Attention Disorders, 11*(6), 737–746.

Where Are the Emotions? How Emotion-Focused Therapy Could Inspire Systemic Practice

Julika Zwack and Leslie Greenberg

The Theoretical Framework of EFT

Emotion-focused therapy (EFT) is based on the assumptions that humans are emotionally organized beings and that emotional change is key to enduring cognitive and behavioural change. In line with neurobiological research (Damasio, 1999), emotions are understood as an evolutionary information processing and problem-solving system that help people survive by offering rapid implicit judgements and action tendencies. Emotions offer messages about threats to our fundamental needs, they help us decode what is going on in our relationships, and signal others about the current relational state we feel we are in. Without emotions, learning seems impossible. Based on previous experience, emotions organize action tendencies in accordance with our needs and goals – much faster than any conscious analysis.

This emotional information processing system evolved due to its adaptivity. However, emotions can also go wrong. They can be misleading, too intense or destructive in their expression. Emotion is not "always right." It should neither be mistaken as the conclusion nor the action itself. Emotional schemes provide information that needs to be listened to and handled in an interplay between bottom-up processing and conscious reflection. Greenberg (2015, p.66) suggests a dialectically constructivist view on emotion: "We construct what we feel by attending to a bodily felt sense and symbolizing it in awareness, and our construction is informed and constrained by what we feel in our bodies." Seen this way, emotion and cognition are inextricably intertwined.

J. Zwack (✉)
Institute of Medical Psychology, Center of Psychosocial Medicine, Heidelberg University Hospital, Heidelberg, Germany
e-mail: Julika.Zwack@med.uni-heidelberg.de

L. Greenberg
Faculty of Health, York University in Toronto, Toronto, ON, Canada

© Springer Nature Switzerland AG 2020
M. Ochs et al. (eds.), *Systemic Research in Individual, Couple, and Family Therapy and Counseling*, European Family Therapy Association Series,
https://doi.org/10.1007/978-3-030-36560-8_14

Working with Emotions: Maps Through the Experiential Territory

EFT assumes that emotions need to be felt to be transformed and to reveal their transforming power. The therapeutic expertise in EFT thus centres around methods to help clients access and express emotions and needs. Since not all emotions are the same, therapists and clients need to differentiate (Greenberg, 2015, p. 73):

- A healthy core feeling, an *adaptive primary emotion*
- A wounded core feeling, a *maladaptive primary emotion*
- A reactive or defensive emotion that obscures a primary feeling, *a secondary emotion*
- An influencing or sometimes manipulative emotion that people use to get something they want, *an instrumental emotion*

Adaptive primary emotions are the main source of emotional intelligence. They represent automatic first responses, in which emotional evaluation, intensity and action tendency fit the situation and prepare for adaptive behaviour. Examples are sadness at loss that reaches out for comfort, fear at threat, anger at violation, hopelessness that lets go of a need that cannot be met.

Maladaptive primary emotions also represent first responses to a given situation. However, they are more a reflection of unresolved past experiences and do not prepare the individual for adaptive action in the current situation. Maladaptive emotions resemble solutions of the past – they might have been adaptive in the original traumatic and aversive circumstances, but no longer help to adapt to the here and now. In a highly nonresponsive and devaluing environment, it can be adaptive to vanish into shame to prevent further rejection, in an abandoning environment to feel sad and fear being alone. In a context of abuse, constant alertness and fear are necessary to protect oneself. If violation of borders and rights is a daily occurrence, anger is a healthy reaction. Being stuck in these emotions of deep worthlessness, shaky insecurity or destructive anger, however, prevents adaptive action in the present. Maladaptive emotions are like unhealed wounds that open again and again without offering a sense of direction.

Secondary emotions act as defences against a more primary feeling. They obscure what is felt deep inside and act as symptoms of emotions that are so far not dealt with. Secondary emotions function to avoid or obscure primary reactions and are often influenced by sociocultural imprints. Women who were told to be submissive might cry when they are angry, men might convert to anger or aggression when they are feeling weak, ashamed or sad. Secondary emotions might also arise from the attempt to protect oneself and important others from feelings that might endanger the relationship. Often, secondary guilt or anxiety can shield off primary anger.

Instrumental emotions are learned expressive behaviours that are – consciously or unconsciously – used to influence or manipulate others. Examples are anger that aims to control the other, submissive shyness to avoid conflict or "crocodile tears" to evoke sympathy.

Whether an emotion is primary or secondary cannot be determined from the type of emotion alone. Sadness, anger, fear, shame and anxiety as well as complex emotions such as guilt, embarrassment, jealousy can each be primary as well as secondary.

Therapeutic Change in EFT

Promoting emotional experience and change presupposes a stable, trusted and safe therapeutic relationship. The therapeutic relationship in EFT is characterized by a high degree of therapist presence, empathic following and a moment-to-moment guiding of emotional processing. This empathic therapeutic relationship is seen curative in itself. Depending on the client's state, marker-guided interventions are used to help to identify, accept, explore and transform emotions. Change evolves as a dynamic self-organizing process and is based on an acceptance and symbolization of what is. As Greenberg (2015) points out: You have to arrive at a place in order to leave it. Using whatever comes up emotionally in the here and now, EFT focuses on experiential instead of conceptual knowledge. Change *emerges* from the bottom-up actualization of primary adaptive emotions, rather than from deliberate actions to reach specific goals.

Within EFT the therapeutic road leads from secondary to primary emotions and from maladaptive to adaptive emotions. This process includes interventions to arrive at core feelings, followed by interventions to move on and transform maladaptive emotions. *Arriving at an emotion* means connecting to its visceral experience, feeling it from the inside rather than gaining intellectual understanding. The EFT therapist will shift clients' attention to the bodily sensations and continuously guide awareness towards internal experience. Using empathic attunement and focusing, the therapist helps the client symbolize feelings and to identify primary emotions beneath secondary reactions. Once arrived at this primary state, therapist and client will ask whether it is a healthy feeling that informs and prepares for adaptive action or a maladaptive reaction that is based on some old wound and needs to be processed further. As Greenberg and Paivio (1997) figured out in their study on affective disorders and childhood maltreatment, two predominant maladaptive core feelings are shame and fear-anxiety. Whereas shame is related to a generalized sense of being worthless ("bad me") fear-anxiety is accompanied by insecurity and fragility – a "weak me" sense of self.

To leave maladaptive emotions, the client is then supported to express accompanying beliefs on self and other. These beliefs ("I am a failure"; "Nobody can be trusted") are not discussed in terms of validity and rationality but used to explore the core emotion schemes that need to be changed. Paradoxically, this guided deepening of maladaptive states stimulates the mobilization of healthier emotions by challenging resilient opponency and offering access to fundamental needs ("What do you need when you feel this?"). Healthy grieving to let go of unmet needs, assertive anger to defend boundaries and right wrongs, self-compassion for the suffered deprivations are some examples of adaptive states that will emerge. It is fundamental to EFT that these emotional changes are not brought about by reason. Instead, shifting clients' attention to the core need that is hidden beneath the maladaptive emotion, is a bottom-up approach to activate different feelings and internal resources ("Changing emotion with emotion"). Access to alternate adaptive emotions is further facilitated by empathic conjectures that address adaptive but subdominant emotions displayed in the client's voice, facial expression, gesture or wording.

Finally, this embodied change is explicated in a new narrative. This may include adding emotions to empty stories ("Feeling what it meant..."), storying unstoried emotions ("Why I am feeling the way I am feeling") or using new emotions to develop new stories ("I deserved better" or "It is not my responsibility") (Angus & Greenberg, 2013). As process-outcome research on the emotion-focused treatment has shown, high emotional arousal plus high reflection on aroused emotion distinguished good and poor outcome cases, indicating the importance of combining arousal and meaning construction (Missirlian, Toukmanian, Warwar, & Greenberg, 2005).

The process described above is supported by *marker-guided interventions* (Greenberg, Rice, & Elliott, 2003) that address specific emotional processing problems. Based on task analysis (Greenberg, 1984) and process research, typical problematic cognitive-emotional states serve as markers for specific interventions that have proven to be effective in problem resolution. Greenberg (2015) differentiates the following tasks: *empathic affirmation* in moments of vulnerable self-disclosure, *experiential focusing* (Gendlin, 1996) to symbolize unclear emotional states, *systematic evocative unfolding* in case of puzzling overreaction to specific events, *two-chair dialogue for self-evaluative splits* (inner critic), *two-chair enactment* to resolve *self-interruptions* and blocked feelings, *empty-chair work* addressing *"unfinished business"* and *compassionate self-soothing* in case of overwhelming emotional suffering from unmet needs.

Research on EFT

Emotion-focused therapies (EFTs) have been shown to be effective in both individual and couples forms of therapy in a number of randomized clinical trials (Elliott, Greenberg, & Lietaer, 2004; Johnson, Hunsley, Greenberg, & Schindler, 1999). A manualized form of emotion-focused therapy of depression, in which specific emotion activation methods were used within the context of an empathic relationship, was found to be highly effective in treating depression in three separate studies (Goldman, Greenberg, & Angus, 2006; Greenberg & Watson, 1998; Watson, Gordon, Stermac, Kalogerakos, & Steckley, 2003). EFT was found to be more effective in reducing interpersonal problems than CBT treatment and highly effective in preventing relapse (77% nonrelapse) (Ellison, Greenberg, Goldman, & Angus, 2009). Emotion-focused therapy for emotional injuries using Empty Chair Dialogue to enact dialogues with the injurer have been found to be superior to psycho-education groups in two studies (Greenberg, Warwar, & Malcolm, 2008; Paivio & Greenberg, 1995). Emotion Focused Trauma Therapy (EFTT) (Paivio & Pascual-Leone, 2009) for adult survivors of childhood abuse has been found effective in treating abuse (Paivio & Nieuwenhuis, 2001; Paivio, Jarry, Chagigiorgis, Hall, & Ralston, 2010).

Emotion-Focused Couple Therapy

The practice of Emotion-Focused Couple Therapy (EFT-C) evolved from its inception as a combination of intrapsychic and systemic/interactional perspectives (Greenberg & Johnson, 1986, 1988) and involved an effort of bringing emotion to a systemic perspective. The aim of EFT-C is to help partners disengage from their negative interactional cycle by having them express the primary vulnerable emotions and unmet needs, which underlie their blaming, controlling, distancing and other hurtful patterns of behaviour. This typically invites empathy and validation from the other partner, which gives way to a new way of relating and serves as an antidote to conflict.

In EFT-C, the focus is on understanding how each partner's emotional experience contributes to the negative interpersonal dynamics in the couple. The tendency to express secondary emotions rather than primary emotions and corresponding needs is what keeps the negative interactional cycle in place. Greenberg & Goldman (2008) conceptualize couple interactions as taking place along two dimensions, of "affiliation" and "influence."

Negative interactional cycles develop when each partner's efforts to manage or shift the other's behaviour inadvertently serve to reinforce the very behaviours that they are hoping will change. For example, on the affiliation dimension, the more one partner pursues for closeness, the more the other withdraws to protect himself/herself, and the more this partner withdraws, the more the other pursues. On the influence dimension, the more controlling one partner behaves, the more the other partner resists his or her influence, and in turn the more resistance this partner shows, the more extreme the first partner becomes in his or her attempts at gaining control.

When working with a couple to identify their negative interactional cycle, the EFT-C therapist frames each partner's problematic behaviours not as personal failings but rather as attempted solutions to problems, which have now become the problem. This framework helps to externalize the blame onto the interaction rather than on the individuals, so that rather than attempting to change one another, the couple's focus shifts towards changing their problematic interactional patterns. Goldman and Greenberg (2013) identify attachment and identity-related needs as being the two fundamental concerns driving negative interactional cycles.

Change in EFT-C is understood to occur, from awareness and expression of primary emotions in the context of negative interactional cycles. This is considered to be the key to transforming the couple's rigid cycle of relating and bringing partners closer together. The EFT-C therapist aims to help each partner realize that what they typically express to each other are secondary or instrumental emotions, which serve to keep them trapped in their negative interactional cycle. Helping partners become aware and express the primary underlying attachment and identity-oriented emotions (e.g. fear underneath the anger/hostility or shame/inadequacy underneath contempt) is at the heart of this approach. Much of the work is spent on understanding each partner's underlying vulnerabilities in the relationship and their sensitivities and there also is a focus on how these may pre-date the couple's union (e.g. feeling sensitive to abandonment or to criticism).

There may be times when a partner's maladaptive emotion schemes especially those of fear and shame stem from unmet childhood needs and/or emotions linked to abandonment (fear) or invalidation (e.g. shame) that cannot be regulated or transformed through a partner's soothing or reassurance, but instead require self-focused work to enhance the capacity to self-soothe. In addition to assisting couples develop proficiency in responding to each other's primary emotions and associated needs, we therefore emphasize that at times, especially in a longer-term therapy, it is helpful to work with self-soothing (Greenberg & Goldman, 2008).

Research on EFT-C

A large number of studies have demonstrated the effectiveness of EFT-C in reducing relationship distress (e.g. Johnson et al. 1999; Greenberg, Warwar, & Malcolm, 2010; Dalgleish et al., 2015). Additional studies have found EFT-C to be effective in promoting forgiveness in couples presenting with unresolved emotional injuries (e.g. Greenberg et al., 2010; Makinen & Johnson, 2006). Moreover, EFT-C has shown success in treating couples presenting with a range of specific challenges, including childhood sexual abuse (MacIntosh & Johnson, 2008), post-traumatic stress disorder (Greenman & Johnson, 2012) and terminal cancer (MacLean, Walton, Rodin, Esplen, & Jones, 2013).

Since the development of EFT-C, there has been a strong research focus aimed at understanding how in-session processes are related to outcome. The first intensive task analyses of couples' conflict resolution in EFT-C revealed that *accessing underlying self-experience* and the *softening* of the critic were central to conflict resolution (Greenberg & Johnson, 1986). This was later confirmed by Johnson and Greenberg (1988), who found that good sessions were characterized by (a) deeper levels of *experiencing* (Klein, Mathieu, Gendlin, & Keisler, 1969) and (b) interactions as "affiliative" (e.g. disclosing, supporting and understanding), (Benjamin, 1974). Moreover, these in-session processes predicted outcome. Recently, vulnerable emotional expression has been linked to greater levels of improvement at *final* outcome among couples seeking to heal from emotional injuries (McKinnon & Greenberg, 2017). Meneses and Greenberg (2014), in studying the resolution of emotional injuries in couples, found that the offending partner's "Expression of Shame" was the strongest predictor of forgiveness post-therapy (accounting for 33% of the variance on the Enright Forgiveness Inventory).

Systemic Therapy: Theoretical Premises and Practical Interventions

Theoretical Framework and Core Interventions of ST

When comparing ST and EFT, we refer to a social-constructivist approach within ST (Bruner, 1990; Gergen & Gergen, 2003) that follows the tradition of Post-Milan/ Heidelberg group as summarized by von Schlippe and Schweitzer (2015).

This systemic tradition is characterized by *context orientation*. It refrains from mono-causal explanations and views problems as the result of self-reinforcing *circular patterns* that create communicative problem systems (Anderson & Goolishian, 1988). Systemic questions (Tomm, 1987a, 1987b, 1988; von Schlippe & Schweitzer, 2015) are used to help clients become aware of the mutual reciprocity of their actions, to challenge existing constructions and evoke alternative meanings that perturbate problem patterns. In many cases, a *genogram* will be worked out jointly that further helps to put a client's problem into a transgenerational perspective (McGoldrick, Gerson, & Petry, 2007). Satir, Banmen, Gerber, and Gomori (1991) introduced *sculpting* as a means to experience the effects of communicative patterns and access possibilities for change in an analogue way.

Another central feature of this systemic branch is its *resource and solution orientation* (de Shazer, 1982), which is rooted within the hypnotherapy of Erickson (1980). Clients' attention is shifted to personal resources and experiences of solution to release approaches that have proven to be effective within the system itself ("When was the last time you were successful at this?"; "What was the last exception to the problem?"). That way, the client is encouraged to learn from himself rather than introducing external advice.

The Therapist-Client Relationship Within ST

The constructivist foundation of ST implicates three kinds of neutrality that coin the therapeutic attitude. *Construct neutrality* lays the foundation for what Cecchin (1993) called irreverence towards ideas – respect towards people. As systemic therapists, we keep in mind that we do not know what a client means by describing himself "depressed," "shy" or "unmotivated." With genuine curiosity, appreciation and open-mindedness, we explore social and individual meaning-making by differentiating descriptions, explanations and evaluations ("What do you do when you feel depressed? If I'd ask your colleague, how would she explain the conflict between the two of you? What does it mean to you when your partner retreats? And once you are sure she doesn't care about you, what do you do then?"). Based on the assumption that current problems always reflect former solutions, systemic therapists will also be guided by *neutrality towards change*. Change includes paying prices – taking social, emotional or material risks. Whether a client is willing to pay that price is his or her choice. The role of the therapist is not to push for change but to guide the client to a conscious decision. This includes exploring the functional aspects of seemingly dysfunctional behaviour ("If there is anything this painful self-rejection is good for – what could this be?" E.g. blaming me instead of others; sticking to the idea "If only I do things right, everything will be fine"). The latter will also be reflected in *reframings* of problematic behaviour and symptoms. Finally, systemic therapists remain neutral towards their own relevance ("Am I the right person? What would you do if there was no such thing as therapy?").

Based on the information generated by systemic exploration, a systemic therapist will develop *hypotheses* concerning the maintenance of intrapersonal as well as interpersonal problem patterns ("The more you/he/she do(es) this, the more/less X will happen"). These hypotheses guide further exploration and are laid open to the client who can then evaluate them in terms of utility – not truth! Systemic intervention fundamentally aims at understanding and disruption of *patterns* – whether they be psychophysiological, communicative, verbal or nonverbal patterns. Therefore, systemic therapists will rather focus on process ("How do you construct, maintain and interrupt problem patterns? What differentiates patterns of success from those of stagnation?") than content ("What exactly happened to whom?").

A Systems Perspective on Emotion

From a systems theory perspective, emotions are perceived body states. Their expression as well as their description is a sociocultural product. Negative emotions help to reorganize the psychic system in case of threat and inconsistency ("immune function of emotions") (Fuchs, 2004). Emotions further serve as an identity-generating process. It is *my* emotion – that helps to distinguish myself from the environment. They indicate threats to social affiliation and serve as an observer's explanatory mechanism for behaviour ("He acts like it because he is disappointed"). Within Luhmann's systems theory, emotions are considered a generalized means of communication (Baecker, 2004). They regulate social interaction and survival in social context by structuring behaviour according to social norms. Emotions can exert manipulative power – "I don't dare to do this since I'm afraid to make you angry," or "I follow your expectation to please you."

When working with emotions, systemic therapy refrains from interpretations that confuse description and explanation ("she denies her feelings"; "he projects his fear on her"). Nevertheless, supporting the psychic system in perceiving and symbolizing embodied experience is highly relevant to broaden naturally selective self-perception and meaning-making. As Lieb (2014, p. 77) clearly states: The distinction between primary and secondary emotions is a descriptive not an explanatory concept that can be fully integrated into systems therapy. A systemic therapist cannot "diagnose" something inside the client, the client himself cannot see – as is presupposed in psychoanalytical interpretation. However, the task is to communicatively connect to the client in a way that stimulates new self- and body perception as well as the expression of so far unsymbolized experience.

Differences that Make a Difference: Comparing ST and EFT

When taking a closer look at EFT and ST, commonalities as well as differences come to mind.

EFT and ST both are *process-oriented* approaches that refrain from positivistic diagnosis and view therapy as a co-constructive process in which therapist and client influence each other in a non-imposing manner. While EFT centres around emotional schemes activated in the here and now, ST focuses on communicative patterns and their effect on relationships. In EFT for couples (Goldman & Greenberg, 2013; Greenberg & Johnson, 1988) both perspectives get combined.

EFT and ST both take a *functional perspective* on symptoms and syndromes: depression, anxiety, panic or generalized insecurity reflect the effect of dysfunctional self-regulation and/or interaction. "The solution is the problem" – this basic systemic premise also refers to instrumental, secondary and maladaptive primary emotions. ST explores functionalities from a cognitive point of view ("I know it might seem a weird question – but if there is anything this depression/bulimia/… is good for, what could it be?"). In contrast EFT aims at an empathic understanding in which secondary and maladaptive emotions can be felt, held and symbolized bottom-up to activate adaptive emotions. This way, we gain access to *implicit* strategies of emotion regulation that maintain the client's problem.

Within couple and family therapy, EFT sheds light on the emotional music that drives the communicative "dance." For systemic therapists, it is therefore helpful to expand their conceptual framework beyond instrumental aspects of emotions. Including secondary and primary maladaptive emotions in their functional analysis of communicative patterns significantly enlarges possibilities for understanding and intervention.

A family therapy is characterized by a highly destructive atmosphere. While one child remains silently withdrawn, the other complains about having to be here, the father resorts to open contempt towards the wife and devaluation of the therapist and the mother tries exculpating herself elaborately. From a systemic as well as an EFT perspective, these communicative behaviours are solutions. People are fighting for their protection and needs in a highly dysfunctional way. With an EFT framework, we might decode contempt and anger as secondary emotions that shield from helplessness, sadness or worthlessness, and interpret submissive insecurity as a maladaptive primary emotion that is triggered by any form of conflict. We then can combine circular questions ("What happens if Karen acts the way she does right now? And how does this reaction of yours probably affect her again? Which good reasons do you assume make him turn to contempt?") with empathic attunement ("When I'm listening to you, I sense this feeling of threat. This need to protect..., like: I want to be safe and unwounded by anyone. Right?").

On a theoretical basis, EFT and ST share the view of *humans as meaning-making systems*, who shape their experience by giving words to it. Both aim at the development of new narratives. While in ST this meaning-making process is considered primarily language based (Grossmann, 2003), EFT sees narratives as driven by emotions. Changing a narrative means changing emotions first. In EFT meaning making and narrative coherence are fundamentally linked with embodied experience. This is particularly evident for traumatic events that shutter one's sense of identity and can only be integrated in a new narrative, if the event is re-experienced emotionally.

Many systemic therapists will probably agree: if a reframing is meant to be more than a relabelling it must resonate emotionally. Triadic questions ("What do you think your son feels, if he looks at his parents?") show the greatest impact if they activate emotions such as empathy, curiosity, surprise or even sometimes shame. Traumatic events, loss, injuries shutter the way we see ourselves not just on a cognitive level, but also affect our bodily felt sense, affect regulation and action tendencies. Developing sound new narratives therefore will often presume becoming aware of and symbolizing emotional schemes activated by the event.

When watching an EFT therapy, one of the first things a systemically trained therapist will wonder about is the relative absence of questions. In EFT, we predominantly find *empathic exploration and conjectures*, combined with *rationales for working with emotions*. In contrast, systemic therapies are marked by an abundance of creative questions (Tomm, 1987a, 1987b, 1988). By answering systemic questions, the client is invited to take an observer perspective. They do not aim at a reproduction of known content but rather invite the client to generate new meanings by shifting the attention to so far unlighted spots of experience and perception.

There are at least three reasons for systemic therapists to become acquainted with empathic exploration as a complementary mode of interviewing. First, questions ask for an answer and thus direct attention towards the therapist. Sometimes however, this other orientation will impede mindful self-awareness as a precondition for new insights. We might end up reflecting on secondary emotions rather than deepening towards primary experience. Second, empathic exploration also draws the therapist's attention to nonverbal expressions of the client's inner landscape. We can see a lot more than we can hear. Empathically connecting to these nonverbal cues ("This sigh just now – what happened inside…?") can reveal highly relevant information. Third, in many cases, the unspeakability of the experienced distress is part of the problem. There simply are no words for the primary loneliness, fear or powerlessness that coined the clients' experience. Asking questions might just replicate this unspeakable void, whereas empathic exploration ("It sounds as if you're saying…") can help clients to find their own symbolizations. Empathic conjectures in EFT are always given in a spirit of careful and open suggestion. They do not represent fixed interpretations ("In truth you feel…"). It is the client who decides on what fits and what doesn't – a constructivist respect that reconnects with systemic principles.

One of the most striking differences between ST and EFT is their *focus on resources/solutions and pain, respectively*. While the focus on positive emotions and events is key to ST, in EFT there's a "pain compass" guiding therapeutic action. While an EFT therapist will ask "What is most painful about it?" a systemically trained therapist might ask "When does or did it hurt less or not at all?" This orientation towards positive feelings can – although helpful in many cases – end up missing central resources, such as informative fear, unexpressed grief or empowering anger.

Systemic intervention is dedicated to making a difference. If a client's survival strategy includes cutting himself off from hurtful but relevant negative emotions, focusing on positive feelings and situations runs the risk of offering "more of the same." People dispose of the resources to solve their problems – this solution-oriented premise should include trust in the self-organizing power of adaptive primary emotions, whether they be "negative" or "positive."

Ben, a 45-year-old man, grew up in a family of four children. He describes a childhood of emotional rejection ("I was primarily seen as a burden to my parents"). From adolescence on he escaped emotionally by using drugs and seeking independence and control in any relationship. He seeks therapy after the birth of his first child when he starts suffering from severe panic attacks and doubts about his fatherhood ("I know it is my child but I somehow can't believe it. I keep thinking of grabbing my stuff and leaving."). He wants to get rid of the symptoms and find a way to stay with his family although he is full of resentment against his wife ("She is not seeing my needs. She just wants me to function her way.").

If we take a simplified and prototype perspective on Ben's case, a first-order resource activation could include searching for reasons to trust in his fatherhood and focusing on situations in which he manages to communicate his needs towards his wife effectively. Following an EFT path, we probably would foster resilient self-organization by helping Ben to feel and express the primary maladaptive sense of worthlessness that is hidden behind the secondary anger and distrust. In an unfinished business work, we might encourage him to express pain and unmet needs towards his parents. We might also activate self-compassion and capacities for self-soothing towards "the child inside him," who still tries to protect himself by maintaining control and distance. Although this path includes a lot of hurtful feelings, it is highly resource oriented, since it supports a second-order solution: Building the capacity to handle the insecurity that comes along with any meaningful relationship in a way that allows for new experiences.

Within the framework of systemic pioneer Virginia Satir (1991, 1993), Ben's communicative style would be described as "Blamer." Satir, with her focus on self-worth-regulation, payed specific attention to the emotions, physiological reactions and sensations underlying communicative styles. She differentiated the dialogue of words from the dialogue of feelings and encouraged therapists to listen beyond words by tuning in to tone of voice, facial expression and clients' posture. Her therapeutic goal of *congruence* refers to a correspondence of feeling, verbal and nonverbal expression of feeling and need-adapted ways to connect to others. Arriving at an (primary) emotion as described by Greenberg (2015) and Greenberg et al. (2003) operationalizes a process Satir et al. (1991) might have had in mind when she invited therapists to learn to be "deep sea divers" to journey with people into their depths and help them discover and own the internal experiences that were out of their awareness, so that they could make congruent and new decisions about them.

What is the goal of ST and EFT respectively – and how is it defined? ST is characterized by *contract orientation*. It is the client who defines "who – wants what – from whom – in what capacity – to what end?" (von Schlippe & Schweitzer, 2015, p.22). Client's expectations are translated into concrete criteria for problem solution

("What would have to happen here for you to make worth the effort?"). This collaborative development of therapeutic goals serves multiple functions. On a relational level it is a signal of empowerment that lifts the client at eye level with the therapist. Exploring the client's expectations also creates a sense of hope ("What will it feel like, once I made the change?"). By developing behavioural operationalizations of good outcomes, ideas for first steps automatically emerge.

In EFT, this contract orientation is replaced by a shared *case formulation* that links the client's symptoms with his emotion regulation strategies (what is the client's core emotion, what caused it and what thoughts and behaviours sustain it). This case formulation is developed bottom-up and presented to the client as a working hypothesis of what is happening to him and what needs to be addressed in therapy. Again, this rationale is a jointly developed picture – not a top-down diagnosis.

As a systemically trained therapist, I [JZ] usually start of by asking for a client's expectations. There are cases, however, in which a case formulation based on hypotheses on implicit emotion regulation strategies effectively supplements directions from systemic contracting.

Maria, a 53-year-old consultant, seeks therapy to get rid of extreme exhaustion and vegetative stress symptoms based on a decade of overwork. When asked for her expectations she wants to learn to say no and to engage in self-care: meeting friends, restricting work to 10 hours a day maximum and searching for a potential partner to overcome a loneliness the work has protected her from feeling. A couple of sessions later, none of the self-care ideas are implemented. Maria seems full of resignation. Empathic exploration of this secondary resignation leads to painful childhood memories. At the age of four the mother went to hospital for several months, Maria was left behind with the clear signal "there's no reason to be sad." During that period and the years following, she tries to survive emotionally by pleasing external expectations and spreading good moods. Loneliness, despair and anger remain covered beneath deep resignation ("There's no use in asking for more"). Maria lacks words for these hurtful memories. It takes several sessions and empathic support to arrive at the primary emotions of loneliness and so far unexpressed anger. She even starts remembering wounds she inflicted on herself as a child to release the pain – the scars of which she has dissociated from for decades.

The EFT case formulation offered to Maria can be summarized like this: There is an almost unbearable core pain of loneliness that has been covered with maladaptive resignation. While this resignation might have been adaptive in the first place by saving fragile relationships, and avoiding an overwhelming pain, it now prevents her from feeling what she needs and acting according to it. Maria learns to be satisfied with less – in taking the role of the affair, in her job when she makes up for four and her friendships in which she gives a lot more than she receives. Feeling and expressing what childhood and later experiences meant to her is – though painful – a precondition to take better care of herself by gaining access to resilient emotions such as grief, self-compassion and anger. Listening to the unexpressed pain inside allows to feel "I deserved and needed better." To feel I deserved better sometimes is a precondition to do better.

As the cases indicate, in EFT, *past events and primary relationships* with care-givers and partners do play a significant role. In contrast, ST primarily focuses on patterns of problem reproduction and disruption in the present. This is partly due to a scepticism, that the past might be good for explanation but not necessarily for change. This certainly holds true if we restrict ourselves to listening to what Angus and Greenberg (2011) call "empty stories" and "same old stories." Within empty stories, clients elaborate on past events with great detail but little or no elaboration of the subjective experience. Same old stories refer to narratives that centre around generalized experiences of stuckness and victimization with a low sense of personal agency. EFT and ST both agree: Simply validating the *content* of these stories ("this must have been intolerable") will not bring any change. However, to make a differ-ence, what is validated and explored is not "what really happened" but the *emo-tional meaning* of these past events ("What did it feel like – listening to these messages? As she looked at you, what was happening inside you?"). That way, cli-ents gain access to their implicit emotional meaning-making processes and learn to take responsibility for their resulting self-protection strategies that guide interaction in the here and now. From a systemic as well as EFT perspective, it is not the early-childhood event that *causes* todays feeling and behaviour. Rather, these experiences shape affect-logic schemes that determine further constructions of reality. The *cause* of today's behaviour is not the past but the *repetition* of patterns that keep the past alive (Lieb, 2014).

Conclusion

Contrasting two complex therapeutic approaches within the scope of this chapter is necessarily reductive and simplifying. Having these limitations in mind, we hope to encourage systemic therapists to look over the EFT fence. EFT offers a concep-tional framework to explore intrapersonal patterns of self-regulation in a non-stigmatizing co-constructive way. It expands our understanding of meaning-making processes and invites us to pay attention to emotionally driven solutions to emo-tional problems. For systemically trained therapists, the space of possible interven-tion is considerably increased if we learn to recognize the emotional function of dysfunctional communication and behaviour – a perspective that has already been emphasized within the work of Satir (1991, 1993). The construct of primary, sec-ondary, maladaptive and adaptive emotions provides a framework that raises new questions. Whether an emotion is productive is no longer determined by its content alone (positive or negative qualities), but also by its novelty ("Is the emotion new or old? Has it been previously blocked and is now freshly expressed or is it the repeti-tion of an old stale emotion that has been expressed numerous times before?"), its intensity ("Is the client experiencing too much or too little emotion?") (Paivio & Greenberg, 2001) and its function ("Is the emotion a sign of distress or a sign of resolving distress?").

Becoming acquainted with the constructs, attitudes and interventions of EFT allows systemic therapists not only to talk about emotion but to work *with* them. "What happens inside of you while you are saying this?" opens the door to transforming emotional resources we might miss out otherwise. EFT further draws our attention to the nonverbal signs of communication. A sigh, a gesture is not only a communicative message towards another person but also a door towards relevant experience and previously unsymbolized information. Expanding the therapist's awareness to nonverbal emotional markers will also help to symbolize prelingual states. As Wittgenstein (1963) put it: The limits of my language mean the limits of my world. Undoubtedly, clients do have expertise for their goals and context – however, there might be relevant information that is embodied but not explicable for them so far. In these cases, empathic exploration and attunement might effectively supplement creative questions.

Neither EFT nor ST mistake the map as the territory. Both approaches are evidence based (for a survey on the effectiveness of ST see Von Sydow, Beher, Schweitzer, & Retzlaff, 2010 and Carr et al., chapter "Research Informed Practice of Systemic Therapy" in this book) and inherently open to reflection and development. EFT is based on process research. It starts off with the question: What brings about change? What differentiates helpful from non-helpful therapeutic processes? Within ST, the constructivist foundation reminds us to constantly reflect the distinctions we make and the realities they create. Sharing fundamental principles of process orientation, functional analysis, social constructivism and narrative theory as well as therapeutic attitudes of deep respect and appreciation, EFT and ST surely have enough in common to connect and enough differences to inspire each other.

References

Anderson, H., & Goolishian, H. A. (1988). Human systems as linguistic systems: Preliminary and evolving ideas about the implications for clinical theory. *Family Process, 27*(4), 371–393.
Angus, L. E., & Greenberg, L. S. (2011). *Working with narrative in emotion-focused therapy: Changing stories, healing lives.* Washington: American Psychological Association.
Angus, L. E., & Greenberg, L. S. (2013). *Working with narrative in emotion-focused therapy: Changing stories, healing lives.* Washington: American Psychological Association.
Baecker, D. (2004). Wozu Gefühle? *Soziale Systeme, 10*(1), 5–20.
Benjamin, L. S. (1974). Structural analysis of social behavior. *Psychological Review, 81*(5), 392.
Bruner, J. (1990). *Acts of meaning.* Cambridge, MA: Harvard University Press.
Cecchin, G. (1993). *Irreverence: A strategy for therapists' survival.* London, UK: Karnac Books.
Dalgleish, T., Johnson, S. M., Burgess, M. M., Lafontaine, M. F., Wiebe, S. A., & Tasca, G. A. (2015). Predicting change in marital satisfaction throughout emotionally focused couple therapy. *Journal of Mairtal and Family Therapy, 41*, 276–291.
Damasio, A. (1999). *The feeling of what happens: Body, emotion and the making of consciousness.* London, UK: Heinemann.
Elliott, R., Greenberg, L., & Lietaer, G. (2004). Research on experiential psychotherapy. In M. Lambert (Ed.), *Bergin & Garfield's handbook of psychotherapy & behavior change* (pp. 493–539). New York, NY: Wiley.

Ellison, J., Greenberg, L., Goldman, R. N., & Angus, L. (2009). Maintenance of gains following experiential therapies for depression. *Journal of Consulting and Clinical Psychology, 77*, 103–112.

Erickson, M. (1980). *The collected papers of Milton H. Erickson on hypnosis*. New York, NY: Irvington.

Fuchs, P. (2004). Wer hat und wozu überhaupt Gefühle? *Soziale Systeme, 10*(1), 89–110.

Gendlin, E. (1996). *Focusing-oriented psychotherapy: A manual of the experiential method. New York Guilford series*. New York, NY: Guilford Press.

Gergen, M., & Gergen, K. J. (2003). *Social construction: A reader*. London, UK: SAGE Publication.

Goldman, R. N., & Greenberg, L. S. (2013). *Emotion-focused couples therapy: The dynamics of emotion, love, and power*. Wahsington: American Psychological Association.

Goldman, R. N., Greenberg, L. S., & Angus, L. (2006). The effects of adding emotion-focused interventions to the client-centered relationship conditions in the treatment of depression. *Psychotherapy Research, 16*, 536–546.

Greenberg, L. (2015). *Emotion focused therapy. Coaching clients to work through their feelings*. Washington: American Psychological Association.

Greenberg, L. J., Warwar, S. H., & Malcolm, W. M. (2008). Differential effects of emotion-focused therapy and psychoeducation in facilitating forgiveness and letting go of emotional injuries. *Journal of Counseling Psychology, 55*(2), 185–196.

Greenberg, L. S. & Goldman, R. N. (2008). Working with identity and self-soothing in emotion-focused therapy for couples. *Family Process, 52*(1).

Greenberg, L., & Johnson, S. M. (1988). *Emotionally focused therapy for couples*. New York, NY: Guilford Press.

Greenberg, L., Rice, L., & Elliott, R. (2003). *The moment by moment process: Facilitating emotional change*. New York, NY: Guilford Press.

Greenberg, L., Warwar, S., & Malcolm, W. (2010). Emotion-focused couples therapy and the facilitation of forgiveness. *Journal of Marital and Family Therapy, 36*(1), 28–42.

Greenberg, L., & Watson, J. (1998). Experiential therapy of depression: Differential effects of client-centered relationship conditions and process experiential interventions. *Psychotherapy Research, 8*(2), 210–224.

Greenberg, L. S. (1984). A task analysis of intrapersonal conflict resolution. In S. G. Toukmainian & D. L. Rennie (Eds.), *Psychotherapy process research: Paradigmatic and narrative approaches* (Vol. 134, pp. 22–50). Newbury Park, CA: Sage Focus Editions.

Greenberg, L. S., & Johnson, S. M. (1986). Affect in marital therapy. *Journal of Marital and Family Therapy, 12*(1), 1–10.

Greenberg, L. S., & Paivio, S. C. (1997). *Working with emotions in psychotherapy: Changing core schemes*. New York, NY: Guilford Press.

Greenberg, L. J., Warwar, S. H., & Malcolm, W. M. (2008). Differential effects of emotion-focused therapy and psychoeducation in facilitating forgiveness and letting go of emotional injuries. *Journal of Counseling Psychology, 55*(2), 185–196.

Greenman, P. S., & Johnson, S. M. (2012). United we stand: emotionally focused therapy for couples in the treatment of posttraumatic stress disorder. *Journal of Clinical Psychology, 68*(5).

Grossmann, K. P. (2003). *Der Fluss des Erzählens. Narrative Formen der Therapie*. Heidelberg, Germany: Carl Auer.

Johnson, S. M., & Greenberg, L. S. (1988). Relating process to outcome in marital therapy. *Journal of Marital and Family Therapy, 14*, 175–183.

Johnson, S. M., Hunsley, J., Greenberg, L., & Schindler, D. (1999). Emotionally focused couples therapy: Status and challenges. *Clinical Psychology: Science and Practice, 6*(1), 67–79.

Klein, M. H., Mathieu, P. L., Gendlin, E. T., & Keisler, D. J. (1969). *The experiencing scale: A research training manual*. Madison, WI: University of Wisconsin Extension Bureau of Audiovisual Instruction.

Lieb, H. (2014). *Störungsspezifische Systemtherapie. Konzepte und Behandlung*. Heidelberg, Germany: Carl Auer.

MacIntosh, H. B., & Johnson, S. M. (2008). Emotionally focused therapy for couples and childhood sexual abuse survivors. *Journal of Marital and Family Therapy, 34*, 298–315.

MacLean, L. M., Walton, T., Rodin, G., Esplen, M. J., & Jones, J. M. (2013). A couple-based intervention for patients and caregivers facing end-stage cancer: Outcomes of a randomized controlled tiral. *Psychooncology, 22*, 28–38.

Makinen, J. A., & Johnson, S. M. (2006). Resolving attachment injuries in couples using emotionally focused therapy: Steps toward forgiveness and reconciliation. *Journal of Consulting and Clinical Psychology, 74*, 1055–1064.

McGoldrick, M., Gerson, R., & Petry, S. (2007). *Genograms: Assessment and intervention.* New York, NY: W.W. Norton.

McKinnon, J. M., & Greenberg, L. S. (2017). Vulnerable emotional expression in emotion-focused therapy for couples: Relating interactional processes to outcome. *Journal of Family and Marital Therapy, 43*, 198–212.

Meneses, C. W., & Greenberg, L. S. (2014). Interpersonal forgiveness in emotion-focused couples' therapy: relating process to outcome. *Journal of Marital and Family Therapy, 40*(1), 49–67.

Missirlian, T., Toukmanian, S., Warwar, S., & Greenberg, L. (2005). Emotional arousal, client perceptual processing, and the working alliance in experiential psychotherapy for depression. *Journal of Consulting and Clinical Psychology, 73*(5), 861–871.

Paivio, S. C., & Greenberg, L. S. (1995). Resolving "unfinished business": Efficacy of experiential therapy using empty-chair dialogue. *Journal of Consulting and Clinical Psychology, 63*, 419–425.

Paivio, S. C., & Greenberg, L. S. (2001). Introduction treating emotion regulation problems. *Journal of Clinical Psychology, 57*, 153–155.

Paivio, S. C., & Nieuwenhuis, J. A. (2001). Efficacy of emotion focused therapy for adult survivors of child abuse: A preliminary study. *Journal of Traumatic Stress, 14*, 115–133.

Paivio, S., & Pascual-Leone, A. (2009). *Emotion-focused therapy for complex trauma: An integrative approach.* Washington: American Psychological Association.

Paivio, S., Jarry, J., Chagigiorgis, H., Hall, I., & Ralston, M. (2010). *Efficacy of two versions of emotion-focused therapy for resolving child abuse trauma. Psychotherapy Research, 20*(3), 353–366.

Satir, V. (1993). *Conjoint family therapy.* Palo Alto, CA: Science and Behavior Books.

Satir, V., Banmen, J., Gerber, J., & Gomori, M. (1991). *The Satir model: Family therapy and beyond.* Palo Alto, CA: Science and Behavior Books.

Shazer, S. D. (1982). *Patterns of brief family therapy: An ecosystemic approach.* New York, NY: Guilford Press.

Tomm, K. (1987a). Interventive interviewing: Part II. Reflexive questioning as a means to enable self healing. *Family Process, 26*, 153–183.

Tomm, K. (1987b). Interventive interviewing: Part I. Strategizing as a fourth guideline for the therapist. *Family Process, 26*, 3–13.

Tomm, K. (1988). Interventive interviewing: Part III. Intending to ask lineal, circular, reflexive or strategic questions? *Family Process, 27*, 1–15.

von Schlippe, A., & Schweitzer, J. (2015). *Systemic interventions.* Göttingen, Germany: Vandenhoeck.

Von Sydow, K., Beher, S., Schweitzer, J., & Retzlaff, R. (2010). The efficacy of systemic therapy with adult patients: A meta-content analysis of 38 randomized controlled trials. *Family Process, 49*(2010), 457–485.

Watson, J. C., Gordon, L. B., Stermac, L., Kalogerakos, F., & Steckley, P. (2003). Comparing the effectiveness of process-experiential with cognitive-behavioral psychotherapy in the treatment of depression. *Journal of Consulting and Clinical Psychology, 71*, 773–781.

Wittgenstein, L. (1963). *Tractatus logico-philosophicus: Logisch-philosophische Abhandlung.* Berlin: Edition suhrkamp.

From Reactivity to Relational Empowerment in Couple Therapy: Insights from Interpersonal Neurobiology

Mona DeKoven Fishbane

What Is Interpersonal Neurobiology?

Years ago, the brain was considered a "black box," mysterious and unknowable. Today, thanks to technological advances such as brain scanners, scientists can observe the human brain as it functions in real time. The technology isn't perfect, and is constantly being improved. But data from fMRI machines and other devices is revealing a great deal about the brain, emotions, and relationships.

Neuroscience data comes not only from brain scanners, but also from research on animals, humans with brain damage, and hormones and neurotransmitters that pulse through the brain and body. Studies are being conducted as well on genetics and epigenetics—the influence of experience and environment on the expression of genes (Meaney, 2010).

Scientists have identified brain processes that affect cognitive, emotional, physical, and interpersonal functioning. Much of this research bears directly on clinical work: for example, how the amygdala sets off the fight-or-flight response and kneejerk reactivity; prefrontal cortex regulation of the amygdala; and the neuroscience of empathy. The action isn't just in the head. There is constant communication between brain and body. Key information is conveyed from gut or heart to brain, shaping emotions (Craig, 2009; Damasio, 2010); and from brain to body, for example, when the amygdala sets off the stress response, getting the heart pumping and limbs ready to fight or flee.

Interpersonal neurobiology (a term coined by Daniel Siegel and Alan Schore) extends the focus beyond the brain-body within the individual, to the circular and recursive interactions of brains, bodies, and relationships. Just as systemic thinking expanded an individual focus to a relational-contextual one, so interpersonal

M. D. Fishbane (✉)
Chicago Center for Family Health, Chicago, IL, USA

© Springer Nature Switzerland AG 2020   265
M. Ochs et al. (eds.), *Systemic Research in Individual, Couple, and Family Therapy and Counseling*, European Family Therapy Association Series,
https://doi.org/10.1007/978-3-030-36560-8_15

neurobiology extends beyond the individual brain, exploring how relationships affect mental and physical health, and the neural-behavioral mechanisms of satisfying or distressed relationships.

Love and Its Discontents

Humans are among the few mammals that form lasting pair bonds. While monogamy may be difficult to sustain, we love to fall in love and maintain secure partnerships. Neuroscientists are studying love and its challenges. Researchers put madly-in-love subjects in the fMRI machine (Aron et al., 2005; Bartels & Zeki, 2000; Fisher, 2004). When looking at a photo of the beloved, the neural reward centers of these lovers become highly activated. Their brains, high on love, look like the brains of people on cocaine. Dopamine is flowing, fueling excitement and anticipation. Other chemicals in the elixir of love include testosterone, fueling lust in both men and women; norepinephrine, focusing on "that special someone," and oxytocin, which facilitates attachment (Feldman, 2012; Fisher, 2004).

Love is blind, Shakespeare tells us. Indeed, neuroscientists have found that in early love, the critical-judgmental parts of the brain tend to be quiet (Zeki, 2007). The beloved is seen through rose-colored glasses. But at some point, critical faculties come back online and the partner is seen, warts and all. Madly-in-love eventually fades to a more sedate version: companionate love. Both passionate and companionate love tend to deteriorate over time (Hatfield, Pilemer, O'Brien, Sprecher, & Le, 2008). For happy couples the shift from passionate love poses a challenge: how to nurture long-term love and preserve and protect their bond. For unhappy couples, the loss of the magic of madly-in-love can pose a crisis. Rather than being bathed in oxytocin-rich loving interactions, they are awash in cortisol, the stress hormone.

A client says, "I still love my wife, but I've fallen out of love with her." He may be missing the high of dopamine and the urgency of testosterone-driven lust that were so abundant early in their relationship. He's also missing her adoring gaze that made him feel so special. He may have an affair or divorce and remarry, looking for the spark and adoration somewhere else. While some second marriages are happier than first ones, the person may end up in a similar bind the next time around; once again, crazy-in-love eventually leads to a saner state, partners take each other for granted, and withdrawal from the dopamine high causes misery.

Mitchell (2003) and Perel (2006) have pointed to the tension between passion—which thrives on mystery and adventure—and secure attachment, which seeks stability and familiarity. The coexistence of these two forces is at times challenging in long-term relationships. Neurobiologically, attachment (supported by oxytocin) and lust (supported by testosterone) can pull in opposite directions (Crespi, 2016; Fisher, 2004).

Given these complexities of long-term love dynamics, developing ways to proactively nurture love is vital for the flourishing of couple bonds. Researchers have identified key components to successful long-term relationships. Learning how to care for each other and regulate one's emotions are key skills for success in love. Interpersonal neurobiology can shed light on the reactive dances of unhappy couples, and point to practices that nourish and enhance love over the long haul. My clinical approach is informed by research from neuroscience, psychology, and relationship science, and integrates wisdom from various therapeutic orientations.

Systemic therapists have a multilevel view of couple and family relationships, exploring individual, interpersonal, and intergenerational factors affecting relational distress. The contexts in which couples live—social systems of support or stress, and wider cultural contexts, the macro level including poverty, marginalization, and oppression—have been addressed in recent years. Interpersonal neurobiology adds another layer to this integrative view: the micro level of processes within brain, body, and relationships (Fishbane, 2013).

Wired to Connect

Humans are social creatures. The child's brain is wired through connection with caregivers (Siegel, 1999). Attachment matters. Nurture and nature (genetics) work together to shape the human being; experience changes the connections between neurons, and even affects the expression of genes (Zhang & Meaney, 2010). Trauma, abuse, neglect, and poverty negatively affect the growing brain (Hackman & Farah, 2009; Perry, 2002). The need for safety and attachment doesn't end in childhood; humans are wired to connect throughout life. Adult love is considered an attachment relationship (Hazan & Shaver, 1987); close relationships and social support are vital for mental and physical health. Happy intimate relationships are associated with better health and longer life, while unhappy relationships and loneliness can be toxic to the body, and being rejected socially triggers pain centers in the brain (Cacioppo & Patrick, 2008; Eisenberger & Lieberman, 2004; Kiecolt-Glaser & Newton, 2001; Kim, Sherman, & Taylor, 2008). The field of psychoneuroimmunology explores the ways bodies and brains are affected by psychological and relational experience. Chronic stress can negatively affect the immune system, increase chronic inflammation, and shorten telomeres, the protective coating on the end of chromosomes, leading to health risks and premature aging (Epel et al., 2004; Kiecolt-Glaser & Glaser, 2010). Much of this damage is caused by chronic elevation of cortisol, the stress hormone. The stakes are very high. Love—and its disappointments—gets under the skin.

Couples co-regulate—or co-dysregulate—each other, for better or worse. People pick up the emotions of those around them—a phenomenon called "emotional contagion" (Hatfield, Cacioppo, & Rapson, 1993). Unhappy couples become more physiologically dysregulated during conflict (Gottman, 2011). Offering clients tools for self-regulation and co-regulation can increase the effectiveness of couple therapy.

Distressed Couples: The Vulnerability Cycle

Many couples come to therapy feeling disempowered and disconnected, caught up in vicious cycles of reactivity. Partners' attempts to reach each other may backfire, as they use tactics of attack/defend or criticize/countercriticize. Legitimate desires for intimacy, support, and affirmation become derailed. In couple therapy the yearnings for closeness lurking underneath the dances of attack/defend are identified, and partners are helped to challenge their own counterproductive behaviors and develop new interactions that promote trust and intimacy (Fishbane, 2013; Johnson, 2004).

Using the Vulnerability Cycle Diagram (Scheinkman & Fishbane, 2004), the therapist and clients together map out the couple's dance of reactivity, including each partner's vulnerabilities and survival strategies. In the process, individual, interpersonal, intergenerational, and larger contextual factors that fuel the impasse are identified. And now we can add neurobiological factors underlying couple reactivity.

Len and Carla's Vulnerability Cycle

Len and Carla are a middle-aged, heterosexual, Caucasian couple with two sons. Len, an attorney in a high-powered law firm, prizes rationality and order. He needs calm when he comes home from work; Carla, a poet and stay-at-home mother, tends to be disorganized. While their older son in college is a star achiever, their younger son Matt, a freshman in high school, has always been more vulnerable and challenging. Like his mother, Matt is disorganized and distractible; he has recently been diagnosed with ADHD. When Len comes home from work and finds chaos at home, his son's coat on the floor and Matt and Carla in the middle of a fight, he gets reactive and blames his wife. Carla feels alone, overburdened, unsupported, and unappreciated (her vulnerabilities) by Len for all she is trying to do to keep Matt focused on his schoolwork. She becomes defensive and angry (her survival strategies) in the face of Len's criticism. For his part, Len feels frightened and overwhelmed (his vulnerabilities) by the emotional intensity and chaos when he walks in the door. He responds with criticism and withdraws from the fray (his survival strategies). But his criticism and withdrawal make Carla feel more alone and unprotected, which fuels her anger, which in turn further fuels Len's anxiety, which leads him to withdraw more. Each one blames the other in a linear fashion. However, their dance is circular, as each one's survival strategy activates the other's vulnerability.

In the beginning of this couple's relationship, trust and intimacy were high. Len adored Carla's free spirit and creativity; Carla cherished Len's solidity and clear thinking. Now, after years of enacting their unhappy dance, trust and intimacy have eroded, and each resents the very qualities in the other that fueled their early love. His orderly rationality and her free-spirited poetic soul once complemented each other; now they are polarizing the couple, fueling a mutually resentful vulnerability cycle.

Vulnerability Cycle

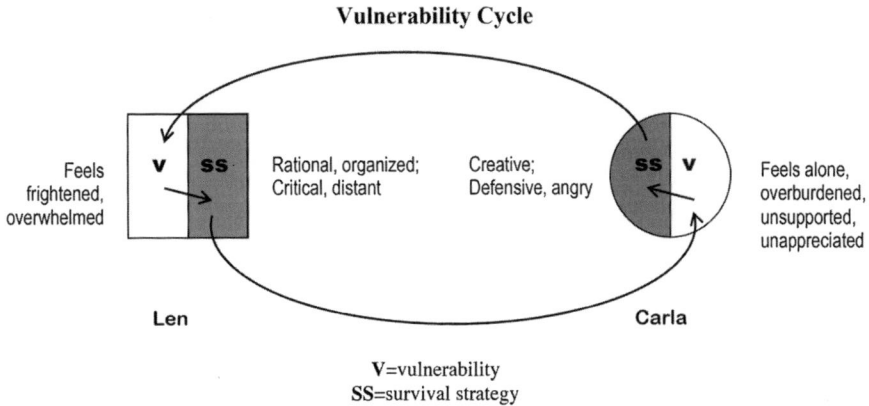

V=vulnerability
SS=survival strategy

Fig. 1 Len and Carla Vulnerability Cycle Diagram

Family-of-Origin Influences on the Couple's Impasse

When Len comes home from work and finds chaos at home, with his wife and son fighting, he feels anxious and overwhelmed. He grew up in a home that was unpredictable and volatile. When Len was 13, his father was hospitalized with bipolar disorder; he would erupt in rages that terrified his son. From an early age Len cultivated a rational, calm demeanor to deal with frightening emotional intensity. When he sees messiness at home and tension between his wife and son, he does not share his anxiety but rather expresses disapproval and withdraws. In the face of his criticism, Carla feels unprotected and unappreciated—much as she felt as a child, a parentified little girl who had to take care of her younger siblings with a critical mother and a distracted, emotionally absent father. Len's disapproval of Carla's parenting triggers painful feelings she had as a child when her mother criticized the way she was taking care of her younger siblings. Carla responds to Len's disapproval with fury, which further threatens Len, who shuts down and shuts Carla out.

Neurobiology of the Vulnerability Cycle

When caught in their impasse, both Len and Carla are driven by their amygdalae; she is in fight mode, he resorts to flight. Their higher brains are not functioning at that moment. Indeed, research shows that when the amygdala is highly activated during stress, the functioning of the higher brain, the prefrontal cortex, is impaired (Arnsten, Raskind, Taylor, & Connor, 2014). We can't think straight when we see red.

In addition to setting off the fight/flight response, the amygdala is involved in encoding and storing old emotional memories (Phelps, 2004). When Len and Carla are hurting each other now, they get a double whammy from their amygdalae. They are activated by the current threat, and also triggered by painful memories from their families of origin. These processes aren't available to their conscious awareness—these partners are just acting instinctively to protect themselves. But the way they do so is backfiring. The therapist helps the couple slow down the action and identify the softer, painful feelings that underlie their reactions. When family-of-origin experiences that inform their current impasse are identified, each partner may do some inter-generational work in the context of couple therapy (Fishbane, 2005, 2013).

Transforming the Vulnerability Cycle: Automaticity -vs. Choice

In this couple's cycle, each partner's reactivity fuels the other's. I offer them techniques to bring prefrontal thoughtfulness to amygdala-driven reactivity, and to step back from their impasse and consider their cycle together, so they can "get meta" to their dance. In this process, they move from being two victims, each blaming the other, to co-authors of their relationship. I encourage empathy and curiosity as they explore the factors fueling their unhappiness. Some couples put their vulnerability cycle diagram on their refrigerator, to remind them, "this is the dance we do together." They are externalizing their dance, and looking at it together as a team.

Much of the time the brain is on autopilot. Humans are emotional, habit-driven creatures, and the subcortical brain is often running the show. The amygdala does its job unbidden; it is constantly scanning for safety or danger, and when it senses danger, it sets in motion the fight or flight (or, in dire situations, freeze) response. This all happens very fast, automatically, beneath awareness. This is to our benefit; think of a time when you were hiking and came across a poisonous snake. Your amygdala probably saved your life and got you out of there. But the amygdala isn't very smart; it doesn't distinguish between scary snake and grumpy spouse. To the amygdala, threat is threat. When Len is critical, Carla feels threatened and lashes back. This is about survival. Len then storms out of the room and shuts Carla out. But his life-saving tactic sends Carla into amygdala overdrive, and she escalates into rage. Gottman (2011) has found that men are more likely to flood emotionally and physi-ologically during conflict, entering a heart-racing state he calls "Diffuse Physiological Arousal," or DPA. He suggests that the tactic of stonewalling, while unproductive interpersonally, serves to calm the man and get him out of the flooded, DPA zone. The relational-neurobiological consequence of this tactic, however, is that a hus-band's stonewalling can send his wife into DPA (Gottman, 2011).

Fortunately, humans are not doomed to be prisoners of the amygdala or of unhappy relational dances. The higher brain allows for choice in responding. But it's not easy to override the amygdala's urgency. To be more adept in those moments of high emotion, it helps to be prepared. I encourage clients—when calm—to iden-tify their higher goals and values so they can "reach for their best self" in moments of relational disappointment or threat. We operationalize their goals, and develop techniques for self-regulation when they are in the emotional fray.

Rethinking Power

Distressed couples are often caught up in power struggles, both partners making a claim for their own position or reality at the expense of the other's. Power is typically construed as the ability to dominate another; this Power Over perspective takes a toll on couple relationships. But relational therapists have begun rethinking power in more complex systemic terms (Fishbane, 2011, 2013, 2015; Goodrich, 1991; Jordan, 2010; Jordan, Kaplan, Miller, Stiver, & Surrey, 1991). In addition to addressing power imbalances and the risk of physical violence and intimidation in couples (Power Over), the therapist can help each partner think about their own goals for personal and relational growth, their ability to live according to their own higher values (Power To), as well as cultivate mutual respect, collaboration, and care in their relationship (Power With). When Len and Carla feel hurt or disconnected from each other, they tend to resort to Power Over tactics. Each feels like a victim of the other, and defends the self with kneejerk reactivity. In this context, they are also victims of their own dysregulated emotional brains. One of the goals of therapy is to facilitate relational empowerment, so clients can develop tools of Power To and Power With. Rather than being victims of each other or of their amygdalae, the couple can become authors of their own best selves and coauthors of their relationship.

Tools for Relational Empowerment: Emotion Regulation

Anger can feel empowering. But when adults have temper tantrums, reacting impulsively rather than responding thoughtfully, they are actually disempowered, driven by the lower brain. I offer clients "tools for relational empowerment." With clients with temper issues, who escalate quickly, going from zero to 100 with little warning, these tools are particularly important. Patrick and Jon have been in a committed relationship for years, but Jon is fed up with Patrick's temper outbursts. Patrick is anxious to improve their relationship and is willing to work on his short fuse. I ask Patrick to tune into the "prodromal cues" from his body before he blows. He notices his teeth clench and his heart beat more rapidly when he starts to get angry; I coach him to pay attention to these cues and do some mindful breathing at that point. Catching his response early in the process, while his prefrontal cortex is still online, Patrick is able to make a different choice. He is no longer the victim of his emotional brain. Both Patrick and Jon are relieved by this change.

Psychologists and neuroscientists are paying a lot of attention to emotion and emotion regulation. Emotion regulation is key to couple well-being. Carla's angry reaction to Len's criticism and Len's subsequent shutdown are signs of emotions unregulated. In that context, each is disempowered in the relationship; neither is getting heard or getting their needs met.

Researchers have identified multiple ways to regulate emotions. For starters, one can name the emotion: Affect labeling quiets the amygdala and heightens prefrontal activity (Creswell, Way, Eisenberger, & Lieberman, 2007). Dan Siegel calls this technique "Name it to tame it" (Siegel & Bryson, 2011). Equally important is pausing when one starts to get upset, and taking a deep breath. This can interrupt the rush to reactivity. The slow exhale of a deep belly breath activates the calming parasympathetic nervous system, which counters the agitation of the sympathetic nervous system.

Another technique for emotion regulation that lowers amygdala reactivity and heightens prefrontal functioning is cognitive reappraisal (Ochsner & Gross, 2005), what therapists call reframing. If your partner leaves her dishes in the sink one morning, you can spin a tale in your head about how selfish she is; this story is likely to rev up your anger and resentment. Or, you can think about all she had to do before she left for work, and instead of resentment, empathy and gratitude will flourish. The stories we tell affect how we feel.

Mindfulness meditation is used in most therapeutic modalities these days. Neuroscientists have found that mindfulness strengthens brain areas involved in attention and attunement to the body, enhances prefrontal regulation of the amygdala, and strengthens the immune system (Davidson & Begley, 2012). Mindfulness is, not surprisingly, associated with happier marriages (Wachs & Cordova, 2007).

Imagery techniques can be helpful tools for self-soothing. Borrowing from Internal Family Systems therapy (Schwartz, 1994), I ask clients to image their hurt inner child, and their good inner parent coming to hold and comfort that child. I've also asked clients to imagine their amygdala all fired up when they are upset; and imagine their wise prefrontal cortex coming in to hold and calm the amygdala. Clients find these visual imagery techniques helpful and empowering. And explaining what part of their brain is heightened when they are agitated is normalizing and de-shaming. A little "neuroeducation" can anchor change in therapy (Fishbane, 2013).

Researchers have begun exploring the interpersonal regulation of emotion. In one study, a woman lying in an fMRI machine waiting for a shock is less stressed— and experiences less pain when the shock comes—if she is holding her husband's hand and they have a good relationship (Coan, Schaefer, & Davidson, 2006). In a subsequent study by Coan and Johnson (Johnson et al., 2013), with insecurely attached couples, the wife doesn't get the benefit of holding her husband's hand. However, after a course of EFT (Emotionally Focused Therapy) treatment, with the couple now securely attached, she gets the hand-holding benefit. In addition to regulating one's own emotions, turning to a beloved partner when stressed can help.

Voice and Empathy

Empathy is soothing when one is upset. Without a compassionate partner response, a person feels alone or disconfirmed. As Judy Jordan (1995) puts it, "Voice implies listening; when I'm with someone who doesn't listen, I lose my voice."

How voice is used in intimate relationships matters. In heterosexual couples, it is usually the wife who brings up issues; Gottman (2011) found that in happier couples, the wife raises her concerns with a soft startup. When she speaks gently, her husband is less likely to have an amygdala-driven defensive reaction. A harsh startup is more likely in unhappy couples.

On the other side of this interaction is the husband. Many men have been socialized by their peer group to be de-skilled in the fine arts of empathy. Len never got the hang of empathy growing up. His peer group of boys didn't cultivate this skill—quite the opposite—and his parents were not equipped to teach him to read emotions—his own or others'. In his family of origin, emotions were associated with his father's bipolar rages, and Len learned to shut down in the face of strong affect—a survival strategy he is using with Carla, to ill effect.

Neuroscientists have identified several components to empathy (Decety & Jackson, 2004). The first step involves resonance—feeling in one's own body what the other is feeling. This information travels from the body to the insula deep inside the brain, ultimately arriving at the prefrontal cortex, where it is named. This process is called Interoception: perceiving within (Craig, 2009). Siegel (1999) has identified an overlap between self-attunement circuits and empathy circuits in the brain. But Len's self-attunement circuits are underdeveloped given his early history and gender socialization, so his ability to attune to Carla is limited. Len works in therapy on the skills of empathy—reading his own body cues, reading his wife's facial expressions, and regulating his anxiety so he can be more present to her. He comes to witness her distress around their son's ADHD and school difficulties with greater compassion. I also encourage Len to become more involved in helping Matt with his schoolwork directly.

The second component of empathy is cognitive—consciously putting oneself into the other's shoes. While Carla is more capable than Len of resonance, her cognitive empathy for him is blocked given her resentment. I help her see his vulnerabilities around chaos and intense emotion given his family-of-origin experiences, and with time she softens and becomes more curious and compassionate toward her husband and his distress with the tumult at home. Her empathy for Len is enhanced as he steps forward to help more and criticize less.

The final two components of empathy according to Decety and Jackson are boundaries between self and other, and self-regulation in the face of the other's pain. If I become overwhelmed by your upset feelings or lose myself in your sorrow, I may become personally distressed rather than empathic, and less inclined to help (Decety & Lamm, 2009).

Eye contact is key for empathy. There are muscles around the eyes dedicated to the expression of emotion, and neurons in the brain dedicated to reading others' emotions. But many couples don't look at each other at all, focusing instead on their smart phones or tablets. Indeed, research shows that empathy has plummeted in the past decade or so (Konrath, O'Brien, & Hsing, 2010). Interventions like the Speaker-Listener technique rely on eye contact to heighten empathic communication.

Scientists are studying gender differences in empathy; hormones and genetics play a role. Testosterone (more abundant in males) is negatively correlated with empathy, while oxytocin (more abundant in females) increases empathy (Zak, 2012). But it's not all biology; gender socialization impacts empathy as well. While females are socialized for attunement and caretaking roles, males are often de-skilled in empathy during their development, encouraged to be tough. In research on empathic accuracy, men's accuracy improved when they were given sufficient motivation. Reading that women find empathic men sexy, the empathic accuracy of (presumably heterosexual) male subjects increased (Thomas & Maio, 2008). Can we motivate our sons with the message: "Real men do empathy"?

Care: Nurturing the Positive

Couples spend a great deal of time in therapy talking about their problems. In recent years, therapists have turned their attention to cultivating the positive as well. Gottman's happy couples create a "culture of positivity," with their 5:1 ratio of positive to negative interactions (Gottman, 2011). Rick Hanson (2016) suggests that it is because the brain is biased toward the negative, with the amygdala ever on the alert for danger, that it takes five positives to outweigh the one negative.

Shelley Taylor (2002), a psychoneuroimmunologist, identifies "Tend and Befriend" behavior, or acts of care and connection, in both animals and humans, particularly females. She notes that Tend and Befriend is as key to survival as fight-or-flight. Tend and Befriend is fueled by oxytocin. In couples, Tend and Befriend behavior includes empathy, generosity, attentiveness, appreciation, and lovemaking. Psychologist Barbara Fredrickson (2013) suggests that love involves "micro-moments of positivity resonance." Neuroscientist Ruth Feldman and colleagues (Feldman, 2012; Schneiderman, Zagoory-Sharon, Leckman, & Feldman, 2012) explore "bio-behavioral synchrony," oxytocin levels, and interactive reciprocity in couples. Beate Ditzen's research (Ditzen et al., 2009) identifies the potentially beneficial impact of oxytocin on couple communication. These studies point to the importance of nurturing love and cultivating positivity.

While some of this research entails administering oxytocin intranasally (where it reaches the brain directly, bypassing the blood-brain barrier), oxytocin is also released naturally. Couple connecting behaviors such as massage, gentle touch, orgasm and empathy can all increase oxytocin and lower cortisol, the stress hormone (Holt-Lunstad, Birmingham, & Light, 2008; Uvnas-Moberg, 2003).

Repair

Love is not a steady state of connection. Rather, it involves an oscillation between connection, disconnection, and repair. How relational hurt is handled makes a big difference. Unhappy couples often get mired in the accuse/defend sequence, which increases their distress; by contrast, happy couples repair well and often (Gottman, 2011).

Guilt feelings prompt the repair process, signaling that one has a conscience, and has acted in a way that violates personal or social norms. Martin Buber (1957) calls this "existential" or "authentic" guilt; without it, one acts like a sociopath. Of course guilt in massive doses—what Buber calls neurotic guilt—can be crippling. Often in unhappy couples each blames the other in order not to feel guilty. And perhaps there is a role for healthy shame as well. Research on forgiveness in couples dealing with infidelity found that the unfaithful partner's experience of shame led to forgiveness in the betrayed partner (Meneses & Greenberg, 2011).

When partners take responsibility for their own part in the relational impasse—not with crippling shame or guilt, but with a healthy sense of personal accountability, revisiting painful moments without reactivity and with compassion can be deeply healing. Holding each other's vulnerabilities with care often increases intimacy. Gottman (2011) suggests that trust is built from repair after hurt in couple relationships. Through mutual understanding and compassionate repair, couples can earn trust and increase intimacy. In a Power With mindset, partners nurture each other and the relationship.

Habits and Change

The human brain is wired for habit. Habits are supported by circuits of neurons that are strengthened through repetition of the habit. These neuronal circuits and habits recursively reinforce each other; Hebb's Theorem, "neurons that fire together wire together," is cited throughout the neuroscience literature (Siegel, 1999). Couples' dances are repeated over and over again; they become automatic as one partner's raised eyebrow prompts defensive anger in the other. Therapists know how hard it is to change these behavioral cycles, so deeply woven into the brain.

The brain is also wired for change. Neuroplasticity, the ability of the brain to change, includes the creation and strengthening of connections between neurons (synaptogenesis); new neurons created from neuronal stem cells (neurogenesis); and the wrapping of myelin around axons, facilitating efficient communication between neurons (myelinogenesis). Neuroplasticity was once thought possible only in the young brain. But research in the past decade or so points to neuroplasticity throughout life (Doidge, 2007). This is good news indeed. Therapists witness the tension between habits and change, as clients struggle to let go of old behaviors and learn new repertoires. Neuroscience offers some insights into how to facilitate neuroplasticity and therapeutic change.

Several factors have been found to promote neuroplasticity in the adult brain. One is physical exercise, which increases blood flow to the brain (Ratey, 2013). I encourage clients to exercise daily, even if only taking a half hour walk. The second factor is paying attention rather than living on autopilot; perhaps this is why mindfulness meditation is so helpful. The third factor is learning new things. Doing same-old, same-old leads to what Lou Cozolino (2008) calls "hardening of the categories." It does not nurture neuroplasticity or relationship plasticity.

The tension between change and no-change in therapy makes sense given the habit-driven brain. When clients are "resistant," I don't engage in power struggles, pathologize their no-change position, or give up hope, but rather work to understand their fears of change. Unproductive relational habits often are based in survival strategies that clients hold dear—and these strategies are reflected in circuits of neurons that have been strengthened over decades. Being asked to change a key survival strategy can feel both difficult and threatening. I honor partners' survival strategies even as I offer them ways to modify or "grow up" these strategies for greater relational success (Fishbane, 2013). The therapist helps each partner author their own change.

Often in therapy one partner is pushing for change while the other is resisting. In Carol Dweck's (2006) terminology, one has a "growth mindset" and the other a "fixed mindset." One partner trying to change the other can backfire and create resentment. No one wants to "be changed" by another—whether that other is the partner or the therapist. Facilitating a shift from a fixed to a growth mindset and helping each partner identify and own their own agenda for change are important therapeutic processes in couple therapy.

To do the hard work of relational change, both partners must feel safe and respected by the therapist. Couples often put the therapist in the position of judge, each partner hoping the therapist will side with them. The therapist must sidestep the judge role, adopting instead a position of "multidirected partiality" (Boszormenyi-Nagy & Spark, 1973) with both partners, holding each one's vulnerabilities and concerns with care. Only then can clients be challenged to grow and change. My office is a "shame-free, blame-free zone"; in this context, partners can risk exploration and growth.

Even when clients do choose change, new habits can be hard to maintain; they need to be practiced over and over before they become wired into the brain. This process, known as "massed practice," was found to be effective with stroke patients re-learning the use of limbs (Taub et al., 2007); it is relevant to all behavior change, which involves brain change. Eventually, the effortful and consciously chosen behaviors will themselves become automatic. But when clients are tired or stressed, the old habits may reappear, as old neural circuits may not completely disappear. Returning to the new practices can get clients back on track; this is important information as therapists and clients work on maintenance of change and relapse prevention.

Proactive Loving

While the rapture of falling in love is delicious, it doesn't usually last. Long-term love is delicate and needs to be cultivated regularly. Rather than being victims of each other, caught up in the blame game, partners can become authors of their own behavior and coauthors of the relationship. And rather than "falling out of love," or waiting for the partner to get it right—both passive positions—I encourage "proactive loving," with each partner working to be their best self in the relationship.

Ethics Meets Neurobiology

A final note: Some people are suspicious of what they see as neurobiological reductionism: My amygdala made me do it! While it's true that we have an amygdala that contributes to reactivity, it's also true that we have a prefrontal cortex that allows us to regulate our emotions and live according to our values. Others are concerned about biological determinism. Genetics do set a blueprint of possibilities, but research shows that how lives are lived shapes both brain and identity, and even affects the expression of genes. The biobehavioral influence is circular. Adding relational neurobiology to a multisystemic discourse doesn't excuse bad behavior. It rather helps clinicians develop tools to facilitate emotion regulation, empathy, responsibility, and care in couple therapy.

References

Arnsten, A. F. T., Raskind, M. A., Taylor, F. B., & Connor, D. F. (2014). The effects of stress exposure on prefrontal cortex: Translating basic research into successful treatments for post-traumatic stress disorder. *Neurobiology of Stress, 1*, 89–99.

Aron, A., Fisher, H., Mashek, D. J., Strong, G., Li, H., & Brown, L. L. (2005). Reward, motivation, and emotion systems associated with early-stage intense romantic love. *Journal of Neurophysiology, 94*, 327–337.

Bartels, A., & Zeki, S. (2000). The neural basis of romantic love. *Neuroreport, 11*, 3829–3834.

Boszormenyi-Nagy, I., & Spark, G. (1973). *Invisible loyalties: Reciprocity in intergenerational family therapy*. New York, NY: Harper & Row.

Buber, M. (1957). Guilt and guilt feelings. *Psychiatry, 20*, 114–129.

Cacioppo, J. T., & Patrick, W. (2008). *Loneliness: Human nature and the need for social connection*. New York, NY: Norton.

Coan, J. A., Schaefer, H. S., & Davidson, R. J. (2006). Lending a hand: Social regulation of the neural response to threat. *Psychological Science, 17*, 1032–1039.

Cozolino, L. (2008). *The healthy aging brain: Sustaining attachment, attaining wisdom*. New York, NY: Norton.

Craig, A. D. (2009). How do you feel—Now? The anterior insula and human awareness. *Nature Reviews Neuroscience, 10*, 59–70.

Crespi, B. J. (2016). Oxytocin, testosterone, and human social cognition. *Biological Reviews, 91*, 390–408.

Creswell, J. D., Way, B. M., Eisenberger, N. I., & Lieberman, M. D. (2007). Neural correlates of dispositional mindfulness during affect labeling. *Psychosomatic Medicine, 69*, 560–565.

Damasio, A. (2010). *Self comes to mind: Constructing the conscious brain*. New York, NY: Pantheon.

Davidson, R. J., & Begley, S. (2012). *The emotional life of your brain*. New York, NY: Hudson Street Press/Penguin.

Decety, J., & Jackson, P. L. (2004). The functional neuroarchitecture of human empathy. *Behavioral and Cognitive Neuroscience Reviews, 3*, 71–100.

Decety, J., & Lamm, C. (2009). Empathy versus personal distress: Recent evidence from social neuroscience. In J. Decety & W. Ickes (Eds.), *The social neuroscience of empathy* (pp. 199–213). Cambridge, MA: MIT Press.

Ditzen, B., Schaer, M., Gabriel, B., Bodenmann, G., Ehlert, U., & Heinrichs, M. (2009). Intranasal oxytocin increases positive communication and reduces cortisol levels during couple conflict. *Biological Psychiatry, 65*, 728–731.

Doidge, N. (2007). *The brain that changes itself*. New York, NY: Viking.

Dweck, C. (2006). *Mindset: The new psychology of success*. New York, NY: Ballantine.

Eisenberger, N. I., & Lieberman, M. D. (2004). Why rejection hurts: A common neural alarm system for physical pain and social pain. *Trends in Cognitive Neurosciences, 8*, 294–299.

Epel, E. S., Blackburn, E. H., Lin, J., Dhabhar, F. S., Adler, N. E., Morrow, J. D., & Cawthon, R. M. (2004). Accelerated telomere shortening in response to life stress. *Proceedings of the National Academy of Sciences USA, 101*, 17312–17315.

Feldman, R. (2012). Oxytocin and social affiliation in humans. *Hormones and Behavior, 61*, 380–391.

Fishbane, M. D. (2005). Differentiation and dialogue in intergenerational relationships. In J. Lebow (Ed.), *Handbook of clinical family therapy* (pp. 543–568). Hoboken, NJ: Wiley.

Fishbane, M. D. (2011). Facilitating relational empowerment in couple therapy. *Family Process, 50*, 337–352.

Fishbane, M. D. (2013). *Loving with the brain in mind: Neurobiology and couple therapy*. New York, NY: Norton.

Fishbane, M. D. (2015). Couple therapy and interpersonal neurobiology. In A. S. Gurman, J. Lebow, & D. K. Snyder (Eds.), *Clinical handbook of couple therapy* (5th ed.). New York, NY: Guilford.

Fisher, H. (2004). *Why we love: The nature and chemistry of romantic love*. New York, NY: Henry Holt.

Fredrickson, B. (2013). *Love 2.0: Finding happiness and health in moments of connection*. New York, NY: Plume.

Goodrich, T. J. (Ed.). (1991). *Women and power: Perspectives for family therapy*. New York, NY: Norton.

Gottman, J. M. (2011). *The science of trust: Emotional attunement for couples*. New York, NY: Norton.

Hackman, D. A., & Farah, M. J. (2009). Socioeconomic status and the developing brain. *Trends in Cognitive Sciences, 13*, 65–73.

Hanson, R. (2016). *Hardwiring happiness: The new brain science of contentment, calm, and confidence*. New York, NY: Harmony.

Hatfield, E., Cacioppo, J. T., & Rapson, R. L. (1993). Emotional contagion. *Current Directions in Psychological Science, 2*, 96–99.

Hatfield, E., Pilemer, J. T., O'Brien, M. U., Sprecher, S., & Le, Y. C. L. (2008). The endurance of love: Passionate and companionate love in newlywed and long-term marriages. *Interpersona, 2*, 35–64.

Hazan, C., & Shaver, P. (1987). Romantic love conceptualized as an attachment process. *Journal of Personality and Social Psychology, 52*, 511–524.

Holt-Lunstad, J., Birmingham, W. A., & Light, K. C. (2008). Influence of a "warm touch" support enhancement intervention among married couples on ambulatory blood pressure, oxytocin, alpha amylase, and cortisol. *Psychosomatic Medicine, 70*, 976–985.

Johnson, S. M. (2004). *The practice of emotionally focused couple therapy: Creating connection* (2nd ed.). New York, NY: Brunner-Routledge.

Johnson, S. M., Moser, M. B., Beckes, L., Smith, A., Dalgleish, T., Halchuk, R., ... Coan, J. A. (2013). Soothing the threatened brain: Leveraging contact comfort with emotionally focused therapy. *PLoS One, 8*(11), 1–10.

Jordan, J. V. (1995). *Family institute conference*. Evanston, IL.

Jordan, J. V. (2010). *Relational-cultural therapy*. Washington, D.C.: American Psychological Association.

Jordan, J. V., Kaplan, A. G., Miller, J. B., Stiver, I. P., & Surrey, J. L. (1991). *Women's growth in connection: Writings from the stone center*. New York, NY: Guilford.

Kiecolt-Glaser, J. K., & Glaser, R. (2010). Psychological stress, telomeres, and telomerase. *Brain, Behavior, & Immunity, 24*, 529–530.

Kiecolt-Glaser, J. K., & Newton, T. L. (2001). Marriage and health: His and hers. *Psychological Bulletin, 127*, 472–503.

Kim, H. S., Sherman, D. K., & Taylor, S. E. (2008). Culture and social support. *American Psychologist, 63*, 518–526.

Konrath, S. H., O'Brien, E. H., & Hsing, C. (2010). Changes in dispositional empathy in American college students over time: A meta-analysis. *Personality and Social Psychology Review, 15*, 180–198.

Meaney, M. J. (2010). Epigenetics and the biological definition of gene x environment interactions. *Child Development, 81*, 41–79.

Meneses, C. W., & Greenberg, L. S. (2011). The construction of a model of the process of couples' forgiveness in emotion-focused therapy for couples. *Journal of Marital and Family Therapy, 37*, 491–502.

Mitchell, S. A. (2003). *Can love last? The fate of romance over time* (Vol. 20, p. 395). New York, NY: Norton.

Ochsner, K. N., & Gross, J. J. (2005). The cognitive control of emotion. *Trends in Cognitive Sciences, 9*, 242–249.

Perel, E. (2006). *Mating in captivity: Reconciling the erotic and the domestic*. New York, NY: Harper.

Perry, B. D. (2002). Childhood experience and the expression of genetic potential: What childhood neglect tells us about nature and nurture. *Brain and Mind, 3*, 79–100.

Phelps, E. A. (2004). Human emotion and memory: Interactions of the amygdala and hippocampal complex. *Current Opinion in Neurobiology, 14*, 198–202.

Ratey, J. (2013). *Spark: The revolutionary new science of exercise and the brain*. New York, NY: Little, Brown.

Scheinkman, M., & Fishbane, M. D. (2004). The vulnerability cycle: Working with impasses in couple therapy. *Family Process, 43*, 279–299.

Schneiderman, I., Zagoory-Sharon, O., Leckman, J. F., & Feldman, R. (2012). Oxytocin during the initial stages of romantic attachment: Relations to couples' interactive reciprocity. *Psychoneuroendocrinology, 37*, 1277–1285.

Schwartz, R. C. (1994). *Internal family systems therapy*. New York, NY: Guilford.

Siegel, D. J. (1999). *The developing mind: How relationships and the brain interact to shape who we are*. New York, NY: Guilford.

Siegel, D. J., & Bryson, T. P. (2011). *The whole-brain child*. New York, NY: Delacorte Press.

Taub, E., Uswatte, G., King, D. K., Morris, D., Crago, J. E., & Chatterjee, A. (2007). A placebo-controlled trial of constraint-induced movement therapy for upper extremity after stroke. *Stroke, 37*, 1045–1049.

Taylor, S. E. (2002). *The tending instinct: Women, men, and the biology of our relationships*. New York, NY: Henry Holt.

Thomas, G., & Maio, G. R. (2008). Man, I feel like a woman: When and how gender-role motivation helps mind-reading. *Journal of Personality and Social Psychology, 95*, 1165–1179.

Uvnas-Moberg, K. (2003). *The oxytocin factor: Tapping the hormone of calm, love, and healing*. Cambridge, MA: Perseus Books.

Wachs, K., & Cordova, J. V. (2007). Mindful relating: Exploring mindfulness and emotion repertoires in intimate relationships. *Journal of Marital and Family Therapy, 3*, 464–481.

Zak, P. (2012). *The moral molecule: The source of love and prosperity*. New York, NY: Dutton.

Zeki, S. (2007). The neurobiology of love. *FEBS Letters, 581*, 2575–2579.

Zhang, T.-Y., & Meaney, M. J. (2010). Epigenetics and the environmental regulation of the genome and its function. *Annual Review of Psychology, 61*, 439–466.

Relationship Distress: Empirical Evidence for a Relational Need Perspective

Lesley L. Verhofstadt, Gilbert M. D. Lemmens, and Gaëlle Vanhee

Introduction

> I had a terrible day at work, but he didn't seem to care about it. It really made me feel sad and angry at the same time. When he asked me when I would start preparing dinner, I became furious and told him to make dinner himself.

> Sometimes, my wife doesn't seem to care about my opinion. Recently, she enthusiastically told me about a trip to the mountains she wanted to organize for the whole family, even though she knows I'm not into hiking. She didn't ask for my opinion and I really felt unheard and hurt. I told her that she was being selfish and I left the room.

These vignettes describe episodes of conflict that typically occur in both distressed and non-distressed couples. Each partner has his or her own goals, needs, or preferences, and these could be conscious or unconscious, general or specific, and short term or long term (Lewin, 1948). Conflict can occur within a couple's relationship because individuals may pursue their goals in a way that interferes with their partner's goals or the goals of both partners may be incompatible with one another. Despite the fact that partners may be largely unaware of these goals, goal or need interference leads to conflict between partners (Bradbury, Rogge, & Lawrence, 2001). Goal interference, need frustration, and conflict between partners are considered an unavoidable part of daily human existence, as a result of partners being highly interdependent and in frequent contact with each other (Bradbury & Karney, 2014).

L. L. Verhofstadt (✉) · G. Vanhee
Department of Experimental Clinical and Health Psychology, Ghent University,
Ghent, Belgium
e-mail: lesley.verhofstadt@ugent.be

G. M. D. Lemmens
Department of Psychiatry, Ghent University Hospital, Ghent, Belgium

Department of Head and Skin – Psychiatry and Medical Psychology, Ghent University,
Ghent, Belgium

© Springer Nature Switzerland AG 2020   281
M. Ochs et al. (eds.), *Systemic Research in Individual, Couple, and Family
Therapy and Counseling*, European Family Therapy Association Series,
https://doi.org/10.1007/978-3-030-36560-8_16

Despite the fact that many theorists and researchers agree that conflict involves some goal interference or goal incompatibility between two parties (Lewin, 1948), there is surprisingly little consensus in the literature about the number and kind of relational needs that matter most within intimate relationships, nor is there consensus on which needs are central in understanding relationship conflict (Vanhee, Lemmens, Moors, Hinnekens, & Verhofstadt, 2018). Furthermore, there is little empirical research on the emotional and behavioral mechanisms underlying the assumed association between need frustration and conflict in couples (see Vanhee, Lemmens, Moors, et al., 2018). In other words, how do partners emotionally react when their needs are unmet within their relationship? Which behaviors – intended to deal with need dissatisfaction or frustration – result from these emotional reactions?

Accordingly, the aim of the present chapter is to develop a better understanding of the origins of relationship conflict in order to provide more evidence-based insights into how conflicts can be addressed in couple therapy. More specifically, an exploration will be made of how partners' frustrated needs for autonomy, competence, and relatedness fuel their emotional reactions toward their partner, as well as their behavioral responses and their general levels of relationship dissatisfaction and conflict. First, a rationale for this need perspective on relationship conflict will be provided. Second, an overview of existing empirical evidence on the associations between our variables of interest will be presented. Next, a series of studies designed to provide an initial test of our predictions will be described. Finally, we consider the major conclusions that can be drawn from this research and some possible theoretical and clinical implications.

A Relational Need Perspective on Conflict: Rationale

Different Perspectives on Relational Needs

In the past few decades, theorists have proposed many ideas to explain fights and arguments between couples (see Vanhee, Lemmens, Moors, et al., 2018; Vanhee, Lemmens, Stas, et al., 2018). These vary from mismatching relational schemas compounded by poor communication skills to an imbalance of costs and benefits (Baldwin, 1992; Clarkin & Miklowitz, 1997; Rusbult, Drigotas, & Verette, 1994). One theory gaining more attention states that conflict and dissatisfaction in a relationship may have its roots in partners' inability to meet one another's needs. In the *couple therapy literature*, some contemporary therapy models consider need fulfillment to be central in intimate relationships. For instance, Sue Johnson's Emotionally Focused Couple Therapy places a firm emphasis on the need for attachment, referring to one's need to feel secure and connected to their partner (Johnson, 2009; see also Bowlby, 1969, 1988; Hazan & Shaver, 1987). Additionally, the fulfillment of partners' needs for identity maintenance (i.e., to be accepted by one's partner as one is) and for attraction and liking (i.e., feeling that one is liked and desired by one's partner) is an important treatment focus in Leslie Greenberg and Rhonda Goldman's Emotion-Focused Couples Therapy (see Greenberg & Goldman, 2008; see also chapter "What are the Emotions? How Emotion-Focused Therapy Could Inspire Systemic Practice" in this book).

The *couple research literature* also documents the role of need fulfillment in intimate relationships. Baumeister and Leary (1995) proposed the need for belonging as one of the most basic needs to be fulfilled in an intimate relationship. Anchored within Interdependence Theory (Kelley & Thibaut, 1978), Drigotas and Rusbult's work (Drigotas & Rusbult, 1992) considered the needs for intimacy, emotional involvement, security, companionship, sex, and self-worth to be essential in intimate relationships (see Le & Agnew, 2001; Le & Farrell, 2009; Lewandowski & Ackerman, 2006). Furthermore, the Self-Expansion Model proposed by Aron and Aron indicates the vital importance of partners' needs for self-expansion or self-improvement within their relationship (Aron & Aron, 1996).

Within the *broader psychological literature*, Self-Determination Theory (SDT) has been one of the most notable approaches to conceptualizing basic psychological needs (Deci & Ryan, 2000). SDT advances the idea that the three needs for autonomy, competence, and relatedness are universal, that is, that they are essential for a person's psychological and physical well-being (Chen et al., 2015; Deci & Ryan, 2000; Ryan & Deci, 2000). Having these needs fulfilled is important in any given social environment, including within intimate relationships (La Guardia & Patrick, 2008).

As illustrated above, there is no theoretical consensus in the literature about the number and kind of relational needs that are central in understanding intimate relationship conflict and distress. A recent review stated that convincing empirical evidence is currently lacking to inform clinicians about the kinds of needs that should be focused upon in couple therapy in order to be effective in alleviating relationship dissatisfaction and instability (Vanhee et al., 2018). Within the current investigation, a focus was taken on partners' needs for autonomy, competence, and relatedness, as stipulated within the SDT framework. The reasons and considerations underpinning this choice will be outlined in the following section.

Partners' Needs for Autonomy, Competence, and Relatedness

First, SDT is the only needs perspective that distinguishes *need satisfaction* and *need frustration* as two separate concepts, rather than conceptualizing them as polar opposites on a scale (Vanhee, Lemmens, Moors, et al., 2018; Vanhee, Lemmens, Stas, et al., 2018; Vansteenkiste & Ryan, 2013). It is essential to create a distinction between need satisfaction and need frustration due to their differential predictive effects; it has been demonstrated that need satisfaction plays a more fundamental role in well-being, while need frustration is seen as a better predictor of malfunction and ill-being (Bartholomew, Ntoumanis, Ryan, Bosch, & Thøgersen-Ntoumani,

2011; Costa, Ntoumanis, & Bartholomew, 2015; Verstuyf, Vansteenkiste, Soenens, Boone, & Mouratidis, 2013). Regarding the specific types of needs, satisfaction of the need for autonomy in intimate relationships describes partners who feel that they have agency over their actions and that they are self-governed and experience psychological freedom in their relationship. When partners feel able to attain their desired goals within the relationship and feel effective in their actions, this satisfies their need for competence. Satisfaction of the need for relatedness means that partners experience a relationship that is mutually loving, stable, and caring. Conversely, frustration of one's need for autonomy occurs when someone feels that their partner is controlling or coercing them to behave in particular ways, against their wishes. A partner's need for competence is frustrated when they are made to feel that they are a failure or in some way inadequate or when their partner makes them doubt their own capabilities. Finally, frustration of one's need for relatedness describes those who feel rejected, lonely, or disliked by their partner (La Guardia & Patrick, 2008). Therefore, need dissatisfaction (i.e., the opposite of need satisfaction) concerns passivity and indifference toward a partner's needs, whereas need frustration refers to a situation where an individual obstructs their partner's needs in an active and direct manner. Need dissatisfaction and need frustration are consequently asymmetrically related to one another; need dissatisfaction is, by definition, covered by need frustration, while the converse is not necessarily true (Vansteenkiste & Ryan, 2013).

Second, SDT provides one of the *most comprehensive* views on relational needs, as many other models deal exclusively with needs that can be captured by only one of the three needs, and in particular the need for relatedness. As a result, the needs for autonomy and competence are often neglected. For example, the needs for intimacy, emotional involvement, security, companionship, and sex, as described by Drigotas and Rusbult (1992), can all be covered by the need for relatedness. Similarly, the need for belonging (Baumeister & Leary, 1995), the need for attachment, and the need for attraction and liking, as described by EFT-C therapists (Greenberg & Goldman, 2008; Johnson, 2004), also fall under the need for relatedness. The need for identity maintenance is described by EFT-C therapists (Greenberg & Goldman, 2008) as a composite of the needs for autonomy and competence. As these examples illustrate, SDT gives equal importance to each of the three needs in a way that the aforementioned perspectives do not.

Finally, cross-cultural replication of the association between well-being and these three needs confirms the *universal importance* of the need for autonomy, competence, and relatedness (Chen et al., 2015). It has been found that the three needs play an equivalent role across different cultures (Chen et al., 2015), despite the fact that, from a cultural relativistic perspective, individualistic cultures teach people to benefit more from the presence of autonomy, while collectivistic cultures teach people to benefit more from the presence of relatedness (Heine, Lehman, Markus, & Kitayama, 1999). This finding gives support to the importance of investigating each of these three needs.

Given these considerations, our research focused on the need for autonomy, competence, and relatedness in intimate relationships. In what follows, an overview is given of the available empirical evidence on the association between the need for autonomy, competence, and relatedness on the one hand and relationship dissatisfaction, conflict frequency, and partners' emotions and behavior during conflict on the other hand.

Relational Needs and Relationship Conflict: Current Empirical Evidence

Relational Needs and Relationship Dissatisfaction

Relationship (dis)satisfaction is defined as partners' subjective evaluation of the positive and negative aspects of their relationship (Fincham, Beach, & Kemp-Fincham, 1997). Conceptually, empirically, and clinically, relationship conflict and relationship dissatisfaction are strongly intertwined (see theory and research from social learning perspectives on intimate relationships; Baucom & Epstein, 1989; Jacobson & Margolin, 1979; see Bradbury & Karney, 2014). Up to this point, studies have demonstrated that greater need satisfaction (i.e., autonomy, competence, and relatedness) is associated with higher levels of relationship satisfaction (Patrick, Knee, Canevello, & Lonsbary, 2007; Uysal, Lin, Knee, & Bush, 2012). There is also preliminary evidence for the dyadic interplay of both partners' levels of need satisfaction in determining relationship satisfaction. More specifically, Patrick et al. (2007) found that one's level of relationship satisfaction was not only predicted by one's own level of need satisfaction but also by one's partner's level of need satisfaction. Moreover, satisfaction of someone's relatedness need has been shown by a longitudinal study to lead to their partner perceiving increased satisfaction with their relationship over time (Hadden, Smith, & Knee, 2013). It has been found that each of the specific SDT needs is a unique predictor of relationship outcomes but that the satisfaction of the need for relatedness is most strongly associated with relational outcomes (Patrick et al., 2007).

Relational Needs and Conflict Frequency

Conflict frequency concerns the number of differences of opinion, disagreements, fights, or arguments experienced by a couple (Canary, Cupach, & Messman, 1995; Kluwer & Johnson, 2007). To the best of our knowledge, only one study examined whether relational need satisfaction shows a link with how often partners disagree. More specifically, Patrick et al. (2007) found that participants whose needs for autonomy, competence, and relatedness were satisfied to a greater extent within their intimate relationship also reported coming into conflict with their partner less frequently. The frequency of conflict reported by an individual was also related to their partner's level of need satisfaction (Patrick et al., 2007), further highlighting the association's dyadic nature.

Relational Needs and Conflict Behavior

The conflict literature devotes much attention to couples' behavior during conflict (Eldridge, 2009), often categorizing the nature of these behaviors as positive versus negative or as constructive versus destructive (Birditt, Brown, Orbuch, & McIlvane, 2010; Fincham & Beach, 1999). Positive/*constructive conflict behaviors* would include listening actively to one's partner, raising issues in a calm and neutral manner, and working to reach agreement. Behaviors such as blaming one's partner, shouting, showing hostility, or interrupting would fall under negative/*destructive conflict behaviors* (Bradbury & Karney, 2014). Withdrawing behaviors, involving a partner disengaging from the interaction either actively or passively, have also been included in this classification (Birditt et al., 2010).

Besides partners' individual conflict behavior, researchers often focus on patterns of behavior that occur within the couple during conflict. These patterns can largely be summarized as three types: mutual constructive behavior (i.e., active and constructive engagement with the discussion by both partners); mutual avoidance (i.e., active or passive withdrawal from the discussion by both partners); and demand-withdrawal (i.e., one partner blames and criticizes the other in pursuit of change, while the other partner either avoids or withdraws from the interaction) (Eldridge, 2009).

Regarding the association with relational need satisfaction, Patrick and colleagues' study (Patrick et al., 2007), focusing on people's responses to conflict, demonstrated that greater satisfaction of each need is associated with responses to conflict that are more constructive and less destructive. The study also found partner effects, showing that those whose partners experience higher levels of need satisfaction respond to conflict in a less destructive way.

Relational Needs and Emotions

As one of the primary functions of emotions is to signal a (mis)match between a person's needs and their environment (Moors, Ellsworth, Scherer, & Frijda, 2013; Scherer & Ellsworth, 2009), negative emotions can be viewed as an alarm system that shows when someone's needs interfere or are not compatible with those of his or her partner (Carver & Scheier, 1990). Additionally, emotions prepare and motivate people to react appropriately to specific circumstances (Keltner & Haidt, 1999; Roseman, 2011). Various therapy models, such as EFT-Cs, follow the same reasoning and place a strong focus on partners' emotions when treating couple conflict and distress (Greenberg & Goldman, 2008; Johnson, 2004). More specifically, EFT-Cs assume that emotions play a mediating role in the association between relational need frustration and relationship conflict and distress.

Regarding the association between emotions and the need for autonomy, competence, and relatedness, one study showed that partners who experience less need satisfaction experience a higher degree of negative emotions and a lower degree of positive emotions (Patrick et al., 2007). These associations have also been demonstrated outside the context of intimate relationships (Reis, Sheldon, Gable, Roscoe,

& Ryan, 2000. Moreover, satisfaction of the needs for competence and relatedness are shown to be related to lower levels of sadness and anger (Tong et al., 2009). The satisfaction of one's competence needs was also found to be related to fewer feelings of fear (Tong et al., 2009).

The association between partners' negative emotions and their conflict behavior has been an important area of investigation in the couple research literature as well (e.g., Gottman, 2011; Verhofstadt, Buysse, De Clercq, & Goodwin, 2005). When negative emotions are divided into hard (i.e., anger or irritation) and soft (i.e., sadness or hurt) categories, more negative communication (i.e., criticism and defensiveness) was found to be related to hard emotions, but the links between soft emotions and more negative communication are far less consistent (Sanford, 2007).

Conclusion

In sum, within different literatures, theoretical associations have been assumed between relational needs on the one hand and relationship conflict and dissatisfaction on the other, with emotions playing a central role (see Vanhee et al., 2018, for a review). The existing evidence on the role of autonomy, relatedness, and competence needs within relationships is promising but also scarce and limited in several respects. The gaps in our knowledge on how autonomy, competence, and relatedness needs relate to relationship conflict, dissatisfaction, and emotions are outlined below, along with how our research aimed to deal with these limitations.

Research Objectives, Predictions, and Study Design

Whereas both the emotion and couple therapy literatures suggest that emotions are important in the relational need-conflict association, specific assumptions are outlined in only a few couple therapy models (Vanhee et al., 2018). More specifically, EFT-Cs assume that (a) couple conflict and relationship distress result from partners being unable to meet each other's needs; (b) unmet needs lead to negative emotions in partners; and (c) negative emotions, accompanying unmet needs, give rise to specific behaviors in partners, resulting in negative interaction cycles between partners over time. However, despite the specificity of these hypotheses, and their centrality in EFT-Cs, research evidence on the interplay between relational needs, emotions, and relationship conflict/dissatisfaction is largely lacking.

Second, the current literature has paid little attention to the distinction between need satisfaction and need frustration. Although there are theoretical grounds by which need (dis)satisfaction may be distinguished from need frustration, up to this point, this difference has only been taken into account by studies outside the intimate relationship context. These empirical studies demonstrate that need satisfaction is a stronger predictor of well-being than need frustration and need frustration is a stronger predictor of ill-being than need satisfaction, which emphasizes the importance of maintaining this distinction. Although a need frustration perspective on relationship conflict would therefore be more appropriate, this perspective has not been adopted by any previous study on intimate relationships.

The third limitation is methodological in nature, as the studies on relational needs in intimate relationships described above have primarily relied on surveys. This is a problem as both motivational and cognitive biases may interfere with reports of participants attempting to recall, interpret, and collect past experiences into current overall impressions of their relationship (Paulhus & Vazire, 2007; Schwartz, Groves, & Schuman, 1998).

Fourth, the studies described above used samples that consisted primarily of partners engaged in relationships of short or average length (mean relationship duration ranged from 1.06 to 3.33 years). A study of long-term relationships has not yet been undertaken, to our knowledge. The generalizability of existing findings is further limited by the fact that most previous studies have tended to use samples consisting of undergraduate (psychology) students.

In order to deal with these shortcomings, we examined in a systematic and rigorous way how relational needs, relationship conflict, dissatisfaction, and emotions relate to each other, using multiple research methods and different samples of partners in a long-term relationship. More specifically, we examined whether (see Fig. 1):

Hypothesis 1. Higher levels of frustration of the need for autonomy, competence, and relatedness are associated with higher levels of relationship dissatisfaction and relationship conflict (higher conflict frequency and lower and higher levels of constructive and destructive conflict behavior, respectively).

Hypothesis 2. Higher levels of frustration of the need for autonomy, competence, and relatedness are associated with higher levels of sadness, fear, and anger.

Hypothesis 3. Sadness, fear, and anger mediate the association between the need for autonomy, competence, and relatedness and relationship conflict (behavior).

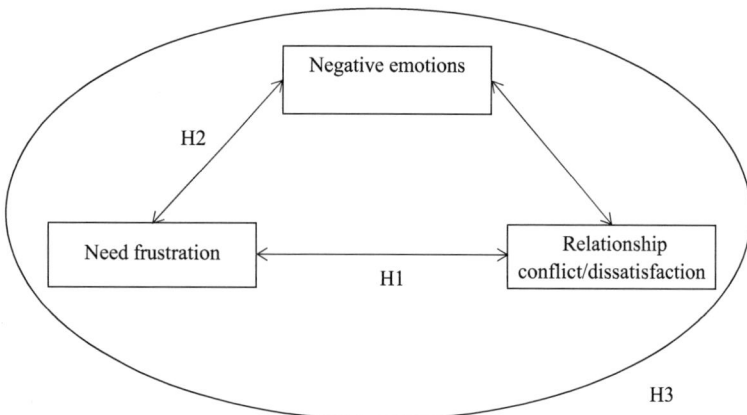

Fig. 1 Hypotheses tested within the current examination

In order to test our predictions, a series of five quantitative studies were conducted. Samples consisted of partners involved in a heterosexual relationship for at least 1 year and married/cohabiting for at least 6 months. The mean age for the men was 38.56 years (ranging from 18 to 77 years), and the mean age for the women was 33.12 years (ranging from 18 to 78 years). The length of their relationships ranged from 1 to 56 years, with an average length of about 14.02 years. Participants were recruited by means of social media and network sampling. Study 1 and Study 2 consisted of cross-sectional, large-scale Internet-based surveys in which 372 individuals (Study 1; Vanhee, Lemmens, & Verhofstadt, 2016) and 230 couples (Study 2; Vanhee, Lemmens, Stas, Loeys, & Verhofstadt, 2018) completed self-report measures on their level of need frustration/satisfaction within their intimate relationship, their level of relationship dissatisfaction, conflict frequency, and conflict behavior. A laboratory-based observational study was then conducted (Study 3) in which 141 couples provided questionnaire data on our variables of interest and participated in a videotaped conflict interaction and video-review task designed to measure partners' interaction-based level of need frustration and corresponding emotions (see Vanhee, Lemmens, & Verhofstadt, in preparation). The videotaped interactions were subsequently coded for the presence of several types of conflict behavior. Within Study 4, a recall-design was used in which 200 participants described a recent self-experienced need-frustrating situation and reported on their level of need-frustration and corresponding emotional and behavioral responses (see Vanhee, Lemmens, Fontaine, Moors, & Verhofstadt, in preparation). Finally, Study 5 used a so-called imagine-design in which 397 participants reported on need frustration and emotional and behavioral responses when presented with hypothetical need-frustrating scenarios (see Vanhee, Lemmens, Fontaine, et al., in preparation).

General Summary of Results and Discussion

Relational Needs and Relationship Conflict and Dissatisfaction (H1)

Regarding *relationship dissatisfaction*, we found that partners' levels of both relational need satisfaction and relational need frustration proved important in explaining their level of (dis)satisfaction in their relationship, thereby confirming both our first hypothesis and the findings of prior investigations (Patrick et al., 2007; Uysal et al., 2012). Although the needs for autonomy, competence, and relatedness all matter equally in intimate relationships according to Self-Determination Theory (Deci & Ryan, 2000), our findings suggested that a person's need for relatedness was most important in evaluating their relationship, followed by their need for autonomy. An association between relationship dissatisfaction and competence needs was not found within our studies. These differential associations are in line with two earlier studies on this subject (Patrick et al., 2007; Uysal et al., 2012).

Moreover, as reported in previous research (Hadden et al., 2013; Patrick et al., 2007), relationship dissatisfaction is affected by the frustration of an individual's partner's relatedness need as much as by their own relatedness frustration, emphasizing the central role of the need for relatedness.

Further, our research generally supported the association between relational need frustration and *relationship conflict*. However, autonomy, competence, and relatedness frustration seemed to play different roles depending on the component of conflict being examined. First, it was found that experiencing higher levels of relatedness frustration was associated with more frequent initiation of conflict. This is in line with Patrick and colleagues' study (Patrick et al., 2007), which also found that relatedness was the strongest correlate of *conflict frequency*. Our findings on relatedness frustration further extend those of this latter study by demonstrating a partner effect in addition to an actor effect (Kenny, Kashy, & Cook, 2006). This means that individuals whose partners experience greater relatedness need frustration also become more frequent initiators of conflict themselves. Second, there was a consistent finding across our studies, and thus methodologies, that greater need frustration was associated with lower levels of *constructive behavior* and higher levels of *destructive behavior*. This was true both regarding behaviors self-reported by partners in general and specific (recalled or hypothetical) need-frustrating situations and during observation of couples' actual conflict interactions. These findings are in line with previous research addressing constructive and destructive responses to conflict more broadly, as self-reported by participants (Patrick et al., 2007). More specifically, a relationship was found between each specific type of need frustration and so-called demanding behavior. These results are in line with the existing conflict literature, which shows that people who want change in either their relationship or their partner typically display behaviors intended to elicit change in their partner, such as pressuring, accusing, or complaining (Heavey, Layne, & Christensen, 1993; Papp, Kouros, & Cummings, 2009), irrespective of the changes required (Verhofstadt et al., 2005). A positive association was also found between need frustration and conflict behavior patterns involving withdrawing behavior (such as mutual avoidance or demand-withdrawal). This might be due to the fact that withdrawing behavior is often seen as the last stage in a cascade that begins with criticizing (i.e., demanding) and escalates to contempt and defensiveness (Gottman, 1994). As such, the relationship between need frustration and withdrawing behavior might be particularly strong when relational needs are frustrated over a longer period of time.

Relational Needs and Negative Emotions (H2)

Our research provides a positive answer to the question of whether the experience of negative emotions in intimate relationships is affected by relational need frustration. These findings coincide with the suggestion of emotion theories that negative feelings function as alarms to signal that an individual's needs interfere or are incompatible with the needs of his or her partner (Carver & Scheier, 1990; Moors et al., 2013; Scherer & Ellsworth, 2009). They also fit with SDT's description of negative feelings as a consequence of people's maladaptive means of coping with need frustration (Vansteenkiste & Ryan, 2013). Additionally, they are in line with previous studies outside a relationship context that have investigated the link between need dissatisfaction and negative emotions (Patrick et al., 2007; Reis et al., 2000). More specifically, it was found that the specific types of need frustration seem to play different roles depending on the type of emotion (sadness, anger, fear) being examined. In particular, we found a robust association between greater frustration of one's relatedness needs and experiencing more *sadness*. The same was true for *anger*, with frustration of the needs for autonomy and competence being the most robust correlates in this case. These results are in line with research dividing feelings into *soft* and *hard* types, which has demonstrated that soft feelings are associated with goals focused on the relationship and hard feelings with goals centered on the self, including protecting oneself from situations leading to harm (Sanford, 2007). These latter goals can encompass the need for autonomy and competence, as autonomy frustration (for instance, feeling controlled by one's partner) and competence frustration (for instance, feeling inferior and unsuccessful by comparison) can be viewed as harming one's identity dimension (i.e., acceptance of who one is; Greenberg & Goldman, 2008). Within the current investigation, feelings of *fear* were found to be less consistently related to partners' need frustration.

Relational Needs, Negative Emotions, and Conflict Behavior (H3)

The third part of our empirical examination involved investigating the roles of negative emotions (i.e., sadness, fear, and anger) as mediators of the association between need frustration (i.e., autonomy, competence, and relatedness) and conflict behavior (i.e., demanding and withdrawing). Before discussing the results of our mediation analyses, it is interesting to consider the link between negative emotions and conflict behavior, as this is the mediation model's final association that is yet to be described, despite it being essential to the mediation. Generally speaking, it can be concluded that higher levels of negative emotions, especially *anger*, were associated with greater instances of destructive conflict behavior and in particular of demanding behavior. Furthermore, we found that higher levels of *fear* were associated with less demanding behavior and more withdrawing behavior. These results confirm previous research that has shown a positive association between hard feelings and higher levels of critical and defensive behavior toward a partner. Previous studies have found that soft feelings, on the other hand, are less consistently associated with destructive communication due to the focus these place on relationship preservation and reparation (Sanford, 2007). Our findings give further support to the literature's prevailing stance on emotions, which tends to associate anger with antagonistic tendencies, such as attempting to induce change by working against or attacking the other person, and fear with tendencies toward distancing or avoiding, which reduce interaction with one's partner (Frijda, 1986; Roseman, 2011). Concerning demanding behavior, these findings are in line with EFT-Cs (Greenberg & Goldman, 2008; Johnson, 2004), in which this is seen as an especially likely result of anger.

In considering an overview of the significant *mediation* models that our studies found, we can conclude that individuals, particularly women, who felt that their autonomy needs were frustrated experienced higher levels of *anger*, which can be viewed as an emotional reaction with a self-protective purpose (Smith & Lazarus, 1990). An association was found in turn between anger and blame, criticism, and placing pressure on a partner to change, which can be viewed as attacking behaviors (Roseman, 2011; Roseman, Wiest, & Swartz, 1994). A similar association was found between frustration of competence and relatedness needs and demanding behavior via the experience of anger in both genders, although the evidence in this case was less robust. These mediation models largely converge with EFT-C's assumptions (Greenberg & Goldman, 2008; Johnson, 2004), which argue that partners' feelings, and in particular reactive feelings such as anger, lead to them enacting destructive behaviors toward a partner, such as demanding and withdrawing behavior, in an attempt to both cope with and protect against their own need frustration.

Implications for Theory and Practice

Our findings demonstrate that conflict can occur when individuals' own relational needs are incompatible or interfere with their partner's needs, which is consistent with the definition of conflict (Lewin, 1948). More specifically, our studies found that the extent to which partners' needs are frustrated corresponds to the frequency with which they initiate conflict with their partner, as well as their feelings, behavior, and interaction with their partner when conflict arises. This proves the relevance of taking a *relational need perspective on conflict*.

Moreover, the present research provides further evidence that the *need for autonomy, competence, and relatedness* is of particular importance in intimate relationships. With a basis in the broader psychological literature, previous research on the psychological needs that Self-Determination Theory describes (SDT; Deci & Ryan, 2000) has predominantly taken place within the context of the workplace, school, parenting, or sports (e.g., Haerens, Aelterman, Vansteenkiste, Soenens, & Van Petegem, 2014; Trépanier, Fernet, & Austan, 2016). Although SDT argues that the fulfillment of these needs is important regardless of the social environment, including in the context of intimate relationships (La Guardia & Patrick, 2008), few attempts had been made to support this theoretical suggestion empirically. Our results, however, also add further nuance to the equal value that SDT places on each specific type of need in an intimate relationship context (La Guardia & Patrick, 2008). Despite the fact that each of these needs contributed in some form to explaining the relational outcomes examined in our investigation (i.e., relationship (dis) satisfaction, conflict frequency, couples' conflict behavior), it was generally found that the *need for relatedness* was the most important correlate of these outcomes. This is logical from a conceptual standpoint, as the key feature to define intimate relationships is interdependence (Bradbury & Karney, 2014). By contrast, the role played by each of the three needs was different, but broadly equally relevant, when it came to predicting the individual outcomes included in our investigation, such as partners' emotions and individuals' varieties of conflict behaviors. Therefore, it would be interesting to reconsider each need's importance while taking into account the differing contexts and outcomes.

Our findings also reinforce SDT's claim that creating a distinction between *need satisfaction* and *need frustration* is important, given that they have differing associations with human functioning and dysfunctioning (Vansteenkiste & Ryan, 2013) and differential roles in relational well-being (i.e., relationship satisfaction), which is distinct from individual well-being (e.g., Bartholomew et al., 2011). With regard to relationship conflict, this research project is the first, to our knowledge, to demonstrate that it is not only partners' passive indifference toward each other's needs (i.e., need dissatisfaction) that affects conflict (see Patrick et al., 2007) but also more active and direct attempts by partners to undermine each other's needs (i.e., need frustration).

The current research used samples consisting of mainly white, heterosexual, middle-class, well-functioning partners or non-distressed couples, and consequently we should exercise caution when using our findings to derive clinical implications. Our findings might nonetheless contribute to a more evidence-based insight into how couple therapists can understand and tackle couples' relationship conflict and relationship dissatisfaction. For instance, relational need frustration is important in intimate relationships as a predictor of partners' levels of dissatisfaction with their relationship, the frequency with which they are likely to initiate conflict with their partner, and their feelings and behavior in conflict situations. Relationship conflict and relationship dissatisfaction are the main reasons for couples seeking therapy, and couple therapists should generally recognize and tackle relational need frustration in order to address these issues. However, as the frustration of each need seems to have differential effects on a relationship, there are implications for the order in which these needs should be addressed by therapists. As the most important correlate of relational outcomes appears to be relatedness frustration, couple therapists should first explore behavior by partners that is cold and rejecting (i.e., the inducers of relatedness frustration) and focus on its reduction. It is nonetheless important that couple therapists pay attention to clients' extreme controlling behaviors (i.e., inducers of autonomy frustration) and vague or unreasonable expectations from partners (i.e., inducers of competence frustration), as frustration of these needs has also been shown to play a role for both genders in intimate relationships. As our findings provide support for a relational need perspective on couple conflict and distress, they also imply (as suggested by an anonymous reviewer of the current chapter) that therapists should reflect on the issue of when and how to start discussing the prospects of "helpful resignation/giving up" need expectations in couples where partners cannot satisfy each other's needs, even if they have tried for a long time.

Furthermore, our results highlight how emotions play an informative role. In line with what has been described by emotion theories (Carver & Scheier, 1990; Moors et al., 2013; Scherer & Ellsworth, 2009), we found that when an individual's needs are incompatible or interfere with those of his or her partner, negative feelings play the role of alarms. More specifically, when partners experience anger, there might be value in exploring the extent to which an individual's needs for autonomy and competence are frustrated by their partner. Although couple therapy sessions represent an environment in which anger is often more present, paying attention to feelings of sadness is also important, as there is a demonstrated link here with partners' frustrated need for relatedness. Partners can also be taught ways to be receptive both to each other's feelings and to the underlying frustrated needs. Destructive behaviors during conflict, such as demanding, are particularly related to feelings of anger, and it is through these emotions that need frustration leads to manifestations of demanding behavior. Couple therapists should use caution with these emotions due to their detrimental associations with conflict behavior. It is important to temper clients' feelings of anger when detected and to convert these feelings into something more constructive.

Finally, concerning EFT-Cs (Greenberg & Goldman, 2008; Johnson, 2004), both our literature review and empirical data found evidence for the broad interpretation of these models' assumptions on the etiology of relationship distress. However, as needs other than those outlined by EFT-Cs may prove to be useful, EFT-C practitioners should consider broadening their view on the needs that couple therapy ought to address (see Vanhee, Lemmens, Moors, et al., 2018; Vanhee, Lemmens, Stas, et al., 2018). Although models of effective couple therapy may not necessarily follow an understanding of the apparent causes of couple distress (Eisler, 2005), establishing empirical links between the etiology and treatment of relationship distress may contribute to emotion-focused therapies increasingly becoming theoretically grounded, research-based therapy approaches (Gurman, 2008; Lebow, 2010; Nef, Philippot, & Verhofstadt, 2012).

References

Aron, E. N., & Aron, A. (1996). Love and expansion of the self: The state of the model. *Personal Relationships, 3*, 45–58. https://doi.org/10.1111/j.1475-6811.1996.tb00103.x

Baldwin, M. W. (1992). Relational schemas and the processing of social information. *Psychological Bulletin, 112*, 461–484. https://doi.org/10.1037/0033-2909.112.3.461

Bartholomew, K. J., Ntoumanis, N., Ryan, R. M., Bosch, J. A., & Thøgersen-Ntoumani, C. (2011). Self-determination theory and diminished functioning: The role of interpersonal control and psychological need thwarting. *Personality and Social Psychology Bulletin, 37*, 1459–1473. https://doi.org/10.1177/0146167211413125

Baucom, D. H., & Epstein, N. (1989). The role of cognitive variables in the assessment and treatment of marital discord. In M. Hersen, R. M. Eisler, & P. M. Miller (Eds.), *Progress in behavior modification* (pp. 223–248). Newbury Park, UK: SAGE.

Baumeister, R., & Leary, M. R. (1995). The need to belong: Desire for interpersonal attachments as a fundamental human motivation. *Psychological Bulletin, 117*, 497–529. https://doi.org/10.1037//0033-2909.117.3.497

Birditt, K. S., Brown, E., Orbuch, T. L., & McIlvane, J. M. (2010). Marital conflict behaviors and implications for divorce over 16 years. *Journal of Marriage and Family, 72*, 1188–1204. https://doi.org/10.1111/j.1741-3737.2010.00758.x

Bowlby, J. (1969). *Attachment and loss: Vol. I. Attachment.* New York, NY: Basic Books.

Bowlby, J. (1988). *A secure base.* New York, NY: Basic Books.

Bradbury, T., Rogge, R., & Lawrence, E. (2001). Reconsidering the role of conflict in marriage. In A. Booth, A. C. Crouter, & M. Clements (Eds.), *Couples in conflict* (pp. 59–81). Mahwah, NJ: Lawrence Erlbaum.

Bradbury, T. N., & Karney, B. R. (2014). *Intimate relationships.* New York, NY: W.W. Norton.

Canary, D. J., Cupach, W. R., & Messman, S. J. (1995). The nature of conflict in close relationships. In D. J. Canary, W. R. Cupach, & S. J. Messman (Eds.), *Relationship conflict* (pp. 1–21). Thousand Oaks, CA: SAGE.

Carver, C. S., & Scheier, M. F. (1990). Origins and functions of positive and negative affect: A control-process view. *Psychological Review, 97*, 19–35. https://doi.org/10.1037/0033-295X.97.1.19

Chen, B., Vansteenkiste, M., Beyers, W., Boone, L., Deci, E. L., Van der Kaap-Deeder, J., et al. (2015). Basic psychological need satisfaction, need frustration, and need strength across four cultures. *Motivation and Emotion, 39*, 216–236. https://doi.org/10.1007/s11031-014-9450-1

Clarkin, J. F., & Miklowitz, D. J. (1997). Marital and family communication difficulties. In T. A. Widiger, A. J. Frances, H. A. Pinkus, R. Ross, M. B. First, & W. Davis (Eds.), *DSM IV sourcebook* (pp. 631–672). Washington, D.C.: American Psychiatric Association Press.

Costa, S., Ntoumanis, N., & Bartholomew, K. J. (2015). Predicting the brighter and darker sides of interpersonal relationships: Does psychological need thwarting matter? *Motivation and Emotion, 39*, 11–24. https://doi.org/10.1007/s11031-014-9427-0

Deci, E. L., & Ryan, R. M. (2000). The "what" and "why" of goal pursuits: Human needs and the self-determination of behavior. *Psychological Inquiry, 11*, 227–268. https://doi.org/10.1207/S15327965PLI1104_01

Drigotas, S. M., & Rusbult, C. E. (1992). Should I stay or should I go? A dependence model of breakups. *Journal of Personality and Social Psychology, 62*, 62–87. https://doi.org/10.1037/0022-3514.62.1.62

Eisler, I. (2005). Editorial. *Journal of Family Therapy, 27*, 307–308. https://doi.org/10.1111/j.1467-6427.2005.0324.x

Eldridge, K. (2009). Conflict patterns. In H. Reis & S. Sprecher (Eds.), *Encyclopedia of human relationships* (pp. 308–311). Thousand Oaks, CA: SAGE.

Fincham, F. D., & Beach, S. R. (1999). Conflict in marriage: Implications for working with couples. *Annual Review of Psychology, 50*, 47–77.

Fincham, F. D., Beach, S. R. H., & Kemp-Fincham, S. I. (1997). Marital quality: A new theoretical perspective. In R. J. Sternberg & M. Hojjat (Eds.), *Satisfaction in close relationships* (pp. 275–304). New York, NY: Guilford.

Frijda, N. H. (1986). *The emotions.* New York, NY: Cambridge University Press.

Gottman, J. M. (1994). *What predicts divorce? The relationship between marital processes and marital outcomes.* Hillsdale, NJ: Lawrence Erlbaum Associates.

Gottman, J. M. (2011). *The science of trust: Emotional attunement for couples.* New York, NY: W. W. Norton.

Greenberg, L., & Goldman, R. N. (2008). *Emotion-focused couples therapy: The dynamics of emotion, love, and power.* Washington, D.C.: American Psychological Association.

Gurman, A. S. (2008). *Clinical handbook of couple therapy* (4th ed.). New York, NY: Guilford Press.

Hadden, B. W., Smith, C. V., & Knee, C. R. (2013). The way I make you feel: How relatedness and compassionate goals promote partner's relationship satisfaction. *The Journal of Positive Psychology, 9*, 155–162. https://doi.org/10.1080/17439760.2013.858272

Haerens, L., Aelterman, N., Vansteenkiste, M., Soenens, B., & Van Petegem, S. (2014). Do perceived autonomy-supportive and controlling teaching relate to physical education students' motivational experiences through unique pathways? Distinguishing between the bright and dark side of motivation. *Psychology of Sport and Exercise, 16*, 26–36. https://doi.org/10.1016/J.PSYCHSPORT.2014.08.013

Hazan, C., & Shaver, P. (1987). Conceptualizing romantic love as an attachment process. *Journal of Personality & Social Psychology, 52,* 511–524. https://doi.org/10.1037/0022-3514.52.3.511

Heavey, C. L., Layne, C., & Christensen, A. (1993). Gender and conflict structure in marital interaction: A replication and extension. *Journal of Consulting and Clinical Psychology, 61,* 16–27. https://doi.org/10.1037/0022-006X.61.1.16

Heine, S. J., Lehman, D. R., Markus, H. R., & Kitayama, S. (1999). Is there a universal need for positive self-regard? *Psychology Review, 106,* 766–794. https://doi.org/10.1037/0033-295x.106.4.766

Jacobson, N. S., & Margolin, G. (1979). *Marital therapy: Strategies based on social learning and behavior exchange principles.* New York, NY: Brunner/Mazel.

Johnson, S. M. (2004). Attachment theory as a guide for healing couple relationships. In W. S. Rholes & J. A. Simpson (Eds.), *Adult attachment: Theory, research, and clinical implications* (pp. 367–387). New York, NY: Guilford Press.

Johnson, S. M. (2009). Attachment and emotionally focused therapy: Perfect partners. In J. Obegi & E. Berant (Eds.), *Attachment theory and research in clinical work with adults* (pp. 410–433). New York, NY: Guilford Press.

Kelley, H. H., & Thibaut, J. E. (1978). *Interpersonal relations: A theory of interdependence.* New York, NY: Wiley.

Keltner, D., & Haidt, J. (1999). Social functions of emotions at four levels of analysis. *Cognition & Emotion, 13,* 505–521. https://doi.org/10.1080/026999399379168

Kenny, D. A., Kashy, D. A., & Cook, W. L. (2006). *Dyadic data analysis.* New York, NY: Guilford Press.

Kluwer, E. S., & Johnson, M. D. (2007). Conflict frequency and relationship quality across the transition to parenthood. *Journal of Marriage and Family, 69,* 1089–1106. https://doi.org/10.1111/j.1741-3737.2007.00434.x

La Guardia, J. G., & Patrick, H. (2008). Self-determination theory as a fundamental theory of close relationships. *Canadian Psychology, 49,* 201–209. https://doi.org/10.1037/a0012760

Le, B., & Agnew, C. R. (2001). Need fulfillment and emotional experience in interdependent romantic relationships. *Journal of Social and Personal Relationships, 18,* 423–440. https://doi.org/10.1177/0265407501183007

Le, B., & Farrell, A. K. (2009). Need fulfilment in relationships. In H. Reis & S. Sprecher (Eds.), *Encyclopedia of human relationships* (pp. 1139–1141). Thousand Oaks, CA: SAGE.

Lebow, J. (2010). What does research have to say about families and psychotherapy? *Clinical Science Insights, 13.* Retrieved from http://www.family-institute.org/research/clinical-science-insights.

Lewandowski, G. W., & Ackerman, R. A. (2006). Something's missing: Need fulfillment and self-expansion as predictors of susceptibility to infidelity. *Journal of Social Psychology, 146,* 389–403. https://doi.org/10.3200/SOCP.146.4.389-403

Lewin, K. (1948). *Resolving social conflicts: Selected papers on group dynamics.* New York, NY: Harper & Row.

Moors, A., Ellsworth, P., Scherer, K. R., & Frijda, N. H. (2013). Appraisal theories of emotion: State of the art and future development. *Emotion Review, 5,* 119–124. https://doi.org/10.1177/1754073912468165

Nef, F., Philippot, P., & Verhofstadt, L. L. (2012). L'approche processuelle en evaluation et intervention cliniques: Une approche psychologique intégrée. *Revue Francophone de Clinique Comportementale et Cognitive, 17,* 4–23. Retrieved from http://rfccc.be/.

Papp, L. M., Kouros, C. D., & Cummings, E. M. (2009). Demand/withdraw patterns in marital conflict in the home. *Personal Relationships, 16,* 285–300. https://doi.org/10.1111/j.1475-6811.2009.01223.x

Patrick, H., Knee, C. R., Canevello, A., & Lonsbary, C. (2007). The role of need fulfillment in relationship functioning and well-being: A self-determination theory perspective. *Journal of Personality and Social Psychology, 92,* 434–457. https://doi.org/10.1037/0022.3514.92.3.434

Paulhus, D. L., & Vazire, S. (2007). The self-report method. In R. W. Robins, R. C. Fraley, & R. F. Krueger (Eds.), *Handbook of research methods in personality psychology* (pp. 224–239). New York, NY: Guilford.

Reis, H. T., Sheldon, K. M., Gable, S. L., Roscoe, J., & Ryan, R. M. (2000). Daily well-being: The role of autonomy, competence, and relatedness. *Personality and Social Psychology Bulletin, 26*, 419–435. https://doi.org/10.1177/0146167200266002

Roseman, I. J. (2011). Emotional behaviors, motivational goals, emotion strategies: Multiple levels of organization integrate variable and consistent responses. *Emotion Review, 3*, 434–443. https://doi.org/10.1177/1754073911410744

Roseman, I. J., Wiest, C., & Swartz, T. S. (1994). Phenomenology, behaviors, and goals differentiate discrete emotions. *Journal of Personality and Social Psychology, 67*, 206–221. https://doi.org/10.1037/0022-3514.67.2.206

Rusbult, C. E., Drigotas, S. M., & Verette, J. (1994). The investment model: A interdependence analysis of commitment processes and relationship maintenance phenomena. In D. J. Canary & L. Stafford (Eds.), *Communication and relational maintenance* (pp. 115–139). San Diego, CA: Academic Press.

Ryan, R. M., & Deci, E. L. (2000). The darker and brighter sides of human existence: Basic psychological needs as a unifying concept. *Psychological Inquiry, 11*, 319–338. https://doi.org/10.1207/S15327965PLI1104_03

Sanford, K. (2007). Hard and soft emotion during conflict: Investigating married couples and other relationships. *Personal Relationships, 14*, 65–90. https://doi.org/10.1111/j.1475-6811.2006.00142.x

Scherer, K. R., & Ellsworth, P. C. (2009). Appraisal theories. In D. Sander & K. R. Scherer (Eds.), *The Oxford companion to emotion and the affective sciences* (pp. 45–49). Oxford, UK: Oxford University Press.

Schwartz, N., Groves, R. M., & Schuman, H. (1998). Survey methods. In D. T. Gilbert, S. Fiske, & G. Lindzey (Eds.), *The handbook of social psychology* (pp. 143–179). Boston, MA: McGraw-Hill.

Smith, C. A., & Lazarus, R. S. (1990). Emotion and adaptation. In L. A. Pervin (Ed.), *Handbook of personality: Theory and research* (pp. 609–637). New York, NY: Guilford Press.

Tong, E. M., Bishop, G. D., Enkelmann, H. C., Diong, S. M., Why, Y. P., Khader, M., & Ang, J. (2009). Emotion and appraisal profiles of the needs for competence and relatedness. *Basic and Applied Social Psychology, 31*, 218–225. https://doi.org/10.1080/01973530903058326

Trépanier, S., Fernet, C., & Austan, S. (2016). Longitudinal relationships between workplace bullying, basic psychological needs, and employee functioning: A simultaneous investigation of psychological need satisfaction and frustration. *European Journal of Work and Organizational Psychology, 25*, 690–706. https://doi.org/10.1080/1359432X.2015.1132200

Uysal, A., Lin, H. L., Knee, C. R., & Bush, A. L. (2012). The association between self- concealment from one's partner and relationship well-being. *Personality and Social Psychology Bulletin, 38*, 39–51. https://doi.org/10.1177/0146167211429331

Vanhee, G., Lemmens, G. M. D., Fontaine, J. R. J., Moors, A., & Verhofstadt, L. L. (in preparation). Need frustration and tendencies to demand or withdraw during conflict: The role of sadness, fear, and anger.

Vanhee, G., Lemmens, G. M. D., Moors, A., Hinnekens, C., & Verhofstadt, L. L. (2018). EFT-C's understanding of couple distress: An overview of evidence from couple and emotion research. *Journal of Family Therapy, 40*(suppl. 1), 24–44.

Vanhee, G., Lemmens, G. M. D., Stas, L., Loeys, T., & Verhofstadt, L. L. (2018). Why are couples fighting? A need frustration perspective on relationship conflict and dissatisfaction. *Journal of Family Therapy, 40*(suppl. 1), 4–23.

Vanhee, G., Lemmens, G. M. D., & Verhofstadt, L. L. (2016). Relationship satisfaction: High need satisfaction or low need frustration? *Social Behavior and Personality, 44*(6), 923–930.

Vanhee, G., Lemmens, G. M. D., & Verhofstadt, L. L. (in preparation). Need frustration and demanding/withdrawing behavior during relationship conflict: An observational study on the role of sadness, fear, and anger.

Vansteenkiste, M., & Ryan, R. M. (2013). On psychological growth and vulnerability: Basic psychological need satisfaction and need frustration as unifying principle. *Journal of Psychotherapy Integration, 23*, 263–280. https://doi.org/10.1037/a0032359

Verhofstadt, L. L., Buysse, A., De Clercq, A., & Goodwin, R. (2005). Emotional arousal and negative affect in marital conflict: The influence of gender, conflict structure, and demand-withdrawal. *European Journal of Social Psychology, 35*, 449–467. https://doi.org/10.1002/ejsp.262

Verstuyf, J., Vansteenkiste, M., Soenens, B., Boone, L., & Mouratidis, A. (2013). Daily ups-and-downs in women's binge eating symptoms: The role of basic psychological needs, general self-control, and emotional eating. *Journal of Social and Clinical Psychology, 32*, 335–361. https://doi.org/10.1521/jscp.2013.32.3.335

Violence in Families: Systemic Practice and Research

Margreet Visser, Justine Van Lawick, Sandra M. Stith, and Chelsea Spencer

Introduction

It is likely that any social worker, couple and family therapist, or counselor will at some point work with a couple who engages in high-conflict behaviors. High-conflict couples can be characterized by destructive communication between partners, fast rates of escalation during conflict, emotional reactivity between partners, unsuccessful conflict resolution skills, as well as the possibility of intimate partner violence in the relationship (Anderson, Palmer, Mutchler, & Baker, 2010). When high conflict and violence occur in a relationship, the partners may choose to work through their differences to end the unhealthy patterns of conflict or violence, or they may choose to break up their partnership, live separately, and get a divorce (if they are married). The purpose of this chapter is to present an overview of two different systemic approaches designed to help couples and families in these situations.

Research has found that couple treatment can be safe and effective in reducing violence and increasing relationship satisfaction for some carefully screened couples (Karakurt, Whiting, Esch, Bolen, & Calabrese, 2016; Stith, McCollum, Amanor-Boadu, & Smith, 2012; Vetere & Cooper, 2001). It is important that systemic clinicians understand the current state of research regarding treating intimate partner violence, as they will work with couples experiencing high conflict and violence who wish to work on their relationship.

M. Visser (✉)
Children's Trauma Center, Kenter Youthcare, Haarlem, The Netherlands

J. Van Lawick
Lorentzhuis, Centrum voor systeemtherapie, opleiding en consultatie, Haarlem, The Netherlands

S. M. Stith · C. Spencer
School of Family Studies and Human Services, Kansas State University, Manhattan, KS, USA

© Springer Nature Switzerland AG 2020
M. Ochs et al. (eds.), *Systemic Research in Individual, Couple, and Family Therapy and Counseling*, European Family Therapy Association Series,
https://doi.org/10.1007/978-3-030-36560-8_17

If high-conflict or violent couples choose to end their relationship, and if these couples have children with one another, it may be especially important for these parents to seek therapeutic services to prevent high conflict after the divorce to aid in their ability to co-parent their children amicably. Even if couples decide to end their relationship after high conflict or violence, a positive co-parenting relationship can aid in the couple's individual levels of adjustment (Katz & Woodin, 2002), as well as the children's adjustment levels after the divorce (Nunes-Costa, Lamela, & Figueiredo, 2009). It is imperative that clinicians have an understanding of working with high-conflict divorcing families, as aiding these parents in positive co-parenting strategies will have positive impacts on all members of the family, especially on the children.

In this chapter, we review the current state of the literature, methodological practices, methodological challenges, future directions for research, and clinical implications derived from our current research on working with violent couples who wish to stay together, as well as high-conflict divorcing parents.

Domestic Violence-Focused Couples Therapy

Brief Introduction

Domestic Violence-Focused Couples Therapy was developed in the United States with funding from the US National Institute of Health. The developers of the program, Stith, McCollum, and Rosen (2011), were faculty in a graduate couple and family therapy program. They had come to believe the prevailing ideology in the United States at that time (the late 1990s) that couples therapy was always dangerous and inappropriate when there had been physical violence in the relationship, yet they continued to find that many couples coming to couples therapy had experienced violence. In fact, other research reported that approximately 36–58% of couples who are seeking therapy services have experienced intimate partner violence in their current relationship (Jose & O'Leary, 2009). They decided to develop and empirically test a systemic treatment program, designed specifically to reduce partner violence, for couples who had experienced partner violence but wanted to stay together.

Inclusion and Exclusion Criteria

When they began to develop the program, Stith, McCollum, and Rosen quickly found that some couples were not appropriate for conjoint treatment. In the first version of their program, they decided to exclude couples with high levels of violence, based on the Revised Conflict Tactics Scale (Straus, Hamby, Boney-McCoy, & Sugarman, 1996). However, they found that some offenders with higher levels of violence (e.g., non-fatal strangulation) took responsibility for their actions and were ready to change and others resorted to power and control to manipulate their partners and took no responsibility for the violence. At the time they were beginning to develop their program, a researcher from the United States, Michael Johnson, developed a typology which they found helpful in screening for appropriateness of conjoint therapy. Johnson reviewed large partner violence data sets and found that there are different types of violence. He suggested that not all high-conflict or violent couples are candidates for couples therapy (such as couples who are experiencing intimate terrorism, which is defined by one partner using violence as a means to exert dominance and control over the other partner; Johnson, 2008). When couples engage in situational violence, which can be described as less severe forms of violence that are often bidirectional in nature, and which are a response to a situation, rather than an attempt to gain power and control over one's partner (Johnson, 2008), therapy may be a suitable option for these couples. Situational violence can be the result of relational conflicts escalating to the point where one or both partners end up acting violently (Stith & McCollum, 2011). Domestic Violence-Focused Couples Therapy was designed for couples experiencing situational violence.

Eventually, the inclusion criteria were identified as couples who voluntarily sought treatment and wanted to try to improve their relationships, and each partner (when screened privately) believed they could speak freely about violence or other struggles in their relationship. Exclusion criteria included couples with large discrepancy on reports of violence they perpetrated and/or received. That is, if a male partner reported on the CTS2 (Straus et al., 1996) that he pushed his wife once, but the female partner reported that her male partner had pushed her, strangled her, raped her, and threatened her with a weapon, the couple would be excluded. We learned over time that if the partner could not safely address the violence perpetrated or received, the treatment could not be delivered safely. We also generally excluded couples in which one partner had serious problems with alcohol or drugs or demonstrated characteristics of intimate terrorism (i.e., extreme levels of power and control).

Overview of Program

During the development phase of the program, some couples were referred after the male partner completed a men's treatment group for batterers, some were referred by protective services because the high levels of conflict put children in the home at risk, and some voluntarily sought help for high conflict. Couples were randomly assigned to a single-couple treatment where co-therapists delivered treatment to one couple or to a multi-couple group where four to six couples participated together with co-therapists. The program consists of 18 weeks, with 6 weeks of primary gender-specific treatment (men only or women only) and 12 weeks of conjoint treatment. Screening is ongoing, where some couples who are screened into the group have been changed to single-couple treatment because of specific issues (e.g., intense grief issues, language challenges where English was not the primary language used at home which led them to struggle with joining in the group).

Each week before the session begins, men and women are separately asked about ongoing physical and psychological violence. Safety is a primary focus throughout the program. At the end of each session, participants (separately) complete a survey about what was helpful and not helpful in the session and about their perception that violence would occur after the session. The therapist reviews the survey before each individual leaves and follows a safety protocol which includes meditation and/or referring to a safe house if either client feels that they are not safe going home together.

Additionally, as part of the research and development of the program, a sub-sample of 16 couples were interviewed 4 times. One female participant, in the research interview said:

> "I mean that's all they emphasized, I mean not all, but that was the major thing they emphasized throughout the program. Feeling safe. Do you feel safe leaving here today? And just feeling safe no matter how heated it got in here." (Lechtenberg et al., 2015, p. 92)
>
>   In some situations where violence is ongoing, couples were referred to a more individualized targeted treatment before beginning conjoint treatment. The overarching model that guides Domestic Violence-Focused Couples Therapy is Solution-Focused Brief Therapy (de Shazer et al., 2007). This therapeutic approach is designed to build on strengths and what is going well. One female participant in her research interview, when asked about the strength focus of the program, said:"You don't want to just have the negatives to focus on and it helps the other person. She [the female therapist] appreciated the things I am doing that are good instead of just the things that are not, that are bad....They always have something positive to say, about what you're doing right or how you're expressing yourself well. I like all that positive, for me, it's the way we all should treat other human beings." (Lechtenberg et al., 2014)

Also, when the intervention was originally developed, the developers planned to exclude participants with problems with alcohol or other drugs, but they quickly learned that the overlap between partner violence was extremely high, so they added a motivational interviewing session (Miller & Rollnick, 2002), based on helping participants decide to make changes in their drinking patterns in week 6 of the program (McCollum, Stith, Strachman Miller, & Ratcliffe, 2011).

The first 6 weeks of the program has a strong psychoeducational component to help couples identify physical, psychological, and sexual violence and to develop their own personal time-out plan, in addition to considering ways that alcohol or other addictive processes might affect their ability to make changes in their relationships. One aspect of the program that is highlighted by many participants as being particularly helpful is the development and use of time-out. One female participant said:

> "We learned time-out. That has been tremendous for us. And when I say timeout to [husband] he now instantly stops...you know...baiting, controlling, fighting, arguing, and it gives me a chance to take a breather, calm down, and we try to get perspective. We're both highly emotional." (Mendez, Horst, Stith, & McCollum, 2014, p. 34)

Another revision of the program based on continued review of systemic research and testing was the inclusion of a strong mindfulness component. Beginning in week 6, before a conjoint session occurs, both partners meet with one co-therapist to practice a mindfulness experience. Mindfulness and other meditation skills have been applied to a variety of mental health problems over the past 20 years, beginning with the development of Mindfulness-Based Stress Reduction (MBSR) by Kabat-Zinn and colleagues (Kabat-Zinn, 1990; Segal, Williams, & Teasdale, 2002). The program developers found that participants often came to the intervention stressed and agitated because of traffic or other events of the day. Beginning the session with a mindfulness activity allowed participants to be more present and more accepting of influence from their partners.

Conjoint Phase of Treatment

After couples complete the first 6 weeks, which are heavily psychoeducational and gender-specific, they begin a 12-week conjoint program. Each session begins with a gender-specific check-in (either one partner with one therapist or the men's group and women's group with separate therapists). In this part of the program, participants are asked to report on what is going well and "what is not going well yet?" Therapists encourage them to share struggles and successes. Next, co-therapists meet for 5 or 10 minutes to determine if the themes in each pre-group meeting are congruent and to determine how the conjoint session will be conducted. For example, if both partners discuss struggles with a child, the session might focus on helping the couple (or couple groups) determines how to reach consensus about a parenting issue. If the co-therapist reports that one partner reports that the other partner has escalated his/her violence but is not comfortable sharing this in a conjoint session, the co-therapists might decide to hold separate sessions. Each partner would be told that they need to work on their own issues for this session. The partner who reported the violence would be helped to activate their safety plan and to increase their feelings of safety. The partner who does not report safety concerns meets with a co-therapist who continues to use a solution-focused approach to determine what he or she needs to do to enhance his or her relationship.

At the end of each conjoint session, therapists meet with each client separately to assess how they feel the session went and to determine what they need to do during the upcoming week to improve their relationship.

Overview of Quantitative Findings

Couples who sought to participate in the program completed a series of quantitative measures before the program began, at the end of treatment, and 6 months after completing treatment. Changes in physical, psychological, and sexual violence were measured by the Revised Conflict Tactics Scale (Straus et al., 1996). We also measured a variety of other relational and individual factors including anger (Novaco Anger Index; Novaco, 1975), differentiation (Differentiation in Couple Relationship Scale; Anderson & Sabatelli, 1992), and relationship satisfaction (Kansas Marital Satisfaction Scale (Schumm, Nichols, Schectman, & Grigsby, 1983).

Both partners in 17 couples who completed single-couple treatment, 26 couples who completed multi-couple group, and 9 couples in the no-treatment comparison group completed all measures. Although the developers of the program planned to randomly assign 1/3 of the couples to the no-treatment group, they found that couples who were randomly assigned to no-treatment sought out treatment in other settings. So, the no-treatment comparison groups were 9 couples who each completed the pre-tests and the follow-up tests but did not choose to (or were not able to) participate in the assigned treatment. Also, the dropout rate was higher in the single-couple treatment condition. Nine more couples completed treatment in the multi-couple treatment program than in the single-couple program. All participants received a financial incentive for completing post-tests. Partners in both treatment conditions reported that their partners were less physically violent after treatment than before, but no significant change occurred in the no-treatment group. Female partners reported that their male partners were less psychologically violent after treatment in both treatment conditions, but no changes were reported in the no-treatment group. Men and women in the multi-couple group reported higher levels of relationship satisfaction, higher levels of self- and partner differentiation, and lower levels of anger. However, only women in the single-couple group reported higher levels of relationship satisfaction. Overall, men reported more positive self-changes in all variables measured in the multi-couple group than in the single-couple treatment. We hypothesized that, at least for men, the opportunity to learn from other men and talk about difficult issues may have been especially beneficial for male clients. For more information on quantitative outcome of research, see Stith, Rosen, McCollum, and Thomsen (2004).

Discussion

Overall, there was a decrease in both physical and psychological violence in couples who participated in either the single-couple format or the multi-couple group format of Domestic Violence-Focused Couples Therapy, whereas there were no statistically significant changes in the couples who received no treatment. At a 2-year follow-up, it was found that all but one participant in the treatment groups reported that their relationship remained violence-free during this period (Stith et al., 2011). These findings strongly suggest that Domestic Violence-Focused Couples Therapy aided in decreasing levels of physical and psychological violence in couples who sought treatment to end the violence in their relationships. There has been a thought that couples that have experienced violence in their relationship are not suitable candidates for therapy, but the success of the Domestic Violence-Focused Couples Therapy suggests that with proper groundwork, there are some couples that can reduce or eliminate the violence in their relationship and then go on to complete traditional couples therapy to improve their relationships.

Couples who had participated in the multi-couple group format of Domestic Violence-Focused Couples Therapy reported higher levels of relationship satisfaction after treatment. Not only did treatment reduce overall levels of violence within the relationship; it also aided in the improvement of relationship satisfaction for these couples. Research has also found that relationship satisfaction has a significant and negative association with intimate partner violence (Stith, Green, Smith, & Ward, 2008). Couples in the group format of the program reported higher levels of self- and partner differentiation. Lower levels of self-differentiation have been found to be associated with intimate partner violence perpetration (Likcani, Stith, Spencer, Webb, & Peterson, 2017). We also found that levels of anger decreased after treatment. Anger and hostility have been linked as risk factors for partner violence (Schweinle & Ickes, 2007). These results suggest that not only did Domestic Violence-Focused Couples Therapy aid in a decrease in overall reports of violence within these relationships but it also aided in increasing individual and relationship changes that could serve as protective factors against violence in the relationship.

Implications

The evaluations conducted throughout the implementation of Domestic Violence-Focused Couples Therapy have aided ongoing changes to treatment and future research. The goal of the research conducted on this treatment was to improve the effectiveness of treatment and further future research endeavors. Some of the important implications to come from this process include:

1. In the beginning of our study, we first decided to exclude couples where there were more severe forms of violence (such as non-fatal strangulation). However, we did find that some of the most successful couples were couples that did engage in these severe forms of violence. This suggests that the perpetrator recognizing the seriousness of their actions and taking responsibility for the severity and seriousness of what they have done may be a stronger indicator of success than the types of violence that have occurred in the relationship.
2. Over the course of treatment, we also found that the honesty surrounding the violence that has occurred in the relationship was also important for success of treatment. If there are large discrepancies between the partners' reports of the types and frequency of violence that has occurred in the relationship, these couples would not be suitable for couple's treatment. This suggests that feeling safe to be open and honesty surrounding discussing the violence is imperative for successful treatment.
3. Throughout treatment, it is also imperative that both partners of the couple feel safe. This includes feeling safe during the session and going home after the session. It is absolutely necessary for clinicians working with couples who have experienced violence in their relationship to continually assess for safety inside and outside of the therapy room.
4. An important suggestion for future research is to include a larger sample, an international sample, and to conduct research designed to identify which aspects

of this program or other systemic programs designed to address partner violence are most important components of effective programs. Future research could also compare DVFCT with treatment-as-usual or batterer intervention program for the offender only.

High-Conflict Families After Divorce

Brief Introduction

Living in divorced families is common (Spruijt & Kormos, 2010) and may be harmful for children (Kelly & Emery, 2003). The average divorce rate in Europe is close to 45% and in the United States about 50% (http://time.com/4575495/divorce-rate-nearly-40-year-low/). International studies indicated that between 8% and 12% of parents continue to be involved in serious conflicts, even 2–3 years after divorce (Kelly & Emery, 2003). In the Netherlands, such data have not yet been collected. The most devastating effect of divorce for children's well-being and adjustment is to be exposed to parental conflict (Amato, 2001; Kelly & Emery, 2003), and the destructiveness of parental conflict increases negative outcomes for the children (Hetherington, 2006; Vandewater & Lansford, 1998). Working with patterns of conflict is part of systemic therapy from the beginning. This is more complicated when parents have a high-conflict divorce, most parents do not want to come together, and stress is extremely high during sessions.

"No Kids in the Middle," which takes a multi-family approach, was developed by Van Lawick and Visser (2015a, 2015b). The program is inspired by Multiple Family Therapy (Asen & Scholz, 2010) and is also trauma informed because the involved children and also the parents often have trauma symptoms. The program was designed to reduce destructive parental conflicts in high-conflict divorce (HCD) families and their damaging influence on children. Parent-Focused Therapy aimed to decrease destructive conflicts, or to make the conflicts more constructive, is needed, to minimize the negative effects of conflicts on children's well-being. Research shows that conflict intensity and escalation are related to (1) negative attributions (Fincham & Bradbury, 1987) (the tendency to make the other parent responsible for all negative situations and expressions of intense negative emotions) (Anderson et al., 2010), (2) parents' lack of acceptance of and/or lack of adjustment to the divorce, (3) perceived social network disapproval of the ongoing co-parenting relationship (Visser et al., 2017), and (4) children's lack of well-being and psychosocial functioning (Amato, 2001; Nunes-Costa et al., 2009).

The ongoing escalation of destructive conflicts between parents suggests that to increase children's well-being, a program was needed that encompasses parental intervention components, and a broader systemic view, in addition to psychoeducation. The developers of this intervention believe that parents need to be stimulated to change their negative attributions toward each other, express less negative emotions, and accept and adjust to the divorce, so that their destructive parental conflicts may decrease. Furthermore, they believe that the social network members have to be involved in the intervention. Such changes may augment the quality of the co-parenting relationship, which, in turn, may have a positive effect on children's well-being. For HCD families, some psychoeducational programs are available, but in an overview of these programs, no published evaluations of the effectiveness of these programs were found (Goodman, Bonds, Sandler, & Braver, 2004). Therefore, Van Lawick and Visser (2015a) sought not only to develop an intervention based on previous research but to test effectiveness of their program and adapt the program based on research findings.

"No Kids in the Middle" takes a multi-family approach and consists of two intake sessions, a network information session, and eight parent treatment sessions and parallel child sessions (sessions of 2 hours). Organizing the children's group in parallel to the parent group has the advantage that the children are continuously "present" in the parent group which serves as a reminder of the main aim for parents, namely, the safety and well-being of the children. At the same time, children are encouraged to share their experiences and to strengthen each other by mutual recognition and advice about handling the stress between parents.

In the intervention, space is made for peer contact between children experiencing HCD, children are given a voice by letting them express how they feel about being a child of parents in conflict, and children are asked to talk about their good experiences with their parents. Parents are asked to participate in experiential exercises that involve empathizing with the position of children and are asked to write a new narrative about the separation in which the co-parent is not demonized, focusing on own behavior instead of the behavior of the other, and parents are encourage to help each other in finding less destructive ways of conflict resolution and formulating what each parent wishes for the children in the future.

The intervention explicitly works to change parents' attributions and feelings for each other's behavior to encourage a more differentiated and nuanced perception, more empathy, acceptance, and perspective-taking of parents for each other. High-conflict couples often show an inability to listen to or empathize with each other in a "psychological climate of endless misery" (Gottman, 1994, p. 47). Rather, they often experience intense feelings of contempt, resentment, and anger and are caught up in a vicious cycle of arguments and competitions (e.g., who is right, proving the other wrong). The goal of "No Kids in the Middle" is not necessarily to achieve reconciliation between parents but to increase parents' acceptance of each other's differences and ways of living and further understanding for each other's circumstances and points of view. Additionally, the program aims to help parents to recognize habituated conflicts and triggers that are heavily loaded with negative affect (e.g., when he smiles like that, he wants to hurt me; he looks at his phone to tell me he doesn't care), which often escalate into full-blown arguments. By identifying these cognitive, emotional, and behavioral patterns and habits, the intervention aims to provide parents with strategies that facilitate stress reduction, de-escalation, and softening of conflict.

The social network members of both parents are also involved in "No Kids in the Middle" by participating in an informational evening at the start of the intervention, by giving parents homework to do with their social network in-between all sessions, and by inviting the network to participate in the evaluation of the treatment (Van Lawick & Visser, 2015a). Central in this intervention is the engagement of therapists, parents and children, and the social networks of both parents in an open dialogue (Van Lawick & Visser, 2015b).

In the context of this chapter, we will summarize the main results of the research project on No Kids in the Middle (Schoemaker, De Kruijff, Visser, Van Lawick, & Finkenauer, 2017). First, we will summarize the findings regarding the children before the intervention focusing on what affected them most in the conflicts and stress between parents. Second, we will summarize the main results of the evaluation study of No Kids in the Middle for parents and children. Third, we will discuss the results and describe the clinical implications and how we have adjusted No Kids in the Middle on the basis of the empirical evidence.

How HCD Affects Children

When 8-year-old Lisa was asked where she lived, she answered: "5 days with mum, in the weekend I am with dad, and if I was two times with dad, I am one weekend with mum."

This illustrates the complicated living arrangements for the children. We wanted to hear their own experiences about being a child of divorced parents that are in high conflict.

So, we asked 142 children (75 boys), coming from 81 families, to fill out a questionnaire about their worries. We used three different questionnaires for the different ages (6–7, 8–11, and 12–18 years). We formulated nine questions about the adaptation of children after the divorce and three questions related to how children experience the conflicts of the parents, and in what situations the conflicts burdened them. We also asked the children if they were worried about their family and with whom they shared their worries.

How do you experience the situation at home? The majority of children mentioned differences in rules in the two households, so that the adaptation when switching from home burdened them (48% of the boys and 79% of the girls), that the stuff that they need for school or sports still are with the other parent (51%), and that parents often complain about bringing children's stuff back and forth (38%). One third of the children had the feeling that they had to choose one of the parents.

Conflicts between parents and children's worries? A majority of children mentioned that they were present when the parents had conflicts (62%) and that parents talked badly about each other (46% mother talking badly about father and 62% father talking badly about mother). More than two thirds of the children (68%) reported concerns about their family.

In which contexts do children feel burdened by the divorce? About half of the children reported that they suffered at home from the divorce, 43% reported difficulties in concentrating at school (especially children 12 years and older), one third also had difficulties during their leisure time (e.g., sports), and a quarter had difficulties in their relationship with grandparents and friends. Some children also reported that they did not suffer from the divorce.

Whom do the children share their worries with? More than half of the children (63%) shared their worries with their mother and best friend (61%). Forty percent also talked with their father about their worries. Also 40% reported that it was helpful to share with teachers. On average, the children discussed their concerns and worries with three to four people, varying from zero to ten persons.

Evaluation of No Kids in the Middle

The evaluation comprised a multicenter study in the Netherlands and Belgium. In this study, we compared questionnaires filled out by parents and children, respectively, at the beginning of the intervention (T1) with questionnaires at the end of the intervention, approximately 12 weeks later (T2). We predicted that, as compared to the beginning of the intervention, parents who participated in the intervention No Kids in the Middle would (a) have less destructive conflicts and become more constructive, (b) make less negative attributions and express less negative emotions toward each other, (c) show more acceptance and be more adjusted after the divorce, and (d) perceive less social network disapproval of the divorce after the intervention. We predicted that, as compared to the beginning of the intervention, children, who participated with their parents in the intervention No Kids in the Middle, would show a higher level of well-being at the end of the intervention.

Participants were 110 parents (54 fathers) and 122 children. The families were referred for intervention at 16 different family treatment centers in the Netherlands and Belgium, because the well-being of their children was threatened by parents' long-lasting conflicts, aggression, and anger surrounding parental decisions. To test changes over time, we used a repeated analysis of variance with time (T1 and T2) as the within-subject factor.

Changes Reported by Parents

Parents reported lower levels of frequency and intensity of problems related to parenting and remaining conflicts became more constructive after completing treatment. No differences between men and women were found. We found no changes in negative attributions, negative feelings, and appreciation toward the other parent after treatment. We did find that parents were more forgiving toward each other and tended to trust each other more. Before the start of the treatment, parents reported a good adjustment to the divorce, we found no change for this variable, but after the intervention, parents accepted the separation more. We also did not find changes in parents' perceived disapproval of the divorce by the social network members.

Changes Reported by Children

Although they were only asked one question about parental conflict, children reported that parents were having less conflict in their presence after treatment. This underlines the results found for the parents. Children described the relationship with both parents as good, as well at T1 as at T2, and the quality did not change. There was a slight tendency that the relationship with mother was becoming better after the intervention. Also, children reported a high quality of life, and they felt that their fundamental needs were met by both parents. These scores did not change over time. However, almost half of the children were at risk for a posttraumatic stress disorder. The posttraumatic stress symptoms were decreased on T2, but not significantly.

Discussion

We found that the conflicts between the parents were less frequent and more constructive after participation in the intervention No Kids in the Middle. Even more important, children reported that parents were having fewer conflicts in their presence. Additionally, we found that parents still disapproved of the other parent and felt good about their own parental adjustment. Also, we found that parents showed more forgiveness toward each other, a tendency to trust each other more, and more acceptance of the divorce after the intervention. These results underline the importance of focusing on positive processes in the intervention. Providers reported additionally that even though parents may not have liked the other parent, parents were more accepting of the differences in their parenting and that they seemed to believe that the other parent was a "good enough" parent for their children. Previous research indicated that couples who have between three and five times more positive than negative interactions had high-quality relationships (Baumeister, Bratslavsky, Finkenauer, & Vohs, 2001; Gottman, 1998). Thus, it appears that our intervention may lead to higher-quality co-parenting relationships. However, because we did not ask about the parent-child relationship changes, we know surprisingly little about the spillover of these positive processes into the parent-child relationship.

We did not find any change in the extent to which parents perceived that their social network disapproved of the other parent. Visser et al. (2017) found that higher levels of perceived social network disapproval were significantly related to more co-parenting conflicts, explained by parents' lower likelihood of forgiving each other. Although No Kids in the Middle involves the social networks of both parents in the intervention, we did not study if the friends and families changed their cognitions and feelings toward the divorce, both parents, or to the co-parenting relationship. Future research, especially qualitative research in which parents, children, and social network members are interviewed about their perception on systemic relationships and possible changes, will be important to further our understanding of the impact of this program and to improve the intervention. HCD families are a difficult group to study, and, as is true with all real-world situations, complexity exists within all levels of the social network and reciprocal influences.

Striking were the results that the children themselves reported a high level of well-being and good relationships with both father and mother, although all families were referred for the intervention because the development and mental health of the children were seriously threatened. However, at the same time, half of the children were at risk for a posttraumatic stress disorder. There are two possible explanations for these results. First, the children told us at the beginning of the intervention that they were worried about their families, they were exposed to parental conflicts, they found it difficult to switch between homes and rules, they found it difficult when one parent talked badly about the other parent, and they had a feeling they had to choose between parents. We have called these problems the "in-between space" for children, that is, the space where children in high-conflict divorces seem to find themselves caught in the middle between their parents. We only asked them about the exposure to parental conflicts, which decreased after the intervention. Unfortunately, we did not ask all the questions concerning the "in-between space" after the intervention. So, it may be that children feel good with both parents, but the stress they experience is related to the "in-between space." Second, we asked children to fill out questionnaires during the first session of the intervention, when parents were also present for treatment. In this way, we hoped children would not be influenced by one parent, as they may have been, if only one of them were present at home. However, we may have underestimated how hopeful the situation may have been for the children to be in the same building with both parents and knowing that parents were motivated to make the situation better for the children. This may have influenced the results for the children positively. Nevertheless, it is also possible that the results reflect children's actual responses. Children in high-conflict divorced families may be in a process of parentification (Hetherington & Elmore, 2003). They may have learned to adjust to their parents' divorce situation and are resilient in acting in the service of family well-being and not to reflect on their own experiences. Their own experiences seem to be mainly affected negatively when they are dependent on or confronted with BOTH parents (e.g., vacation organization, school, performances, and graduation ceremony). Although moderate levels of parentification may contribute to greater early maturity and resilience among children in divorced families, excessive levels of parentification are associated with behavior problems, low self-esteem, and low social competence. Later in life, parentificated children may evaluate toward a greater consideration for oneself and a repositioning within the families (Van Parys, Bonnewyn, Hooghe, De Mol, & Rober, 2015). So, children may have a good quality of life with both parents, and may experience a good relationship with both parents at this moment, but may develop all kinds of problems later in life associated with being too responsible and emotionally available for their parents during childhood.

The number of children who were at high risk for a posttraumatic stress disorder was as high as in a sample of children exposed to child abuse (Alisic et al., 2014). The number of children at risk for PTSD was decreased after the intervention, but this was not a significant result. This result may be explained that there was also a group of children who were not at risk for PTSD before the intervention, but they were after the intervention. It is known that some children experience PTSD in a delayed reaction when the context becomes less stressful (Andrews, Brewin, Philpott, & Stewart, 2007).

Clinical Implications

In our project, No Kids in the Middle, the evaluation research influenced our practice, and the clinical practice leads to new questions for research. We hope this will be an ongoing process that helps us to improve both practice and research continuously. The research outcomes described in this chapter have implications for our intervention and for other potential interventions for families experiencing HCD.

The findings provided support for the overall intervention, and future research should be conducted to determine which components might be most crucial in leading to which outcomes. In addition, the research also helped us to focus more on some crucial issues in treatment:

1. We used results from our conversations with parents and children to guide attention to the space in between the parents and their networks.
2. As a result of the children's reports, the program of the children's group is more structured in relation to the issues and worries children have mentioned.
3. We have also learned from the children about their resilience and have adapted the program to encourage children to exchange experiences about how to handle the stress.
4. As we began to realize the importance of reducing stress between parents, we began to focus more on stimulating positive processes where parents can accept the differences between them and forgive each other. To create a more positive context, we now start the session with a short warming-up activity with parents and children together. This creates a warm and soft start of each session.
5. The outcome that parents can forgive each other better after the intervention but do not necessarily like each other more helped us to understand that many divorced parents caught in high-conflict processes do differ in many essential ways, about many issues. To ask them to be a better team can confront them more with the differences and can make conflicts worse. To accept the divorce and the differences and let go of the need to change the other can lower the stress. So we focus more on acceptance of the differences and the divorce.
6. The research showed how important the role of the network is in the process of forgiving. So we reach out to the network more.

The clinical experiences will raise new research questions, qualitative and quantitative. We hope to find resources to go on with this ongoing developmental process.

Conclusion

In this chapter, we have discussed two treatment modalities clinicians may use when working with high-conflict couples, as well as the research supporting the effectiveness of these treatments. There are times where clinicians will work with couples where there is violence within the intimate relationship, and these couples wish to stay together. Domestic Violence-Focused Couples Therapy is a resource for helping these couples end the violence in their relationship. However, if these couples make the choice to end their partnership, it still may be useful for clinicians to work with these couples after the dissolution of their relationship, especially if they have children with one another. No Kids in the Middle is a resource for helping these individuals to find a child-focused way of parenting with one another. It is important to note that the research conducted on these programs has guided, and continues to guide, the development of these programs. Future research may look into integrating these two modalities of treatment for couples experiencing violence in their relationships but also having children together.

References

Alisic, E., Zalta, A. K., Van Wesel, F., Larsen, S. E., Hafstad, G. S., Hassanpour, K., & Smid, G. E. (2014). Rates of post-traumatic stress disorder in trauma-exposed children and adolescents: Meta-analysis. *British Journal of Psychiatry, 204*(5), 335–340.

Amato, P. R. (2001). Children of divorce in the 1990s: An update of the Amato and Keith (1991) meta-analysis. *Journal of Family Psychology, 15*, 355–370.

Anderson, S. A., Palmer, K. L., Mutchler, M. S., & Baker, L. K. (2010). Defining high conflict. *American Journal of Family Therapy, 39*(1), 11–27.

Anderson, S. R., & Sabatelli, R. M. (1992). The differentiation in the family systems scale (DIFS). *American Journal of Family Therapy, 20*, 77–89.

Andrews, B., Brewin, C. R., Philpott, R., & Stewart, L. (2007). Delayed-onset posttraumatic stress disorder: A systematic review of the evidence. *American Journal of Psychiatry, 164*(9), 1319–1326.

Asen, E., & Scholz, M. (2010). *Multi-family therapy. Concepts and techniques.* Oxford, UK: Taylor and Francis.

Baumeister, R. F., Bratslavsky, E., Finkenauer, C., & Vohs, K. D. (2001). Bad is stronger than good. *Review of General Psychology, 5*(4), 323–370.

Fincham, E. D., & Bradbury, T. N. (1987). Cognitive processes and conflict in close relationships: An attribution-efficacy model. *Journal of Personality and Social Psychology, 53*(6), 1106–1118.

Goodman, M., Bonds, D., Sandler, I., & Braver, S. (2004). Parent psychoeducational programs and reducing the negative effects of interparental conflict following divorce. *Family Court Review, 42*(2), 263–279. https://doi.org/10.1111/j.174-1617.2004.tb00648.x

Gottman, J. M. (1994). Why marriages fail. *Family Therapy Networker, 18*(1), 41–48.

Gottman, J. M. (1998). Psychology and the study of marital processes. *Annual Review of Psychology, 49*(1), 169–197.

Hetherington, E. M. (2006). The influence of conflict, marital problem solving and parenting on children's adjustment in nondivorced, divorced and remarried families. In A. Clarke-Stewart & J. Dunn (Eds.), *Families count: Effects on child and adolescent development. The Jacobs Foundation series on adolescence* (pp. 203–237). New York: Cambridge University Press.

Hetherington, E. M., & Elmore, A. M. (2003). Risk and resilience in children coping with their parents' divorce and remarriage. In S. S. Luthar (Ed.), *Resilience and vulnerability. Adaptation in the context of childhood adversities*. Cambridge, UK: Cambridge University Press.

Johnson, M. P. (2008). *A typology of domestic violence: Intimate terrorism, violent resistance, and situational couple violence*. Lebanon, NH: Northeastern Press.

Jose, A., & O'Leary, K. D. (2009). Prevalence of partner aggression in representative and clinic samples. In K. D. O'Leary & E. M. Woodin (Eds.), *Psychological and physical aggression in couples: Causes and interventions* (pp. 15–35). Washington, DC: American Psychological Association.

Kabat-Zinn, J. (1990). *Full catastrophe living: Using the wisdom of your body and mind to face stress, pain and illness*. New York: Delacorte.

Karakurt, G., Whiting, K., Esch, C. V., Bolen, S. D., & Calabrese, J. R. (2016). Couples therapy for intimate partner violence: A systematic review and meta-analysis. *Journal of Marital and Family Therapy, 42*(4), 567–583.

Katz, I. F., & Woodin, E. M. (2002). Hostility, hostile detachment, and conflict engagement in marriages: Effects on child and family functioning. *Child Development, 73*, 636–651.

Kelly, J. B., & Emery, R. E. (2003). Children's adjustment following divorce: Risk and resilience perspectives. *Family Relations, 52*(4), 352–362. https://doi.org/10.1111/j.1741-3729.2003.00352

Lechtenberg, M., Stith, S., Horst, K., Mendez, M., Minner, J., Dominguez, M., … McCollum, E. (2015). Gender differences in experiences with couples treatment for IPV. *Contemporary Family Therapy, 37*(2), 89–100.

Lechtenberg, M., Stith, S., Horst, K., Mendez, M., Minner, J., Dominguez, M. & McCollum, E. (2014). Gender Differences in Experiences with Couples Treatment for IPV. Contemporary Family Therapy, 1–12.

Likcani, A., Stith, S. M., Spencer, C., Webb, F., & Peterson, F. R. (2017). Differentiation and intimate partner violence. *American Journal of Family Therapy, 45*(5), 235–249. https://doi.org/1 0.1080/01926187.2017.1365663

McCollum, E. E., Stith, S. M., Strachman Miller, M., & Ratcliffe, G. C. (2011). Including a brief substance abuse motivational intervention in a couples treatment program for intimate partner violence. *Journal of Family Psychotherapy, 22*, 216–231.

Mendez, M., Horst, K., Stith, S. M., & McCollum, E. E. (2014). Couples treatment for intimate partner violence: Clients' reports of changes during therapy. *Partner Abuse, 5*, 21–40.

Miller, W. R., & Rollnick, S. (2002). *Motivational interviewing: Preparing people for change* (2nd ed.). New York: Guilford.

Novaco, R. W. (1975). Anger control: *The development and evaluation of an experimental treatment*. Lexington.

Nunes-Costa, R. A., Lamela, D. J., & Figueiredo, B. F. (2009). Psychosocial adjustment and physical health in children of divorce. *Jornal de Pediatria, 85*(5), 385–396.

Schoemaker, K., de Kruijff, A., Visser, M., van Lawick, J., & Finkenauer, C. (2017). *Vechtscheidingen. Beleving en ervaringen van ouders en Kinderen en verandering na Kinderen uit de Knel. Onderzoeksrapport*. Academische Werkplaats aanpak Kindermishandeling: Amsterdam.

Schumm, W. R., Nichols, C. W., Schectman, K. L., & Grigsby, C. C. (1983). Characteristics of the Kansas marital satisfaction scale by a sample of 84 married mothers. *Psychological Reports, 53*, 567–572.

Schweinle, W. E., & Ickes, W. (2007). The role of men's critical/rejecting over attribution bias, affect, and attentional disengagement in marital aggression. *Journal of Social and Clinical Psychology, 26*, 173–198.

Segal, Z. V., Williams, J. M. G., & Teasdale, J. D. (2002). *Mindfulness-based cognitive therapy for depression: A new approach to preventing relapse*. New York: Guilford Press.

de Shazer, S., Dolan, Y., Korman, H., McCollum, E., Trepper, T., & Berg, I. K. (2007). *Haworth brief therapy series. More than miracles: The state of the art of solution-focused brief therapy*. Haworth Press.

Spruijt, E., & Kormos, H. (2010). *Handboek scheiden en de kinderen [Handbook of divorce and the children]*. Houten, The Netherlands: Bohn Stafleu van Loghum.

Stith, S. M., Green, N. M., Smith, D. B., & Ward, D. B. (2008). Marital satisfaction and marital discord as risk markers for intimate partner violence: A meta-analytic review. *Journal of Family Violence, 23*(3), 149–160.

Stith, S. M., McCollum, E., Amanor-Boadu, Y., & Smith, D. (2012). Systemic perspectives on intimate partner violence treatment. *Journal of Marital and Family Therapy, 38*(1), 220–240. https://doi.org/10.1111/j.1752.0606.2011.00245.x

Stith, S. M., McCollum, E. E., & Rosen, K. H. (2011). *Couples treatment for domestic violence: Finding safe solutions*. Washington, DC: American Psychological Association.

Stith, S. M., & McCollum, E. E. (2011). Conjoint treatment of couples who have experienced intimate partner violence. *Aggression and Violent Behavior, 16*(4), 312–318.

Stith, S. M., Rosen, K. H., McCollum, E. E., & Thomsen, C. J. (2004). Treating intimate partner violence within intact couple relationships: Outcomes of multi-couple versus individual couple therapy. *Journal of Marital and Family Therapy, 30*(3), 305–318.

Straus, M. A., Hamby, S. L., Boney-McCoy, S., & Sugarman, D. B. (1996). The revised conflict tactics scales (CTS2): Development and preliminary psychometric data. *Journal of Family Issues, 17*, 283–316.

Van Lawick, J., & Visser, M. (2015a). *Kinderen uit de Knel. Een interventie voor gezinnen verwikkeld in een vechtscheiding*. Amsterdam: SWP.

Van Lawick, J., & Visser, M. (2015b). No kids in the middle: Dialogical and creative work with parents and children in the context of high conflict divorces. *Australian and New Zealand Journal of Family Therapy, 36*(1), 33–50.

Van Parys, H., Bonnewyn, A., Hooghe, A., De Mol, J., & Rober, P. (2015). Toward understanding the child's experience in the process of parentification: Young adults' reflections on growing up with a depressed parent. *Journal of Marital and Family Therapy, 42*(4), 522–536. https://doi.org/10.1111/jmft.12087

Vandewater, E. A., & Lansford, J. E. (1998). Influences of family structure and parental conflict on children's well-being. *Family Relations, 47*, 323–330. https://doi.org/10.2307/585263

Vetere, A., & Cooper, J. (2001). Working systemically with family violence: Risk, responsibility and collaboration. *Journal of Family Therapy, 23*, 378–396.

Visser, M., Finkenauer, C., Schoemaker, K., Kluwer, E., van der Rijken, R., van Lawick, J., … Lamers-Winkelman, F. (2017). I'll never forgive you: High conflict divorce, social network, and co-parenting conflicts. *Journal of Child and Family Studies, 26*, 1–12.

Part IV
Improving Therapy Quality by Feedback: Training and Publication

Research-Informed Practice of Systemic Therapy

Alan Carr, Martin Pinquart, and Markus W. Haun

Introduction

This chapter presents a summary of important research results and the implications of these for research-informed practice of systemic therapy. It addresses the following key questions:

- How effective is systemic therapy in general?
- What sorts of systemic therapy work best for specific sorts of clinical problems?
- Is systemic therapy cost-effective?
- What common processes characterize effective systemic therapy?
- What are the potential negative effects of systemic therapy?

How Effective Is Systemic Therapy?

Systemic therapy can be defined as a form of psychotherapy that treats a wide range of psychosocial problems and psychiatric disorders within the context of the social systems the individuals live in and focuses on the interpersonal relations and

A. Carr
School of Psychology, University College Dublin, and Clanwilliam Institute Dublin, Dublin, Ireland

M. Pinquart
Department of Psychology, Philipps University, Marburg, Germany

M. W. Haun (✉)
Department of General Internal Medicine and Psychosomatics, Heidelberg University, Heidelberg, Germany
e-mail: markus.haun@med.uni-heidelberg.de

© Springer Nature Switzerland AG 2020
M. Ochs et al. (eds.), *Systemic Research in Individual, Couple, and Family Therapy and Counseling*, European Family Therapy Association Series,
https://doi.org/10.1007/978-3-030-36560-8_18

interactions, social constructions of realities, and recursive causality between symptoms and interactions (Retzlaff, von Sydow, Beher, Haun, & Schweitzer, 2013; von Sydow, Beher, Schweitzer, Retzlaff, 2010; von Sydow, Retzlaff, Beher, Haun, & Schweitzer, 2013). A main goal of systemic therapy is to mobilize the strengths of interpersonal relations and to change the conditions of the social system that contributed to the development and maintenance of the symptoms of the individual (Stratton, 2016). Systemic approaches are resource-oriented and solution-focused, and the therapy takes place in a short time frame (e.g. de Shazer & Dolan, 2007). The term systemic therapy overlaps with the terms couple therapy and family therapy because systemic therapy is often conducted with couples or families. However, systemic therapy can, in principle, also be offered as individual therapy, group therapy, or multifamily group therapy (e.g. Lemmens, Eisler, Buysse, Heene, & Demyttenaere, 2009), and some couple and family therapies are grounded in psychodynamic, cognitive-behavioural, or other theories rather than in a primary systemic orientation (Shadish & Baldwin, 2003).

The first comprehensive reviews of the evidence base for couple and family therapy date back to the 1970s (e.g. Gurman & Kniskern, 1978a, 1978b) and the earliest meta-analyses to the 1980s and early 1990s (Hazelrigg, Cooper, & Borduin, 1987; Markus, Lange, & Pettigrew, 1990; Shadish et al., 1993). These showed conclusively that couple and family therapy worked for a range of problems and was as effective or in some cases more effective than individual therapy. The late William Shadish conducted the most influential early meta-analyses of couple and family therapy (e.g. Shadish & Baldwin, 2003; Shadish et al., 1993). In his ground-breaking first major meta-analysis of 163 trials of couple and family therapy involving thousands of cases, he concluded that the average treated case fared better after treatment than 73% of cases in control groups, and this is equivalent to a treatment success rate of 65% (Shadish et al., 1993). Shadish and Baldwin (2003) reviewed 20 meta-analyses of marital and family interventions for a wide range of child- and adult-focused problems. The average effect size across all meta-analyses was $d = 0.65$ standard deviation units after therapy and $d = 0.52$ at 6–12 months of follow-up. These results show that, overall, the average treated family fared better after therapy and at follow-up. However, these meta-analyses included marital and family interventions that were based on very different approaches, including cognitive-behavioural therapy and psychodynamic therapy. Shadish et al. (1993) even reported that, when compared against an untreated control condition, the included 14 systemic intervention studies produced smaller improvements at post-test (of $d = 0.28$) than couple and family therapy in general ($d = 0.51$).

Since 1993, the number of controlled studies on the effects of systemic therapy has increased considerably. This is reflected in reviews by Retzlaff, von Sydow, and colleagues in Germany (Retzlaff et al., 2013; von Sydow et al., 2010, 2013), Stratton (2016) in the UK, and contributors to special issues of the *Journal of Marital and Family Therapy* on systemic therapy effectiveness in the USA (Pinsof & Wynne, 1995; Sprenkle, 2002, 2012). Carr has documented the growing evidence base for family therapy in general and systemic family therapy in particular in a pair of review papers. These have been updated three times since they were first published in 2000 (Carr, 2000a, 2000b, 2009a, 2009b, 2014a, 2014b, 2018a, 2018b).

Two recent meta-analyses examined the effects of systemic therapy on adults (Pinquart, Oslejsek, & Teubert, 2016) as well as children and adolescents (Riedinger, Pinquart, & Teubert, 2017). Other meta-analyses addressed the effects of individual systemic approaches, such as brief strategic family therapy (BSFT; Baldwin, Christian, Berkeljon, Shadish, & Bean, 2012; Lindström et al., 2013), multidimensional family therapy (MDFT; Baldwin et al., 2012; Filges, Andersen, & Jørgensen, 2018; van der Pol et al., 2017), multisystemic therapy (MST; Baldwin et al., 2012; Curtis, Ronan, & Borduin, 2004; Littell, Campbell, Green, & Toews, 2005; van der Stouwe, Asscher, Stams, Deković, & van der Laan, 2014), and solution-focused brief therapy (SFBT; Kim, 2008; Kim et al., 2015; Schmit, Schmit, & Lenz, 2016; Stams, Dekovic, Buist, & de Vries, 2006; Zhang, Franklin, Currin-McCulloch, Park, & Kim, 2018). We first summarize the updated results of the two broad meta-analyses that combined results from randomized controlled trials across different systemic approaches. Both meta-analyses included only studies with participants being diagnosed with a mental disorder according to the International Classification of Diseases (ICD) or the *Diagnostic and Statistical Manual of Mental Disorders* (DSM) or with participants likely fulfilling this criterion (e.g. scores above the clinical cut-off in a screening instrument for mental disorders). Change in the core symptoms of the disorder was the assessed outcome variable.

The meta-analysis by Riedinger et al. (2017) included 59 papers from 56 randomized controlled trials (RCTs) with children and adolescents that were published between 1973 and 2014. As an additional 6 papers have become available after submission of this meta-analysis (Agras et al., 2014; Dakof et al., 2015; Fonagy et al., 2018; Humayun, et al., 2017; Löfholm, Olsson, Sundell, & Hansson, 2009; Santisteban et al., 2015), we present updated computations based on 65 papers. When compared against an untreated control group, young people treated with systemic therapy showed moderate improvements of their core symptoms at post-test ($d = 0.59$) and small improvements at follow-up about 11 months after completion of the treatment ($d = 0.27$). When compared against an active alternative treatment, young people treated with systemic therapy showed, on average, significantly stronger improvements of core symptoms at post-test ($d = 0.30$) and follow-up ($d = 0.25$). Sufficient numbers of studies for illness-specific analyses were only available for studies that compared systemic therapy with an alternative treatment. As shown in Fig. 1, young people with conduct disorders/oppositional defiant disorders (CD/ODD; $d = 0.27$) and substance use disorders (SUD; $d = 0.33$) showed stronger improvements of their symptoms at post-test after systemic therapy. At follow-up, young people with CD/ODD ($d = 0.29$), depression ($d = 0.41$), SUD ($d = 0.22$), and eating disorders ($d = 0.30$) showed a stronger decline of core symptoms after systemic treatment than after an alternative treatment. The treatment effects did not vary by child age, but studies were lacking on families with younger children (<5 years). Higher numbers of sessions were associated with stronger improvements at follow-up.

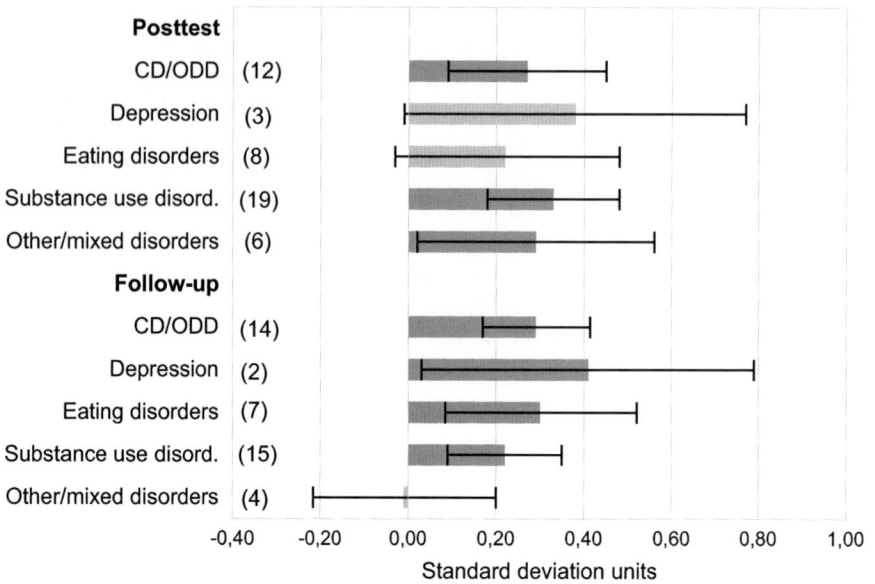

Fig. 1 Weighted mean improvements of symptoms of children and adolescents after receipt of systemic therapy compared to an alternative treatment. Note: Numbers in brackets represent the number of included studies. Error bars show the 95% confidence interval (CI) of the mean effect size. Dark bars indicate statistically significant effects

The meta-analysis by Pinquart et al. (2016) included 45 papers that described results of 37 independent RCTs on systemic therapy with adults published up to 2014. As an additional 5 papers became available in an updated electronic search (Castelnuovo, Manzoni, Villa, Cesa, & Molinari, 2011; Dashtizadeh, Sajedi, Nazari, Davarniya, & Shakaram, 2015; Han et al., 2015; Kim, Brook, & Akin, 2018; Zhang, Zhang, Song, Han, & Xu, 2017), we present an updated meta-analysis of the results from 50 papers. Separate analyses were computed for three different study designs. When compared with patients who did not receive an active treatment, patients treated with systemic therapy showed stronger improvements of their core symptoms at post-test ($d = 0.68$) and follow-up ($d = 0.52$). When compared against an alternative psychological treatment, patients treated with systemic therapy showed, on average, stronger improvements of their core symptoms at post-test ($d = 0.22$), although between-group differences were not statistically significant at follow-up ($d = 0.14$). Finally, patients who received systemic therapy plus psychotropic drugs showed stronger improvements at post-test ($d = 0.77$) and follow-up ($d = 0.87$) than those treated with psychotropic drugs alone. As effect sizes did not differ between studies comparing systemic therapy against a no-treatment control condition and systemic therapy plus medication against medication, both groups of studies were combined in the illness-specific analyses. Analyses indicated that patients who received systemic therapy showed stronger improvements of their symptoms at post-test in the case of eating disorders ($d = 1.43$), depression ($d = 0.47$), obsessive-

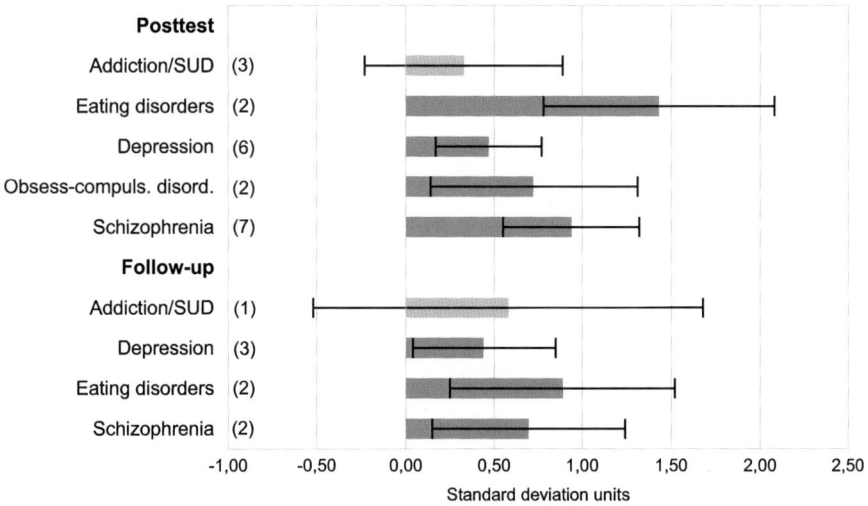

Fig. 2 Weighted mean improvements of symptoms of adults after receipt of systemic therapy in studies with control groups receiving no alternative active treatment. Note: Numbers in brackets represent the number of included studies. Error bars show the 95% CI of the mean effect size

compulsive disorder ($d = 0.72$), and schizophrenia ($d = 0.94$) than patients who did not receive an alternative active treatment (Fig. 2). Effects on depression ($d = 0.44$), eating disorders ($d = 0.89$), and schizophrenia ($d = 0.70$) were maintained at the follow-up. Studies that compared systemic therapy with an alternative active treatment found significantly stronger effects of systemic therapy on anxiety disorders at post-test ($d = 0.40$). Effects of systemic and alternative treatments at post-test did not differ significantly for addiction/SUD, eating disorders, and depression. Similarly, no significant between-group differences were found for the four illness groups at follow-up. In addition, the meta-analysis found stronger effects in more recent studies and larger long-term effects if manualized treatments were used.

In sum, these meta-analyses show empirical evidence for positive effects of systemic therapy on (older) children and adolescents as well as adults. Systemic therapy is at least as effective as individual therapy and for some problems more effective. The observed small differences between effects of systemic therapy and of other active treatments should not be surprising as a number of common psychotherapeutic factors works across different kinds of psychotherapy (e.g. Cuijpers et al., 2013; Wampold et al., 1997). Illness-specific analyses from randomized controlled trials provide evidence for effects of systemic therapy on anxiety disorders (in adults), CD/ODD (in children/adolescents), depression (in children/adolescents and adults), eating disorders (in children/adolescents and adults), obsessive-compulsive disorders (in adults), schizophrenia (in adults), and substance use disorders/addiction (in adolescents). Systemic interventions combined with medication are more effective than medication alone for disorders normally treated with medication alone, such as depression and psychosis. Gains made during systemic therapy are sustained at follow-up. Nonetheless, the numbers of RCTs on individual disorders are limited, and RCTs are lacking for some conditions in particular age groups, such as anxiety disorders in children and adolescents.

Most of the available RCTs did not report the number of responders, such as individuals who do no longer meet the criteria of a mental disorder at post-test. Based on the available d-scores, the binomial effect size display (Rosenthal & Rubin, 1982) gives a rough estimation of success rates if success is defined as improvement above the median change of the total sample. The observed mean improvements of $d = 0.59$ (in children and adolescents) and $d = 0.68$ (in adults) at post-test compared to an untreated control group translate to 64% (systemic therapy) versus 36% success (control group) in children and adolescents and to 66% (systemic therapy) versus 34% success (control group) in adults. The differences are smaller when compared against active alternative psychological treatments (57.7% vs. 42.3% in children/adolescents and 55.5% vs. 44.5% in adults).

What Kinds of Systemic Therapy Work for Specific Sorts of Clinical Problems?

While the two cited meta-analyses provide support for efficacy of systemic therapy in general, a number of approaches exist under the umbrella of systemic therapy with some of them targeting a particular group of psychological symptoms and disorders. Meta-analyses have been published on five approaches. Treatment manuals giving detailed guidance on the delivery of empirically supported approaches to systemic treatment for specific problems identified are marked with an asterisk in the reference list at the end of this chapter.

Brief strategic family therapy (BSFT) is a manual-based family therapy approach concerned with identifying and ameliorating patterns of interaction in the family system that are presumed to be directly related to adolescent drug usage (Szapocznik, Duff, Schwartz, Muir, & Brown, 2015; Szapocznik, Hervis, & Schwartz, 2002). It relies primarily on structural family theory (i.e. how the structure of the family influences young people's behaviour) and strategic family theory (i.e. problem-focused and pragmatic treatment methods). A meta-analysis by Lindstrøm et al. (2013) integrated the results of three studies that compared BSFT to community treatment programmes, group treatment, and minimum contact comparison. On average, BSFT did not produce larger effects than the control conditions ($d = 0.04$), although one of the three included studies found a significant but small effect of BSFT on marijuana use when compared against a group intervention that provided information on negative effects of drug use and encouraged problem-solving (Santisteban et al., 2003) . Similarly, a meta-analysis by Baldwin et al. (2012) did not find significantly stronger effects of BSFT on a summary measure of delinquency, conduct problems, and substance use when compared against treatment as usual ($d = 0.09$, based on one study) and alternative active treatments ($d = 0.11$, based on three studies). Moderate improvements were found when comparing BSFT against attention placebo control conditions ($d = 0.68$, based on three studies), but the mean effect size did not reach statistical significance because of limited test power.

Functional family therapy (FFT) is a strength-based intervention that has been developed for treating families of juvenile delinquents. It combines family systems theory with social learning approaches with the goal to improve family relationships and develop positive behaviours of the individual family members (Alexander, Waldron, Robbins, & Neeb, 2013; Sexton, 2011, 2015). The meta-analysis by Baldwin et al. (2012) found small but nonsignificant effects of FFT on a summary measure of delinquency, conduct problems, and substance abuse when compared with an alternative treatment ($d = 0.29$, based on three studies). However, test power was not sufficient for identifying small differences between the effects of systemic and alternative treatments.

Multidimensional family therapy (MDFT) is a manualized, evidence-based, intensive intervention programme with assessment and treatment modules focusing on four areas, (a) adolescents' substance use disorder, delinquency, and comorbid psychopathology, (b) parents' child-rearing skills and personal functioning, (c) communication and relationships between adolescents and their parents, and (d) interactions between family members and key social systems (Liddle, 2002, 2015). Baldwin et al. (2012) found slightly stronger improvements in a summary measure of delinquency, conduct problems, and substance use after MDFT compared to an alternative treatment ($d = 0.22$, based on four studies). However, the difference did not reach statistical significance, probably because of limited statistical power. More differentiated results for these outcomes were provided in a recent meta-analysis by van der Pol et al. (2017). Again, MDFT was compared against other active treatments (such as cognitive-behavioural or group therapy). MDFT was more effective in ameliorating problems in the areas of delinquency ($d = 0.21$, based on five studies), externalizing problems ($d = 0.17$, based on five studies), internalizing problems ($d = 0.30$, based on five studies), and substance abuse ($d = 0.25$, based on eight studies). In addition, MDFT had a small positive effect on family functioning ($d = 0.25$). Based on five controlled studies, Filges et al. (2018) found significantly greater improvements in substance abuse problems in families who engaged in MDFT compared to other treatments ($d = 0.31$ to 0.35). Treatment effects were maintained at the 12-month follow-up ($d = 0.25$ to 0.27).

Multisystemic therapy (MST) is a multifaceted, short-term, home-, and community-based intervention for juvenile delinquents and juveniles with social, emotional, and behavioural problems (Henggeler, Schoenwald, Bordin, Rowland, & Cunningham, 2009; Schoenwald, Henggeler, & Rowland, 2015). A first meta-analysis by Curtis et al. (2004) on delinquent, abused, and neglected young people and youth at risk for psychiatric hospitalization found moderate effects of MST on criminal/delinquent activities ($d = 0.50$, based on seven studies) and family functioning ($d = 0.57$–0.76, based on five studies). Shortly after publication of the first meta-analysis, Littell et al. (2005) analysed the effects of MST on three indicators of externalizing problems. Effects of MST on self-reported delinquency ($d = 0.21$, based on three studies), summary measures of externalizing problems ($d = 0.18$, based on two studies), and numbers of arrests or convictions ($d = 0.16$, based on five studies) did not reach statistical significance, probably due to restricted test power. A later meta-analysis by Baldwin et al. (2012) found statistically significant small effects of MST on a summary measure of delinquency, conduct problems, and substance use when compared against treatment as usual ($d = 0.22$, based on ten studies) and a moderate marginally significant effect when compared against an alternative active treatment ($d = 0.57$, based on two studies). Based on 22 controlled studies, the most recent meta-analysis on effects of MST in antisocial, conduct-disordered, and/or delinquent juveniles found, on average, significant small effects on delinquency ($d = 0.20$) and psychopathology ($d = 0.27$; van der Stouwe et al., 2014). Further analyses showed that significant effects were only found when the participants consisted of offenders (and had more severe initial externalizing problems) and when the average age of the assessed young people was below 15 years.

Solution-focused brief therapy (SFBT) is a short-term, strength-based intervention which focuses on creating client-generated solutions to problems. Specifically, SFBT helps clients explore resources and past successes and identify goals and future hopes as opposed to focusing predominantly on present and past problems (de Shazer & Dolan, 2007). Kim (2008) conducted the first meta-analysis of SFBT. It included 22 RCTs and quasi-experimental studies with heterogeneous samples, such as participants of family therapy, student populations, or patients in orthopaedic rehabilitation. Kim (2008) found statistically significant small improvements in internalizing symptoms ($d = 0.26$, based on 12 studies), while changes in externalizing problems ($d = 0.13$, based on 9 studies) and family relationship outcomes ($d = 0.26$, based on 8 studies) were not significant. A more recent meta-analysis on SFBT by Schmit et al. (2016) included 26 quasi-experimental and experimental studies. Significant small effects on internalizing symptoms were found in comparison with an active control condition ($d = 0.24$, based on 12 studies) and with an untreated control group ($d = 0.31$, based on 14 studies). While studies from Western countries found, on average, small effects of SFBT, a meta-analysis on nine studies done in China found large effects of SFBT on internalizing problems ($d = 1.26$; Kim et al., 2015). Six included Chinese studies compared SFBT with an untreated control group and three studies with treatment as usual. All but one of the Chinese studies involved additional counselling services along with SFBT which might have contributed to the above-average intervention effects. Finally, a meta-analysis by Zhang et al. (2018) synthesized results of RCTs on SFBT in medical settings such as burn rehabilitation, orthopaedic rehabilitation, or treatment of paediatric obesity. An overall significant effect of SFBT was found for health-related psychosocial outcomes (e.g. adjustment to illness; $d = 0.34$) and a nearly significant outcome for health-related behavioural outcomes (such as adherence, $d = 0.28$).

In sum, available meta-analyses provide support for greater improvements after MDFT (with regard to internalizing problems, externalizing problems, and substance abuse), MST (regarding externalizing problems and substance abuse), and SFBT (regarding internalizing problems and adjustment to physical illness) when compared against alternative active treatments and/or untreated control conditions. In addition, BSFT and FFT were found to produce similar changes in externalizing problems and substance abuse to alternative treatments, but the number of controlled studies is still limited for BSFT and FFT. The overall pattern of meta-analytic results suggests that MST, MDFT, and SFBT are marginally more effective than FFT and BSFT. There are, however, alternative explanations for this finding. Both FFT and BSFT may have been compared in RCTs to more potent alternative treatments than were used as comparators in trials of MST, MDFT, and SFBT. Also, studies in which BSFT was compared to placebo control conditions yielded medium to large effect sizes, but these were not significant as the studies were statistically underpowered. Most meta-analyses on specific models of systemic therapy found, on average, small improvements in a statistical sense, although large effects of SFBT have been observed in China (Kim et al., 2015). Small between-group differences are not surprising if two active treatments are compared, for example, due to common psychotherapeutic factors, such as the therapeutic alliance and empathy. In addition, most meta-analyses included participants in the subclinical range which reduced the size of possible symptom improvements.

While meta-analytic evidence is available for the effects of five specific models of systemic therapy, other systemic approaches have been assessed in a few controlled studies. For example, the Maudsley model has been found to be effective for both anorexia and bulimia nervosa in adolescents (Eisler et al., 2015; Le Grange & Lock, 2007; Lock & Le Grange, 2013), and systemic couple therapy has been found to reduce adult depression (Jones & Asen, 1999). While most available meta-analyses focused on the effects of systemic therapy on a range of psychological symptoms or disorders, systemic therapy has been shown to be effective in addressing severely dysfunctional family relationships, such as child abuse and neglect (MST: Brunk, Henggeler, & Whelan, 1987) and domestic violence (solution-focused couple therapy: Stith, McCollum, & Rosen, 2011).

These research findings have important implications for clinical practice. They let us know what we can tell clients to expect when they attend systemic therapy for help with common child- and adult-focused problems. At any rate, systemic therapy tends to help at least as much or more than other alternative treatments.

Is Systemic Therapy Cost-Effective?

It is important for practising clinicians to let service funders as well as clients know that systemic therapy is effective. However, it is also useful for clinicians to let service funders know the economic benefits of funding a family therapy service. In a series of 22 studies conducted over 20 years, Russell Crane has shown that family therapy is more cost-effective than individual therapy and systemic therapy leads to medical cost offsets (Crane & Christenson, 2014; see Table 1 for an overview). Medical cost offsets occurred because people, who engaged in family therapy, particularly frequent health service users, used fewer medical services after family therapy. Large US databases involving over 250,000 cases of routine systemic therapy were used for these studies. Cases included families of people diagnosed with

Table 1 Studies on cost-effectiveness of systemic therapy identified by Crane and Christenson (2014)

Health maintenance organization (HMO)

Western United States' HMO serving 180,00 subscribers

Sample	*Conditions/comparisons*	*Results for health-care use*
Law and Crane (2000)		
n = 292, average age 30 years, middle income, Caucasian individuals	(a) Marital/couples therapy (b) Family therapy identified patient (c) Family therapy other patient (d) Individual therapy; (e) No-therapy comparison group	Significant reductions: 1. By 21.5% 1 year after psychotherapy started for family therapy group (n = 172) vs. 10% reduction for individual therapy group (n = 60) 2. Family therapy participant who was not the identified patient group (n = 60) also showed a reduction of 30% in health-care use after 1 year
Law, Crane, and Berge (2003)		
High utilizers of health care (n = 65) within the sample of Law and Crane (2000)	(a) Individual therapy (n = 22) (b) Marital therapy (n = 15) (c) Family therapy (n = 28)	1. Groups (a), (b), and (c) reduced health-care use by 50% 2. Family therapy other patients reduced health-care use by 57% 3. Largest reduction by participants in 'conjoint' therapy (50–57% reduction) 4. Individual therapy participants reduced health-care use by 48%
Crane, Wood, Law, and Schaalje (2004)		
197 clients, 13 providers (marriage and family therapists, n = 4; psychologists, n = 2; clinical social workers, n = 7; range age providers 37–47 years)	Relationship between therapist characteristic (age, gender, profession, etc.) and medical use of their clients	Logistic regression analysis supports the argument that psychotherapy in general contributed to reductions in health-care use more than specific therapist characteristics or provider type
Crane and Christenson (2008)		
Sample of Law and Crane (2000)	Therapy modalities	1. 78% reduction in urgent care visits 2. 56% reduction in laboratory/X-ray visits 3. 68% reduction in health screening visits (T1–T2) by MFT participants
Kansas Medicaid data		
300,000 beneficiaries, administered at state level, funded at federal level, lower-income children and families		

Sample	Conditions/comparisons	Results for costs
Crane, Hillin, and Jakubowski (2005)		
Youth, n = 3753; mostly male (81%), Caucasian (73%), mean age 14.4 years	Comprehensive services (e.g. case management and pharmacological intervention), along with one of three types of therapy: (a) In-office family therapy (n = 164) (b) In-office individual therapy (n = 3086) (c) In-home family therapy (n = 503)	1. Over the 2.5-year follow-up period, the cost of health care was: (a) 16,260 USD for the in-office individual therapy group, (b) 11,116 USD for the in-office family therapy group, and (c) 1622 USD for the in-home family therapy group 2. Compared to health-care costs for individual therapy group, (a) 32% lower costs for in-office family therapy, (b) 85% lower costs for in-home family therapy
Christenson, Crane, Bell, Beer, and Hillin (2014)		
Patients diagnosed with schizophrenia (n = 164), mostly male (55%), Caucasian (90%), mean age 30 years	Structural equation models related to the cost of treating patients	1. 1st model: limited direct effects for family intervention (e.g. reductions in hospitalization costs) 2. 2nd model: direct and indirect effects (e.g. reducing hospitalizations by increasing medication compliance); significant indirect relationship between family intervention and general medical costs (~586 USD for each session) Better fit for 2nd model.
Cigna data		
A large national health insurance company with over nine million members; Cigna initially provided cost data for all psychotherapy services in the United States and Puerto Rico during a 4-year period (2001–2004), producing a sample that included 490,000 unique patients; majority female (60%), average age 32 years		

Sample	Conditions/comparisons	Results
Crane and Payne (2011)		
	Providers: (a) marital and family therapists (MFTs), (b) master's level nurses, (c) social workers, (d) professional counsellors (PCs), (e) psychologists, and (f) physicians (MDs)	Total cost of therapy: 1. Family therapy alone more cost-effective than individual therapy or 'mixed' therapy 2. 85% of patients required only a single episode of care 3. Services provided by PCs were the least expensive 4. MFT: 86.6% success rate, 13.4% recidivism rate, best among providers

(continued)

Table 1 (continued)

Hamilton, Moore, Crane, and Payne (2011)

N = 434,317	(a) Provider type (b) Individual/family therapy (c) Diagnosis	Dropout rates: 1. MFT: lowest dropout rates for individuals 2. Lowest dropout rate for individual therapy 3. Lowest dropout rates for patients with mood and anxiety disorders; highest dropout rates among schizophrenia and substance abuse disorders

Moore, Hamilton, Crane, and Fawcett (2011)

31,488 men, 36,333 women	Examine more specifically whether having a MFT license affected outcomes in family therapy Provider types (e.g. MFTs, MDs, nurses, social workers)	1. Lowest dropout rates: licensed MFT 2. MFT more cost-effective than nurses, MDs, psychologists; less cost-effective than social workers and PCs

Moore and Crane (2014)

3315 patients, who participated in psychotherapy for relational problems (parent–child; partner relation)	Providers: (a) psychologists, (b) PCs, (c) MFTs, (d) social workers	1. No higher recidivism rate for patients who received individual therapy than for those who participated in family therapy 2. Couple therapy relatively brief intervention, 280 USD for an episode of care, 8.43% recidivism

Chiang (2011)

2000 patients	Therapy modality (individual vs. family therapy)	1. Family therapy more cost-effective due to lower recidivism rates and lower total treatment costs 2. Higher dropout rates for family therapy than for individual therapy

Morgan, Crane, Moore, and Eggett (2013)

14,000 patients with substance abuse disorder receiving individual and family therapy		1. Family therapy uses 2.41 sessions, individual therapy 3.38 sessions, and mixed therapy 6.40 sessions 2. Cost for one treatment episode: 124.55 USD for family therapy; 170 USD for individual therapy; 319.55 USD for mixed therapy 3. Recidivism rate lowest for family therapy (8.9%) and mixed therapy (9.5%) and highest for individual therapy (12%)

Fawcett and Crane (2013)

Sample	Conditions/comparisons	Outcome/results
230 men, 189 women, who had received treatment for sexual dysfunction	Provider type (psychologists, social workers, MFTs, PCs) and modality (individual therapy, family therapy, mixed therapy)	1. Average number of sessions: 7 2. Marriage/family therapists used family and mixed modalities more often than other provider types 3. Mixed therapy lower dropout rates

Crane et al. (2012)

149 patients with somatoform disorder	The same as in Fawcett, D., and Crane, D. R. (2013)	1. Somatoform disorder patients experienced higher than average recidivism and participated in more session (regardless of provider type) 2. No significant difference in total cost or dropout between the various professions

Crane et al. (2013)

164,667 patients with depression	Age, gender, modality, and provider type	1. MFT services: lowest recidivism rates 2. MFT services least costly

Training clinic data

Student training clinic that provides opportunities for clinical training for master's and doctoral students at a large university located in the Western United States; couples and families who requested psychotherapy services, students from marriage/family therapy, clinical psychology and social work programmes as providers; prospective data

Sample	Conditions/comparisons	Outcome/results
Jakubowski et al. (2008)		
60% female, 94% Caucasian; average 31 years, 6 months of medical records for 130 clients	1. Comparison of medical record to self-reported medical use 2. Family members' report on health-care use of their spouses	1. Medical record and self-reported health-care use highly correlated 2. Spouses were able to report their partners and their children's health-care use
Crane, Christenson, Shaw, Fawcett, and Marshall (2010)		
Biopsychosocial measures administered to parents ($n = 60$)		Children's health-care use: parent's marital cohesion and life satisfaction strongest correlates, accounts for 46% variance in health care use (best subset regression)

(continued)

Table 1 (continued)

Christenson, Crane, Hafen, Hamilton, and Schaalje (2011)

110 participants seeking services for relationship problems, 66% female, 96% Caucasian, average 31 years; additionally: $n = 40$ participants as a subsample from Law, Crane, and Berge (2003)	Biopsychosocial measures administered to their parents (for $n = 60$)	Children's health-care use: 1. Variables accounting for most variance: 'informational support', 'somatization' 2. 'Hostility' highest correlate among high utilizer group from Law et al. (2003)

Christenson, Crane, Law, Schaalje, and Marshall (under review)

56 participants, 96% Caucasian, diverse annual income ranging from 2500 USD to 100,000 USD		Health-care use: (1) MFT participants showed significant (44%) decrease in health-care use between T1 and T2; light uptick in health-care use from T2 to T3; overall 33% decrease between T1 and T3; (2) 58% decrease in health-care use for patients who reported an improvement in general family functioning after treatment, whereas patients without improvement showed no decrease in health-care use

schizophrenia, depression, sexual disorders, somatoform disorder, substance misuse, relationship problems, and other disorders.

A couple of examples illustrate how systemic therapy leads to reduced overall costs for society. Interventions such as FFT, MST, and multidimensional treatment foster care have been shown to be very cost-effective for conduct disorders and substance misuse because they save a lot of money that would be spent on residential care or detention of juvenile offenders and costs to society associated with crime and court involvement (Savignac, 2009).

The main message for service funders is that systemic and family therapy work and cost less than other interventions. For most common child, adolescent, and adult mental health problems or adjustment problems associated with physical illnesses, the success rate is as good as that of other psychotherapies. However, systemic therapy is more cost-effective than individual therapy. It leads to greater medical cost offsets. The funds spent on providing systemic therapy are considerably less than the costs of medical consultations, tests, and hospitalization that would occur if clients did not engage in systemic or family therapy.

What Common Processes Characterize Effective Systemic Therapy?

Certain common processes or factors are shared by effective systemic therapy practices (Carr, 2012, Lebow, 2014). These relate to the structure of therapy; the role of the therapeutic alliance; the focus of the therapy contract; the value of models and manuals; the practices associated with the engagement phase, middle phase, and disengagement phase of treatment; and the importance of measurement. These processes may be incorporated into research-informed family therapy practice. The model from the book – *Family Therapy: Concepts Process and Practice* (Carr, 2000c, 2006, 2012) – is an example of a research-informed approach to the practice of family therapy. What follows are some comments on each of the processes listed above.

Structure of Therapy

The following comments refer to family therapy in general and systemic therapy in particular. In research-informed family and systemic therapy, therapists and families meet regularly. However, meetings are not confined to conjoint family sessions. Therapists may also meet with family subsystems (e.g. with parents alone or adolescents alone) or with members of the wider system (e.g. with other involved professionals from health and social services, education or probation agencies, or the extended family). Therapy is relatively brief spanning 3–6 months and involving

6–20 sessions. Therapy typically progresses through three phases: the engagement phase, the middle phase, and the disengagement phase. Therapy sessions are guided by the five-part session model. These five parts include (1) planning (alone or with a team or supervisor), (2) meeting with clients, (3) taking a break from the meeting with clients to review progress and plan an end-of-session intervention, (4) reconvening the meeting with clients to provide feedback and an end-of-session intervention, and (5) reviewing the session (alone or with a team or a supervisor). Clients are often explicitly invited to do 'homework' between sessions to continue work that occurred in sessions and facilitate problem resolution.

These features of the structure of therapy (therapy duration, system members attending sessions, stages of therapy, session structure, and homework) are central to empirically supported models of systemic therapy, notably BSFT (Szapocznik et al., 2002, 2015), FFT (Alexander et al., 2013; Sexton, 2011, 2015), MDFT (Liddle, 2002, 2015), and MST (Henggeler et al., 2009; Schoenwald et al., 2015). The evidence base for these models has been reviewed in an earlier section of this chapter. There are few studies of the relationship between features of the structure of therapy and outcome of systemic therapy. However, there are exceptions. For example, in an RCT, Lock, Agras, Bryson, and Kraemer (2005) found that extending the duration of family therapy beyond 6 months to 1 year did not result in better outcomes for adolescent anorexia nervosa. There is also research on other types of therapy about the relationship between some of the features of therapy structure and therapy outcome. For example, in a meta-analysis of studies of cognitive-behavioural therapy, Kazantzis, Whittington, and Dattilio (2010) found a significant effect of therapeutic homework on outcome ($d = 0.48$).

Therapeutic Alliances

In research-informed family therapy, therapists prioritize facilitating strong alliances within the treatment system and reducing negativity. Therapists facilitate alliances between themselves and family members; between family members; and, where appropriate, between family members and members of the wider system (e.g. other involved professionals from health and social services, education and probation agencies, and the extended family). Warmth, empathy, respect, curiosity, optimism, a focus on strengths and solutions, an openness to all viewpoints, and an acceptance that differing viewpoints may lead to conflicts that can be resolved are some of the more important strategies used to create and maintain positive therapeutic alliances with members of families and wider systems. In a meta-analysis of 24 trials of couple and family therapy, Friedlander, Escudero, Heatherington, and Diamond (2011) found a correlation of $r = 0.26$ between the therapeutic alliance and outcome in systemic therapy. This small-to-medium effect size is similar to that for individual adult psychotherapy.

Focus of the Therapy

In research-informed family therapy, within the therapy contract, and in subsequent therapy sessions, there is an explicit focus on resolving the main presenting problem, rather than on broader goals such as personal growth, or an unfocused exploration of family issues. Therapy goals are usually explicit and relate directly to the main presenting problem, for example, weight restoration in anorexia; reducing drug or alcohol use where substance use is the main problem; improving mood and activity in depression; decreasing panic and avoidance in anxiety disorders; increasing prosocial behaviour in disruptive behaviour disorders; and so forth.

These features on the focus of therapy are central to empirically supported models of systemic therapy notably the Maudsley model for treating adolescent eating disorders (Eisler et al., 2015; Le Grange & Lock, 2007; Lock & Le Grange, 2013), systemic couple therapy for depression (Jones & Asen, 1999), BSFT (Szapocznik et al., 2002, 2015), FFT (Alexander et al., 2013; Sexton, 2011, 2015), MDFT (Liddle, 2002, 2015), and MST (Henggeler et al., 2009; Schoenwald, Henggeler, & Rowland, 2015). The evidence base for these models has been reviewed in an earlier section of this chapter. There are few studies of the relationship between therapeutic focus and outcome of systemic therapy. However, there are exceptions. For example, in an RCT, Agras et al. (2014) compared the effectiveness of the problem-focused Maudsley model of family therapy for anorexia and generic systemic family therapy which was not problem-focused. They found that both were equally effective in terms of symptom remission, but the Maudsley model led to significantly faster weight gain early in treatment, fewer days in hospital, and lower treatment costs.

Models and Manuals

In research-informed systemic and family therapy, treatment is guided by models of how problems develop and are resolved. These are typically multifactorial models. They may specify the role of a wide range of factors that cause and maintain problems and that contribute to the resolution of presenting problems. Some models point to ways in which family processes inadvertently maintain presenting problems. However, research-informed systemic and family therapy invariably highlights the value of the family as a therapeutic resource. That is, a central position is accorded to the critical role of the family in problem resolution. Technical aspects of therapy are guided by the flexible use of guidelines set out in therapy manuals. Manuals outline principles of practice and specific therapeutic techniques that therapists may use during therapy to help families work towards resolution of presenting problems. The principles of practice and specific therapeutic techniques given in therapy manuals are typically informed by multifactorial models of how presenting problems develop and are resolved.

Engagement Phase

The overall effectiveness of treatment depends to a large extent on initially engaging families in the therapeutic process, and facilitating commitment to therapy goals, while concurrently conducting a thorough assessment and comprehensive formulation of the presenting problem and the system within which it occurs. In the engagement phase, in research-informed family therapy, therapists typically have goals in the domains of content and process. In the content domain, they aim to assess the presenting problem, the multiple factors involved in its development and potential resolution, and the family's strengths and vulnerabilities. This assessment will lead to the construction of a formulation or hypothesis about why the problem developed and possible solutions. This formulation typically affords an important role to multiple factors especially relational factors in the resolution of the presenting problems. This formulation will be informed by relevant theory and research. In the process domain, the main goal in the first phase of treatment is to engage family members in therapy and establish co-operative working alliances with family members. Across many empirically supported models of family therapy, there is a remarkable consistency in strategies that are used to promote engagement. Reframing and psychoeducation are widely used in the engagement phase to help families arrive at a more useful formulation of their presenting problems.

Middle Phase

In the middle phase, the aim in research-informed systemic and family therapy is to help families achieve therapeutic goals and resolve presenting problems. The specific therapeutic strategies used in the middle phase are usually informed by the therapeutic model and manual but also fine-tuned and guided by a formulation or hypothesis developed during the engagement phase. A wide range of therapeutic techniques are used in research-informed family therapy to help families achieve therapeutic goals and resolve presenting problems. A useful way to classify these many techniques is to distinguish between (1) those that focus on family behaviour, or what families do; (2) those that focus on family narratives, or what families believe; and (3) those that address broader contextual factors that affect problem-related behaviour patterns and narratives. These broader contextual factors include personal and family history, the wider system which may contain other involved professionals and the extended family, and psychobiological characteristics of family members.

Middle phase interventions focusing on behaviour In the middle phase, examples of interventions that aim to disrupt problem-maintaining behaviour patterns include enhancing communication skills, problem-solving and solution-finding skills, and specific problem-relevant skills.

Middle phase interventions focusing on beliefs In the middle phase of research-informed systemic and family therapy, examples of interventions that aim to transform narratives that keep families stuck in problem-maintaining behaviour patterns include reframing, validating multiple perspectives, highlighting strengths and exceptions, and addressing ambivalence about therapeutic change.

Middle phase interventions focusing on contexts In the middle phase of research-informed family therapy, there are many interventions that aim to address contextual factors (including developmental factors, the wider system, and psychobiological characteristics) that keep families stuck in problem-maintaining behaviour patterns and that subserve problem-maintaining narratives. What follows are some examples. Where unresolved developmental factors are contributing significantly to the presenting problem, therapists may help clients address developmental issues or family-of-origin issues. Where stresses or lack of coordination within the wider social system is contributing significantly to the presenting problem, therapists may hold network meetings with schools, health and social services, and probation agencies. Where psychobiological characteristics such as vulnerability to mental or physical health problems (e.g. psychosis or diabetes) are contributing significantly to the presenting problem, therapists may offer detailed psychoeducation and interventions to facilitate adherence to medication and illness management regimes.

In the middle phase of research-informed systemic and family therapy, the overarching principles for good practice are to keep focused on resolving the presenting problem (and avoid being side-tracked into addressing other issues), matching the intervention to client needs, and letting families know that you are optimistic about recovery and prepared to 'go the distance'.

Disengagement Phase

In the disengagement phase, the aim in research-informed systemic and family therapy is to prepare families to autonomously manage their difficulties in future. The key interventions in this therapeutic phase include reviewing lessons learned in therapy, relapse prevention planning, and fading out sessions.

Measurement

In research-informed systemic and family therapy, before and after treatment (or at regular intervals), measurements are made to evaluate progress. The most important thing to measure is the presenting problem or symptom, even if just on a 10-point scale. Other constructs that may usefully be measured include family functioning, the therapeutic alliance, and treatment fidelity or adherence to a particular therapy model. Reviews of family therapy measures have been provided by Hamilton and Carr (2016) as well as Lebow and Stroud (2012). We have found Peter Stratton's brief version of the SCORE (Systemic Clinical Outcome in Routine Evaluation) a very useful measure (Carr & Stratton, 2017). It assesses overall family adjustment; family strengths, difficulties, and communication; and the severity and impact of the presenting problem.

What Are the Potential Negative Effects of Systemic Therapy?

On the General Risk of Harm from Psychological Therapies

To differentiate (a) between negative effects and unavoidable negative developments of the disorder or negative life events and (b) ambiguous treatment effects, that are therapeutic and negative at the same time (e.g. temporary destabilization during therapy or a divorce), often constitutes a major challenge in psychotherapy (Linden, 2013). Hence, according to Linden (2013), all unwanted events should be evaluated concerning their causation by the applied therapy and the question whether this therapy was conducted correctly. Three potential scenarios should be contemplated:

- If the event was not caused by the therapy, it may be immanent to the therapeutic process (e.g. unavoidable temporary destabilization) or to the characteristics of the disorders itself (lack of therapeutic efficacy – 'not all patients may be "cured"').
- If the event was caused by the treatment and the treatment was applied insufficiently, this would constitute a malpractice situation.
- If the event was caused by the treatment, but the treatment was adequate, one would face a true adverse treatment reaction.

It is important to acknowledge that all three scenarios above may entail non-response to psychotherapy and/or deterioration of the disorder. To date, this classification has not yet been applied in empirical investigations, so that most current findings are not differentiated concerning unavoidable unwanted events, malpractice situations, or adverse treatment reactions. Investigators in clinical trials often do not monitor or report negative psychotherapy effects (Cuijpers, Reijnders, Karyotaki, de Wit, & Ebert, 2018; Duggan, Parry, McMurran, Davidson, & Dennis, 2014; Jonsson, Alaie, Parling, & Arnberg, 2014). Recently, it was shown that only 6% of all trials comparing psychotherapy with a control condition reported deterioration rates (Cuijpers et al., 2018). However, psychotherapists have highlighted negative effects in routine practice (Castonguay, Boswell, Constantino, Goldfried, & Hill, 2010). There is also some evidence that therapists may have major difficulties in predicting and/or acknowledging failures and deterioration during the treatment course (Kächele & Schachter, 2014; Lambert, 2011; Linden, 2013). If deterioration is detected by therapists, it is rarely discussed with the patient or in supervision (Hardy et al., 2017).

From the patients' perspective, results for patient-reported outcomes (PROs) indicate that between 5 and 10% of patients deteriorate following therapy – a figure that can be regarded as a proxy of negative patient experiences, although deterioration on PROs is not necessarily linked with a negative therapy experience (Cahill, Barkham, & Stiles, 2010; Hardy et al., 2017). More recently, according to the largest survey of this kind to date, 1 in 20 psychological therapy service users in England had experienced 'lasting bad effects from the treatment' (Crawford et al., 2016). Specifically, the authors explicitly asked whether the effect was related to the treatment (malpractice situation or adverse treatment reaction according to self-report) and differentiated the longer-lasting effects from 'upsetting experiences' during therapy. They also found that insufficient information about the nature of the psychotherapy and/or rationale for the interventions but not the number of therapy sessions was associated with lasting bad effects.

Current recommendations for the assessment of negative psychotherapy effects include (1) raising awareness in therapists, (2) addressing both positive and negative effects when obtaining informed consent, and (3) focusing on systematic clinical real-time monitoring for unwanted events (Parry, Crawford, & Duggan, 2016). Unwanted negative psychotherapy effects may comprise emergence of new symptoms, deterioration of existing symptoms, lack of improvement or deterioration of illness, prolongation of treatment, patient's non-adherence, strains in the patient-therapist relationship, very good patient-therapist relationship, therapy dependency, strains or changes in family relations, strains or changes in work relations, any change in the life circumstances of the patient, and stigmatization (Linden & Schermuly-Haupt, 2014). Above all, therapists should always monitor the therapeutic process towards unwanted events and, if applicable, determine their relatedness to the (type of) therapy and its conduct.

Potential Adverse Treatment Reactions of Systemic Therapy

From a theoretical point of view, there are a few contraindications which have to be considered when offering systemic therapy to patients (Schweitzer & Schlippe, 2015). These include (a) absence of a motivational consensus among the clients in couples and family setting, (b) risk that disclosure during sessions may provoke/reinforce violence between partners/within the family, and (c) therapist's lack of an appropriate qualification for working with couples and families. Both population-based and clinical trial data on potential adverse treatment reactions specific to systemic therapy are scarce. According to the survey by Crawford et al. (2016), 4% of patients who had undergone solution-focused therapy reported lasting negative effects which is comparable to the findings for cognitive-behavioural therapy (4%) and humanistic therapy (3%) and somewhat lower compared to psychodynamic therapy (9%). The rate of 4% of patients reporting negative effects subsequent to solution-focused therapy corresponds with the recently reported 4% median deterioration in the therapy groups of clinical trials (Cuijpers et al., 2018).

A specific characteristic of systemic therapy concerns the nature of the therapeutic alliance. Since the therapeutic relationship is usually built up in the context of a low-frequency long-term therapy, one may assume that some patients who aim for and/or are in the need of an intensive, high-frequency process that supports intimate disclosure (e.g. experiences of shame) and extensive biographical work might not gain the optimal benefit from systemic therapy (Braverman, 1990; Schweitzer & Schlippe, 2015). However, against the background of the robust evidence base for systemic therapy from meta-analyses, this hypothesis of an ecological fallacy has to be evaluated empirically in future research.

At any rate, meta-analytic data from clinical trials indicates that average dropout rates are significantly lower in systemic therapy than in alternative active treatments (15% vs. 23%; risk ratio = 0.64; 95% confidence interval = 0.50–0.82) (Pinquart et al., 2016). One explanation may be the systemic constructionist philosophical stance characteristic of systemic therapy which on a practical level is reflected on (a) the explicit contracting at the beginning of each therapy, (b) the encouragement of decision-making, and (c) the continuous patient feedback generated through circular questioning. All in all, therapeutic processes as laid out in systemic therapy account for clear information of patients, clarity about sessions and progress, as well as management of patient expectations throughout the course of the therapy, which all have been identified as key elements in the prevention of negative psychotherapy effects (Crawford et al., 2016).

Conclusions

This chapter addressed five key questions and outlined the implications of answers to these questions for the research-informed practice of systemic therapy. The short answer to the first question – How effective is systemic therapy? – is that the success rates of systemic therapy are similar or higher than those of alternative treatments. Therapists may let clients know about this when forming a treatment contract. The second question was: What sorts of systemic therapy work best for specific sorts of clinical problems? For both young people and adults, there is evidence for the effectiveness of specific systemic interventions. Randomized controlled trials provide evidence for effects of systemic therapy on alcohol and drug problems (adolescents), adjustment to chronic illness, anxiety disorders (in adults), CD/ODD (in children/adolescents), depression (in children/adolescents and adults), eating disorders (in children/adolescents and adults), obsessive-compulsive disorders (in adults), and schizophrenia (in adults). There is evidence for the effectiveness of systemic interventions for child abuse and neglect as well as intimate partner violence in adults. With regard to individual systemic approaches, there is strongest empirical support for effects of MDFT, MST, and SFBT. Treatment manuals giving detailed guidance on the delivery of evidence-based systemic

treatment for specific child- and adult-focused problems are marked with an asterisk in the reference list at the end of this chapter. Systemic interventions combined
with medication are more effective than medication alone for disorders normally
treated with medication alone. The short answer to the third question – Is systemic
therapy cost-effective? – is that systemic therapy is more cost-effective than individual therapy and leads to medical cost offsets because people who engage in
systemic therapy, particularly frequent health service users, use fewer medical services after family therapy. Therapists may inform service funders of this. The
fourth question was: What common processes characterize effective systemic therapy? These processes relate to the structure of therapy; the role of the therapeutic
alliance; the focus of the therapy contract; the value of models and manuals; the
practices associated with the engagement phase, middle phase, and disengagement
phase of treatment; and the importance of measurement. Finally, the short answer
to the fifth question –What are potential negative effects of systemic therapy? – is
that there is no empirical data on specific adverse treatment reactions to systemic
therapy. However, the rate of patients with long-lasting negative effects following
solution-focused therapy is comparable to the one for cognitive-behavioural as
well as humanistic therapy. We hope that our answers to the above five key questions serve to inform system practice in primary care, counselling/therapeutic services, and organizational and corporate contexts. Systemic therapy can make a
very significant contribution to alleviating suffering, enhancing well-being, and
making the world a better place to be.

References[1]

Agras, W. S., Lock, J., Brandt, H., Bryson, S. W., Dodge, E., Halmi, K. A., ... Woodside, B. (2014).
   Comparison of 2 family therapies for adolescent anorexia nervosa: A randomized parallel trial.
   JAMA Psychiatry, 71, 1279–1286. https://doi.org/10.1001/jamapsychiatry.2014.1025
∗Alexander, J., Waldron, H., Robbins, M., & Neeb, A. (2013). *Functional family therapy for ado-
   lescent behaviour problems.* Washington, D.C.: American Psychological Association.
Baldwin, S. A., Christian, S., Berkeljon, A., Shadish, W. R., & Bean, R. (2012). The effects of
   family therapies for adolescent delinquency and substance abuse: A meta-analysis. *Journal of
   Marital and Family Therapy, 38*, 281–304. https://doi.org/10.1111/j.1752-0606.2011.00248.x
Braverman, S. (1990). Long-term family therapy: A developmental approach. *Contemporary
   Family Therapy, 12*, 129–138. https://doi.org/10.1007/BF00892491
Brunk, M., Henggeler, S., & Whelan, J. (1987). Comparison of multisystemic therapy and parent
   training in the brief treatment of child abuse and neglect. *Journal of Consulting and Clinical
   Psychology, 55*, 171–178. https://doi.org/10.1037/0022-006X.55.2.171
Cahill, J., Barkham, M., & Stiles, W. B. (2010). Systematic review of practice-based research on
   psychological therapies in routine clinic settings. *British Journal of Clinical Psychology, 49*,
   421–453. https://doi.org/10.1348/014466509X470789

---

[1] Treatment manuals detailing empirically supported approaches to systemic treatment for specific
problems are marked with an asterisk in the reference list.

Carr, A. (2000a). Evidence-based practice in family therapy and systemic consultation, I. child-focused problems. *Journal of Family Therapy, 22,* 29–59. https://doi.org/10.1111/1467-6427.00137

Carr, A. (2000b). Evidence-based practice in family therapy and systemic consultation. II. Adult-focused problems. *Journal of Family Therapy, 22,* 273–295. https://doi.org/10.1111/1467-6427.00152

Carr, A. (2000c). *Family therapy: Concepts, process and practice.* Chichester, UK: Wiley.

Carr, A. (2006). *Family therapy: Concepts, process and practice* (2nd ed.). Chichester, UK: Wiley.

Carr, A. (2009a). The effectiveness of family therapy and systemic interventions for child-focused problems. *Journal of Family Therapy, 31,* 3–45. https://doi.org/10.1111/j.1467-6427.2008.00451.x

Carr, A. (2009b). The effectiveness of family therapy and systemic interventions for adult-focused problems. *Journal of Family Therapy, 31,* 46–74. https://doi.org/10.1111/j.1467-6427.2008.00452.x

∗Carr, A. (2012). *Family therapy: Concepts, process and practice* (3rd ed.). Chichester, UK: Wiley.

Carr, A. (2014a). The evidence-base for family therapy and systemic interventions for child-focused problems. *Journal of Family Therapy, 36,* 107–157. https://doi.org/10.1111/1467-6427.12032

Carr, A. (2014b). The evidence-base for couple therapy, family therapy and systemic interventions for adult-focused problems. *Journal of Family Therapy, 36,* 158–194. https://doi.org/10.1111/1467-6427.12033

Carr, A. (2018a). Family therapy and systemic interventions for child-focused problems: The current evidence base. *Journal of Family Therapy., 41,* 153. https://doi.org/10.1111/1467-6427.12226

Carr, A. (2018b). Couple therapy, family therapy and systemic interventions for adult-focused problems: The current evidence base. *Journal of Family Therapy, 41,* 492. https://doi.org/10.1111/1467-6427.12225

Carr, A., & Stratton, P. (2017). SCORE family assessment questionnaire: A decade of progress. *Family Process, 56*(2), 285–301. https://doi.org/10.1111/famp.12280.

Castelnuovo, G., Manzoni, G. M., Villa, V., Cesa, G. L., & Molinari, E. (2011). Brief strategic therapy vs cognitive behavioral therapy for the inpatient and telephone-based outpatient treatment of binge eating disorder: The STRATOB randomized controlled clinical trial. *Clinical Practice & Epidemiology in Mental Health, 7,* 29–37. https://doi.org/10.2174/1745017901107010029

Castonguay, L. G., Boswell, J. F., Constantino, M. J., Goldfried, M. R., & Hill, C. E. (2010). Training implications of harmful effects of psychological treatments. *American Psychologist, 65,* 34–49. https://doi.org/10.1037/a0017330

Chiang, F. F. (2011). *The cost effectiveness of individual and family therapy for schizophrenia in managed care.* (Unpublished master's thesis). Brigham Young University, Provo, UT.

Christenson, J. D., Crane, D. R., Bell, K. M., Beer, A. R., & Hillin, H. H. (2014). Family intervention and health care costs for Kansas Medicaid patients with schizophrenia. *Journal of Marital and Family Therapy, 40,* 272–286. https://doi.org/10.1111/jmft.1202.

Christenson, J. D., Crane, D. R., Hafen, M., Hamilton, S., & Schaalje, G. B. (2011). Predictors of health care use among individuals seeking therapy for marital and family problems: An exploratory study. *Contemporary Family Therapy: An International Journal, 33,* 441–460. https://doi.org/10.1007/s10591-011-9159-1

Christenson, J. D., Crane, D. R., Law, D. D., Schaalje, B., & Marshall, E. (under review). The effect of marital and family therapy on health care use.

Crane, D. R., & Christenson, J. D. (2008). The medical offset effect: Patterns in outpatient services reduction for high utilizers of health care. *Contemporary Family Therapy: An International Journal, 30,* 127–138. https://doi.org/10.1007/s10591-008-9058-2.

Crane, D. R., & Christenson, J. D. (2014). A summary report of cost-effectiveness: Recognizing the value of family therapy in health care. In J. Hodgson, A. Lamson, T. Mendenhall, & R. Crane (Eds.), *Medical family therapy: Advanced applications* (pp. 419–436). Cham, Switzerland: Springer. https://doi.org/10.1007/978-3-319-03482-9

Crane, D. R., Christenson, J. D., Dobbs, S. M., Schaalje, G. B., Moore, A. M., Pedal, F. F. C., ... Marshall, E. S. (2013). Costs of treating depression with individual versus family therapy. *Journal of Marital and Family Therapy, 39*, 457–469. https://doi.org/10.1111/j.1752-0606.2012.00326.x

Crane, D. R., Christenson, J. D., Shaw, A. L., Fawcett, D., & Marshall, E. S. (2010). Predictors of health care use for children of marriage and family therapy clients. *Journal of Couple and Relationship Therapy, 9*, 277–292. https://doi.org/10.1080/15332691.2010.515530

Crane, D. R., Hillin, H., & Jakubowski, S. (2005). Costs of treating conduct disordered Medicaid youth with and without family therapy. *The American Journal of Family Therapy, 33*, 403–413. https://doi.org/10.1080/01926180500276810

Crane, D. R., Morton, L. B., Fawcett, D., Moore, A. M., Larson, J., & Sandberg, J. (2012). Somatoform disorder: Treatment utilization and cost by mental health professions. *Contemporary Family Therapy: An International Journal, 34*, 322–333. https://doi.org/10.1007/s10591-012-9182-x.

Crane, D. R., & Payne, S. H. (2011). Individual and family therapy in managed care: Comparing the costs of treatment by the mental health professions. *Journal of Marital and Family Therapy, 37*, 273–289. https://doi.org/10.1111/j.1752-0606.2009.00170.x

Crane, D. R., Wood, N. D., Law, D. D., & Schaalje, B. (2004). The relationship between therapist characteristics and decreased medical utilization: An exploratory study. *Contemporary Family Therapy: An International Journal, 26*, 61–69. https://doi.org/10.1023/B:COFT.0000016912.25239.52.

Crawford, M. J., Thana, L., Farquharson, L., Palmer, L., Hancock, E., Bassett, P., ... Parry, G. D. (2016). Patient experience of negative effects of psychological treatment: Results of a national survey. *British Journal of Psychiatry, 208*, 260–265. https://doi.org/10.1192/bjp.bp.114.162628

Cuijpers, P., Berking, M., Andersson, G., Quigley, L., Kleiboer, A., & Dobson, K. S. (2013). A meta-analysis of cognitive-behavioural therapy for adult depression, alone and in comparison with other treatments. *Canadian Journal of Psychiatry, 58*, 376–385. https://doi.org/10.1177/070674371305800702

Cuijpers, P., Reijnders, M., Karyotaki, E., de Wit, L., & Ebert, D. D. (2018). Negative effects of psychotherapies for adult depression: A meta-analysis of deterioration rates. *Journal of Affective Disorders, 239*, 138–145. https://doi.org/10.1016/j.jad.2018.05.050

Curtis, N. M., Ronan, K. R., & Borduin, C. M. (2004). Multisystemic treatment: A meta-analysis of outcome studies. *Journal of Family Psychology, 18*, 411–419. https://doi.org/10.1037/0893-3200.18.3.411

Dakof, G. A., Henderson, C. E., Rowe, C. L., Boustani, M., Greenbaum, P. E., Wang, W., . . . Liddle, H. A. (2015). A randomized clinical trial of family therapy in juvenile drug court. Journal of Family Psychology, 29, 232–241. doi:https://doi.org/10.1037/fam0000053.

Dashtizadeh, N., Sajedi, H., Nazari, A. M., Davarniya, R., & Shakaram, M. (2015). Effectiveness of solution-focused brief therapy (SFBT) on reducing symptoms of depression in women [in Farsi]. *Journal of Clinical Nursing and Midwifery, 4*, 67–78.

Duggan, C., Parry, G., McMurran, M., Davidson, K., & Dennis, J. (2014). The recording of adverse events from psychological treatments in clinical trials: Evidence from a review of NIHR-funded trials. *Trials, 15*, 335. https://doi.org/10.1186/1745-6215-15-335

Eisler, I., Le Grange, D., & Lock, J. (2015). Treating adolescents with eating disorders. In T. Sexton & J. Lebow (Eds.), *Handbook of family therapy* (4th ed., pp. 387–406). New York, NY: Routledge.

Fawcett, D., & Crane, D. R. (2013). The influence of profession and therapy type on the treatment of sexual dysfunctions. *Journal of Sex & Marital Therapy, 39*, 453–465. https://doi.org/10.1080/0092623X.2012.665814

Filges, T., Andersen, D., & Jørgensen, A.-M. K. (2018). Effects of Multidimensional Family Therapy (MDFT) on nonopioid drug abuse: A systematic review and meta-analysis. *Research on Social Work Practice, 28*, 68–83. https://doi.org/10.1177/1049731515608241

Fonagy, P., Butler, S., Cottrell, D., Scott, S., Pilling, S., Eisler, I., ... Goodyer, I. M. (2018). Multisystemic therapy versus management as usual in the treatment of adolescent antisocial behaviour (START): A pragmatic, randomised controlled, superiority trial. *Lancet Psychiatry*, 5, 119–133. https://doi.org/10.1016/S2215-0366(18)30001-4

Friedlander, M. L., Escudero, V., Heatherington, L., & Diamond, G. M. (2011). Alliance in couple and family therapy. *Psychotherapy, 48*, 25–33. https://doi.org/10.1037/a0022060

Gurman, A. S., & Kniskern, D. P. (1978a). Research on marital and family therapy: Progress, perspective, and prospect. In S. L. Garfield & A. E. Bergin (Eds.), *Handbook of psychotherapy and behaviour change* (pp. 817–902). New York, NY: Wiley.

Gurman, A. S., & Kniskern, D. P. (1978b). Deterioration in marital and family therapy: Empirical, clinical, and conceptual issues. *Family Process, 17*, 3–20. https://doi.org/10.1111/j.1545-5300.1978.00003.x

Hamilton, E., & Carr, A. (2016). Systematic review of self-report family assessment measures. *Family Process, 55*, 16–30. https://doi.org/10.1111/famp.12200

Hamilton, S., Moore, A. M., Crane, D. R., & Payne, S. H. (2011). Psychotherapy dropouts: Differences by modality, license, and DSM-IV diagnosis. *Journal of Marital and Family Therapy, 37*, 333–343. https://doi.org/10.1111/j.1752-0606.2010.00204.x

Han, H., Zhang, H., Zhang, H., Gao, X., Zhang, W., & Zhang, S. (2015). Study on the curative effect of eszopiclone tablets combined with systemic family therapy for generalized anxiety disorder and its effect on the social and cognitive function [in Chinese]. *Chinese Journal of Practical Nervous Diseases, 23*, 15.

Hardy, G. E., Bishop-Edwards, L., Chambers, E., Connell, J., Dent-Brown, K., Kothari, G., … Parry, G. D. (2017). Risk factors for negative experiences during psychotherapy. *Psychotherapy Research, 29*, 403. https://doi.org/10.1080/10503307.2017.1393575. [Epub ahead of print].

Hazelrigg, M., Cooper, H., & Borduin, C. (1987). Evaluating the effectiveness of family therapies: An integrative review and analysis. *Psychological Bulletin, 101*, 428–442.

*Henggeler, S., Schoenwald, S., Bordin, C., Rowland, M., & Cunningham, P. (2009). *Multisystemic therapy for antisocial behaviour in children and adolescents* (2nd ed.). New York, NY: Guilford.

Humayun, S., Herlitz, L., Chesnokov, M., Doolan, M., Landau, S., & Scott, S. (2017). Randomized controlled trial of functional family therapy for offending and antisocial behavior in UK youth. *Journal of Child Psychology and Psychiatry, 58*, 1023–1032. https://doi.org/10.1111/jcpp.12743

Jakubowski, S. F., Crane, D. R., Christenson, J. D., Miller, R. B., Marshall, E. S., & Hafen, M. (2008). Marriage and family therapy research in health care: Investigating the accuracy of self and family reports of medical use. *The American Journal of Family Therapy, 36*, 437–448. https://doi.org/10.1080/01926180701441320

*Jones, E., & Asen, E. (1999). *Systemic couples therapy for depression*. London, UK: Karnac.

Jonsson, U., Alaie, I., Parling, T., & Arnberg, F. K. (2014). Reporting of harms in randomized controlled trials of psychological interventions for mental and behavioral disorders: A review of current practice. *Contemporary Clinical Trials, 38*, 1–8. https://doi.org/10.1016/j.cct.2014.02.005

Kächele, H., & Schachter, J. (2014). On side effects, destructive processes, and negative outcomes in psychoanalytic therapies: Why is it difficult for psychoanalysts to acknowledge and address treatment failures? *Contemporary Psychoanalysis, 50*, 233–258. https://doi.org/10.1080/00107530.2014.880321

Kazantzis, N., Whittington, C., & Dattilio, F. (2010). Meta-analysis of homework effects in cognitive and behavioral therapy: A replication and extension. *Clinical Psychology: Science and Practice, 17*, 144–156. https://doi.org/10.1111/j.1468-2850.2010.01204.x

Kim, J. S. (2008). Examining the effectiveness of solution-focused brief therapy: A meta-analysis. *Research on Social Work Practice, 18*, 107–116. https://doi.org/10.1177/1049731507307807

Kim, J. S., Brook, J., & Akin, B. A. (2018). Solution-focused brief therapy with substance-using individuals: A randomized controlled trial study. *Research on Social Work Practice, 28*, 452–462. https://doi.org/10.1177/1049731516650517

Kim, J. S., Franklin, C., Zhang, Y., Liu, X., Qu, Y., & Chen, H. (2015). Solution-focused brief therapy in China: A meta-analysis. *Journal of Ethnic & Cultural Diversity in Social Work, 24*, 187–201. https://doi.org/10.1080/15313204.2014.991983

Lambert, M. J. (2011). What have we learned about treatment failure in empirically supported treatments? Some suggestions for practice. *Cognitive and Behavioral Practice, 18*, 413–420. https://doi.org/10.1016/j.cbpra.2011.02.002

Law, D. D., & Crane, D. R. (2000). The influence of marital and family therapy on health care utilization in a health maintenance organization. *Journal of Marital and Family Therapy, 26*, 281–291. https://doi.org/10.1111/j.1752-0606.2000.tb00298.x

Law, D. D., Crane, D. R., & Berge, J. (2003). The influence of marital and family therapy on high utilizers of health care. *Journal of Marital and Family Therapy, 29*, 353–363. https://doi.org/10.1111/j.1752-0606.2000.tb00298.x.

*Le Grange, D., & Locke, J. (2007). *Treating bulimia in adolescents. A family-based approach.* New York, NY: Guilford.

Lebow, J. (2014). *Couple and family therapy: An integrative map of the territory.* Washington, D.C.: American Psychological Association.

Lebow, J., & Stroud, C. (2012). Assessment of effective couple and family functioning: Prevailing models and instruments. In F. Walsh (Ed.), *Normal family processes: Growing diversity and complexity* (pp. 501–528). New York, NY/London, UK: Guilford.

Lemmens, G. M. D., Eisler, I., Buysse, A., Heene, E., & Demyttenaere, K. (2009). The effects on mood of adjunctive single-family and multi-family group therapy in the treatment of hospitalized patients with major depression. *Psychotherapy and Psychosomatics, 78*, 98–105. https://doi.org/10.1159/000201935

Liddle, H. (2015). Multidimensional family therapy. In T. Sexton & J. Lebow (Eds.), *Handbook of family therapy* (4th ed., pp. 231–249). New York, NY: Routledge.

*Liddle, H. A. (2002). *Multidimensional family therapy treatment (MDFT) for adolescent cannabis users: Vol. 5 Cannabis Youth Treatment (CYT) manual series.* Rockville, MD: Centre for Substance Abuse Treatment, Substance Abuse and Mental Health Services Administration. Available at http://lib.adai.washington.edu/clearinghouse/downloads/Multidimensional-Family-Therapy-for-Adolescent-Cannabis-Users-207.pdf

Linden, M. (2013). How to define, find and classify side effects in psychotherapy: From unwanted events to adverse treatment reactions. *Clinical Psychology & Psychotherapy, 20*, 286–296. https://doi.org/10.1002/cpp.1765

Linden, M., & Schermuly-Haupt, M.-L. (2014). Definition, assessment and rate of psychotherapy side effects. *World Psychiatry, 13*, 306–309. https://doi.org/10.1002/wps.20153

Lindstrøm, M., Saidj, M., Kowalski, K., Filges, T., Rasmussen, P. S., & Jørgensen, A.-M. K. (2013). Brief Strategic Family Therapy (BSFT) for young people in treatment for non-opioid drug use. *Campbell Systematic Reviews, 7*, 1–95. https://doi.org/10.4073/csr.2013.7.

Littell, J. H., Campbell, M., Green, S., & Toews, B. (2005). Multisystemic therapy for social, emotional, and behavioral problems in youth aged 10–17. *Cochrane Database of Systematic Reviews, 4*, 1–42. https://doi.org/10.1002/14651858.CD004797.pub4.

Lock, J., Agras, W. S., Bryson, S., & Kraemer, H. C. (2005). A comparison of short- and long-term family therapy for adolescent anorexia nervosa. *Journal of the American Academy of Child & Adolescent Psychiatry, 44*, 632–639. https://doi.org/10.1097/01.chi.0000161647.82775.0a

*Lock, J. & Le Grange, D. (2013). *Treatment manual for anorexia nervosa. A family based approach* (2nd ed.). New York, NY: Guilford.

Löfholm, C. A., Olsson, T., Sundell, K., & Hansson, K. (2009). Multisystemic therapy with conduct-disordered young people: Stability of treatment outcomes two years after intake. *Evidence & Policy, 5*, 373–397. https://doi.org/10.1332/174426409X478752

Markus, E., Lange, A., & Pettigrew, T. F. (1990). Effectiveness of family therapy: A meta-analysis. *Journal of Family Therapy, 12*, 205–221.

Moore, A. M., & Crane, D. R. (2014). Relational diagnosis and psychotherapy treatment cost effectiveness. *Contemporary Family Therapy, 36*, 281–299. https://doi.org/10.1007/s10591-013-9277-z

Moore, A. M., Hamilton, S., Crane, D. R., & Fawcett, D. (2011). The influence of professional license type on the outcome of family therapy. *The American Journal of Family Therapy, 39*, 149–161. https://doi.org/10.1080/01926187.2010.530186

Morgan, T. B., Crane, D. R., Moore, A. M., & Eggett, D. L. (2013). The cost of treating substance use disorders: Individual versus family therapy. *Journal of Family Therapy, 35*, 2–23. https://doi.org/10.1111/j.1467-6427.2012.00589.x

Parry, G. D., Crawford, M. J., & Duggan, C. (2016). Iatrogenic harm from psychological therapies – Time to move on. *The British Journal of Psychiatry, 208*, 210–212. https://doi.org/10.1192/bjp.bp.115.163618

Pinquart, M., Oslejsek, B., & Teubert, D. (2016). Efficacy of systemic therapy on adults with mental disorders: A meta-analysis. *Psychotherapy Research, 26*, 241–257. https://doi.org/10.1080/10503307.2014.935830

Pinsof, W., & Wynne, L. (Eds.) (1995). *Family therapy effectiveness: current research and theory.* Special issue on research of the *Journal of Marital and Family Therapy*, Volume 21, Number 4. Alexandria, VA: The American Association for Marriage and Family Therapy.

Retzlaff, R., von Sydow, K., Beher, S., Haun, M. W., & Schweitzer, J. (2013). The efficacy of systemic therapy for internalizing and other disorders of childhood and adolescence: A systematic review of 38 randomized trials. *Family Process, 52*, 619–652. https://doi.org/10.1111/famp.12041

Riedinger, V., Pinquart, M., & Teubert, D. (2017). Effects of systemic therapy on mental health of children and adolescents: A meta-analysis. *Journal of Clinical Child & Adolescent Psychology, 46*, 880–894. https://doi.org/10.1080/15374416.2015.1063427

Rosenthal, R., & Rubin, D. B. (1982). A simple, general purpose display of magnitude of experimental effect. *Journal of Educational Psychology, 74*, 166–169. https://doi.org/10.1037/0022-0663.74.2.166

Santisteban, D. A., Mena, M. P., Muir, J., McCabe, B. E., Abalo, C., & Cummings, A. M. (2015). The efficacy of two adolescent substance abuse treatments and the impact of comorbid depression: Results of a small randomized controlled trial. *Psychiatric Rehabilitation Journal, 38*, 55–64. https://doi.org/10.1037/prj0000106

Santisteban, D. A., Perez-Vidal, A., Coatsworth, J. D., Kurtines, W. M., Schwartz, S. J., LaPerriere, A., & Szapocnik, J. (2003). Efficacy of brief strategic family therapy in modifying Hispanic adolescent behavior problems and substance use. *Journal of Family Psychology, 17*, 121–133. https://doi.org/10.1037/0893-3200.17.1.121

Savignac, J. (2009). *Families, youth and delinquency: The state of knowledge, and family-based juvenile delinquency prevention programs.* Ottawa, ON: National Crime Prevention Centre.

Schmit, E. L., Schmit, M. K., & Lenz, S. (2016). Meta-analysis of solution-focused brief therapy for treating symptoms of internalizing disorders. *Counseling Outcome Research and Evaluation, 7*, 21–39. https://doi.org/10.1177/2150137815623836

Schoenwald, S., Henggeler, S., & Rowland, M. (2015). Multisystemic therapy. In T. Sexton & J. Lebow (Eds.), *Handbook of family therapy* (4th ed., pp. 271–285). New York, NY: Routledge.

Schweitzer, J., & von Schlippe, A. (2015). *Lehrbuch der systemischen Therapie und Beratung II: das störungsspezifische Wissen* (Vol. 2). Göttingen, Germany: Vandenhoeck & Ruprecht.

*Sexton, T. (2011). *Functional family therapy in clinical practice.* New York, NY: Routledge

Sexton, T. (2015). Functional family therapy. In T. Sexton & J. Lebow (Eds.), *Handbook of family therapy* (4th ed., pp. 250–270). New York, NY: Routledge.

Shadish, W. R., & Baldwin, S. A. (2003). Meta-analysis of MFT interventions. *Journal of Marital and Family Therapy, 29*, 547–570. https://doi.org/10.1111/j.1752-0606.2003.tb01694.x

Shadish, W. R., Montgomery, L. M., Wilson, P., Wilson, M. R., Bright, I., & Okwumabua, T. (1993). Effects of family and marital psychotherapies: A meta-analysis. *Journal of Consulting and Clinical Psychology, 61*, 992–1002.

Shazer, D., & Dolan, Y. (2007). *More than miracles: The state of the art of solution-focused brief therapy.* Binghamton, NY: Haworth Press.

Sprenkle, D. (Ed.). (2002). *Effectiveness research in marital and family therapy.* Alexandria, VA: American Association for Marital and Family Therapy.

Sprenkle, D. (Ed.) (2012). Special issue on research of the *Journal of Marital and Family Therapy*, Volume 38, Number 1. Alexandria, VA: The American Association for Marriage and Family Therapy.

Stams, G. J., Dekovic, M., Buist, K., & de Vries, L. (2006). Effectiviteit van oplossingsgerichte korte therapie: Een meta-analyse [Efficacy of solution-focused brief therapy: A meta-analysis]. *Gedragstherapie, 39*, 81–94.

*Stith, S., McCollum, E., & Rosen, K. (2011). *Couples therapy for domestic violence. Finding safe solutions*. Washington, D.C.: American Psychological Association.

Stratton, P. (2016). *The evidence base of family therapy and systemic practice*. Warrington, Cheshire: Association for Family Therapy, UK.

Szapocznik, J., Duff, J., Schwartz, D., Muir, J., & Brown, C. (2015). Brief strategic family therapy treatment for behaviour problem youth: Theory, intervention, research and implementation. In T. Sexton & J. Lebow (Eds.), *Handbook of family therapy* (4th ed., pp. 286–304). New York, NY: Routledge.

*Szapocznik, J., Hervis, O., & Schwartz, S. (2002). Brief strategic family therapy for adolescent drug abuse. Rockville, MD: National Institute for Drug Abuse. Available at http://archives. drugabuse.gov/TXManuals/BSFT/BSFTIndex.html

van der Pol, T. J. M., Hoeve, M., Noom, M. J., Stams, G. J. J. M., Doreleijers, T. A. H., van Domburgh, L., & Vermeiren, R. R. J. M. (2017). The effectiveness of multidimensional family therapy in treating adolescents with multiple behavior problems – A meta-analysis. *Journal of Child Psychology and Psychiatry, 58*, 532–545. https://doi.org/10.1111/jcpp.12685.

van der Stouwe, T., Asscher, J. J., Stams, G. J. M. S., Deković, M., & van der Laan, P. H. (2014). The effectiveness of Multisystemic Therapy (MST): A meta-analysis. *Clinical Psychology Review, 34*, 468–481. https://doi.org/10.1016/j.cpr.2014.06.006

von Sydow, K., Beher, S., Schweitzer, J., & Retzlaff, R. (2010). The efficacy of systemic therapy with adult patients: A meta-content analysis of 38 randomized controlled trials. *Family Process, 49*, 457–485. https://doi.org/10.1111/j.1545-5300.2010.01334.x

von Sydow, K., Retzlaff, R., Beher, S., Haun, M. W., & Schweitzer, J. (2013). The efficacy of systemic therapy for childhood and adolescent externalizing disorders: A systematic review of 47 RCTs. *Family Process, 52*, 576–618. https://doi.org/10.1111/famp.12047.

Wampold, B. E., Mondin, G. W., Moody, M., Stich, F., Benson, K., & Ahn, H.-n. (1997). A meta-analysis of outcome studies comparing bona fide psychotherapies: Empirically, "all must have prizes.". *Psychological Bulletin, 122*, 203–215. https://doi.org/10.1037/0033-2909.122.3.203

Zhang, A., Franklin, C., Currin-McCulloch, J., Park, S., & Kim, J. (2018). The effectiveness of strength-based, solution-focused brief therapy in medical settings: A systematic review and meta-analysis of randomized controlled trials. *Journal of Behavioral Medicine, 41*, 139–151. https://doi.org/10.1007/s10865-017-9888-1

Zhang, W., Zhang, J., Song, W., Han, H., & Xu, L. (2017). A randomized single-blind controlled study of systemic family therapy on 186 patients with schizophrenia [in Chinese]. *Chinese Journal of Clinicians, 11*, 7.

The Effectiveness of Three Psychotherapies of Different Type and Length in the Treatment of Patients Suffering from Anxiety Disorders

Paul Knekt, Olavi Lindfors, Erkki Heinonen, Timo Maljanen, Esa Virtala, and Tommi Härkänen

Highlights

- Persons with non-comorbid anxiety disorder are a group of patients for whom short-term and cost-effective treatments can be applied.
- Short-term psychodynamic psychotherapy which is not anxiety disorder specific may be less effective than solution-focused therapy and long-term psychodynamic psychotherapy for these patients.
- A subgroup of patients with non-comorbid anxiety disorder require additional therapy for gaining remission.

Introduction

For a patient with a given mental disorder, determining the optimal type and duration of psychotherapy often requires considering multiple factors, with psychiatric comorbidity being one of the most common (Laaksonen, Lindfors, Knekt, & Aalberg, 2012; Newby, McKinnon, Kuyken, Gilbody, & Dalgleish, 2015). Theoretical (Gabbard, Gunderson, & Fonagy, 2002; Perry & Bond, 2009) and empirical (Falkenstrom, Grant, Broberg, & Sandell, 2007; Sandell et al., 2000) grounds suggest long-term therapies facilitate psychological growth, adaptation, and symptom reduction even years after treatment termination, which may be needed in the treatment of patients with relatively enduring and more severe problems as typically reflected in psychiatric comorbidity. Accordingly, it has been

P. Knekt (✉) · O. Lindfors · E. Heinonen · E. Virtala · T. Härkänen
Finnish Institute for Health and Welfare, Helsinki, Finland
e-mail: paul.knekt@thl.fi

T. Maljanen
Social Insurance Institution, Helsinki, Finland

© Springer Nature Switzerland AG 2020
M. Ochs et al. (eds.), *Systemic Research in Individual, Couple, and Family Therapy and Counseling*, European Family Therapy Association Series,
https://doi.org/10.1007/978-3-030-36560-8_19

shown that long-term psychodynamic psychotherapy more effectively reduces symptoms and improves work ability than short-term psychotherapies in the treatment of patients with "complex" mental disorders consisting of the comorbid conditions of depression, anxiety, and/or personality pathology (Knekt et al., 2016; Leichsenring & Rabung, 2011). In patient groups with lesser psychiatric severity, dysfunction, and psychological complexity, the superiority of LPP in comparison to less intensive and shorter therapies may not be as apparent.

Offering the least intensive intervention required for recovery is also among the principles of stepped care treatment guidelines (National Institute for Health and Care Excellence (NICE), 2011). However, since comorbidity is often the rule rather than the exception (Newby et al., 2015), it is highly relevant both for clinical decision-making and organizing services to identify the patient groups where the effectiveness of short-term therapy is likely to be as effective as long-term therapy.

The prevalent first-line psychotherapeutic treatments recommended for patients with some anxiety disorder are cognitive-behavioral short-term therapies, supported by higher-level evidence than other short- or long-term therapies, in which there is a lack of clinical trials (Bandelow, Lichte, Rudolf, Wiltink, & Beutel, 2014). Psychodynamic therapies, which in treatment recommendations are usually considered second-line options, stress the importance of early conflictual relationship experiences, characterized often by conscious and unconscious fears of abandonment. These are understood to result in avoiding certain experiences and avoiding the expression of one's feelings and wishes and thus create the foundation for clinical anxiety symptoms (Busch, Milrod, Singer, & Aronson, 2011; Luborsky, 1984). In short-term psychodynamic psychotherapy (SPP), the aim of exploring intensively a dynamically central conflictual problem area is to facilitate emotional insight and self-understanding by linking past experiences to the present anxiety symptoms, while in LPP, a wider scope of related problems can be worked through (Gabbard, 1992, 2004) suggesting that SPP may better suffice for patients with milder symptoms. Recent findings based on the effectiveness of diverse short-term therapies in routine care, i.e., in treating patients with lesser psychiatric complexity, have shown relatively good results of psychodynamic brief therapies, comparable to cognitive therapies using a more directive orientation (Holmqvist, Strom, & Foldemo, 2014), whereas little is known of comparative effects of other treatment orientations during a long-term follow-up.

In contrast to the psychodynamic psychotherapies, the outcome of solution-focused therapy (SFT), to our knowledge, has not previously been studied in a clinical trial, in comparison to other psychotherapeutic treatment models in the treatment of anxiety disorders. In a patient population with depressive and/or anxiety disorders, the outcomes of SFT have been comparable to those treated by SPP during a long-term follow-up (Knekt, Lindfors, Sares-Jäske, Virtala, & Härkänen, 2013). One randomized trial has suggested that a specific resource-oriented focus, based on SFT principles, is associated with greater reduction of psychiatric symptoms by the end of therapy in patients with social anxiety disorder when treated by a combined model of SFT and cognitive therapy (CT) versus traditional CT, whereas in more long-term follow-up, no differences in outcome were seen (Willutzki, Neumann, Haas, & Schulte, 2004; Willutzki, Teismann, & Schulte, 2012). SFT does not base its technique on assumptions regarding the etiology of the disorder. Instead, it focuses on identifying exceptions in encountering the problem, and/or examples of dealing with it effectively, thereby enhancing the person's resources to find new practical solutions in his or her situation (de Shazer et al., 1986; Trepper et al., 2014). SFT also differs from psychodynamic psychotherapies in being carried out with lesser frequency, as it is not predicated on an intense patient-therapist relationship as part of the treatment strategy. This therapy might thus especially suffice for persons with anxiety disorders only, for whom symptom severity and personality-related problems are milder than in complex anxiety and depressive disorder (Penninx et al., 2011).

There is still is a lack of information on the effectiveness of short-term therapies having a different theoretical conception in comparison with long-term therapies in patients with relatively benign disorder. We therefore decided to compare the clinical outcomes of SPP and SFT with that of LPP during a 5-year follow-up in the specific diagnostic group of patients suffering from anxiety disorders as their only axis I mental disorder.

Methods

Subjects and Study Design

Outpatients from psychiatric services in the Helsinki region, aged 20–46 years, and having long-standing (>1 year) depressive or anxiety disorders causing work dysfunction were considered eligible for the Helsinki Psychotherapy Study (HPS) (Knekt & Lindfors, 2004). Patients with psychotic disorder, severe personality disorder, adjustment disorder, bipolar disorder, or substance abuse were excluded. A total of 459 eligible patients were referred to the study between June 1994 and June 2000. Of these, 133 refused to participate. Using a randomized design, the remaining 326 patients were assigned to 1 of 3 treatment groups: solution-focused therapy (SFT, $N = 97$) and short-term psychodynamic (SPP, $N = 101$) and long-term psychodynamic psychotherapy (LPP, $N = 128$). Patients gave written informed consent, and the study was approved by the Helsinki University Central Hospital's ethics council.

At baseline, 50 patients (SFT, $N = 13$; SPP, $N = 22$; LPP, $N = 15$) suffered from non-comorbid anxiety disorders, i.e., having no other axis I disorders (Table 1). The most usual anxiety disorder diagnoses were social phobia and anxiety disorder not otherwise specified (NOS). Altogether 20% of the patients had non-severe personality disorder on axis II, most usually of the NOS type. At baseline, the mean level of psychiatric symptoms of the patients was in the clinical range (Knekt & Lindfors, 2004). In comparison to the HPS patients with depressive and comorbid axis I disorders, the anxiety disorder patients had lesser psychiatric severity and dysfunction. Of the participants, one allocated to SFT, one to SPP, and four to LPP did not receive the treatment (Fig. 1). Of the patients starting the assigned therapy, none assigned to SFT, two to SPP, and three to LPP discontinued the treatment prematurely. The patients were mainly women (66%), and the mean age of the patients was 32 years (SD = 6).

Of the patients allocated to the therapy, the participation rate in the assessments was high, being 76% at the 5-year follow-up point. The participation, however, varied considerably between therapies (i.e., SFT 77%, SPP 68%, and LPP 87%).

Table 1 Number of axis I and II diagnoses among patients with anxiety disorders only, by therapy group

	Therapy group		
Diagnosis	SFT	SPP	LPP
Axis I			
Social phobia	4	5	6
Generalized anxiety disorder	2	3	0
Panic disorder	2	3	2
Specific phobia	1	2	1
Obsessive-compulsive disorder	1	1	0
NOS	3	8	6
Any anxiety disorders	13	22	15
Axis II			
Cluster B personality	1	0	0
Cluster C personality	0	1	0
NOS	1	6	2
Any axis II disorder	2	7	2
No axis II diagnosis	11	15	13

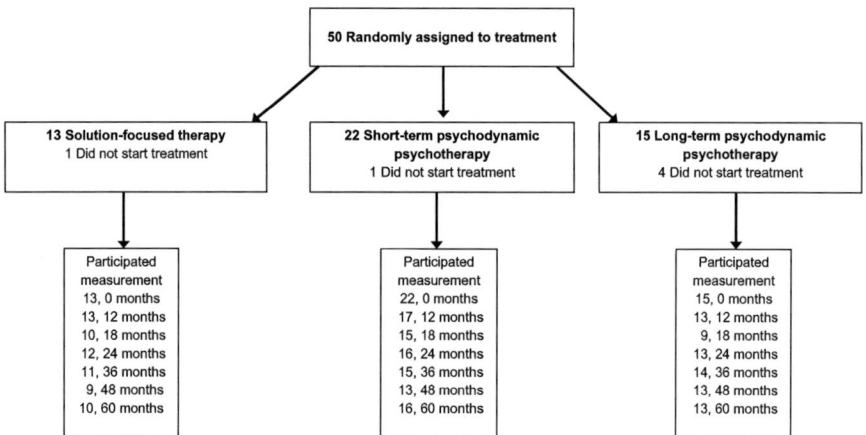

Fig. 1 Flow chart of the patients with anxiety disorder

Therapies and Therapists

SFT (de Shazer et al., 1986) included 12 therapy sessions and SPP (Malan, 1976) 20 therapy sessions, with both therapies lasting about half a year. The frequency of therapy sessions differed between these short-term therapies, being once a week in SPP and once every second or third week in SFT. LPP was open-ended, lasting about 3 years and consisting of about 240 sessions, with a frequency of usually twice a week (Gabbard, 2004). Only SFT was manualized. The psychodynamic therapies were conducted in accordance with clinical practice, where the therapists might modify their interventions according to the patient's needs within the respective frameworks. All the therapists had received standard training and were experienced: The mean number of years of work experience was 9 in the short-term and over 15 years in the long-term therapies.

Assessments

Psychiatric diagnoses on axes I and II (American Psychiatric Association, 1994) were assessed at baseline using a semi-structured interview (Knekt & Lindfors, 2004).

The outcome measures, covering different measures of psychiatric symptoms, work ability, need for treatment (auxiliary treatment), and remission, were administered prior to the start of treatment and at 6 pre-chosen time points (i.e., 1, 1.5, 2, 3, 4, and 5 years) during a 5-year follow-up from the start of treatment.

The assessment of psychiatric symptoms and work ability were based on self-report questionnaires. Psychiatric symptoms were assessed using the Symptom Checklist (SCL-90) (Derogatis, Lipman, & Covi, 1973) and the Beck Depression Inventory (BDI) (Beck, Steer, & Carbin, 1988; Beck, Ward, Mendelson, Mock, & Erbaugh, 1961). Work ability was assessed using the Perceived Psychological Functioning (PPF) (Lehtinen et al., 1991), the Work-subscale (SAS-Work) of the Social Adjustment Scale (SAS-SR) (Weissman & Bothwell, 1976), and the Work Ability Index (WAI) (Ilmarinen, Tuomi, & Klockars, 1997; Tuomi, Ilmarinen, Jahkola, Katajarinne, & Tulkki, 1998), with the question on current employment status collected by a single item included in a follow-up questionnaire developed in the project.

Information on the use of psychotropic medication (antidepressant, anxiolytic, neuroleptic, and psychiatric combination medication), additional psychotherapy (individual short-term or long-term, group, couple, or family, or others), and hospitalization for psychiatric reasons were continuously assessed during the 5-year follow-up using questionnaires and nationwide public health registers (Knekt et al., 2011). Remission from psychiatric symptoms (measured by SCL) at every measurement point of the follow-up was defined as a 50% reduction of symptoms in comparison to the baseline level or a measurement value lower than the remission level (i.e., SCL-90-ANX < 0.9, SCL-DEP < 0.9, and SCL-GSI < 0.9) (Holi, Marttunen, & Aalberg, 2003) and simultaneously a lack of considerable auxiliary treatment (use of psychotropic medication for at least 6 months, psychotherapy for at least 20 sessions, or hospitalization due to psychiatric reason) at the measurement point.

The direct costs taken into account in this study due to the treatment of mental disorders comprised costs accruing from (1) protocol-based and additional SFT, SPP, and LPP sessions; (2) auxiliary psychotherapy sessions (individual short- or long-term therapy, group, couple, or family therapy, or others), reflecting the insufficiency of the protocol-based therapies; (3) outpatient visits due to mental disorders; (4) psychotropic medication; (5) inpatient care due to mental disorders; and (6) travelling due to therapy visits (Maljanen et al., 2016).

Primary measures were SCL-90-GSI, WAI, remission from psychiatric symptoms (measured by SCL), and direct costs.

Statistical Methods

The effectiveness of the three therapies was studied in a design with repeated mea-surements of the outcome variables mainly using "intention-to-treat" (ITT) analyses (Härkänen et al., 2016; Härkänen, Knekt, Virtala, & Lindfors, 2005; Knekt, Lindfors, Härkänen, et al., 2008). Linear mixed models were used (Verbeke & Molenberghs, 1997), and model-adjusted statistics using predictive margins were calculated for different time points and treatment groups (Graubard & Korn, 1999; Lee, 1981). The delta method was used for calculating confidence intervals (Migon & Gamerman, 1999). Statistical significance was tested using the Wald test.

The basic model included the main effects of follow-up time, the treatment group, and the first-order interaction of time and treatment group. A full model was also adjusted for the specific diagnoses of anxiety disorders and personality disor-ders. Both models were further adjusted for the baseline level of each outcome measure in a completed model. The results of the full model were presented when the model could be estimated.

The costs of the three therapy groups were compared by calculating the annual mean costs as well as the mean costs for the whole 5-year follow-up period. The costs were not discounted (Maljanen et al., 2016).

The statistical analyses were performed using SAS software 9.3 (SAS Institute Inc., 2011).

Results

Psychiatric Symptoms and Work Ability

Changes in *psychiatric symptoms* during the 5-year follow-up are presented in Table 2. A statistically significant decrease from baseline to the end of the follow-up was seen in all measures and in all therapy groups. The average change in the four psychiatric symptom measures varied from 52.6% to 75.6%, from 29.0% to 53.0%, and from 48.5% to 65.0% for the SFT, SPP, and LPP groups, respectively. During the first year of follow-up, no statistically significant differences in the outcomes between the three therapies were noted. During the following 3 years, psychiatric symptoms were statistically significantly more effectively reduced in LPP and SFT than in SPP for all symptom measures considered. For the primary measure SCL-90-GSI, the mean difference between SPP and SFT was 39.7% (95% confidence inter-val (CI) = 4.8, 74.7) and between SPP and LPP 47.7% (CI = 13.4, 81.9) at the 4-year of follow-up point. No significant differences in symptom reduction were seen between LPP and SFT.

Changes in *work ability* are presented in Table 3. All three measures were signifi-cantly improved during follow-up for all three therapy groups. The average changes varied from 16.2% to 25.5%, from 9.2% to 15.7%, and from 9.3% to 19.1%, for SFT,

Table 2 The effectiveness of short- and long-term psychotherapy on psychiatric symptoms during the 5-year follow-up: the ITT model

Variable	Follow-up (years)	SFT N	SFT Mean	SPP N	SPP Mean	LPP N	LPP Mean	Mean difference[a] SPP-SFT	SPP-LPP	LPP-SFT
SCL-90-GSI	0	13	1.11	21	1.13	15	1.09			
	1	12	0.59	16	0.82	11	0.73	0.23	0.05	0.18
	1.5	10	0.39	15	0.84	9	0.66	**0.46**[b]	0.13	0.34
	2	11	0.65	15	0.93	11	0.73	0.33	0.15	0.18
	3	10	0.67	15	0.84	10	0.58	0.15	0.21	−0.06
	4	9	0.47	13	0.76	12	0.36	**0.30**[b]	**0.36**[b]	−0.06
	5	10	0.51	15	0.71	13	0.44	0.23	0.28	−0.06
Change (%)	0–5		53.7[c]		37.0[c]		60.1[c]			
SCL-90-DEP	0	13	1.61	21	1.55	15	1.46			
	1	12	0.83	16	1.13	11	0.86	0.34	0.14	0.20
	1.5	10	0.60	15	1.16	9	0.88	**0.61**[b]	0.16	0.45
	2	11	0.91	15	1.31	11	0.98	0.44	0.24	0.19
	3	10	0.96	15	1.08	10	0.81	0.23	0.22	0.01
	4	9	0.73	13	1.06	12	0.47	0.37	**0.48**[b]	−0.11
	5	10	0.76	15	1.10	13	0.75	0.40	0.29	0.11
Change (%)	0–5		52.6[c]		29.0[c]		48.5[c]			
SCL-90-ANX	0	13	1.30	21	1.36	15	1.14			
	1	12	0.66	16	0.85	11	0.58	0.21	0.15	0.06
	1.5	10	0.47	15	0.91	9	0.65	**0.48**[b]	0.12	0.37
	2	11	0.44	15	1.03	11	0.69	**0.57**[b]	0.20	0.37
	3	10	0.68	15	0.96	10	0.48	0.30	0.36	−0.06
	4	9	0.36	13	0.64	12	0.38	0.34	0.19	0.15
	5	10	0.43	15	0.64	13	0.40	0.26	0.18	0.08
Change (%)	0–5		66.8[c]		53.0[c]		65.0[c]			
BDI	0	13	14.4	22	13.7	15	11.2			
	1	12	6.5	16	8.2	11	6.9	2.2	0.20	2.0
	1.5	10	3.8	15	9.3	9	6.1	5.9	2.4	3.5
	2	11	4.1	15	9.8	11	5.6	**6.1**[b]	3.5	2.6
	3	10	6.5	15	8.5	11	2.3	2.2	**5.3**[b]	−3.1
	4	9	5.4	13	6.9	12	2.6	1.5	3.4	−1.9
	5	10	3.5	15	7.2	13	4.3	3.7	2.2	1.5
Change (%)	0–5		75.6[c]		47.0[c]		61.5[c]			

[a]Difference further adjusted for baseline of respective outcome variable
[b]A statistically significant difference occurred between the therapy groups
[c]A statistically significant change occurred between baseline and the 5-year follow-up point

SPP, and LPP, respectively. SPP showed statistically significantly less improvement than SFT at some time points for the outcome measures SAS-Work and the primary measure WAI. At the end of follow-up, WAI was 12.0% (CI = 9.2, 23.0) more improved in the SFT group than in the SPP group.

Table 3 The effectiveness of short- and long-term psychotherapy on work ability during the 5-year follow-up: the ITT model

Variable	Follow-up (years)	SFT		SPP		LPP		Mean difference[a]		
		N	Mean	N	Mean	N	Mean	SPP-SFT	SPP-LPP	LPP-SFT
PPF	0	13	22.3	22	22.0	15	22.6			
	1	12	18.5	16	19.4	10	19.7	0.97	−0.75	1.73
	2	11	18.1	15	20.8	10	18.8	2.98	1.68	1.30
	3	10	17.9	15	19.8	9	16.4	2.04	2.76	−0.72
	4	9	16.9	13	18.5	9	17.6	1.26	0.80	0.46
	5	9	18.2	14	18.5	13	18.3	0.92	0.10	0.82
Change (%)	0–5		18.7[c]		15.7[c]		19.1[c]			
SAS-Work	0	13	1.92	22	1.82	15	1.96			
	1	11	1.68	16	1.84	10	1.82	0.21	0.07	0.14
	2	11	1.63	15	1.86	10	1.77	0.30	0.13	0.17
	3	10	1.70	15	1.73	10	1.62	0.10	0.16	−0.06
	4	9	1.40	13	1.63	9	1.50	**0.28**[b]	0.23	0.05
	5	10	1.61	14	1.58	13	1.67	0.03	−0.02	0.05
Change (%)	0–5		16.2		13.3[c]		14.7[c]			
WAI	0	13	35.5	22	36.1	15	38.4			
	1	12	40.3	16	39.2	10	39.3	−1.15	0.24	−1.39
	2	11	44.3	15	38.5	10	41.0	**−5.14**[b]	−2.10	−3.04
	3	10	42.5	15	38.7	9	41.8	−3.61	−3.02	−0.58
	4	9	42.9	13	40.3	9	42.1	−2.11	−1.97	−0.13
	5	10	44.3	14	39.3	13	42.0	**−4.70**[b]	−2.98	−1.72
Change (%)	0–5		25.5[c]		9.2		9.3			

[a]Difference further adjusted for baseline of respective outcome variable
[b]A statistically significant difference occurred between the therapy groups
[c]A statistically significant change occurred between baseline and the 5-year follow-up point

Need for Treatment

At the end of follow-up, the use of auxiliary psychiatric treatment (psychotropic medication, psychotherapy, or hospitalization) was relatively low (i.e., 9% in the SFT and 36% in the SPP and the LPP groups) (Fig. 2a). This difference between SFT and the psychodynamic psychotherapies was mainly due to statistically significantly greater use of psychotropic medication in the psychodynamic therapy groups (i.e., 0%, 32%, and 34% in the SFT, SPP, and LPP groups, respectively) (Fig. 2b). The patients receiving LPP used no auxiliary therapy during the 2 last years of follow-up (Fig. 2c). One hospitalization for psychiatric reasons was observed in the SPP group during the second to fourth year of follow-up.

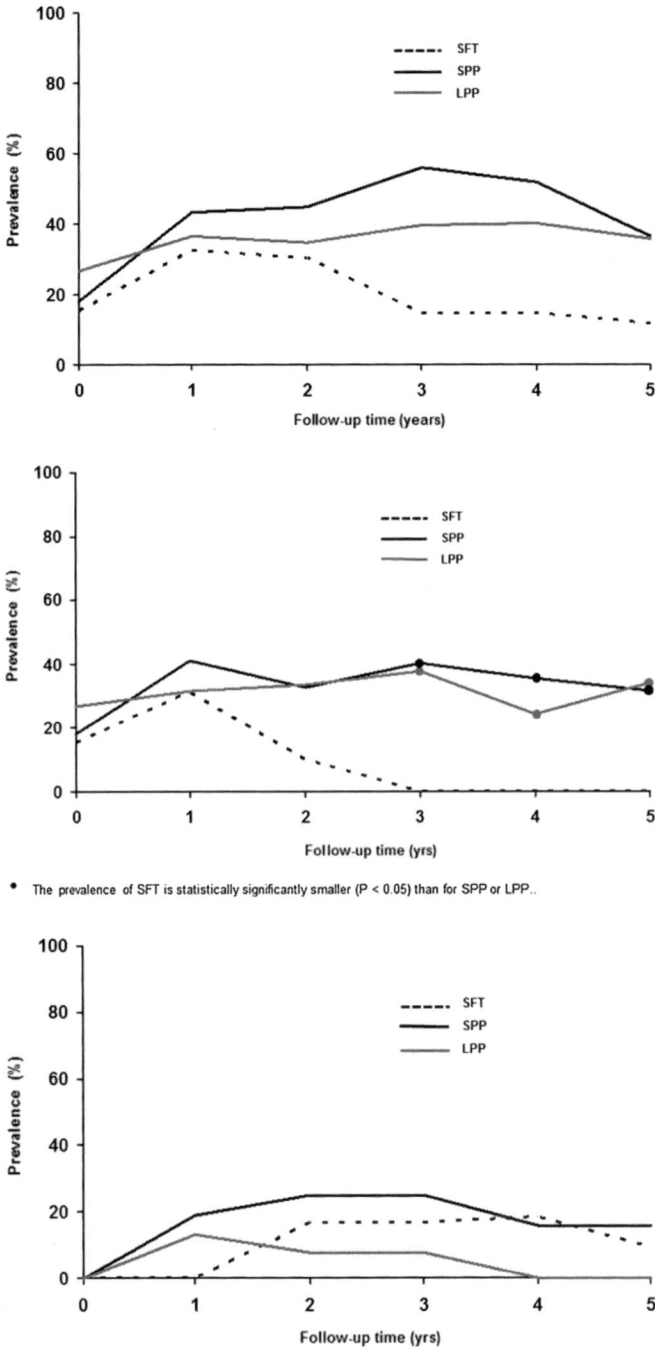

Fig. 2 (**a**) Prevalence of auxiliary psychiatric treatment (i.e., psychotropic medication, additional psychotherapy, and hospitalization for psychiatric reasons) during the 5-year follow-up. (**b**) Prevalence of psychotropic medication during the 5-year follow-up. (**c**) Prevalence of auxiliary psychotherapy during the 5-year follow-up

Study of the cumulative auxiliary use of therapy during the entire follow-up showed twice as many therapy users in the SPP (35%) as in the SFT (17%), although no statistical significance was reached (Table 4). The mean number of auxiliary therapy sessions was seven- to tenfold in the short-term therapy groups in comparison to LPP (Table 5).

Table 4 Cumulative prevalence (%) of auxiliary therapy at the 5-year follow-up point

Therapy	N	n	%	P-value*
All				
SPP	20	7	35	0.45
LPP	15	3	20	
SFT	12	2	17	
Short-term				
SPP	20	2	10	0.55
LPP	15	1	7	
SFT	12	0	0	
Long-term				
SPP	20	5	25	0.26
LPP	15	1	7	
SFT	12	1	8	

N = number of patients at risk (N = 47) after exclusion of those with missing data (N = 3)
n = number of patients receiving auxiliary therapy (n = 12)
*P-value for difference between therapy groups

Table 5 Cumulative mean number of sessions among users of auxiliary therapy at the 5-year follow-up point

Therapy group	N	Mean	Range	P-value*
All				
SPP	7	142	24–520	0.46
LPP	3	20	3–31	
SFT	2	209	14–404	
Short-term				
SPP	2	28	24–32	0.91
LPP	1	27	–	
SFT	0	–	–	
Long-term				
SPP	5	188	42–520	0.46
LPP	1	31	–	
SFT	1	404	–	

N = number of patients receiving auxiliary therapy (N = 12) after exclusion of those with missing data (N = 3)
*P-value for difference between therapy groups

Remission

The remission rate increased in all therapy groups and for all three outcome measures (Table 6). There was significantly less improvement in SPP in comparison to SFT and LPP in several measurement points. SFT gave about 40% higher prevalence of remission from psychiatric symptoms than SPP during three consecutive years of follow-up; the prevalence differences between SFT and SPP were 0.42, 0.47, and 0.39 for the second, third, and fourth follow-up year, respectively. No significant differences were seen between SFT and LPP. The remission rates at the end of follow-up did not statistically significantly differ between the three therapy groups (78%, 56%, and 75%, for SFT, SPP, and LPP, respectively).

Cost-Effectiveness

The average total undiscounted direct costs of persons belonging to the LPP group (EUR 19755) were approximatively three times as high as those of persons belonging to the SFT group (EUR 6314) or SPP group (EUR 6265). This significant difference

Table 6 Prevalence of remission by therapy group and year of follow-up: the ITT model

Remission variable[a]	Follow-up (years)	SFT		SPP		LPP		Mean difference[b]		
		N	Prev.	N	Prev.	N	Prev.	SPP-SFT	SPP-LPP	LPP-SFT
General symptoms	0	13	0.31	21	0.24	15	0.33			
	1	12	0.75	16	0.58	11	0.45	−0.24	0.08	0.31
	2	11	0.83	15	0.45	11	0.67	−0.42	−0.23	−0.19
	3	10	0.74	15	0.22	10	0.64	−0.47[c]	−0.32	−0.15
	4	9	0.72	13	0.30	12	0.76	−0.39[c]	−0.41[c]	0.02
	5	10	0.78	15	0.56	13	0.75	−0.22	−0.16	−0.06
Depression	0	13	0.23	21	0.24	15	0.13			
	1	12	0.48	16	0.30	11	0.49	−0.21	−0.17	−0.04
	2	11	0.73	15	0.09	11	0.68	−0.67[c]	−0.56[c]	−0.12
	3	10	0.63	15	0.21	10	0.53	−0.45[c]	−0.30	−0.15
	4	9	0.68	13	0.22	12	0.67	−0.51[c]	−0.48[c]	−0.03
	5	10	0.51	15	0.41	13	0.64	−0.13	−0.21	0.08
Anxiety	0	13	0.29	21	0.24	15	0.21			
	1	12	0.81	16	0.60	11	0.68	−0.23	−0.11	−0.12
	2	11	0.81	15	0.57	11	0.67	−0.22	−0.09	−0.13
	3	10	0.58	15	0.37	10	0.64	−0.17	−0.26	0.09
	4	9	0.80	13	0.42	12	0.76	−0.34	−0.33	−0.02
	5	10	0.78	15	0.62	13	0.67	−0.16	−0.06	−0.11

[a]The remission variables were based on respective symptom variables, SCL-90-GSI, SCL-90-DEP and SCL-90-ANX, and use of considerable auxiliary treatment
[b]Difference further adjusted for baseline of respective outcome variable
[c]A statistically significant difference occurred between the therapy groups

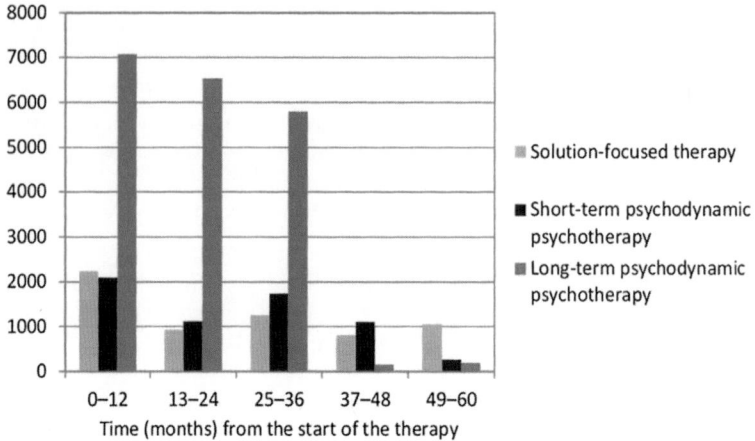

Fig. 3 The mean annual total undiscounted direct costs (EUR) during the 5-year follow-up period

was mainly due to the greater total costs of the LPP sessions. The cost difference between SFT and SPP was small, and in both groups, the main cost driver was auxiliary psychotherapy. The costs of all groups were highest when the study therapies were in progress, i.e., during the first year in the SFT and SPP groups and during the first 3 years in the LPP group (Fig. 3). After LPP had been terminated, the costs of the LPP group decreased remarkably, and during the fourth and fifth year, they were somewhat smaller than those of the SFT or SPP patients. Because of the small differences in effectiveness of SFT and LPP, the former can be considered more cost-effective.

Discussion

General Findings

This study compared the outcomes of two short-term therapies and long-term psychodynamic psychotherapy (LPP) among patients with anxiety disorders as the only axis I mental disorder. The main finding was that SFT, the least intensive therapy with the lowest number of sessions of the therapies studied, appeared to produce outcomes comparable with LPP, the most intensive and longest therapy. This new finding demonstrates the potential of a resource-oriented approach in the treatment of patients with anxiety disorders only. It is in line with the claim that resource-oriented therapeutic models may be needed to challenge the more traditional psychotherapeutic deficit models that concentrate on working with underlying conflicts or changing developmentally based maladaptive thinking and behavior (Priebe, Omer, Giacco, & Slade, 2014). Whereas a previous study on patients with social anxiety disorder with relatively frequent comorbidities found no additional long-term benefit of a resource-oriented focus when comparing a combined SFT-CT to traditional CT (Willutzki et al., 2012), our study suggests that the lack of comorbidity of anxiety disorder patients may increase the potential of SFT in the long run. The results suggesting inability of LPP to show benefits significantly greater than SFT in symptoms and work ability indicate that the theoretical and therapeutic model behind it – based on identifying, exploring, and working through developmentally induced vulnerability to anxiety – is not essential to achieving sustained changes in this less complex patient group, at least on these outcome domains (Gabbard, 1992). Greater benefits might, however, be expressed in other outcome domains (Gibbons et al., 2009; Lindfors et al., 2015).

No differences between the groups emerged during the first year after the treatments started. These findings differ from those observed in the total sample of the Helsinki Psychotherapy Study, where SFT and SPP both produced faster decreases in symptoms and increase in work ability than LPP (Knekt, Lindfors, Härkänen, et al., 2008; Knekt, Lindfors, Laaksonen, et al., 2008). Thus it may be that anxiety patients with relatively benign intrapsychic and interpersonal problems (Knekt & Lindfors, 2004) did not, even in LPP, engage in or need thorough exploration of such problems during the first year of therapy as patients with more heterogeneous problems – for whom, in turn, an intense treatment such as LPP often prolongs the experience of early reduction of manifest symptoms, albeit leading to greater long-term symptom reduction and more improved work ability (Knekt et al., 2013).

Our study also gave preliminary evidence of potentially greater benefits of SFT in contrast to SPP in this patient group. As a previous meta-analysis indicated that the effectiveness of SPP in the treatment of anxiety disorders does not differ from that of alternative therapies (Keefe, McCarthy, Dinger, Zilcha-Mano, & Barber, 2014), our preliminary finding indicates the need for further research to understand more deeply what specific treatment strategies and aspects of the therapy process of SFT were considered by the patients as more helpful than in SPP. The fact that SPP has only recently been developed as a manualized treatment for anxiety disorders (Busch et al., 2011; Leichsenring et al., 2014) and has shown comparable effectiveness to cognitive therapy (Leichsenring et al., 2014; Leichsenring, Beutel, & Leibing, 2007) may account for the poorer response of SPP in this study, since here a non-manualized model was used. Furthermore, the exclusion of patients with comorbid depressive disorders and the relatively lower severity of interpersonal problems of these patients in comparison to the HPS total sample (Knekt & Lindfors, 2004) may account for the outcome differences found between SPP and SFT (Wiltink et al., 2016). In line with our findings and the hypotheses that the lack of comorbidity and specific anxiety-related technique may be relevant for the differences found between SFT and SPP, Rakowska (2011) has shown that a variation of solution-focused therapy, brief strategic therapy, was more effective in reducing symptoms of anxiety in comparison to minimal supportive therapy in patients with anxiety disorder only but not in those with comorbidity.

Additional differences were observed between both of the psychodynamic therapies and SFT in the use of additional psychiatric treatment. Remarkably, no patients were on psychotropic medication in the SFT group at the final 5-year follow-up, in contrast to about a third of patients in SPP and LPP. These differences may be due to the SFT approach, which strongly guides the patient to rely on his/her own decision-making abilities and expertise rather than following the medical deficit model (de Shazer, 1985) and corresponding pharmacological help. It may also be due to other unknown differences in therapists' advice and patients' treatment-seeking behavior after the therapies.

A strong argument, from the societal perspective, for SFT for having potential as a cost-effective treatment in treating patients with anxiety disorders was its overall effectiveness, comparable to LPP, but with significantly lower costs. In case these findings can be replicated and generalized, an average net cost saving during the 5-year follow-up of more than EUR 13,000 per patient in comparison to LPP suggests that the brief resource-oriented model of SFT might be a favorable option from an economic and public health perspective and that LPP would apparently be more appropriate for patients with more complex disorders.

The majority of treatment guidelines based on clinical trials on the effectiveness of psychotherapies for anxiety disorders highlight the beneficial effects of brief cognitive-behavioral treatment (CBT) models, including exposure techniques (Cuijpers et al., 2016) and recently also suggest comparable effects of low-dose Internet-based vs. face-to-face therapy programs (Anderson, Cuijpers, Carlbring, Riper, & Hedman, 2014). There are thus several options of potentially cost-effective short-term treatments for this patient group and accordingly a need for additional studies comparing the effectiveness of the CBT treatments with SFT and with the more recent applications of SPP and other short-term therapy modalities while covering outcomes more comprehensively (Knekt et al., 2015).

Methodological Considerations

A strength of this randomized clinical trial comparing the outcomes of short- and long-term psychotherapy was the exceptionally long follow-up, with ten repeated measurements of the outcome variables during a 5-year follow-up. The inclusion of information about the use of auxiliary treatment during the entire follow-up is also of importance, as it gave the possibility to evaluate the net remission from psychiatric symptoms.

The main limitation of this study is the fact that only 50 patients with anxiety disorders as the only axis I disorder were included in this study. Given the small number of patients, divided into three therapy groups (SFT = 13, SPP = 21, LPP = 15), the associations or lack of them may be due to chance findings. Additionally, the fact that every fourth of the patients randomized to LPP did not start the treatment compared to the average 5% in the short-term therapy groups – although initial preference for short- vs. long-term therapy was rarely mentioned – may potentially bias the results despite the difference being taken into account in the statistical analyses as a potential confounding factor. Thus no firm conclusion about a lack of differences in the effectiveness of SFT and LPP can be made.

Due to the small number of patients, those with personality disorder could not be excluded, which may have favored LPP, which is often considered necessary for working through pervasive personality-related problems (Leichsenring & Rabung, 2011; Lindfors et al., 2015). Similarly, due to the small number of patients, it was not possible to separately investigate the effects of the therapies in different anxiety disorder subgroups. However, adjustment for differences in anxiety and personality disorders performed apparently has excluded the possibility for bias.

The focus of this study on patients with anxiety disorders as the only axis I disorder is based on a disorder-specific approach that has long been the dominant approach in psychiatric research (Newby et al., 2015). However, it has practical limitations, such as not considering the high degree of comorbidity of different anxiety disorders (Andrews, Slade, & Issakidis, 2002) or the comorbidity of anxiety and depressive disorder, which is generally between 30% and 80% (Brown, Campbell, Lehman, Grisham, & Mancill, 2001; Moffitt et al., 2007), being 28% in the HPS total sample (Knekt & Lindfors, 2004). Therefore, as comorbidity is associated with greater severity and a poorer prognosis, a more complete picture of the potential of SFT, SPP, and LPP in the treatment of anxiety disorders as a whole needs to be complemented by studies of comorbid conditions. Furthermore, unavoidable general weaknesses in this study were that, for ethical reasons, it was not possible to measure effectiveness using a control group; the lack of manuals for the psychodynamic therapies used, and the lack of blindness in the assessments (Knekt, Lindfors, Härkänen, et al., 2008).

Moreover, because of the randomized design and patient selection based initially on the presence of a mood or an anxiety disorder and at least moderate level of symptoms, different patients' psychological suitability for the different therapies could not be taken into account when allocating the therapies. This possibly underestimated especially the effectiveness of the short-term therapies, which may require a considered selection of patients who are capable of recovering with brief treatment (Laaksonen et al., 2012).

This study suggests that SFT is more cost-effective than psychodynamic psychotherapies, being either as costly as SPP but more effective or as effective as LPP but less costly in the treatment of patients suffering from non-comorbid anxiety disorders. The therapy alone, however, does not guarantee remission. The incomplete effect of the therapy may be compensated for by additive therapy or use of psychiatric medication. To obtain deeper insight into which type of therapy to use, further research should be carried out as well in large-scale effectiveness studies as in naturalistic studies aiming at identifying individual suitability factors, which would inform on the optimal type and length of psychotherapy.

Acknowledgements This study was supported by a grant from the Academy of Finland (grant no. 138876); the Finnish Cultural Foundation; the Deutsche Gesellschaft für Systemische Therapie, Betratung und Familietherapie (DGSF); and the Systemische Gesellschaft (SG). The foundations had no role in the design, analysis or writing of this article.

The statistical analyses were carried out by Mr. Julius Rissanen.

References

American Psychiatric Association. (1994). *Diagnostic and statistical manual of mental disorders DSM-IV* (4th ed.). Washington, DC: APA.

Anderson, G., Cuijpers, P., Carlbring, P., Riper, H., & Hedman, E. (2014). Guided Internet-based vs. face-to-face cognitive behavior therapy for psychiatric and somatic disorders: A systematic review and meta-analysis. *World Psychiatry, 13*, 288–295.

Andrews, G., Slade, T., & Issakidis, C. (2002). Deconstructing current comorbidity: Data from the Australian National Survey of mental health and well-being. *British Journal of Psychiatry, 181*, 306–314.

Bandelow, B., Lichte, T., Rudolf, S., Wiltink, J., & Beutel, M. E. (2014). The diagnosis and treatment recommendations for anxiety disorders. *Deutsches Ärzteblatt International, 111*, 473–480.

Beck, A. T., Steer, R. A., & Carbin, M. G. (1988). Psychometric properties of the beck depression inventory: Twenty-five years of evaluation. *Clinical Psychology Review, 8*, 77–100.

Beck, A. T., Ward, C. H., Mendelson, M., Mock, J., & Erbaugh, J. (1961). An inventory for measuring depression. *Archives of General Psychiatry, 4*, 561–571.

Brown, T. A., Campbell, L. A., Lehman, C. L., Grisham, J. R., & Mancill, R. B. (2001). Current and lifetime comorbidity of the DSM-IV anxiety and mood disorders in a large clinical sample. *Journal of Abnormal Psychology, 110*, 585–599.

Busch, F. N., Milrod, B. L., Singer, M. B., & Aronson, A. B. (2011). *Manual of panic focused psychodynamic psychotherapy – extended range* (1st ed.). New York: Routledge.

Cuijpers, P., Gentili, C., Banos, R. M., Garcia-Campayo, J., Botella, C., & Cristea, I. A. (2016). Relative effects of cognitive and behavioral therapies on generalized anxiety disorder, social anxiety disorder and panic disorder: A meta-analysis. *Journal of Anxiety Disorders, 43*, 79–89.

de Shazer, S., 1985. Keys to solution in brief therapy. W. W. Norton & Company, New York.

de Shazer, S., Berg, I. K., Lipchik, E., Nunnally, E., Molnar, A., Gingerich, W., & Weiner-Davis, M. (1986). Brief therapy: Focused solution development. *Family Process, 25*, 207–221.

Derogatis, L. R., Lipman, R. S., & Covi, L. (1973). SCL-90: An outpatient psychiatric rating scale- -preliminary report. *Psychopharmacology Bulletin, 9*, 13–28.

Falkenstrom, F., Grant, J., Broberg, J., & Sandell, R. (2007). Self-analysis and post-termination improvement after psychoanalysis and long-term psychotherapy. *Journal of the American Psychoanalytic Association, 55*, 629–674.

Gabbard, G. O. (1992). Psychodynamics of panic disorder and social phobia. *Bulletin of the Menninger Clinic, 56*, A3–A13.

Gabbard, G. O. (2004). *Long-term psychodynamic psychotherapy: A basic text* (1st ed.). Arlington, VA: American Psychiatric Publishing.

Gabbard, G. O., Gunderson, J. G., & Fonagy, P. (2002). The place of psychoanalytic treatments within psychiatry. *Archives of General Psychiatry, 59*, 505–510.

Gibbons, M. B., Crits-Christoph, P., Barber, J. P., Wiltsey Stirman, S., Gallop, R., Goldstein, L. A., … Ring-Kurtz, S. (2009). Unique and common mechanisms of change across cognitive and dynamic psychotherapies. *Journal of Consulting and Clinical Psychology, 77*, 801–813.

Graubard, B. I., & Korn, E. L. (1999). Predictive margins with survey data. *Biometrics, 55*, 652–659.

Härkänen, T., Arjas, E., Laaksonen, M. A., Lindfors, O., Haukka, J., & Knekt, P. (2016). Estimating efficacy in the presence of non-ignorable non-trial interventions in the Helsinki Psychotherapy Study. *Statistical Methods in Medical Research, 25*, 885–901.

Härkänen, T., Knekt, P., Virtala, E., & Lindfors, O. (2005). A case study in comparing therapies involving informative drop-out, non-ignorable non-compliance and repeated measurements. *Statistics in Medicine, 24*, 3773–3787.

Holi, M. M., Marttunen, M., & Aalberg, V. (2003). Comparison of the GHQ-36, the GHQ-12 and the SCL-90 as psychiatric screening instruments in the Finnish population. *Nordic Journal of Psychiatry, 57*, 233–238.

Holmqvist, R., Strom, T., & Foldemo, A. (2014). The effects of psychological treatment in primary care in Sweden--a practice-based study. *Nordic Journal of Psychiatry, 68*, 204–212.

Ilmarinen, J., Tuomi, K., & Klockars, M. (1997). Changes in the work ability of active employees over an 11-year period. *Scandinavian Journal of Work, Environment & Health, 23*(Suppl 1), 49–57.

Keefe, J. R., McCarthy, K. S., Dinger, U., Zilcha-Mano, S., & Barber, J. P. (2014). A meta-analytic review of psychodynamic therapies for anxiety disorders. *Clinical Psychology Review, 34*, 309–323.

Knekt, P., Heinonen, E., Härkäpää, K., Järvikoski, A., Virtala, E., Rissanen, J., et al. (2015). Randomized trial on the effectiveness of long- and short-term psychotherapy on psychosocial functioning and quality of life during a 5-year follow-up. *Psychiatry Research, 229*, 381–388.

Knekt, P., Lindfors, O., (2004). A randomized trial of the effect of four forms of psychotherapy on depressive and anxiety disorders: Design, methods, and results on the effectiveness of short-term psychodynamic psychotherapy and solution-focused therapy during a one-year follow-up, studies in social security and health; 77. Helsinki, Finland: Social Insurance Institution.

Knekt, P., Lindfors, O., Härkänen, T., Välikoski, M., Virtala, E., Laaksonen, M. A., et al. (2008). Randomized trial on the effectiveness of long-and short-term psychodynamic psychotherapy and solution-focused therapy on psychiatric symptoms during a 3-year follow-up. *Psychological Medicine, 38*, 689–703.

Knekt, P., Lindfors, O., Laaksonen, M. A., Raitasalo, R., Haaramo, P., Järvikoski, A., et al. (2008). Effectiveness of short-term and long-term psychotherapy on work ability and functional capacity--a randomized clinical trial on depressive and anxiety disorders. *Journal of Affective Disorders, 107*, 95–106.

Knekt, P., Lindfors, O., Renlund, C., Sares-Jäske, L., Laaksonen, M. A., & Virtala, E. (2011). Use of auxiliary psychiatric treatment during a 5-year follow-up among patients receiving short- or long-term psychotherapy. *Journal of Affective Disorders, 135*, 221–230.

Knekt, P., Lindfors, O., Sares-Jäske, L., Virtala, E., & Härkänen, T. (2013). Randomized trial on the effectiveness of long- and short-term psychotherapy on psychiatric symptoms and working ability during a 5-year follow-up. *Nordic Journal of Psychiatry, 67*, 59–68.

Knekt, P., Virtala, E., Härkänen, T., Vaarama, M., Lehtonen, J., & Lindfors, O. (2016). The outcome of short- and long-term psychotherapy 10 years after start of treatment. *Psychological Medicine, 46*, 1175–1188.

Laaksonen, M. A., Lindfors, O., Knekt, P., & Aalberg, V. (2012). Suitability for psychotherapy scale (SPS) and its reliability, validity, and prediction. *British Journal of Clinical Psychology, 51*, 351–375.

Lee, J. (1981). Covariance adjustment of rates based on the multiple logistic regression model. *Journal of Chronic Diseases, 34*, 415–426.

Lehtinen, V., Joukamaa, M., Jyrkinen, T., Lahtela, K., Raitasalo, R., & Aromaa, A. (1991). *Suomalaisten aikuisten mielenterveys ja mielenterveyden häiriöt. (In Finnish with an English summary: Mental health and mental disorders in Finnish adults)*. Helsinki and Turku: Kansaneläkelaitoksen julkaisuja AL:33.

Leichsenring, F., Beutel, M., & Leibing, E. (2007). Psychodynamic psychotherapy for social phobia: A treatment manual based on supportive-expressive therapy. *Bulletin of the Menninger Clinic, 71*, 56–83.

Leichsenring, F., & Rabung, S. (2011). Long-term psychodynamic psychotherapy in complex mental disorders: Update of a meta-analysis. *British Journal of Psychiatry, 199*, 15–22.

Leichsenring, F., Salzer, S., Beutel, M. E., Herpertz, S., Hiller, W., Hoyer, J., ... Leibing, E. (2014). Long-term outcome of psychodynamic therapy and cognitive-behavioral therapy in social anxiety disorder. *American Journal of Psychiatry, 171*, 1074–1082.

Lindfors, O., Knekt, P., Heinonen, E., Härkänen, T., Virtala, E., & Helsinki Psychotherapy Study Group. (2015). The effectiveness of short- and long-term psychotherapy on personality functioning during a 5-year follow-up. *Journal of Affective Disorders, 173*, 31–38.

Luborsky, L. (1984). *Principles of psychoanalytic psychotherapy: A manual for supportive-expressive treatment*. New York: Basic Books.

Malan, D. (1976). *The frontier of brief psychotherapy: An example of the convergence of research and clinical practice.* New York: Plenum Medical Book Co.

Maljanen, T., Knekt, P., Lindfors, O., Virtala, E., Tillman, P., Härkänen, T., & Helsinki Psychotherapy Study Group (2016). The cost-effectiveness of short-term and long-term psychotherapy in the treatment of depressive and anxiety disorders during a 5-year follow-up. *Journal of Affective Disorders, 190*, 254–263.

Migon, H., & Gamerman, D. (1999). *Statistical inference: An integrated approach.* London: Arnold.

Moffitt, T. E., Harrington, H., Caspi, A., Kim-Cohen, J., Goldberg, D., Gregory, A. M., & Poulton, R. (2007). Depression and generalized anxiety disorder: Cumulative and sequential comorbidity in a birth cohort followed prospectively to age 32 years. *Archives of General Psychiatry, 64*, 651–660.

National Institute for Health and Care Excellence (NICE). (2011). NICE guidelines: Generalised anxiety disorder and panic disorder in adults: management.

Newby, J. M., McKinnon, A., Kuyken, W., Gilbody, S., & Dalgleish, T. (2015). Systematic review and meta-analysis of transdiagnostic psychological treatments for anxiety and depressive disorders in adulthood. *Clinical Psychology Review, 40*, 91–110.

Penninx, B. W., Nolen, W. A., Lamers, F., Zitman, F. G., Smit, J. H., Spinhoven, P., … Beekman, A. T. (2011). Two-year course of depressive and anxiety disorders: Results from the Netherlands Study of Depression and Anxiety (NESDA). *Journal of Affective Disorders, 133*, 76–85.

Perry, J. C., & Bond, M. (2009). The sequence of recovery in long-term dynamic psychotherapy. *Journal of Nervous and Mental Disease, 197*, 930–937.

Priebe, S., Omer, S., Giacco, D., & Slade, M. (2014). Resource-oriented therapeutic models in psychiatry: Conceptual review. *British Journal of Psychiatry, 204*, 256–261.

Rakowska, J. M. (2011). Brief strategic therapy in patients with social phobia with or without personality disorder. *Psychotherapy Research, 21*, 462–471.

Sandell, R., Blomberg, J., Lazar, A., Carlsson, J., Broberg, J., & Schubert, J. (2000). Varieties of long-term outcome among patients in psychoanalysis and long-term psychotherapy. A review of findings in the Stockholm Outcome of Psychoanalysis and Psychotherapy Project (STOPP). *International Journal of Psychoanalysis, 81*, 921–942.

SAS Institute Inc (Ed.). (2011). *SAS/STAT ® 9.3: User's guide* (2nd ed.). Cary, NC: SAS Institute Inc..

Trepper, T. S., McCollum, E. E., De Jong, P., Korman, H., Gingerich, W., & Franklin, C. (2014). *Solution-focused therapy treatment manual for working with individuals.* In: Kim, J. S. (Ed.) Solution-focused brief therapy: a multicultural approach (pp. 14–31). Los Angeles: Sage.

Tuomi, K., Ilmarinen, J., Jahkola, A., Katajarinne, L., & Tulkki, A. (1998). *Work ability index* (2nd ed.). Helsinki, Finland: Finnish Institute of Occupational Health.

Verbeke, G., & Molenberghs, G. (1997). *Linear mixed models in practice: A SAS-oriented approach, lecture notes in statistics.* New York: Springer.

Weissman, M. M., & Bothwell, S. (1976). Assessment of social adjustment by patient self-report. *Archives of General Psychiatry, 33*, 1111–1115.

Willutzki, U., Neumann, B., Haas, H., & Schulte, D. (2004). Zur Psychotherapie sozialer Ängste: Kognitive Verhaltenstherapie im Vergleich zu einem kombiniert resourceorientierten Vorgehen. *Zeitschrift für Klinische Psychologie und Psychotherapie, 33*, 42–50.

Willutzki, U., Teismann, T., & Schulte, D. (2012). Psychotherapy for social anxiety disorder: Long-term effectiveness of resource-oriented cognitive-behavioral therapy and cognitive therapy in social anxiety disorder. *Journal of Clinical Psychology, 68*, 581–591.

Wiltink, J., Hoyer, J., Beutel, M. E., Ruckes, C., Herpertz, S., Joraschky, P., … Leichsenring, F. (2016). Do patient characteristics predict outcome of psychodynamic psychotherapy for social anxiety disorder? *PLoS One, 11*, e0147165.

The SCORE in Europe: Measuring Effectiveness, Assisting Therapy

Peter Stratton, Alan Carr, and Luigi Schepisi

Introduction

There are powerful demands on us to adapt our practices according to what evidence shows to be effective, and so we should. Unfortunately the research method that has become dominant, the randomised control trial (RCT), is clearly not generally appropriate for systemic family therapy. RCTs require an unequivocally diagnosed condition and two standardised treatments with patients allocated randomly to one or the other (think blue versus red pills). In the real world, systemic couple and family therapy (SCFT) clinics, like some other therapies, see a great variety of clients, many of whom do not have a DSM-type diagnosis; we discover the problems during treatment not at referral; and we treat people in their relationships, not diagnoses.

Even so, many researchers have managed to accumulate convincing evidence primarily using the RCT paradigm. In 2005 AFT sponsored the first report which collated the published evidence base of systemic family therapy. Since that time, especially while I (PS) was funded as the AFT "Academic and Research Development Officer", we have undertaken various initiatives to make the evidence base available while exploring the reasons for its limitations. The third version of the report

P. Stratton (✉)
Leeds Institute of Health Sciences (LIHS), University of Leeds, Leeds, UK

A. Carr
School of Psychology, University College Dublin, and Clanwilliam Institute Dublin, Dublin, Ireland

L. Schepisi
Centro di Studi e di Applicazione della Psicologia Relazionale, Prato, Italy

© Springer Nature Switzerland AG 2020
M. Ochs et al. (eds.), *Systemic Research in Individual, Couple, and Family Therapy and Counseling*, European Family Therapy Association Series,
https://doi.org/10.1007/978-3-030-36560-8_20

(Stratton, 2016) is based on a good number of recent high-quality systematic reviews of the evidence base, several by our German colleagues, and is available on the AFT website.

A different approach was a comprehensive survey of the 225 outcome studies published in English in the decade 2000–2009 (Stratton et al., 2015). Seventy-three per cent of the studies claimed to be RCTs although only 21% met our full criteria for sound randomisation. So family therapy researchers are engaging with the dominant paradigm but with some difficulty. Most relevant here is that we found a complete lack of coherence in the measures used to evaluate effectiveness with only a small proportion of researchers using a systemic measure. This lack of consistency partly arises from the variety of practice in our field so that researchers adopt measures that are specific to the conditions they are investigating. But a consequence is to make comparisons between studies extremely difficult. Also, the absence of a measure that is suitable for the nature of general SCFT practice while being compatible with systemic thinking may be one factor in the reluctance of many practitioners to routinely use outcome measures.

Development of the SCORE Index of Family Functioning and Change

In 2004 a group of practising systemic therapists with a research orientation came together to see whether we could create a suitable outcome measure. We started from a belief that across the whole range of reasons that people came for family therapy, the ways family members operated their relationships would be central to what the therapy would achieve. So we wanted a tool to provide a robust measure of family relationships at the start and at subsequent points in therapy.

The rationale for SCORE (Stratton, Bland, Janes, & Lask, 2010) argues that lasting therapeutic change in an individual client or a couple will generally be indicated by an improvement in their close relationships and will need healthy relationships in order to be sustained. It is a stance that is explicit in systemically based treatments for individuals, couples, and families. We would see it as applying to clients in any form of counselling or psychotherapy, but it is not yet seen as a priority in therapies that developed out of working with individuals. Measures should contain language that reflects the culture and experience of the client group, and it should focus on interactional processes within the family rather than general evaluative statements. We have reported substantial testing out of SCORE at different stages of its development with therapists, clients, and the general public. The fact that it has been possible to achieve culturally sensitive versions in 22 different languages speaks, we believe, to our careful work in generating items that would be relevant across different cultural groups (Stratton & Low, 2020).

In summary:

- We wanted a measure based on self-report (the family being the only expert on how it lives its life).
- Which indicated a selection of the more important aspects of relational life at home.
- That would be relevant for a very wide range of families and referrals.
- In the process, being informative about how family members see their lives together while making differences between family members explicit and visible.

After substantial psychometric development, we published the SCORE in 2010. This was achieved by the SCORE team, initially of Julia Bland (Chair), Peter Stratton, Judith Lask, Chris Evans, and Emma Janes, while many others have contributed at various stages. The main financial support was provided by AFT with contributions from EFTA and UKCP, plus a research grant from the South London and Maudsley Trust. The processes of development are already well described in the literature and have resulted in three main versions: the SCORE-40 and the SCORE-15 (Stratton et al., 2010) and the SCORE-28 (Cahill, O'Reilly, Carr, Dooley, & Stratton, 2010).

Development of the SCORE-40

The first version of SCORE to be made available included 40 items describing family interactions, rated on a 6-point Likert scale in terms of how well they describe the respondent's current family. SCORE items were based on substantial reviews of the existing literature with a large number of items generated and retained if they appeared to assess the quality of family life, functionality of family relationships, and change from beginning to end of therapy. The refinement of the SCORE item pool, leading to the SCORE-40, was informed by expert clinician and service user feedback obtained in a series of preliminary small-scale qualitative and quantitative studies.

Starting in 2006, the SCORE-40 and a set of demographic items were administered to 510 individuals in 228 consecutively referred families before attending therapy or during the early stage of therapy at 15 NHS clinical sites in the UK. Families were attending couple or family therapy for adult- or child-focused mental health problems. Data were also available for 126 non-clinical cases from preliminary studies mentioned above.

Analyses of these data showed that the SCORE-40 achieved good internal consistency reliability; it discriminated between clinical and non-clinical cases; all 40 items correlated with the scale total and with the family's ratings of the severity and impact of the main clinical problems. Factor analysis indicated that the items fitted a three-factor structure with factors assessing family strengths, difficulties, and communication. We concluded that every question in the SCORE-40 was viable as an indicator of family functioning. All of the questions related significantly to different measures and elicited variability in responses, with none being answered at an extreme by a significant number of respondents. We concluded that the SCORE-40 is a viable instrument with clear psychometric properties. Ratings provided by the respondents indicated a high level of acceptability of all of the items (Stratton et al., 2010).

However, the full version with 40 scored items is too long for most clinical situations, so we proceeded to use the existing data to create a shorter version while retaining most of the power of SCORE-40. A 15-item version was derived by the original team. At the same time, Alan Carr and his team were working with the SCORE-40 using their own procedures and criteria and established a 28-item version (see below). Initially a six-point Likert response format was used for SCORE items. However, this was replaced in the SCORE-15 with a five-point response format in light of results of Webster's (2008) study of distributions of ratings made on SCORE item six-point Likert scales in data from non-clinical samples. She found that the first two scale points were not independently informative. Negligible information was lost by reducing item Likert scales from six to five points. In Irish studies conducted by Alan Carr's group, the six-point response format was used throughout development of their shorter versions and so has been retained. In UK and other European studies, five-point Likert scales have been used.

Versions of SCORE for Clinical Use

Development of the SCORE-15

The SCORE-15 (see Fig. 1) was developed by selecting those items that had high correlations with the SCORE total and families' ratings of problem severity or ratings of problem impact. We used multivariate statistical analyses to guide the elimination of those that duplicated the content of another item or had an exceptionally high correlation with another item; those that did not discriminate strongly between clinical and non-clinical cases; and those that were judged by the therapist-researchers to be less clinically useful and less likely to change during therapy. The processes are described in Stratton et al. (2010).

There were three main results concerning the psychometric properties of the SCORE-15. It showed good internal consistency reliability; a three-factor structure with factors assessing family strengths, difficulties, and communication; and criterion validity insofar as its total scores explained 95 per cent of the variance in the SCORE-40 total.

Site Code☐☐☐ Family Number ☐☐☐ Family Position ....

Describing your family   Date....................

We would like you to tell us about how you see your family at the moment. So we are asking for YOUR view of your family.

When people say 'your family' they often mean the people who live in your house. **But we want you to choose who you want to count as the family you are going to describe.**

For each item, make your choice by putting ☑ in just one of the boxes numbered 1 to 5. If a statement was "We are always fighting each other" and you felt this was not especially true of your family, you would put a tick in box 4 for "Describes us: not well".

		✓	

Do not think for too long about any question, but do try to tick one of the boxes for each question.

For each line, would you say **this describes our family**:	1. Describes us: Very well	2. Describes us: Well	3. Describes us: Partly	4. Describes us: Not well	5. Describes us: Not at all
1) In my family we talk to each other about things which matter to us					
2) People often don't tell each other the truth in my family					
3) Each of us gets listened to in our family					
4) It feels risky to disagree in our family					
5) We find it hard to deal with everyday problems					
6) We trust each other					
7) It feels miserable in our family					
8) When people in my family get angry they ignore each other on purpose					
9) We seem to go from one crisis to another in my family					
10) When one of us is upset they get looked after within the family					
11) Things always seem to go wrong for my family					
12) People in the family are nasty to each other					
13) People in my family interfere too much in each other's lives					
14) In my family we blame each other when things go wrong					
15) We are good at finding new ways to deal with things that are difficult					
	1.	2.	3.	4.	5.

Now please turn over and tell us a bit more about your family.

SCORE-15 © Association for Family Therapy www.aft.org.uk

Fig. 1 The SCORE-15

Development of the SCORE-28

In parallel with the development of the SCORE-15, Alan Carr's group in Dublin derived a 28-item version using a new mixed sample ($N = 791$) to complete the SCORE-40 along with a number of established measures of personal and family adjustment (Cahill et al., 2010). Procedures similar to those described above for the SCORE-15 indicated 28 items which met the criteria and fitted the 3 factors. The SCORE-28 total and subscales correlated highly with the FAD General Functioning Scale and moderately with the other measures. The SCORE-28 includes 14 of the SCORE-15 items and retains the original 6-point Likert scale. It is therefore possible to define a 29-item version of well-tested items from which both the SCORE-15 and the SCORE-28 statistics can be derived.

Evaluating the Clinical Versions

The achievements of the many researchers who have used SCORE during 10 years of experience are described in detail by Carr and Stratton (2017), with an accompanying YouTube video. This article offers the best overview of the work so far. We have become convinced that the SCORE is an appropriate basis for indicating general effects of SCFT.

A new UK sample of 584 participants from 239 families attending 20 NHS adult and child and adolescent mental health services and private or training institutes completed the SCORE-15 (Stratton et al., 2014). At the first session (Time 1), 515 (88%) participants completed the SCORE-15, and 247 (42% of the sample) completed it again at the start of the fourth session (Time 2). Participants also described their family qualitatively and completed items on the main challenges to their family, how well they were dealing with these, and their view of the usefulness of family therapy. For each family at Time 2, therapists rated their perception of change in the family on a four-point scale and made a judgement about the helpfulness of the therapy on a visual analogue scale.

The SCORE-15 was found to be acceptable to participants with strong consistency and reliability. Change over only three sessions of systemic therapy was highly statistically significant. Further validation is provided by improvements in quantified scores correlating significantly with the independent measures provided by both the family members and their therapists. The paper concludes that "The SCORE-15 is a proven measure of therapy and of therapeutic change in family functioning. It is therefore a routinely usable tool applicable to service evaluation, quality improvement, and to support clinical practice" (Stratton et al., 2014, p. 3).

Alan Carr's team report a series of studies of the SCORE-28. Cahill et al. (2010) and Cahill, O'Reilly, Carr, Dooley, and Stratton (2013) found that the SCORE-28 replicates the three factor scales that assess family strengths, difficulties, and communication. The SCORE-28 total and subscales were shown to have good internal consistency and test-retest reliability, while overall the instrument showed good construct validity (O'Hanrahan et al., 2017). The SCORE-28 total and subscales correlated highly with the FAD General Functioning Scale and moderately with the GARF, KMS, KPS, SWLS, MHI-5, and SDQ. The SCORE-28 therefore has the same statistical strengths as the SCORE-15 and will provide a more detailed account of family interactions, and possibly a more stable measure, for those situations in which the increased length is acceptable. Typically the 15-item version is completed in about 5 minutes, while many users need less time at a second or third presentation.

Fay, Carr, O'Reilly, Cahill, Dooley, Guerin, and Stratton (2013) report a national random sample obtained with a random digit dialling telephone survey using computer-assisted telephone interviewing with a stratified national random sample. Four hundred three adults living in the Republic of Ireland and Northern Ireland completed the SCORE-29 (which contained all items from the SCORE-15 and SCORE-28) and brief measures of family and personal adjustment. The response rate was 21%. This study had four main findings. First, for the totals on the SCORE-28 and SCORE-15, the 90th percentile points for parents in the national random sample were 2.86 and 2.92, respectively. The article also reported norms for 457 young adults and 132 adolescents from convenience samples described in the paper by Cahill et al. (2010). For young adults, the 90th percentile points were 3.58 and 3.62 for the totals on the SCORE-28 and SCORE-15, respectively. For totals on the SCORE-28 and SCORE-15, the 90th percentile points were 4.18 and 4.29, respectively, for adolescents. These 90th percentile points may be used as clinical cut-off scores since only 10% of families obtain scores higher than these.

Developments for European Translations

As the SCORE-15 became established, we wanted to make it available both internationally and for use with families from linguistic minorities who might struggle with the English. Judith Lask and Reenee Singh have taken the lead in the translation process, and with the support of the EFTA Research Committee, we have 22 versions translated according to a rigorous but culturally sensitive protocol. Apart from the extensive research with the English language versions in the UK and Ireland, so far the most substantial successful applications have been in Portugal, Italy, Poland, Spain, and Germany. We have learned much about the ways SCORE has been used through conversations with users in many different countries, through many email queries, and through surveys. Researchers from these countries participated in the symposium at the ISR, Heidelberg, 2017 which provided an overview of the current state of SCORE research in Europe. The symposium "Clinical and Research Experiences Across Europe Using the SCORE as an Indicator of Family Functioning" was chaired by Peter Stratton and Alan Carr.

For the first presentation, Alan Carr reported on six of the research studies conducted by the team at University College Dublin. In addition to those described above, O'Hanrahan et al. (2017) validated the SCORE-15 and SCORE-28 with adult mental health service users, and Cassells et al. (2015) used the SCORE to assess outcome in a controlled trial of Positive Systemic Practice for families of adolescents with psychological problems. Hartnett, Carr, and Sexton (2016) used the SCORE to assess outcome in a randomised controlled trial of Functional Family Therapy for families of adolescents with conduct problems. The SCORE − 28 and SCORE-15 were reported as reliable, valid, and sensitive to the change arising from systemic therapy. Carr concluded that they can be used to assess families of children with disabilities, chronic illness, and mental health problems, adolescents, young adults, and adult mental health service users. Norms may be used to detect families with clinically significant difficulties and to show when families in therapy have recovered.

A valuable addition to our understanding of how SCORE translations work was provided for the symposium by Margarida Vilaça, Anna Paula Relvas, and Roberto Pereira with "SCORE-15 Portuguese and Spanish Agreement: Validation studies in the Iberian Peninsula". The highly productive group in Portugal have been comparing the 15- and 28-item versions, finding comparable validity, and concluding that the SCORE-15 is more practical for clinical use, without any significant loss of power (Vilaca, Relvas, & Stratton, 2017).

Results of the Portuguese (Vilaça, Stratton, Sousa, & Relvas, 2015) and Spanish (Rivas & Pereira) validation analyses indicate respectable psychometric properties in both countries, as the comparative studies (Relvas, Vilaça. Rivas, & Pereira, 2015) suggest that both versions function in a similar way. Considering those findings and the historical, cultural, and economic proximity between the two countries, a SCORE-15 Iberian Agreement was established in order to promote its study and practice in the Iberian Peninsula context. The results of the SCORE-15 Iberian version validation analysis, based on a sample of Portuguese and Spanish participants, from clinical and community contexts found overall consistency between the two countries (Rivas & Pereira, 2015). There were however interesting differences at a more detailed level. For example, the Spanish version showed higher reference values in the clinical sample (family communication and family difficulties), as well as higher cut-off points than the Portuguese and Irish versions. There were higher values in Portugal for the reliability dimension of family communication and less therapeutic improvement in the family strengths dimension in Portugal.

Barbara Jozefik and Bogdan de Barbaro have led the SCORE research in Poland, and Feliks Matusiak, Barbara Jozefik, and Aleksandra Katarzyna Tomasiewicz described this work. While they found the now expected quantitative changes between first and last sessions, they also carried out a qualitative analysis of the responses to the open-ended questions, using the Consensual Qualitative Research method – a version modified for simple qualitative data (CQR-M). The results indicate a change in the participants' narratives regarding family and problem (Matusiak, Józefik, Wolska, Ulasińska, & Stratton, submitted).

In these data, the items that had formed a third factor of "communication difficulties" became combined with those of "overwhelmed by difficulties" except for item 13 "people in my family interfere too much in each other's lives" which were loaded with "strengths and adaptability". SCORE totals improved significantly from first to fourth sessions and very substantially by the final sessions. However, a number of completed forms were much reduced by the later session (see Table 1). There were highly statistically significant correlations of the changes from first to fourth session on the SCORE total with the self-ratings of severity of the problem and successful coping. There was no significant change in patients' assessment of the usefulness of therapy. Encountering these differences from data collected with the English versions raises questions about whether they are primarily cultural differences or differences in how therapy is practised in Poland, an issues discussed in detail by Stratton and Low (2020).

The group from Krakow also carried out one of the first rigorous analyses of the qualitative material provided in the second part of SCORE (Matusiak et al., submitted). Responses from 28 families to the 2 qualitative items inviting descriptions of the family and a statement of the main problem created interesting differences

Table 1 Current major European projects: numbers of non-clinical SCORE-15 and of clinical SCORE-15 completed at (I), 4th (II), and final (III) sessions

Country	Source	Non-clinical	Clinical I	II	III
Belgium	Report to EFTA (2016)	115			
Czech Republic	Report to EFTA (2017)	148	48	21	
Finland	Report to EFTA (2013)		54	27	4
Germany 1 (Nordhausen)	Report to EFTA (2014)	80	240		
Germany 2 (Schwerin)	Report to EFTA (2017)		184		112
Greece	Report to EFTA (2017)	50 (families)	115 (families)	35 (families)	35 (families)
Ireland 1	Fay et al. (2013)	403			
Ireland 2	Hamilton, Carr, Cahill, Cassells, and Hartnett (2015)		701	433	
Ireland 3	O'Hanrahan et al. (2017)		199		
Italy	Presented at ISR, Heidelberg (2017)	264	660	299	94
Poland	Report to EFTA (2016)	42	679	337	125
Poland II	Presented at ISR, Heidelberg (2017)		332[a]	202[a]	85[a]
Portugal	Vilaça et al. (2015)	482	136		
Portugal II	Report to EFTA (2016)	406	146	77	50
Spain	Report to EFTA (2016–2017)	85	506	238	60
Sweden	Report to EFTA (2018)	70 (families)	152 (families)		
UK	Stratton et al. (2014)		584	247	

[a]They are part of the above groups

between first and last session. The "Consensual Qualitative Research Methodology" when applied to these descriptions generated five categories. For example, positively rated "Descriptions of the family as a whole" increased from 32% preceding the first session to 44% after the last session. Meanwhile descriptions of the problem through symptoms and diagnosis dropped from 41% to 21%. These certainly appear to be the changes we would hope SCFT would achieve.

In the final presentation of the symposium, Luigi Schepisi and Daniele Paolini reported on "The Use of SCORE-15 in Italy: Some Potential Research and Clinical Applications". Their data showed reliable change from first to fourth sessions but with almost as many family members (7%) deteriorating as improved (9%). At the final administration, 20% significantly improved, but there were still 7% whose SCORE totals deteriorated. However, in common with experience in other countries, the numbers of completed SCOREs substantially decreased (see Table 1): session 1, $N = 660$; session 4, $N = 299$; final session, $N = 93$. Mainly for this reason, as they explained in their report, "...we should consider that data we collected at the 4th session and at the end of the therapy are still preliminary". Therefore, further questionnaires are absolutely needed to be administered in order to draw any conclusions on this subject.

The Italian researchers also analysed the descriptive answers. Comparing the description of the family made by family members with their definition of the problem, the most frequent combinations (categories) were:

1. *Coherent:* There is something negative within the family (e.g. "my family is unstable, or, has sunk") and the problem being defined as a family one (e.g. "inability to solve our problems").
2. *Guilty:* Negative family ("absurd or confused"), but individual problem ("the negativity of my mother").
3. *Scapegoat:* The family as a whole is positive ("it is a beautiful family"), while one member is problematic ("my child's breakdown").
4. *Incoherent:* The family is positive ("we are a very close family"), while there is a family issue ("there is a great distance between us").

Taking the fourth category "incoherent" as an example, it is proposed that a therapist must bring this apparent incoherence into therapy, not only by saying "why is it that your family, that you define very close, has a problem with distance?", but much more interesting is to ask the family member "how might this being close one to each other in your family help you to overcome your feeling of distance?"

By reformulating the questions, we switch from family's problems to family's resources, which is an approach that a growing number of family therapists like to use. Moreover, SCORE, in all its parts, allows the family to identify its resources, besides its problems. For instance, we have the strengths scale in the questionnaire or the question "how are you managing as a family" following "how severe is your problem" .

Currently Luigi Schepisi is leading the EFTA Research Committee project to compile data on usage throughout Europe. Data at the time of writing from major contributors are presented in Table 1.

To summarise, the following countries have already published the results of the studies carried out on the use of SCORE-15: Ireland, Poland, Portugal, Spain, and the UK. As far as we know, research groups in Italy and Sweden are both working to publish their findings. Generally, in all of these studies, SCORE-15 showed good internal consistency reliability, as well as a three-factor structure with factors assessing family strengths, difficulties, and communication (e.g. Jozefik, Matusiak, Wolska, & Ulasińska, 2015; Rivas & Pereira, 2015 ; Vilaça et al., 2015); similarly, results were obtained that showed significant differences between non-clinical and clinical samples (e.g. Hamilton et al., 2015; Stratton et al., 2010; Vilaça et al., 2015). Moreover, the ability to detect clinical improvement has been reported in several studies (e.g. Hamilton et al., 2015; Jozefik et al., 2015; Stratton et al., 2014). However, as reported below, in many of the centres involved, there were difficulties in obtaining the three questionnaires to be provided by the same person in the three different stages of therapy. For this reason, it would be appropriate, in our opinion, to implement more detailed studies on the outcome of therapy.

Keeping in mind Carr and Stratton's article on the use of SCORE over the past 10 years (Carr & Stratton, 2017), we would like to discuss another aspect that emerges from the administration of SCORE-15 to members of families in therapy. We are referring here to how the SCORE can be considered as a further source of information, which can be added to and integrated with those that come from everything that actually happens during the session with family members. This is particularly interesting, of course, when a therapist decides to use SCORE to support the process of therapy. In fact, as reported below, 75% of therapists seem to be doing this.

It should be emphasised that the information that comes from SCORE has to do with, and allows us to work on, differences, of which the most obvious are those between family members. These differences are generally found in all parts of the questionnaire, both in the responses to the 15 items and in the so-called open questions. Sometimes they are so strong that it seems that each family member was not describing the same family. Even at the end of therapy, they quite often give discordant results in the indicators associated with the outcome of the therapy. Sometimes, as our Polish colleagues showed in their presentation, it has been found more useful to use the position/role of family members in their families (all the fathers, all the mothers, all the children, all the patients), rather than the family they belong to, as a grouping variable. We could therefore conclude that differences between members of the same family challenge data analysis. From a certain point of view, it would be much easier if a hypothetical "official spokesperson" of the family could answer questions and make judgements on behalf of everyone. At the same time, the emergence of multiple voices within the family, even discordant among themselves, is instead a very specific feature of the families we meet in therapy. Therefore, using an instrument that sensitively detects such differences allows us to preserve this variety and to relate with the family in a more appropriate manner.

We should emphasise now the differences between the responses of the same person to the different parts of the questionnaire. Stratton et al. (2014), for instance, measured the correlation between the score on the three SCORE scales and the score given to the "problem severity" or to the "problem impact". As mentioned above, Schepisi and Paolini have proposed to compare the answers given to the two open questions of SCORE by the same family member. In the above example has been highlighted the possible clinical use of two discordant responses to SCORE ("we are a very close family" and/but "there is a great distance between us"), as, during the session, the therapist can constructively use discordant words or gestures from a family member. And it is just for this peculiar characteristic, perhaps, that SCORE is especially powerful as a clinical instrument as well as a research tool.

Limitations and Feedback in Use

The very particular form of the SCORE creates both constraints and affordances in its use as a research instrument:

- When used in everyday clinical practice, most centres achieve high rates of satisfactorily completed forms at the start of therapy but a substantial reduction at session 4 and far fewer at the final session. Apart from the unreliability of statistics with the smaller numbers, there is the risk that people who complete the SCORE at all three occasions may be unrepresentative.
- SCORE may only be relevant as an outcome measure for those clinical situations where close relationships are relevant (in at least one of the many ways they can be).
- There can be an issue because of the attractiveness to therapists of using the SCORE interactively with families. It is often clinically valuable but difficult to do without interfering in the research process. Luigi Schepisi's suggestion is for therapists to focus in the session on the descriptive material provided by the family after the ratings as this avoids "contaminating" the 15 ratings. However, Wolpert (2013), in her role as one of the UK's most senior therapy researchers, has argued that when research or measurement objectives conflict with clinical considerations, priority must always be given to optimising the therapy.

In various web discussions and surveys, while most comments are positive and encouraging, we sometimes hear concerns such as:

We find SCORE-15 to be cumbersome to administer so we no longer use it.

The logistics are also challenging at times when all family members are unable to attend regularly, keeping track and ensuring relevant questionnaires are completed.

A survey of UK users generated some challenging comments among the more common positives:

What Would Be Your Thoughts About Starting to Use SCORE?
- It was short and family oriented but also seemed problem focused.
- It is time to have a good reliable measure in our own field that can reflect the complexity of families and change.

- I had mixed feelings and was pleased to have the opportunity to give it a go as part of the research without having to commit to using it.
- I was enthusiastic about using a systemic outcome measure, but not confident in explaining its purpose and obtaining consent for the research.
- I thought it might interrupt the engagement process.

Experiences with Using SCORE-15
- The "tick" columns are cumbersome, and the headings for each column are too long.
- It allows me to see which families are best suited to a systemic approach of therapy.
- I work in an area where literacy levels are extremely low and many families found it really hard to understand.
- My concerns about the effect on engagement didn't seem to be borne out.
- Clients with medical/illness understandings react negatively to be asked about family relationships.
- SCORE needs to be used in conjunction with tools that measure symptom change.

What Were Your Clients' Feelings About Whether an Outcome Measure Would Affect the Therapy?
- They appreciated being able to give feedback that acknowledges change.
- This has improved as I have become better at administering it.
- Clients generally felt fairly neutral about the effect on therapy.

Therapeutic Uses of SCORE

As we had been focused on being able to measure outcome, the extent to which SCORE has been used to support the process of therapy has been both surprising and gratifying. A survey of EFTA users found that while most (88%) used it to measure outcomes, 75% also used SCORE to support the process of therapy. A typical comment is "SCORE helps to verbalise issues and it makes it easier to check with clients what they are talking about, a useful discussion starter". We in fact had an indication from a qualitative study in which an early version was trialled by nine experienced therapists. Their enthusiasm for using it clinically led us to conclude "The findings indicate that the uses of SCORE as a potential therapeutic tool have perhaps been underestimated and should be considered further, particularly as therapists need to feel that there is some benefit for their practice to be derived from participating in research" (Stratton, McGovern, Wetherell, & Farrington, 2006, p. 206).

Therapists may choose to talk with the family about their answers on the SCORE items. Through repeated presentations, it is also used to evaluate the course of therapy, indicate where there are changes, and suggest issues that it is important to bring into focus.

Some uses of SCORE with families that have been suggested were:

- Pre-treatment information and screening.
- Discussing those items that are most significant for clients.
- Informing the therapist of major areas of change, and of no change, between sessions.
- Reconsider the way therapy is being conducted when SCORE indicates deterioration.
- A context for discussions of the usefulness of therapy.
- Using the items to alert family members to disregarded aspects of their home life.
- Presenting families with scores that have changed during therapy and those that have not.
- Checking for differences between therapist and client perceptions.

We invite therapists who have found other ways that SCORE has helped their practice, to put a description on the Google discussion group (at the end of this chapter) for others to try.

Looking to the Future

With SCORE now established and available, we have a great opportunity to develop it further. At the time of writing, we are in the process of setting up new teams to take SCORE forward. One focus, arising from the AFT "Big Research Conversation" in March 2017, is to take on new research-based initiatives. We will link with the broader Research Activation Group (RAG) that is also being formed and also with the EFTA Research Committee project on SCORE being led by Peter Stratton and Luigi Schepisi. Some of these initiatives could be to develop extensions to the SCORE suite of measures, while others may pick up some of the many suggestions that have been made for research projects using SCORE. As we offer our current suggestions, please do consider whether you might become involved with one of them or want to suggest a new way that SCORE could be used to generate evidence about, or even to answer, one of your questions.

Concluding Discussion: Extending the Usefulness of SCORE

A priority is to build on the innovative work by Teh, Lask, and Stratton (2017) in producing a version for use with LGBT couples. While most couples are happy to work with the wording of SCORE about "my family", some are not, and this varies by country. In Greece, for example, a couple without children do not describe themselves as a family. Furthermore, the existing items, while certainly usable by couples, may be missing some of the most significant interactional issues when the household consists of a couple. Should a new couple's SCORE have the same ratio-nale: of ratings of particular forms of interaction? We already have a team within RAG (see above) working on a general couple version and suggesting examples that would indicate the quality and functionality of the relationship. As in current SCORE, these would not be general evaluative statements but more concrete descriptions of aspects of interaction. And they need to be applicable across cultures and sub-cultures.

Originally SCORE was developed to be readily comprehensible by children of 12 years or older. We did find that younger children often wanted to participate and were able to do so. But Tom Jewell (2013) developed a version specifically for chil-dren from 7 years upwards. Clinicians have reported that it is sometimes appropriate to use this version with young people up to the age of 16. We have in the past tried to encourage the development of a version for adults with learning disability. It has proved difficult to progress with this, but it may be that a small enthusiastic team could achieve this important objective. And should we consider a version for use in systemic consultations to organisations and work teams? Is the rationale of concrete indicators of interpersonal interactions applicable in the workplace?

Another project could be to pull together all of the ways that SCORE has been used clinically and create a small manual for use in training and established practice.

Several users have built SCORE into their NHS software, but we have not got a generic IT version that we can make available to all practitioners. There are organ-isations who would readily do this, but they would need to charge for each use, and we are determined to keep to the principle of SCORE being free to use.

Exploiting the Research Possibilities for SCORE to Help Answer Some Important Questions

The availability and proven functionality of SCORE raises many possibilities of research, and we are hoping that the new teams will find practitioners who are inter-ested to take one of them on, perhaps through a vehicle of a practitioner research network (Stratton, 2008). It is important to remember that because SCORE has been found to provide an incisive account of crucial family interactions, it can be used for research outside of the context of therapeutic outcomes. Particularly the SCORE-40.

Here we can just offer summary headings, but the EFTA Research Committee and/or RAG will be happy to explore any of them with you if you are interested:

Relationship of SCOREs to events in therapy.
In what circumstances is SFT most effective?
Relationship to nature of problem.
Use for screening potential clients.
Interview families whose SCOREs have changed, about their perceptions of why these specific changes occurred (+ or -), or when there has been no change in SCORE totals but therapists judge there was change.

Effect on outcome of feeding back to family in session.

Collecting a very large sample via social media.

At follow-up, have therapist and family complete the SCORE. Compare their perceptions. Feed the comparison back to them. What changes as a result?

Enhance our criteria for significant change and clinical cut-offs.

Explore relationship with well-being, happiness, demographics, the GRRAACCES, etc.

Use as an intervention in community/ non-clinical samples to find out whether, when a family does the SCORE, this orients them to be more alert to how they are operating their relationships. It is quite a common response in our non-clinical participants for them to say it made them think about aspects of their family life that they had not been noticing.

Non-clinical samples have been based on a single member from each family. A sample in which SCORE is provided by all family members would allow us to examine whether they are more similar to each other in their responses than families who come for family therapy.

As exemplified by the symposium, SCORE has been found to be robust for use in different cultural contexts when using our culturally sensitive translation protocol (Stratton & Low, 2020). Beyond Europe: to put together data from different countries. Compare and combine. Examine the transportability of translations. For example, the Portuguese version has been successfully used in the very different context of Angola. Would the Spanish translation work just as well in South American countries? Does the Mandarin version work the same for Chinese families in Leeds as it does in Shanghai?

And we have a great wealth of existing data, from our 2 original UK samples of 500 people each as well as all that have been gathered since. We could examine whether family members who filled in the SCORE independently give similar scores. We have the independent family descriptions and ratings and the expectations about therapy waiting to be analysed thematically and related to the quantitative data.

Finally, we could research therapist views about self-report outcome measures before starting and after using SCORE.

As you can see, there are so many exciting opportunities that SCORE opens up,

See full information, with videos, on the AFT website www.aft.org.uk; join our discussions by emailing to aftSCORE+subscribe@googlegroups.com; and/or contact Peter Stratton at p.m.stratton@ntlworld.com.

References

Cahill, P., O'Reilly, K., Carr, A., Dooley, B., & Stratton, P. (2010). Validation of a 28-item version of the systemic clinical outcome and routine evaluation in an Irish context: The SCORE-28. *Journal of Family Therapy., 32*, 210–231.

Cahill, P., O'Reilly, K., Carr, A., Dooley, B., & Stratton, P. (2013). Systemic clinical outcome and routine evaluation- 28 (SCORE-28). In C. Simmons & P. Lehmann (Eds.), *Tools for strengths-based assessment and evaluation* (pp. 447–450). New York, NY: Springer.

Carr, A., & Stratton, P. (2017). The score family assessment questionnaire: A decade of progress. *Family Process, 56*, 285–301. https://doi.org/10.1111/famp.12280

Cassells, C., Carr, A., Forrest, M., Fry, J., Beirne, F., Casey, T., et al. (2015). Positive systemic practice: A controlled trial of family therapy for adolescent emotional and behavioral problems in Ireland. *Journal of Family Therapy, 37*, 429–449. https://doi.org/10.1111/1467-6427.12038

Fay, D., Carr, A., O'Reilly, K., Cahill, P., Dooley, B., Guerin, S., & Stratton, P. (2013). Irish norms for the SCORE-15 and 28 from a national telephone survey. *Journal of Family Therapy, 35*, 24–42.

Hamilton, E., Carr, A., Cahill, P., Cassells, C., & Hartnett, D. (2015). Psychometric properties and responsiveness to change of 15- and 28-item versions of the SCORE: A family assessment questionnaire. *Family Process, 54*, 454–463. https://doi.org/10.1111/famp.12117

Hartnett, D., Carr, A., & Sexton, T. (2016). The effectiveness of Functional Family Therapy in reducing mental health risk and family adjustment difficulties in an Irish Context. *Family Process, 55*(2), 287–304. https://doi.org/10.1111/famp.12195

Jewell, T., Carr, A., Stratton, P., Lask, J., & Eisler, I. (2013). Development of a children's version of the SCORE index of family function and change. *Family Process, 52*(4), 673–684. https://doi.org/10.1111/famp.12044

Jozefik, B., Matusiak, F., Wolska, M., & Ulasińska, R. (2015). Family therapy process—Works on the Polish version of SCORE-15 tool. *Psychiatria Polska*, www.psychiatriapolska.pl. doi:https://doi.org/10.12740/PP/OnlineFirst/42894

Matusiak, F., Józefik, B., Wolska, M., Ulasińska, R., & Stratton, P. (submitted). *A quantitative and qualitative analysis of changes in systemic family therapy: Results of the polish clinical version of the SCORE – 15 questionnaire. Psychiatria Polska.*

O'Hanrahan, K., Daly White, M., Carr, A., Cahill, P., Keenleyside, M., Fitzhenry, M., … Browne, S. (2017). Validation of 28 and 15 item versions of the SCORE family assessment questionnaire with adult mental health service users. *Journal of Family Therapy, 39*, 4–20. https://doi.org/10.1111/1467-6427.12107

Relvas, A. P., Vilaça, M., Rivas, G., & Pereira, R. (2015). SCORE-15: Datos portugueses y españoles. Communication presented at the III Iberian Congress of Family Therapy, Cáceres, Spain.

Rivas, G., & Pereira, R. (2015). *Validación de una escala de evaluación familiar: adaptación del score-15 con normas en español*. III Congreso Ibérico de Terapia Familiar, Caceres.

Stratton, P. (2008). Practitioner Research Network in Action: Constructing an outcome measure for therapy with relational systems. *The Psychotherapist, 38*, 15–16.

Stratton, P. (2016). *The evidence base of family therapy and systemic practice*. Association for Family Therapy, UK. Online copy available at www.aft.org.uk

Stratton, P., Bland, J., Janes, E., & Lask, J. (2010). Developing a practicable outcome measure for systemic family therapy: The SCORE. *Journal of Family Therapy., 32*, 232–258.

Stratton, P., Lask, J., Bland, J., Nowotny, E., Evans, C., Singh, R., … Peppiatt, A. (2014). Validation of the SCORE-15 Index of Family Functioning and Change in detecting therapeutic improvement early in therapy. *Journal of Family Therapy, 36*, 3–19. https://doi.org/10.1111/1467-6427.12022

Stratton, P., & Low, D. (2020) Culturally sensitive measures of systemic family therapy. In K. S. Wampler, M. Rastogi, & R. Singh, (Eds) *Handbook of systemic family therapy* (Vol. 4). *Systemic family therapy and global health issues.* John Wiley and Sons.

Stratton, P., McGovern, M., Wetherell, A., & Farrington, C. (2006). Family therapy practitioners researching the reactions of practitioners to an outcome measure. *Australian and New Zealand Journal of Family Therapy, 27*, 199–207.

Stratton, P., Silver, E., Nascimento, N., McDonnell, L., Powell, G., & Nowotny, E. (2015). Couples and family therapy in the previous decade – What does the evidence tell us? *Contemporary Family Therapy, 27*, 1–12. https://doi.org/10.1007/s10591-014-9314-6

Teh, Y. Y., Lask, J., & Stratton, P. (2017). From family to relational SCORE-15: An alternative adult version of a systemic self-report measure for couples and LGB people. *Journal of Family Therapy, 39*, 21–40. https://doi.org/10.1111/1467-6427.12103

Vilaca, M., Relvas, A. P., & Stratton, P. (2017). A Portuguese translation of the Systemic Clinical Outcome and Routine Evaluation (SCORE): The psychometric properties of the 15- and 28-item versions. *Journal of Family Therapy, 40*, 537–556. https://doi.org/10.1111/1467-6427.12197

Vilaça, M., Stratton, P., Sousa, B., & Relvas, A. P. (2015). The 15-item systemic clinical outcome and routine evaluation (SCORE-15) scale: Portuguese Validation Studies. *The Spanish Journal of Psychology, 18*(E87), 1–10. https://doi.org/10.1017/sjp.2015.95

Wolpert, M. (2013). Uses and abuses of Patient Reported Outcome Measures (PROMs): Potential iatrogenic impact of PROMs implementation and how it can be mitigated. *Administration and Policy in Mental Health and Mental Health Services Research.* https://doi.org/10.1007/s10488-013-0509-1. Open access at Springerlink.com

The Idiographic Voice in a Nomothetic World: Why Client Feedback Is Essential in Our Professional Knowledge

Terje Tilden

There is an ongoing struggle about knowledge. The new phrase "alternative facts" goes to the core of a relativism claiming that "everything is equally valid." Some typical phenomena in the current "post-factual era" are several alternative movements that challenge science in a variety of areas, e.g., creationists demand at least as much recognition as Darwinists, and climate skeptics dismiss the UN climate panel. Additionally, there are several attempts to gag the free press through allegations that they spread "fake news." Hence, uncertainty may grow about what kind of knowledge is reliable. As part of this concern, we may be tempted to seek knowledge that confirms what we already believe, something that is contradictory to the principles of science.

Realizing that knowledge is under such pressure should inspire us professionals to speak up. As professionals, we are expected to relate to knowledge very explicitly. However, simply claiming that our work is knowledge-based or evidence-based becomes meaningless unless we reflect upon how different types and levels of knowledge relate to and influence our daily work. Because the development and growth of couple and family therapy (CFT) has partly been a postmodern movement in opposition to established mainstream psychiatry and psychology, acknowledged ways to establish knowledge (i.e. epistemology) have been addressed: "postmodernism offers an ideological critique or skepticism of the authority and certainty of inherited knowledge" (Anderson, 2016, p. 182). Anderson further argues that our perception of truth and reality is socially created through language within a particular culture and is therefore only one of multiple perspectives. Even though this point of view is appealing for treatment purposes (e.g., every voice in a family has the same right to be heard), it could reveal a concern about relativism in our professional field. Relativism defined as "(a) a theory that knowledge is relative to the

T. Tilden (✉)
Modum Bad, Vikersund, Norway
e-mail: tilden@modum-bad.no

© Springer Nature Switzerland AG 2020 385
M. Ochs et al. (eds.), *Systemic Research in Individual, Couple, and Family Therapy and Counseling*, European Family Therapy Association Series,
https://doi.org/10.1007/978-3-030-36560-8_21

limited nature of the mind and the conditions of knowing, and (b) a view that ethical truths depend on the individuals and groups holding them" (Merriam-Webster Online Dictionary) may imply that professionals can feel free to pick and choose from ideologies, treatment philosophies, and approaches far away from bona fide treatments and in doing so may legitimize quackery. Clearly, there are certain ideologies (e.g., Fascism, Nazism) that cannot be compatible with being a CFT clinician. Similarly, astrology and clairvoyance are examples of knowledge not accepted by the scientific community. In other words, "everything is *not* equally valid." For this reason, we have an obligation in our professional field to be clear about certain norms and criteria for what is accepted as a bona fide treatment approach, followed by ethical guidelines for the professional. And as part of this clarity, we need to be conscious of our knowledge references such as ontology and epistemology so that professionals achieve insight into how knowledge is produced, as this enhances our ability to critically consider the quality of the knowledge we encounter (Pinsof & Lebow, 2005). This aim is challenged by the unfortunate gap between clinical practice and research that to some extent has been extended by the postmodern critique of established research methodology (Heatherington, Friedlander, Diamond, Escudero, & Pinsof, 2015; Pinsof & Wynne, 2000). As a result, a considerable group of systemic CFT therapists do not see research-based knowledge produced within the traditional research frameworks as helpful (Anderson, 2016). Thus, the risk is that professionals perceive different scientific ways of producing knowledge as dichotomous. The perspective in this chapter is rather that different types of knowledge are complementary as long as established norms for epistemology are followed. The links between levels and types of knowledge in our field will be clarified, something that should increase our ability to make wise use of the available knowledge to help our clients. In particular, client feedback will be addressed as one crucial means to narrow the gap between systemic practice and systemic research.

User Involvement as a Goal and as a Means

User involvement is closely associated with the term empowerment (WHO, 1986) that is defined as part of health promotion entailing a process through which people gain greater control over decisions and actions affecting their health. The background of this effort may stem in particular from the troubled history of psychiatry exemplified by the film One Flew Over the Cuckoo's Nest (1975) that illustrates how power within a professional regime becomes suppressive and disrespectful of individuals. Empowerment and user involvement offer one way of reducing the risk of this happening again. The aim is instead to put into practice the ideals of human rights and the respect for each individual's autonomy and integrity.

Reflecting the Norwegian ideals of democracy, justice, and equity, user involvement was established as a client right in Norwegian legislation in 1999. Accordingly, professionals are legally committed to ensure that the client's right to be informed and involved in his or her own treatment-relevant decision-making is respected and realized (Oanes, Karlson, & Borg, 2017). As a consequence, similar instructions are given in several white papers that provide guidelines and recommendations from the governmental offices that professionals must follow. Similarly, the same objective is included in the professions' ethical guidelines, establishing a blend of political and professional values that are to be put into practice.

One book that created – at least in Norway – elevated emphasis on user involvement was Duncan, Miller, and Sparks (2000) *The Heroic Client*, whose publication was perfectly timed in light of the launching of the user involvement act the previous year. A Norwegian book, *The Client: The Forgotten Therapist [Klienten – den glemte terapeut]* (Ulvestad & Henriksen, 2007), adapted these ideas into a Norwegian CFT context. These authors also noted research suggesting that it is the client's assessment of therapeutic alliance – not the therapist's – that predicts outcome (Hannan et al., 2005), implying that therapists have a distinctly limited capacity to assess therapy progress. As a result, "asking the one who this is about" – namely, the client – became a new paradigm that was followed by implementation of several systematic ways of making use of standardized feedback instruments and procedures as part of clinical practice. Because the CFT theory of feedback within self-regulating systems (see, e.g., Rohrbaugh, 2014) already had paved the way for this objective in the training of CFT professionals, the rationale for implementing the use of systematic feedback procedures in CFT was established. (For further reading on this development in Norway, see Tilden & Wampold, eds., 2017.)

However, despite the consensus on empowerment and user involvement, *how* this is implemented in daily clinical practice is less clear, and one may assume that there is great variety. In this chapter, it is argued that a concrete and viable way to ensure user involvement is to establish regular, systematic, and frequent feedback procedures in clinical practice. Whether this can be defined as evidence-based practice is discussed in the following pages.

The Claim for Evidence

An old English saying claims that "The proof of the pudding is in the eating," meaning that to be sure of the result, we need to try something out, see what happens, and learn from the experience. Thus new knowledge is earned, for instance, whether we can trust that the "pudding's" ingredients are indicative of good outcome. As a compass for our professional activity, we therefore need some kind of proof or evidence, and research is one way to establish such knowledge. However, some quite similar conceptions of evidence may confuse, hence they will be clarified in the following pages.

Evidence-based treatments – EBT (also called *empirically supported treatments – EST* – Duncan & Reese, 2013; Wampold & Imel, 2015) – is a concept adopted from the medical model that regards randomized controlled trials (RCTs) as the knowledge with highest credibility. To be top graded (level 1 = the treatment works very well), the evidence needs support from at least two large-scale RCTs, and these should not be conducted by the treatment developers. The requirements for evidence support are gradually reduced in the next four levels. The aim is to establish solid knowledge based on level 1 and level 2 evidence supporting the recommendation of a particular method of treatment for a specific disorder. A therapist can then check on an evidence list which treatment is suggested for which disorder and, if there are more than one recommended, decide which method to choose, follow the instructions (manual) in the treatment of the client, and finally document this in the client's records. Even though this procedure satisfies the criteria of evidence-based work, the pitfall is how significant we may consider the method in relation to outcome: If the client improves, it is easy to give credit to the method. If there is unsuccessful outcome, the tempting interpretation is that this had nothing to do with the method, the therapist, or service, since everything was done according to the manual, i.e., the treatment was evidence-based. The conclusion therefore points at the client: He or she was not motivated or ready for treatment. This is an example of the negative implications of expertise within traditional psychiatry and psychology to which systemic CFT is in opposition.

There are several good reasons for making use of the EBT approach, such as ensuring the highest level of quality of available treatment that can be offered to clients. This also relates to the Hippocratic Oath that as therapists we have an obligation not to cause harm to our clients. Part of promoting increased client rights is the client's right to legally sue the therapist and service if the client feels mistreated. Services and professionals therefore become increasingly more careful, making sure we have the needed documentation for our assessments so that the criteria for the choice of treatment are manifestly met.

Another good reason for EBT is that user involvement implies transparency by making the lists of evidence-based treatments available to the public. Hence, clients are able to check the list themselves, searching for the treatment that has the best evidence, thus enhancing their competence in collaboration with the therapist.

For bureaucrats, the EBT way to offer psychotherapy is in line with the New Public Management (NPM) that entails a higher level of standardized approaches ("treatment packages") in which public health services are increasingly regarded as profitable businesses. "Cost-effectiveness" is the primary rationale, so that public money on professional services can be spent wisely to optimally benefit as many clients as possible. Hence, public treatment services need to achieve a certain level of successful outcomes and numbers of clients treated to stay in business. This implies thorough documentation and reports to the service owner or governmental offices before the service is reimbursed from public insurance. In Norway (and presumably in many other Western countries as well), NPM causes, however, a difficult debate, because professionals feel they gradually lose their professional autonomy or worse they feel they are not appreciated by the authorities to make professional judgments in their effort to tailor the treatment to each client's unique profile. This dilemma will be discussed more in detail later.

As a reaction to such negative effects of EBT (reinforced by the criticism of NPM), the American Psychological Association declared evidence-based practice (EBP) to be "the integration of the best available research with clinical expertise in the context of patient characteristics, culture, and preferences" (APA Task Force, 2006, p. 273). In contrast to the EBT, EBP does not consider one source of knowledge as superior to another: There is not one defined gold standard of research methodology, but rather "different methodologies are required to answer different research questions, including effectiveness studies, process research, single-subject designs, case studies, and qualitative methodologies" (Duncan & Reese, 2013, p. 491). In particular, it is emphasized that the client's knowledge about himself or herself (values, preferences, culture, theory of change, etc.) must be included in the clinician's daily work in line with the user involvement goal mentioned above. Further, EBP to a stronger degree than EBT targets the process-outcome research that seeks to learn more about the *why* and *what* of an effective treatment and also emphasizes the *who*, meaning, for instance, the therapist's clinical expertise on facilitative interpersonal skills (FIS – Anderson, Ogles, Patterson, Lambert, & Vermeersch, 2009; Wampold & Imel, 2015). Evidence within EBP is therefore considered from a much broader perspective than within EBT, holding that treatment outcome is related to a variety of contextual and relational factors, not just associated with picking the right method.

In transforming the EBP principles into clinical practice, the concept of distinguishing between different *levels of evidence* (Gullestad, 2001; Howard, Moras, Brill, Martinovich, & Lutz, 1996) is helpful. The *efficacy* level informs the clinician about knowledge derived from RCTs and summarized in meta-analyses. According to this evidence, the therapist should inform the client that a treatment or set of treatments are generally more effective than others for his or her specific distress or disorder. The next level is called *effectiveness* and relates to whether the recommended treatment at the efficacy level also is found effective in naturalistic settings. Hence, the therapist should then let the client know: "Studies from regular therapy settings show that the recommended treatment is also experienced as useful by clients with the same problems you have." These two levels can be labeled as *nomothetic knowledge* because they aim to capture some general phenomena on a group level that should be relevant as a treatment recommendation for clients with similar characteristics. Nomothetic knowledge is typically based on quantitative data that are collected from many respondents and are analyzed using statistical computer programs. Thirdly, even though the therapist has searched through this nomothetic knowledge addressing a recommended treatment of choice, if one exists, the therapist cannot be assured that this treatment will help *this* particular client. Hence, the therapist needs to say to the client: "Based on the research recommendations, this specific treatment approach is what I would suggest we go for. However, we will not know whether this will fit *you*. So, if you agree to try this approach it is important that you let me know whether this treatment is helpful and meaningful for you. If not, we will figure out something else to try." This level of evidence is by Gullestad (2001) and Howard et al. (1996) called *efficiency* and is by definition an *idiographic level of knowledge* as opposed to the nomothetic level. Idiographic knowledge is typically focused on examining the individual event or person and their individual and distinctive characteristics and prerequisites. Thus, nomothetic evidence needs to be weighed against the client's own experience, theory of change, and so forth (idiographic evidence). One may assume that clients seek professional help partly because their own idiographic knowledge has not been sufficient for them to over-come their problems. Thus, nomothetic knowledge is welcomed. In other words, idiographic and nomothetic types of knowledge are mutually complementary, and we should therefore be aware of how they are to be integrated into EBP.

One empirical rationale that supports the need to ask for the client's idiographic knowledge is suggested by Walfish, McAlister, O'Donnell, and Lambert (2012), who found that therapists are unreliable in predicting the outcome of their own therapy: Therapists showed poor judgment in identifying clients that were deterio-rating during therapy, as they only managed to predict 2.5% of those who actually got worse. This "self-assessment bias" finding suggests that as therapists, we are not successful in a true assessment of therapy progress when we rely upon our profes-sional judgment alone. Furthermore, attempts have been made to compare the use of statistical algorithms with therapists' predictions in calculating expected therapy development, and it was found that the algorithms were more reliable than the thera-pists' judgment (Hannan et al., 2005). The conclusion from these studies is that as professionals we need some kind of aid to achieve a better understanding of how our clients develop. And because the most reliable information comes from the client, we need to find systematic ways to be informed by the client during therapy. The use of standardized and frequent feedback systems is one promising means to realize this goal.

Studies of the use of feedback have so far suggested that it is associated with better outcomes, shorter treatment time, and lower risk of dropout than when no feedback was used (Gondek, Edbrooke-Childs, Fink, Deighton, & Wolpert, 2016). The most robust finding from a meta-analysis shows that using feedback is an important tool for detecting signs early in the process when therapy is not heading in the desired direction and whether there is a risk of dropout (Shimokawa, Lambert, & Smart, 2010). Because this should serve as an alarm signal for the therapist dur-ing therapy, it could give the therapist and client an opportunity to evaluate and make adjustments that can lead to the desired goals. Such a realization of user involvement will assumingly also enhance the working alliance between the client and therapist. When the therapist and client both experience collaboration in sharing that feedback information is useful, this has been associated with improved out-come (Lutz, De Jong, & Rubel, 2015). Good outcome is also associated with thera-pists having good professional self-esteem combined with his or her uncertainty whether his or her professional work with the client is successful, and as a conse-quence, feedback is requested (Nissen-Lie, Monsen, Ulleberg, & Rønnestad, 2013). In summary, research supports how user involvement via feedback works as an important source of knowledge in psychotherapy.

One may argue that compared to EBT, the EBP has taken a great leap toward a more systemic understanding of psychotherapy. The use of feedback seems in par-ticular to be of vital importance in this transformation. Because research on feed-back also shows that it is associated with successful outcomes to the same degree as well tested methods, feedback can be defined as evidence-based practice (McHugh

& Barlow, 2012). This development seems to answer the call from Lambert, Garfield, and Bergin (2004):

> A necessary and productive direction for psychotherapy researchers involves methods of monitoring patient treatment response in real time and modifying ongoing treatment when its intended positive impact fails to materialize. We call for more such research and encourage those in the field to give special consideration to engaging in this "patient-focused" or "outcome-focused" research. (p. 818)

Even though EBP includes several research methodologies (Duncan & Reese, 2013, p. 491), the call from Lambert et al. (2004) addresses even more distinctly how research can be integrated with regular clinical work: something that has been labeled as practice-based evidence (PBE – Holmquist, Phillips, & Barkham, 2015). Compared to efficacy and effectiveness research, PBE emphasizes "a bottom-up model whereby routine data are used at an individual level and locally within the service but then also accumulated across services and used to generate a higher-order evidence base" (Holmquist et al., 2015, p. 22). Another phrase for this is practice-oriented research (POR – Castonguay & Muran, 2015), describing the use of feedback as a way to collect data for both clinical and research purposes (also called routine outcome monitoring – ROM). This approach implies in particular the possibility of studying session-to-session development of change, identifying change trajectories that may vary for different persons or groups with specific characteristics. This way, psychotherapy research has the capacity to target the *why* and *what* and also the *who* (Duncan & Reese, 2013, p. 291–292) in its effort to create a more idiographically tailored clinical practice. Using sophisticated statistical analyses on data collected frequently enables addressing mechanisms of change, which will increase our knowledge of what makes psychotherapy work. These analyses further allow us to follow the individual client's change *compared with the group* included in the study ("between-client variation") as well as investigating the individual client's change *compared to himself or herself* at an earlier timepoint ("within-client variation" – Hoffart, 2017). Interestingly, such statistical approaches actually address the needed link between nomothetic and idiographic knowledge that should pave the way ahead because of its clinical relevance: The PBE research's objective is in accord with therapists' main focus, namely, on following the individual client's change based on his or her individual situation, prerequisites, and goals. This idiographic level, supplemented by the use of quantitative and qualitative research designs (nomothetic level), should together create more knowledge on change mechanisms. In conclusion, feedback (ROM) appears to work as a needed link between nomothetic and idiographic knowledge by reducing the gap between clinical practice and research. This endeavor represents a willingness to integrate research procedures and clinical practice so that the therapist and the client become empirically informed in their joint effort to optimize the treatment outcome.

Feedback Promoting User Involvement

Feedback (ROM) means that the client frequently responds to therapy-related questions in a standardized and systematic way, for example, on an online questionnaire. A report based on client answers is fed back to the therapist informing him or her about progression (outcome goals, such as symptom burden) and process (therapeutic relationship, including alliance) as experienced by the client before, during, or after each therapy session. If it appears that the therapy is not proceeding in the desired direction, this information should be an important basis for evaluating the way the therapist and client so far have worked, assessing whether the work should be adjusted. In other words, ROM can be an equally important auxiliary tool for a psychotherapist as somatic test answers are for the physician's assessment and choice of appropriate patient treatment. ROM information that includes risk areas such as suicide and violence threats, as well as substance abuse and maltreatment, can contribute to the implementation of life-saving and preventive actions.

The user involvement is enhanced especially when the therapist shares the ROM information with the client and follows that sharing by inviting the client to interpret and reflect on his or her own answers. The theory of feedback indicates that if the feedback differs from what one expects or has set as goals, it is a motivation for change (Scheier & Carver, 2003). When the client at the start of treatment answers questions about, for example, symptom distress, this becomes a client-defined starting point that can act as an evaluation anchor: If a score of a depression burden during the course of therapy shows a reduction (e.g., with the value 12) in symptoms compared to the starting point (e.g., value 19), this difference (i.e., 7) can work as a specific and concrete achieved change score. Clients may be unfamiliar with typical topics in therapy such as recognizing and talking about feelings, cognitions, memories, perceptions, and relations. Because of the abstract nature of these topics, the client may more easily relate to a concrete number or graph symbolizing a level or change of the abstract phenomena. In particular, when the numbers and graphs indicate a change, this observation may evoke the client's recognition of how this change can be manifest in his or her bodily sensations, etc. This client may therefore learn via ROM-created numbers and graphs to be more aware of feelings, thoughts, and relationships and become more self-observing, earning more consciousness of and curiosity about his or her own important therapeutic process, viz., the term "psychological mindedness." The therapist should in particular emphasize for the client how his or her scoring on ROM is associated with the client's efforts in therapy. This is important because attributing change to one's own efforts is found to be associated with faster and more lasting recovery (Wampold & Imel, 2015). If the ROM procedure includes the use of electronic platforms like PC, Mac, tablets, and cell phone devices that now are familiar for the majority of people, this could create a bridge between the familiar (i.e., electronic devices) and the unfamiliar (i.e., therapy). If the therapist acts clumsily and apparently struggles to make use of the electronic device, the client may offer himself or herself to help out, creating a better balance in the therapy room by the client demonstrating competence that is appreciated by the therapist. This way ROM can contribute to the needed sorting work that often is essential in psychotherapy, for instance, in identifying and categorizing feelings, thoughts, and experiences (Zahl-Olsen & Oanes, 2017). Another experience is that using ROM in itself entails a common focus and language, something that forms a basis for favorable therapeutic dialogues that increase the client's ownership and responsibility in therapy (Sundet, 2017). Finally, this example illustrates feedback procedures as psychoeducation – A female client in her 50s asked the therapist: "Now I have been answering the same questions over and over again. Does it mean they are important?" Therapist: "Yes, we do believe they are." Client: "OK."

Empirically Informed Therapy: The New Wave?

The abovementioned gap in our field between clinical work and research (Heatherington et al., 2015; Pinsof & Wynne, 2000) implies that research-based knowledge, for example, which therapeutic approach is found to be the most promising for a certain psychiatric disorder, is rarely known and used by clinicians. And the opposite way around; clinicians are rarely directly involved in research in a way that is perceived as relevant to their clinical practice. Clinicians may be asked by researchers to facilitate research to be conducted in their clinical unit, research that represents change in the daily clinical routines. Hence, clinicians often perceive research as a "top-down" activity that little affects their performance as therapists, or worse, that research protocols force them to act in ways they don't believe benefit treatment. Further, the research community's "tribal language" also contributes an undesired distance between the two fields. This is unfortunate as both fields ideally should benefit from each other's contributions. The abovementioned "practice-oriented research" (POR; Castonguay & Muran, 2015) within a "practice-based evidence" (PBE – Holmquist et al., 2015) paradigm is rather a "bottom-up" approach that does not impede the normal conduct of therapy. A PBE approach that stands side by side with the more established concept of EBP (ibid.) is promising with respect to reducing the gap between clinical practice and research and as a way to resolve the dichotomy that may exist between paradigms in the field. Interestingly, several research components are found useful clinically. For instance, asking clients systematically about their perception of process and progress, testing one's clinical hypotheses, and inviting a shared interpretation of results, all demonstrate that research applies directly to clinical use.

The integrated use of ROM and POR in clinical practice should pave the way for a new type of psychotherapy practice that to a greater extent informs the therapist directly through feedback from the client so that therapy becomes empirically informed. This approach will likely influence the relationship between the therapist and clients, especially when the therapist uses the ROM information as a conversation tool, for instance, by inviting the clients to interpret their own results. This way the client may enter a more active and empowered position in a therapy that truly is user involvement and collaboration as the best means of achieving the client's goals.

Professional Autonomy

One characteristic of being a professional is the trust given by authorities, stakeholders, leaders, and the public to the professional to make autonomous assessments and decisions within a defined delegated area. As mentioned, the influence of NPM (New Public Management) in our field, characterized by the introduction of a business model of how to run public services in human care and treatment, e.g., by the use of concepts like "financial control," "value for the money," and "documentation of effectiveness," has by many professionals in our field been considered alien. The more strict governmental documentation requirements in Norway are by many therapists perceived as inappropriate interference with professionals' performance, resulting in a feeling that their autonomy is under pressure (Ekeland, Aurdal, & Skjelten, 2014). These therapists question the extent that the governmental system should be involved in regulating clinical decisions on which treatment should be offered: for whom, when, within which level of care, duration, etc. These professionals claim that the governmental criterion of only including evidence-based treatments in their guidelines excludes those treatments not yet empirically tested. But not being empirically tested does not mean the treatment is not working. In essence, this governmental regulation feels unfair to many therapists who in their clinical practice experience that their treatment approach is working, even though it does not appear on the governmental EBT lists. While there is solid agreement about the golden principle of ensuring that clients receive the best available professional help, it should be questioned what kind of knowledge has formed the basis for developing the governmental EBT list that distinguishes between accepted and non-accepted treatments (Utvåg, Steinkopf, & Holgersen, 2014). For the purposes here, this issue highlights a question whether the single client's treatment trajectory (which by definition is at an idiographic level) can be predicted precisely based on research knowledge collected on a nomothetic level. With reference to the above-mentioned EBP (APA Task Force, 2006), employing three sources of knowledge interpreted with the use of three levels of evidence (Gullestad, 2001; Howard et al., 1996), the EBT implies only making use of one source of knowledge and one level of evidence. Still, to what extent is EBT really a threat to professional autonomy? Interestingly, this dilemma seems to be solved by the use of EBP! Norwegian psychologists (Utvåg et al., 2014) have explored and discussed the concern of losing professional autonomy as a result of what is regulated by Norwegian legislation and governmental guidelines. Their conclusion was that if research knowledge and/or clinical experience in line with EBT comes in conflict with the client's preferences and values, the latter – based on feedback from the client – should have priority, as stated by the user involvement act. Because the therapist in such a situation is the one to weigh these different and conflicting interests against each other, this actually strengthens the therapist's discretion, which is an important aspect of autonomy. Therefore, EBP will win against EBT by safeguarding important elements embedded in the role of a therapist while at the same time strengthening the voice of the client. By systematically inviting feedback from the clients via ROM, this information adds to the knowledge needed for the therapist to work in agreement with EBP. In conclusion, the principles of EBP in combination with the awareness of the different levels of evidence appear to create the best guarantee for maintenance of professional autonomy.

Professional Transparency and Deliberate Practice

Another subject that may be related to professional autonomy – particularly in psychotherapy – is the therapist's ability to work alone together with one or more clients in confidentiality behind a closed door showing a "Do Not Disturb" sign. In such circumstances, it is rare for psychotherapists to give access to other professionals to what happens inside this room during therapy sessions. At one extreme, we know that abuse occurs where therapists do not respect the client's integrity and intimate borders. Sadly, such violations illustrate how risky a "therapeutic" relationship may be: Linguistically, "therapist" is too close to "the rapist." More commonly – we must assume – no violations of the client's intimate borders occur, but research points to the risk that therapy will not be helpful to a considerable portion of clients, estimating approximately 40% will remain unchanged and about 10% will deteriorate after psychotherapy (Shimokawa et al., 2010). ROM is particularly beneficial in revealing these trajectories as treatment unfolds, enabling the therapist and client to discover early signs of no change, deterioration, or risk for dropout followed by an evaluation and adjustment of the therapy (Shimokawa et al., 2010). However, because of the previously mentioned "self-assessment bias" (Walfish et al., 2012), therapists may wrongly believe that they are able to identify unsuccessful therapies during the course of treatment, and so may not see the need for feedback.

Another factor affecting the utility of ROM is that it should be implemented in a climate of transparency at the clinical unit. Transparency implies that therapists also share their feedback from clients with colleagues and supervisors or consultants. In particular, transparency of unsuccessful cases has the highest learning potential as it addresses which areas the therapist needs to improve, for example, by skills training. Such self-disclosure may be unusual within a professional culture of confidentiality. And therapists may resist it because admitting unsuccessful outcomes is usually associated with shame: "My colleagues must think I'm not a good therapist!" "If my boss sees my feedback results, my salary may be reduced!" Such challenges are often associated with "Big Brother is watching you" and have been experienced several places where feedback has been implemented (Boswell, Kraus, Miller, & Lambert, 2015; Tilden, 2017). Such natural resistance needs to be addressed through a deliberate effort to change the work culture toward a more transparent climate. The leader of the job context needs therefore to be clear about the desired goal, introducing the use of ROM as a standard procedure that is included in job requirements. Presenting this as "the way we do it here" in a job interview will prepare the candidate for a culture of transparency that characterizes this particular workplace. We have seen that this approach seems to be much easier to introduce to young therapists who see this as a great potential for learning in line with the concept of "deliberate practice" – for instance, in how to improve one's facilitative interpersonal skills (FIS – Anderson et al., 2009; Wampold & Imel, 2015). A prerequisite for a successful culture of transparency is the overarching attitude that constructive critique is given within a climate of caring and that revealing our errors should be the first step toward improving our skills. Making professional supervision or consultation inclusive of a therapist's ROM data will eventually create a more relaxed atmosphere where curiosity and a desire to learn more from each other will dominate rather than anxiety and fear of being judged and disparaged. Again, a culture of transparency should not be conceived as a threat against professional autonomy; it is rather another way to conduct oneself professionally.

Closing Remarks

This chapter has been built on the premise that the use of valid and recognized knowledge is crucial for the quality of our clinical practice. Externally, this practice legitimates our professional relationships with policymakers, stakeholders, governmental bureaucracy, funding agencies, and other neighboring professional fields, and last but far from least, it helps establish a trustworthy relationship with our clients. In particular, clients need to perceive the professional helper as credible, as one who represents competence by explaining the problems, as well as creating expectations for improvement (Wampold & Imel, 2015). This external legitimacy is crucial for our field, or else we risk becoming marginalized in relation to other comparable fields.

Internally, we need some well-defined criteria on the kind and levels of knowledge (epistemology and paradigms) that are valid within our own field and are also accepted by the scientific community. If only a few approaches are recognized within our field without understanding and acceptance within the greater scientific community, this position may be characterized as self-nurture with the risk of starvation and obliteration as a distinct professional field in the long run. In light of CFT being under pressure from stronger professions, we need to interact with others in order to grow and demonstrate our relevance and contributions as part of the service systems that are offered to the public. Therefore we need to play by the rules, and by doing so, we also have the best chance to have impact on the rules, if we think they should be changed.

Within our field, there has been a tendency to choose camps, for instance, whether you belong to a positivistic or social constructionist tradition of knowledge. This can risk creating and sustaining a less communicative and productive practitioner-researcher gap. Even though there may be several dilemmas in combining the use of different knowledge approaches, the established principles of EBP and the levels of evidence presented in this chapter work as a frame from which several knowledge approaches can be integrated because they are mutually complementary. As emphasized, nomothetic knowledge offered from research blended with idiographic knowledge from the client suggests that clinical practice becomes empirically informed.

We must assume that we as humans are more similar than we are different. Hence we need to make use of the existing nomothetic knowledge when there is a significant chance that this knowledge will be helpful for the individual. At the same time, every person is unique, demanding that treatment needs to be tailored according to this individual's background, values, preferences, problems, and goals. For this reason, idiographic knowledge is necessary, and we should welcome the use of ROM systems that are easily accessible tools in therapy to collect this crucial information. In conclusion, nomothetic and idiographic knowledge cannot work isolated from each other in our field; they both benefit in an interdependent, mutually nourishing exchange.

References

American Psychological Association Presidential Task Force on Evidence Based Practice. (2006). Evidence-based practice in psychology. *American Psychologist, 61*, 271–285. https://doi.org/10.1037/0003-066X.61.4.271

Anderson, H. (2016). Postmodern/poststructural/social construction therapies. In T. L. Sexton & J. Lebow (Eds.), *Handbook of family therapy* (pp. 182–204). New York, NY: Routledge.

Anderson, T., Ogles, B. M., Patterson, C. L., Lambert, M. J., & Vermeersch, D. A. (2009). Therapist effects: Facilitative interpersonal skills as a predictor of therapist success. *Journal of Clinical Psychology, 65*(7), 755–768. https://doi.org/10.1002/jclp.20583

Boswell, J. F., Kraus, D. R., Miller, S. D., & Lambert, M. J. (2015). Implementing routine outcome monitoring in clinical practice: Benefits, challenges, and solutions. *Psychotherapy Research, 25*, 6–19.

Castonguay, L. G., & Muran, C. (2015). Fostering collaboration between researchers and clinicians through building practice-oriented research: An introduction. *Psychotherapy Research, 25*, 1–5.

Duncan, B., Miller, S., & Sparks, J. (2000). *The heroic client.* San Francisco, CA: Jossey-Bass Publishers.

Duncan, B. L., & Reese, R. J. (2013). Empirically supported treatments, evidence-based treatments, and evidence-based practice. In I. B. Winer (Ed.), *Handbook of psychology* (2nd ed., pp. 489–513). Hoboken, NJ: Wiely.

Ekeland, T.-J., Aurdal, Å., & Skjelten, I. M. (2014). Når staten vil være terapeut. *Fokus på familien, 42*, 139–156.

Gondek, D., Edbrooke-Childs, J., Fink, E., Deighton, J., & Wolpert, M. (2016). Feedback from outcome measures and treatment effectiveness, treatment efficiency, and collaborative practice: A systematic review. *Administration and Policy in Mental Health and Mental Health Services Research, 43*, 325–343. https://doi.org/10.1007/s10488-015-0710-5

Gullestad, S. E. (2001). Hva er evidensbasert psykoterapi? *Tidsskrift for Norsk Psykologforening, 38*, 942–951. ISSN 0332-6470.

Hannan, C., Lambert, M. J., Harmon, C., Nielsen, S. L., Smart, D. W., Shimokawa, K., & Sutton, S. W. (2005). A lab test and algorithms for identifying clients at risk for treatment failure. *Journal of Clinical Psychology: In Session, 61*, 155–163. https://doi.org/10.2002/jclp.20108

Heatherington, L., Friedlander, M. L., Diamond, G. M., Escudero, V., & Pinsof, W. M. (2015). 25 years of systemic therapies research: Progress and promise. *Psychotherapy Research, 25*, 348–364.

Hoffart, A. (2017). Terapiforskningen trenger en ideografisk vending. *Tidsskrift for Norsk Psykologforening, 54*(2), 210–212.

Holmquist, R., Phillips, B., & Barkham, M. (2015). Developing practice-based evidence: Benefits, challenges, and tensions. *Psychotherapy Research, 25*, 20–31. https://doi.org/10.1080/105033 07.2013.861093

Howard, K. I., Moras, K., Brill, P. L., Martinovich, Z., & Lutz, W. (1996). Evaluation of psychotherapy. Efficacy, effectiveness and client progress. *American Psychologist, 51*, 1059–1064.

Lambert, M. J., Garfield, S. L., & Bergin, A. E. (2004). Overview, trends, and future issues. In M. J. Lambert (Ed.), *Bergin and Garfield's handbook of psychotherapy and behavior change* (5th ed., pp. 805–821). New York, NY: Wiley.

Lutz, W., De Jong, K., & Rubel, J. (2015). Patient-focused and feedback research in psychotherapy: Where are we and where do we want to go? *Psychotherapy Research, 25*(6), 625–632. https://doi.org/10.1080/10503307.2015.1079661

McHugh, R. K., & Barlow, D. H. (2012). *Dissemination and implementation of evidence-based psychological interventions*. New York, NY: Oxford University Press.

Nissen-Lie, H. A., Monsen, J. T., Ulleberg, P., & Rønnestad, M. H. (2013). Psychotherapists' self-reports of their interpersonal functioning and difficulties in practice as predictors of patient outcome. *Psychotherapy Research, 23*(1), 86–104. https://doi.org/10.1080/10503307.2012.7 35775

Oanes, C. J., Karlson, B., & Borg, M. (2017). User involvement in therapy: Couples' and family therapists' lived experiences with the inclusion of a feedback procedure in clinical practice. *Australian & New Zealand Journal of Family Therapy, 38*, 451–463. https://doi.org/10.1002/ anzf.1232

One Flew Over the Cuckoo's Nest. (1975). American comedy-drama film directed by Miloš Forman, based on the 1962 novel *One Flew Over the Cuckoo's Nest* by Ken Kesey.

Pinsof, W. M., & Lebow, J. L. (2005). A scientific paradigm for family psychology. In W. M. Pinsof & J. L. Lebow (Eds.), *Family psychology. The art of science* (pp. 3–19). New York, NY: Oxford.

Pinsof, W. M., & Wynne, L. C. (2000). Toward progress research: Closing the gap between family therapy practice and research. *Journal of Marital & Family Therapy, 26*, 1–8.

Rohrbaugh, M. J. (2014). Old wine in new bottles. Decanting systemic family process research in the era of evidence-based practice. *Family Process, 53*, 434–444.

Scheier, M. F., & Carver, C. S. (2003). Goals and confidence as self-regulatory elements underlying health and illness behavior. In L. D. Cameron & H. Leventhal (Eds.), *The self-regulation of health and illness behavior* (pp. 17–41). London, UK: Taylor Francis.

Shimokawa, K., Lambert, M. J., & Smart, D. (2010). Enhancing treatment outcome of patients at risk of treatment failure: Meta-analytic and mega-analytic review of a psychotherapy quality assurance system. *Journal of Consulting and Clinical Psychology, 78*, 298–311. https://doi. org/10.1037/a0019247

Sundet, R. (2017). Feedback as means to enhance client-therapist interaction in therapy. In T. Tilden & B. E. Wampold (Eds.), *Routine outcome monitoring in couple and family therapy. The empirically informed therapist* (pp. 121–142). Cham, Switzerland: Springer.

Tilden, T. (2017). How can I know whether my efforts are helpful for the client? Implementing feedback in Norway. In T. Tilden & B. E. Wampold (Eds.), *Routine outcome monitoring in couple and family therapy. The empirically informed therapist* (pp. 3–13). Cham, Switzerland: Springer.

Tilden, T., & Wampold, B. E. (Eds.). (2017). *Routine outcome monitoring in couple and family therapy. The empirically informed therapist*. Cham, Switzerland: Springer.

Ulvestad, A. K., & Henriksen, A. K. (2007). I skyggen av elfenbenstårnet. In A. K. Ulvestad, A. K. Henriksen, A.-G. Tuseth, & T. Fjeldstad (Eds.), *Klienten – den glemte terapeut. Brukerstyring i psykisk helsearbeid* (pp. 20–27). Oslo, Norway: Gyldendal Akademisk.

Utvåg, K. M., Steinkopf, S., & Holgersen, H. (2014). Vilkår for klinisk autonomi og dens betydning for praksis. *Tidsskrift for Norsk Psykologforening, 51*, 861–867.

Walfish, S., McAlister, B., O'Donnell, P., & Lambert, M. J. (2012). An investigation of self-assessment bias in mental health providers. *Psychological Reports, 110*(2), 639–644. https://doi.org/10.2466/02.07.17.pr0.110.2.639-644

Wampold, B. E., & Imel, Z. E. (2015). *The great psychotherapy debate: The research evidence for what works in psychotherapy* (2nd ed.). New York, NY: Routledge.

WHO. (1986). http://www.who.int/healthpromotion/about/HPR%20Glossary%201998.pdf. Retrieved from internet April 26. 2018.

Zahl-Olsen, R., & Oanes, C. J. (2017). An anthill of questions that made me prepare for the first session. In T. Tilden & B. E. Wampold (Eds.), *Routine outcome monitoring in couple and family therapy. The empirically informed therapist* (pp. 121–142). Cham, Switzerland: Springer.

Therapeutic-Factor-Oriented Skill-Building in Systemic Counselling: Productively Conjoining Attitude and Method

Petra Bauer and Marc Weinhardt

Introduction

In the last decade, there has been renewed research into therapeutic or common factors behind counselling and therapy. This research has regularly come to the conclusion that the success of counselling and therapy must be considered far more methodologically invariant than previously assumed (Lambert, Bergin, & Garfield, 2013; Wampold & Imel, 2015): when other influences are sufficiently controlled for, different counselling and therapy methods (in the following, we shall refer generally to counselling) exhibit a very similar degree of efficacy. Moreover, the proportion of the overall outcome which results from specific methodological practices is considerably smaller than is often assumed; estimates vary in a range from 10 to 20% (Lambert, Bergin, & Garfield, 2013; Pfammatter & Tschacher, 2012; Vossler, 2014; Wampold & Imel, 2015). As a result, in this field of research, the question of influences is shifted from examining the efficacy of individual methods to studying the efficacy of the professionals who, as one common explanation goes, use these methods with differing levels of productivity to implement successful support processes. From this point of view, methods are mainly seen as instruments for achieving the successful professionalisation of (prospective) counsellors. The key question raised here is that of how to achieve therapeutic-factor-oriented skill-building aimed especially at these common factors. It should be made clear from the start that this piece is specifically not intended to question the importance of training counsellors using consistent theories and methods: after all, the abstract

P. Bauer
Institute of Educational Sciences, Department of Social Pedagogy, Tübingen University, Tübingen, Germany

M. Weinhardt (✉)
School of Professional Studies, Darmstadt Protestant University of Applied Sciences, Darmstadt, Germany
e-mail: Marc.Weinhardt@eh-darmstadt.de

© Springer Nature Switzerland AG 2020
M. Ochs et al. (eds.), *Systemic Research in Individual, Couple, and Family Therapy and Counseling*, European Family Therapy Association Series,
https://doi.org/10.1007/978-3-030-36560-8_22

factors identified by research into therapeutic factors cannot be directly instrumen-talised or taught. These factors which are reconstructed in the research are in fact correlates of highly implicit, abstract knowledge and ability which experts generate situationally through their counselling processes. This type of knowledge is not directly accessible to teachers – a familiar problem in helping professions which is also known in other fields (Neuweg, 2015) and which, if ignored, would lead to efficacy being disastrously mistaken for learnability (Weinhardt, 2016). Just as before, techniques and methods can and must be taught within a theoretically con-sistent learning environment, at first geared towards cognitive understanding and then becoming increasingly routine until they are finally habitualised as profes-sional expertise which produces the efficacy subsequently identified in the research. As each subject requires different means of acquiring this form of expertise, and different educational pathways to achieve that goal, professionalisation processes must be oriented towards therapeutic factors, while the professionals' various learning and education processes must necessarily be subject-specific. In the fol-lowing contribution, we thus focus on issues around developing therapeutic-factor-oriented systemic skills in the light of subject-oriented professionalisation, examining two topics in particular: firstly the difference between attitude and method – one of the standard main distinctions made in research into therapeutic factors – and secondly a stage in professionalisation processes which has until now been somewhat overlooked, the early stages during which students acquire exper-tise. To this end, we use performance-oriented data from a study which has been running for 10 years: a simulated psychosocial counselling environment which enables students to gain experience in counselling with trained simulation clients in a highly realistic learning environment.[1]

Attitude and Method as Central Didactic Concepts for Learning Counselling

The terms "attitude" and "method" both describe dimensions of counselling skills[2] which are considered fundamental to the shape of counselling processes whatever the method applied (Weinhardt, 2016). On close inspection, differences between these two dimensions do, however, soon become apparent both in terms of the weight given to each by the different counselling concepts and in terms of the exact

---

[1] Some parts of the following chapter are taken from an earlier publication: "Über die Schwierigkeit, Neugier, Offenheit und Anerkennung zu lehren und zu lernen." In: Zipperle, M., Bauer, P., Stauber, B., Treptow, R. (eds.): *Vermitteln. Eine Aufgabe von Theorie und Praxis Sozialer Arbeit* (pp. 205–216). Wiesbaden: VS.

[2] We use the term "method" as employed in the German-speaking discussion among social work-ers: methods are a "well-founded, knowledge-based set of instructions providing a planned, struc-tured means of achieving a goal" (Galuske & Müller, 2012, p. 588) and, in this broader sense, mediate between theoretical concepts on one hand and specific techniques on the other.

content of those dimensions. Systemic counselling can be viewed as an approach which is relevant in many fields of counselling, and attitude can certainly be said to be a significant aspect of skill-building in systemic therapy and counselling (von Schlippe & Schweizer, 2016). Nonetheless, for a long time, training and continuing education in systemic counselling seemed to be characterised by teaching specific techniques (e.g. for asking questions) and methodological concepts. By contrast, less attention was paid to the question of how prospective professionals could be taught an essential attitude of curiosity, openness and acknowledging other people as a constitutive basis for their work. The finding is thus all the more interesting that, even in extremely specialised counselling settings (e.g. at advice centres or in hospitals), this vague, indefinable factor of attitude repeatedly comes to the fore: even in such environments, studies of the efficacy of individual factors, assessed by technological means, persistently churn out the findings of "Lambert's pie" (Lambert et al., 2013). For two decades, this pie chart has shown that relationship-forming, motivation and other relatively soft, unclear determinants play the greatest role in the efficacy of counselling. In the following, we will show that a scientific examination of students' counselling skills similarly reveals a generalist factor that is difficult to pin down, expressed in their counselling as an attitude of attentive curiosity, openness and acknowledgement in the relationship which the students form with clients and people seeking advice.[3] It can be described as a generalist factor as it covers various aspects of the way the relationship is established, all of which together, however, are of great importance when it comes to making measurable progress in the development of counselling skills. In the following, when we speak of developing counselling skills, we are referring to a learning concept which involves students being taught initial counselling approaches based on systemic concepts. Thematically, the focus is on counselling for psychosocial problems. In the German-speaking counselling landscape, this type of psychosocial counselling is a form of professional support which has expanded rapidly in recent years, diverging into highly disparate institutional manifestations (Bauer & Weinhardt, 2014). Various types of counselling are available which specialise in individual problems, such as addiction counselling or debt counselling, alongside a range of broader range of services such as social counselling or family counselling. Conceptually, professional psychosocial counselling has moved strongly away from everyday forms of counselling such as giving advice, etc. Instead, it sees itself as a sophisticated, scientifically backed form of discussion during which clients are guided and accompanied through processes of gaining self-understanding. Great importance is attached to the clients' autonomy and to carefully constructing the counselling process (Nestmann & Sickendiek, 2018).

There is no doubt within the scientific community, or in most fields of practice, that this specific professionalised form of counselling has to be learned so precisely. In German-speaking countries, counselling has not yet been able to develop

---

[3]We do not directly analyse this generalised factor with regard to outcome-oriented efficacy; instead, we are interested in the role it plays in developing counselling skills, with the question of whether efficacy acts as a benchmark for skills always, of course, being implicit.

independently either as an academic discipline or as a profession (Strasser, 2015). Qualifications in psychosocial counselling are mainly gained through specialised continuing education curricula which are often privately run. More rarely, in recent years, some postgraduate degree courses in counselling have become available at masteral level. Counselling courses frequently draw upon one or more therapeutic procedures and, accordingly, teach counselling skills as a "slimmed down" therapy. By contrast, in the English-speaking world, counselling is already taught on first-cycle degree courses and up to doctoral level and involves qualifications which are equivalent to a medical licence.

Becoming a skilled counsellor hinges upon various aspects: not only different realms of knowledge (relating to specific fields and problems or about structuring the process and directing the conversation) but also skills (intervention methods and techniques) and the ability to form an appropriate therapeutic relationship. Until now, however, academics studying how counselling is learnt have paid little attention to the extent to which developing this kind of relationship in particular can actually be taught or learned at all. Focusing on this brings back a classic pedagogical question: can skills in forming a relationship of this kind be taught at all; if so, how, and could such teaching even become a function of higher education? Or is the ability to form a therapeutic relationship simply a correlate of a well-suited personality, as expressed in the traditional topos of the "born teacher" and passed down through time as the prevalent understanding of the profession to this day? Within the broader question of how professionality can develop at institutes of higher education, in the following section, we will present a model which empirically describes the fundamental structure of counselling skill and the far-reaching role of a generalised ability to establish the counselling relationship. In particular, we will discuss the extent to which a professional therapeutic relationship conceptualised in this manner can be taught and learned. Our discussion is based on the assumption that some parts of this "diffuse" element of professional practice and forming a viable working relationship can be taught and learned but that other parts do seem to be incorporated, personality-related factors resulting from an individual's socialisation, making changes much harder to trigger in the context of higher education.

Professionalisation and Skill-Building at Degree Level with Regard to Therapeutic Attitude

If it is assumed that counselling, or at least major aspects of it, can be learned and developed as a profession, then even the early stages of acquiring skills in higher education are of interest. Even looking beyond the realm of counselling skills, the emerging interplay of previous experience, personality traits and growing stockpiles of knowledge is particularly clear in higher education endeavours aimed at professionalisation (e.g. see Bauer, 2014; Becker-Lenz & Müller, 2008). This assumption can also be tied in with the question of the extent to which the basic elements of a counsellor's essential attitude and the relationship established as a result can be acquired, developed and built upon in the context of higher education (Bauer & Weinhardt, 2016; Weinhardt, 2015).

In the following, when we speak of an attitude geared towards establishing a professional therapeutic relationship, there is a lack of clarity behind this terminology which can only be resolved to a limited extent even in this article. Though the term "attitude" is used as a matter of course in many therapeutic concepts and procedures, there has as yet been no systematic examination of how therapeutic methods differ with respect to the attitudes they consider appropriate (for an example of the central aspects of a systemic essential attitude, see Barthelmess (2016). There seems to be even less clarity regarding the question of what attitudes might be generally appropriate for counselling in all its facets and institutional settings. As a result, the following can only get us slightly closer to answering this question that is central to how counselling is learned.

In the context of research into therapy, attitude can initially be described as the "contribution" which the therapist makes to the ongoing relationship (Staats, 2017, p. 26), leaving aside the fact that it can very much be seen as problematic to focus on individual aspects of an intersubjective session. Person-centred therapy concepts especially have focused firmly on the type of attitude that leads to a relationship which brings about change in therapy and counselling and how this attitude can be achieved in the here and now of the actual relationship (Kriz, 2014, p. 200ff.). As Kriz (ibid., p. 200) puts it, the classic triad of genuineness, unconditional positive regard and empathic understanding form "three aspects of an attitude in the therapist" which are the central "core conditions" of the therapeutic process. Rogers himself worked for decades on the question of how that attitude can be learned. One central means seems to be lesson plans aimed largely at students regulating their own learning process and undergoing personal growth (Kunze-Pletat, 2018), which, however, only appears feasible to a limited extent within higher education.

Preß and Gmelch (2014) propose a definition of therapeutic attitude which is more closely aligned to behaviourist concepts. A semantic analysis involving 40 interviews with psychotherapists (both trainees and experts with many years of experience) indicates that attitude is universally seen as a "relatively stable characteristic over time", something approaching a personality trait (Preß and Gmelch, 2014, p. 360). However, the meanings ascribed to the term by practitioners do not make it clear whether it refers to people's outlooks, normative tendencies or aspects of empathy and interest (ibid.). Based on their semantic analysis, the two authors propose that attitude should be seen as a component which is based on cognitive structures and is expressed in specific therapy-related ways: this defines the "therapeutic attitude as the way in which psychotherapists' beliefs, outlooks and values are manifested in their reactions in the context of psychotherapy" (ibid.). Attitudes are thus based on an individual's personal philosophy regarding therapy and contribute to specific assumptions about how therapy works and a certain view of clients. If one defines the term following the approach set out here, this, too, underlines the difficulty of learning attitude. All that can be offered is rather vague references to the need for continuous self-reflection in the context of therapeutic training.

Drawing upon the basic principles of the theory of professionalism, attitude can also be described as the development of a professional habitus based not only on object-related knowledge but also on central maxims and values of professional practice and concepts for establishing a relationship while mediating between specific and non-specific roles (Becker-Lenz, et al. 2009, 2011, 2012).

From this point of view based on the theory of professionalism, the way in which therapists approach and deal with clients can be described as the expression of an ingrained (habitualised and thus strongly incorporated) attitude seen among (prospective) professionals and comprising central values such as clients' autonomy in coping with their lives (Becker-Lenz and Müller, 2009, p. 201). The specific subject of these investigations was how an attitude of this kind, with an ethical and moral basis, develops on social work degree courses. However, almost all the findings indicate that courses offering qualifications in social work fields are not or only rarely able to guarantee that a specific professional ethos and corresponding habitus will be formed. This comes across even more clearly when one addresses the aspect of how to shape the professional relationship from the point of view of the theory of professionalism. Here, too, there is a great deal of evidence that degree courses, if at all, only inadequately teach the abilities required to form a viable working alliance or cement those abilities through habitualisation.

While this focus on the professional ethos also strongly emphasises the role of the professional, approaches coming from interaction theory place greater stress on the intersubjective mechanisms which characterise professional relationships in the field of counselling and therapy. Here, the relationship between the client and professional is regarded as key to a professional working alliance (Welter-Enderlin & Hildenbrand, 2004; regarding counselling, see also Stimmer, 2013) – a working alliance that is especially characterised by a conflicting mix of role-like and diffuse elements to the relationship. These definitions from the theory of professionalism provide only a very rough outline of what is a very complex mission when the therapist is working on a specific situation and case. On one hand, that mission involves tackling role-related requirements and tasks against the background of institutional responsibility and making them transparent to the client in an appropriate manner (Bauer, 2014). On the other hand, it means opening up to an interpersonal encounter in which the professional is seen and approached as a whole person, and thus all kinds of aspects of their personality come into effect. This means that "establishing a relationship that is seen as helpful, working through assumptions and projections that are destructive for the relationship, understanding and feeling understood, working through unprocessed biographical traumas and conflicts, opening up to emotions and affects which have been shut out" are elementary mechanisms for effective therapy which are required in order to unlock potential actions and means of effecting change (Frommer, 2014, p. 117). The professionality inherent in the way the counsellor shapes this kind of working relationship is then evident, for example, in his or her reflections on transference phenomena – which can be extreme and take the form of acting out (Becker-Lenz and Müller, 2009, 209). On one hand, reflection on these mechanisms, which come from psychoanalytic theory and are considered to effect emotional change, involves self-reflectively pinpointing one's own role in the situation that forms and develops during interaction with clients. On the other hand, however, it equally involves reflecting on feelings which have been triggered and risen to attention in the context of the relational patterns reproduced by the client. Above all, it is necessary to separate one's own experience from that of others and at the same time to observe one's own involvement in the relationship sensitively, rather than immediately acting out (Staats, 2017).

That means that even the establishment of a counselling relationship – similar to explicitly therapeutic settings – does not just come down to communication skills or social competency (Stimmer, 2013) but also includes an ability to interrelate that is acquired from a person's life experiences and involves therapists not only succeeding in creating a trusting setting and approaching the client with a sense of curiosity and appreciation but also, when faced with what can be incredibly difficult stories of suffering, "not evading the issues but also not being overwhelmed by them" (Levold, 2004, p. 4).

These approaches taken from the theory of professionalism can be used to pin down once more what it is that should be seen as a central challenge for learning processes, especially among students and in the setting of an institute of higher education. As Levold (ibid.) emphasises, a "kind of authenticity paradox" comes about. If professionals' establishment of a therapeutic relationship is understood as part of a strongly habitualised proceeding, then it is all about a "slow and gradual process of inscribing social and cultural forms and practices into an individual process of psychological and physical development" (ibid.). This means that the habitus is deeply intertwined with the experiences of the respective person and with their existence, however, that is physically mediated, placing systematic limits on the extent to which these aspects of the relationship can be trained: "Developing therapeutic expertise is thus a highly personal process tied to the development of a therapeutic personality and a corresponding habitus" (ibid.).

Countless studies have shown that, as yet, most degree courses in counselling can neither provide a sufficient conceptual basis for this form of professionally establishing a relationship nor enable it to become suitably habitualised. This conclusion is also underlined by the results of studies dealing with the connection between biographical development patterns and professionals' self-understanding, showing that the acquisition of knowledge within higher education depends strongly on propensities which are formed biographically and related to personality. It is thus sometimes the case that this knowledge does not seem to have educational effects in the sense of transforming learners' relationships with themselves and the world around them (Koller, 2012), but instead remains superficial (Harter & Lauinger, 2016; Weinhardt, 2014a).

A Performance-Oriented Approach to Learning Counselling at Institutes of Higher Education

With all this in mind, in the following, we present the results of a study investigating counselling skill acquisition processes at institutes of higher education (Weinhardt 2013, 2014a, 2014b). This study was designed to generate knowledge both about educational processes and about potential instructional innovations within higher education. The study forms part of the research activities at the Counselling Research Section, which mainly looks into learning and education processes among prospective counsellors in the early stages of acquiring their expertise. One part of the study is based on a performance-oriented approach which involves gathering data on and making accessible counselling activities as they occur in various kinds of simulation settings. To this end, different simulation environments were developed for different methods and forms of counselling – in the case of online counselling, for example, analytically condensed test cases from real counselling consultations. A counselling laboratory is available for research into counselling processes, where learners can hold video-recorded counselling sessions with trained simulation clients on typical counselling issues known from social work. The findings reported below are from a sub-study within this line of research.

The video-recorded conversations act both as the basis for student-specific learning materials (often sparking processes of education and reflection extending well beyond the context of the seminar) and as research data. Data on the video-recorded counselling sessions is coded by a team of trained raters using a highly inference coding instrument: the TBKS (Tübinger Beratungskompetenz-Skala; Tübingen Counselling Skills Scale) (Weinhardt, 2014b). The TBKS is an adapted version of the US Counseling Skills Scale (Eriksen & McAuliffe, 2003, 2006), translated into German. It operationalises counsellor competency using six skills: shows interest and appreciation (SIA), explores problems (EXP), deepens the session (D), encourages change (ENC), develops counsellor/therapeutic relationship (REL) and structures the session (STR). The scale is formulated based on competency using specifically operationalised steps. The tool was developed as an empirically viable solution for measuring counselling skills in research, teaching and practice. Analysing video-recorded counselling sessions using the TBKS thus helps measure the level and scope of counselling skills based on these six dimensions and show how they change over time. When this is done, a strong spotlight is cast, for example, on the role of the biographical phase during which students are taught and learn counselling. Another aspect highlighted is the significance of prior practical experience for students learning counselling (Weinhardt, 2014a, 2014b). For the present contribution, we are interested in another aspect, namely, elucidating the structure of consulting competency (Weinhardt & Kelava, 2016). The question of what elements make up counselling competency and what factors determine it can be answered using structural equation modelling based on what is now an extensive body of TBKS data. For this purpose, three models were formulated following standard presuppositions used in the theory of professionalism (Fig. 1). These were transformed into structural equation models using the TBKS data and checked for fits with the empirical data.

Model 1 postulates a simple structure (CC (counselling competency)), which is also posited by the original authors of the Counseling Skills Scale (Eriksen & McAuliffe, 2003, 2006). Here, counselling ability is understood as a one-dimensional, domain-specific construct on which the various variables covered by the TBKS depend. Model 2 postulates a two-factor structure for describing counselling ability, namely, the ability to form relationships on the one hand (IAR (interest, appreciation and relationship)) and the ability to carry out techniques and methods (TM) on the other. Finally, Model 3 also postulates a two-factor structure,

Model 1	Model 2	Model 3
N=206	N=206	N=206
χ2/DF= 8.66, p=.00	χ2/DF=4.07, p=.02	χ2/DF=1.16, p=.128
CFI=.93	CFI=.97	CFI=.99
RMSEA=.19	RMSEA=.12	RMSEA=.02
SRMR = .0416	SRMR = .0289	SRMR=.0114

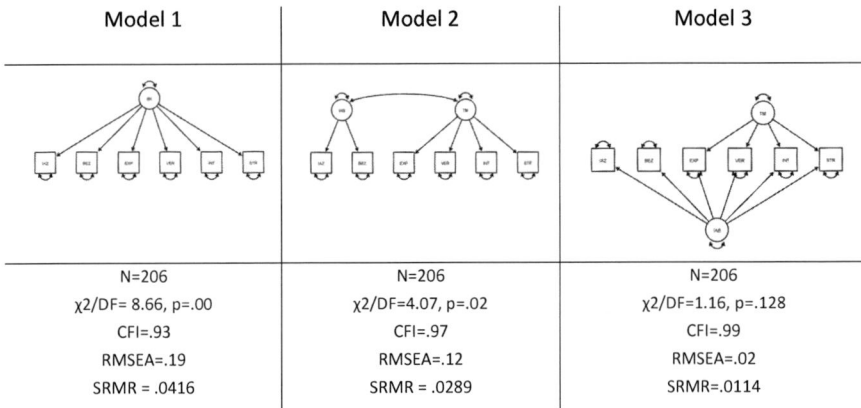

Fig. 1 Elucidating the structure of counselling skills

the difference being a hierarchical ("nested") factor structure which assumes that counselling techniques and methods (TM) are also always subject to the general IAR factor. At this juncture, we limit ourselves to reports on the standard fit indices (Hu & Bentler, 1995) and the resulting comparison of the model. It can be seen that the models can be ranked: Model 1 fits worst and Model 3 fits the data best. Model 3 is also the only one to fulfil the usual criteria for goodness of fit; it thus best represents the structure of counselling skills among the 206 student counsellors investigated here. Thus, these findings support the assumption that the basis for counselling competency is a fundamental ability to form relationships, on which the use of techniques and methods is based. This is an interesting result, which – generalised somewhat – offers a good explanation of the cited well-known phenomena from counselling research and practice. It is, for example, in line with the theory: not just the findings of common factor research into counselling and psychotherapy but also programmatic descriptions of counselling (Vossler, 2014), which postulate a general construct of successful relationship-forming along with techniques and methods based on that construct. In Model 3, these can be summed up concisely as techniques and methods (TM). A model of this kind also offers a logical explanation for the well-documented efficacy demonstrated by some laypeople and counselling novices (Strasser, 2006): their ability to establish a relationship (IAR) already happens to be strong (e.g. due to favourable biographical and personal preconditions), though their ability to carry out techniques and methods (TM) is still underdeveloped due to the lack of any training in counselling. As a result, they are very much capable of going through entire counselling processes but come up against typical limits in complex cases, the typical quality of which can often be described as "congenial failure" or "peaceful stagnation".

Reflections on the Therapeutic-Factor-Oriented Acquisition of Counselling Skills from the Angle of Didactics: Subject-Centred Professionalisation Instead of Method Training

This finding sheds new light on old lines of discourse relating to the nature of counselling skills. Counselling expertise has always been discussed in terms of the relation between attitude and method, frequently in the form of crudely drawn dichotomy and exaggeration, as found, for example, in the conventional social stereotypes of the unmethodological do-gooder or the technocratic social engineer. The "nested factor" model postulated here can be taken as an indication that the generalist factor is inseparable from counselling techniques and methods: no complex questioning and intervention techniques can be applied without a working alliance based on a professional session, with a strong relationship that offers not only the client but also the professional self-efficacy, meaning-making and confidence. It is striking how closely the programmatic desiderata from the literature on counselling coincide with the findings of research into therapeutic factors as, for example, presented by Wampold and Imel with regard to the contextual model (Wampold & Imel, 2015; Weinhardt, 2018), findings which, with a high degree of face validity, could be transferred to the contextual model which they developed, as specified below for the case of systemic counselling.

What does this now imply in terms of a targeted didactic design for learning and educational processes for aspiring systemic counsellors? Following the example of the considerations from the theory of professionalism, outlined above, by assuming that the ability to form relationships has a habitual component, then there is – as Levold (2004) calls it – a kind of "authenticity paradox". What needs to be done is to produce something in professional practice, the essence of which develops naturally in a habitualised form through a combination of personal and professional experiences over the course of a person's occupational socialisation: "One aspect of the social construction of personality seems to lie in successfully being able to – and having to – successfully conceal from others and indeed oneself the fact that it is socially constructed. We are dealing here with a slow and gradual process of inscribing social and cultural forms and practices into an individual process of mental and physical development" (ibid.).

How can such complex processes be integrated, reproduced and operationalised to structure processes of learning and education, following the principles of didactics? Taking on board the thoughts developed here about efficacy leads to a model (Fig. 2) which, in the context of our research work, we call the model of subject-centred professionalisation (Bauer et al., 2017) and which we use in the following to develop some further lines of thought (for a detailed study of systemic counselling, see Weinhardt, 2017, 2018).

To begin, this model shows how complex the situation is at the outset in terms of the individual learner on one hand (see the examples in the box on the right) and the structural demands made in professionalisation schemes on the other – even though this model only lists the most important factors found in the research into

structural requirements, e.g.

- curriculum
- classroom formats/social learning forms
- exams/assessment
- working/practicum conditions
- embedding of work and education in the lifeworld
- ...

accumulation, interpretation and knowledge formation
as subjective, professional development task in the mode of deliberate practice

individual requirements, e.g.

- previous knowledge
- previous experience
- career motives
- self-efficacy beliefs
- epistemic beliefs about counseling/therapy
- ...

common factor indicators
(e.g. relationship, attitude, self-efficacy, routinization, creating social significance ...)

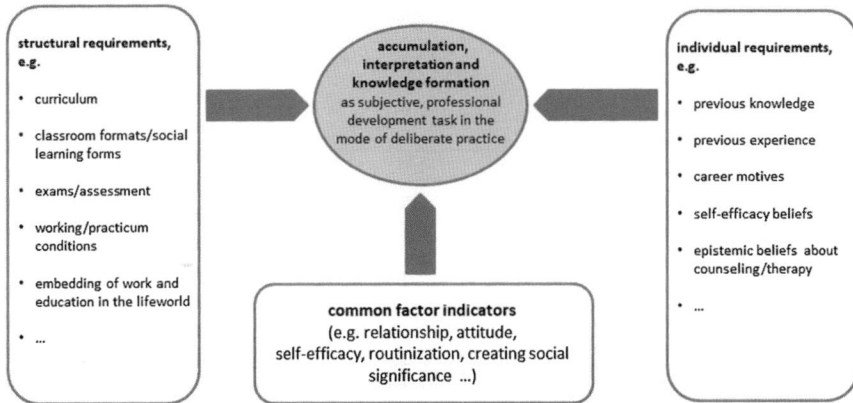

Fig. 2 Subject-centred professionalisation. (Simplified adaptation of Weinhardt, 2018)

professionalisation. The tug of war which comes to light between structural and personal aspects thus makes it clear that professionalisation oriented towards therapeutic factors must be constructed (or reconstructed) as an extremely subjective process of learning and education revolving around describing and dealing with developmental tasks specific to the profession. These developmental tasks differ greatly from one another, but focus on one aim which applies to all learners: providing successful systemic counselling. The criterion for assessment must therefore always be the extent to which a person's existing skills can already be used to bring the indicators for therapeutic factors into play. The model thus makes it possible to work on the question of who must and can learn from or with whom to advance to the next stage of their own professionalisation.

Numerous tried-and-tested instruments are available for working on this type of subject-centred programme and are already being used in many fields of work in education. On the level of self-assessment and reflection on initial requirements, for example, portfolio work has proved its worth, an instrument which is gaining additional momentum through the digitisation of the (higher) education system (Boos, Krämer, & Kricke, 2016; Bräuer, 2016; Nore, 2014; Paikar-Megaiz, 2015; Papadopoulou, 2015). This means systematically collecting materials relevant to training and repeatedly examining and assessing them with regard to learning aims and educational goals. A portfolio of this kind can be defined very broadly or according to standardised guidelines, e.g. including an appraisal of a counsellor's own place of work, the results of supervision being carried out or especially relevant aha experiences (critical incidents) from daily counselling practice. The central point is that the portfolio belongs to the learner, though this does not mean it cannot be integrated into skills-based testing formats at specific points. A portfolio of this type is a material correlate of the idea that in education, as elsewhere, the most important work goes on between lessons. Another topic which is largely put in second place within the teaching of counselling and therapy is the use of e-learning in the light of subject-centred professionalisation. This means far more than simply providing texts on learning websites: instructional videos, knowledge tests with individual feedback or even the chance to use e-learning tools and guiding criteria to reflect upon one's own video-recorded counselling work alone, with peers or teachers, at any time or place and at one's own speed, offers as yet untapped potential for the acquisition of counselling/therapy skills. It is thus possible for everyone to learn the same thing, but each in a different order and at an effective pace. Seen in this way, subject-centred professionalisation is more than just adding elements of reflection or specially adapting to individual learners' needs. Instead, learners are required to actively change their processes of learning and education, meaning that they are prepared by the very nature of things for the key elements of lifelong learning: maintaining curiosity, creating ways of developing a passion for the subject, and thus expanding their own counselling expertise. In the research into the formation of knowledge and the generation of expertise, this approach is known as "deliberate practice" (Ericsson, Krampe, & Tesch-Römer, 1993; Wampold, 2017), which emphasises the close interlinking of the three basic elements of knowledge acquisition, practice and reflection following the ideally suitable approach in each case. This makes it possible to acquire empirically supported professional experience by means of continuous reflection, backed by knowledge, especially on experiences which are confusing and initially seem difficult to slot in (Buchholz, 2007).

Though this type of model promises to be able to make professionalisation processes more targeted, the primary tenet of long-term developments, well known from research into expertise, applies: gathering professional experience takes time and patience (Strasser, 2014) and does not lead to success through practice alone (Goldberg et al., 2016; Owen, Wampold, Kopta, Rousmaniere, & Miller, 2016; Tracey, Wampold, Lichtenberg, & Goodyear, 2014). Instead, it must be integrated lastingly, from an early stage, in the form of deliberate practice (Rousmaniere & Miller, 2017).

With regard to our focus on the early stages of expertise, as found among students, an examination of current conditions at universities and other institutes of higher education, as well as practice later on, shows that significant changes have taken place in this field in particular. Drastic cuts in the length of courses, compressing the course content into a shorter learning time, cutting back on practical elements of courses and the practice of putting graduates at an early stage of their career into potentially overwhelming jobs all fly in the face of these central components of acquiring professionalised knowledge. One major and hitherto underappreciated contribution made by change-factor-oriented research is thus that it places greater emphasis on professionalisation from the educational perspective.

Bibliography

Barthelmess, M. (2016). *Die systemische Haltung. Was systemisches Arbeiten im Kern ausmacht.* Heidelberg, Germany: Vandenhoeck & Ruprecht.

Bauer, P. (2014). "Den Anfang gestalten ....". Beraterische Erstgespräche von Beratungsnovizen. In P. Bauer & M. Weinhardt (Eds.), *Perspektiven sozialpädagogischer Beratung. Empirische Befunde und aktuelle Entwicklungen* (pp. 232–251). Weinheim, Germany: Beltz.

Bauer, P., & Weinhardt, M. (Eds.). (2014). *Perspektiven sozialpädagogischer Beratung. Empirische Befunde und aktuelle Entwicklungen*. Weinheim, Germany: Beltz.

Bauer, P., & Weinhardt, M. (2016). *Professionalisierungs- und Kompetenzentwicklungsprozesse in der sozialpädagogischen Beratung*. Baltmannsweiler, Germany: Schneider Hohengehren.

Bauer, P., Weinhardt, M., Carfagno, K., Christ, A., Kniep, K., Thomas, M. & Urban, M. (2017). *Posterpräsentation ProfiL – Professionalisierung durch Beratung im Lehramtsstudium*. Tübingen: Abschlusstagung der DFG-Forschergruppe "Analyse und Förderung effektiver Lehr- Lernprozesse". https://www.researchgate.net/publication/316687708_ProfiL_-_Professionalisierung_durch_Beratung_im_Lehramtsstudium

Becker-Lenz, R., & Müller, S. (2008). *Der professionelle Habitus in der Sozialen Arbeit. Grundlage eines Professionsideals*. Frankfurt am Main, Germany: Peter Lang.

Becker-Lenz, R., & Müller, S. (2009). *Der professionelle Habitus in der Sozialen Arbeit. Grundlagen eines Professionsideals*. Bern, Swiss: Peter Lang.

Boos, M., Krämer, A., & Kricke, M. (Eds.). (2016). *Portfolioarbeit phasenübergreifend gestalten. Konzepte, Ideen und Anregungen aus der LehrerInnenbildung*. Münster, Germany: Waxmann.

Bräuer, G. (2016). *Das Portfolio als Reflexionsmedium für Lehrende und Studierende*. Opladen: Verlag Barbara Budrich.

Buchholz, M. (2007). Entwicklungsdynamik psychotherapeutischer Kompetenzen. In: *Psychotherapeutenjournal 6*(4), 373–382.

Engel, F., Nestmann, F., & Sickendiek, U. (2018). Beratung – alte Selbstverständnisse und neue Entwicklungen. In S. Rietmann & M. Sawatzki (Eds.), *Zukunft der Beratung, Soziale Arbeit als Wohlfahrtsproduktion* (pp. 83–115). Wiesbaden, Germany: VS.

Ericsson, K. A., Krampe, R. T., & Tesch-Römer, C. (1993). The role of deliberate practice in the acquisition of expert performance. *Psychological Review, 100*(3), 463.

Eriksen, K., & McAuliffe, G. (2003). A measure of counselor competency. *Counselor Education and Supervision, 43*(2), 120–133.

Eriksen, K., & McAuliffe, G. (2006). Constructive development and counselor competence. *Counselor Education and Supervision, 45*(3), 180–192.

Frommer, J. (2014). Therapie als Fallarbeit: Über einige Grundprobleme und Paradoxien professionellen Handelns in der Medizin. In J. R. Bergmann, U. Dausenschön-Gay, & F. Oberzaucher (Eds.), *der Fall. Studien zur epistemischen Praxis professionellen Handelns*. Bielefeld, Germany: Transcript.

Galuske, M., & Müller, W. C. (2012). Handlungsformen in der Sozialen Arbeit Geschichte und Entwicklung. In W. Thole (Ed.), *Grundriss Soziale Arbeit* (pp. 587–610). Wiesbaden, Germany: VS.

Goldberg, S. B., Rousmaniere, T., Miller, S. D., Whipple, J., Nielsen, S. L., Hoyt, W. T., & Wampold, B. E. (2016). Do psychotherapists improve with time and experience? A longitudinal analysis of outcomes in a clinical setting. *Journal of Counseling Psychology, 63*(1), 1–11.

Harter, K., & Lauinger, F. (2016). Die Bedeutung der Biographie beim Lernen von Beratung. In: P. Bauer und M. Weinhardt (Hg.): Professionalisierungs- und Kompetenzentwicklungsprozesse in der sozialpädagogischen Beratung. Baltmannsweiler, Germany: Schneider Hohengehren, 92–105.

Hu, L.-T., & Bentler, P. M. (1995). Evaluating model fit. In R. H. Hoyle (Ed.), *Structural equation modeling* (pp. 76–99). Thousand Oaks, CA: Sage.

Kunze-Pletat, D. (2018). Personzentrierte Erwachsenenpädagogik. Die pädagogische Beziehung als Mittelpunkt im Lehr-Lern-Prozess. Wiesbaden, Germany: VS.

Lambert, M. J., Bergin, A. E., & Garfield, S. L. (Eds.). (2013). *Bergin and Garfield's handbook of psychotherapy and behavior change*. Hoboken, NJ: Wiley.

Levold, T. (2004). Therapeutenpersönlichkeit zwischen Rolle und Identität. *Systeme, 18*, 41–51.

Nestmann, F., & Sickendiek, U. (2018). Beratung. In: H.-U. Otto, H. Thiersch, R. Treptow und H. Ziegler (Hg.): Handbuch Soziale Arbeit. Grundlagen der Sozialarbeit und Sozialpädagogik. München, Germany: Reinhardt, 153–163.

Neuweg, G. H. (2015). *Das Schweigen der Könner. Gesammelte Schriften zum impliziten Wissen*. Münster, Germany: Waxmann.

Nore, H. (2014). *Bridging the gap between work and education in vocational education and training. A study of Norwegian apprenticeship training offices and e-portfolio systems.* Bremen, Germany: University of Bremen.

Owen, J., Wampold, B. E., Kopta, M., Rousmaniere, T., & Miller, S. D. (2016). As good as it gets? Therapy outcomes of trainees over time. *Journal of Counseling Psychology, 63*(1), 12–19.

Paikar-Megaiz, A. (2015). *E-Portfolio- und Social Networking-Systeme zur Unterstützung des lebenslangen Lernens.* Munich, Germany: University Library.

Papadopoulou, C.-O. (2015). *The use of the learning portfolio in foreign language teacher education. The promotion of learner autonomy.* Hamburg, Germany: Kovač.

Pfammatter, M., & Tschacher, W. (2012). Wirkfaktoren der Psychotherapie - eine Übersicht und Standortbestimmung. *Zeitschrift für Psychiatrie, Psychologie und Psychotherapie, 60*(1), 67–76.

Preß, H., & Gmelch, M. (2014). Die „therapeutische Haltung". Vorschlag eines Arbeitsbegriffs und einer klientenorientierten Variante. In: *Psychotherapeutenjournal 13*(4), 358–366.

Rousmaniere, T., & Miller, S. D. (Eds.). (2017). *Cycle of excellence.* New York, NY: Wiley.

Staats, H. (2017). Die therapeutische Beziehung – Spielarten und verwandte Konzepte. Göttingen, Germany: Vandenhoeck & Ruprecht.

Stimmer, F. (2013). Verständigungsorientiert methodisch handeln in der Fokussierten Beratung. In: K. Blaha, C. Meyer, H. Colla und S. Müller-Teusler (Hg.): Die Person als Organon in der Sozialen Arbeit: Erzieherpersönlichkeit und qualifiziertes Handeln. Wiesbaden, Germany: VS, 211–236.

Strasser, J. (2006). Erfahrung und Wissen in der Beratung. Theoretische und empirische Analysen zum Entstehen professionellen Wissens in der Erziehungsberatung. Göttingen, Germany: Cuvillier.

Strasser, J. (2014). Reflexion von Erfahrungen und Fehlern. Eine Voraussetzung für die berufliche Wissensentwicklung von Beraterinnen und Beratern. In: P. Bauer und M. Weinhardt (Hg.): Perspektiven sozialpädagogischer Beratung. Empirische Befunde und aktuelle Entwicklungen. Weinheim, Germany: Beltz, 196–213.

Strasser, J., & Gruber, H. (2015). Learning processes in the professional development of mental health counselors: knowledge restructuring and illness script formation. In: *Advances in Health Sciences Education 20*(2), 515–530.

Tracey, T. J., Wampold, B. E., Lichtenberg, J. W., & Goodyear, R. K. (2014). Expertise in psychotherapy. An elusive goal? *Am Psychol, 69*(3), 218–229. https://doi.org/10.1037/a0035099

von Schlippe, A., & Schweizer, J. (2016). *Lehrbuch der systemischen Therapie und Beratung. Das Grundlagenwissen.* Heidelberg, Germany: Vandenhoeck & Ruprecht.

Vossler, A. (2014). Beratungs- und Therapieforschung im Überblick. In P. Bauer & M. Weinhardt (Eds.), *Perspektiven sozialpädagogischer Beratung. Empirische Befunde und aktuelle Entwicklungen* (pp. 269–285). Beltz: Weinheim.

Wampold, B. E. (2017). What should we practice?: Using deliberate practice to improve supervision and training. In T. Rousmaniere & S. D. Miller (Eds.), *Cycle of excellence* (pp. 49–65). New York, NY: John Wiley & Sons.

Wampold, B. E., & Imel, Z. E. (2015). *The great psychotherapy debate. The evidence for what makes psychotherapy work.* New York, NY: Routledge.

Weinhardt, M. (2013). Methodenkompetenzerwerb im Studium? – Chancen und Grenzen der Methodenausbildung an der Hochschule am Beispiel psychosozialer Beratung. In: Sozialmagazin 11/12, 60–69.

Weinhardt, M. (2014a). Beraterische Basisqualifikation im Studium? Eine qualitative Längsschnittstudie zum Beratungskompetenzerwerb an der Hochschule. *Kontext, 45*(1), 85–101.

Weinhardt, M. (2014b). Kompetenzentwicklung in der psychosozialen Beratung am Beispiel von Studierenden der Erziehungswissenschaft. In P. Bauer & M. Weinhardt (Eds.), *Perspektiven sozialpädagogischer Beratung. Empirische Befunde und aktuelle Entwicklungen* (pp. 214–231). Beltz: Weinheim, Germany.

Weinhardt, M. (2015). *Beratungskompetenzerwerb. Pilotstudien aus der Arbeitsstelle für Beratungsforschung*. Weinheim, Germany: Beltz.

Weinhardt, M. (2016). *Methodenintegration in Beratung und Therapie: die fatale Verwechslung von Wirksamkeit und Lernbarkeit*, blog article. https://marcweinhardt.de/?p=962

Weinhardt, M. (2017). Subjektorientierte Professionalisierung, Lebenslanges Lernen und der EQR/DQR in der Systemischen Fort- und Weiterbildung. *Kontext, 47*(3), 262–227.

Weinhardt, M. (2018). *Kompetenzorientiert systemisch beraten lernen. Eine Gebrauchsanweisung für die eigene Professionalisierung*. Heidelberg, Germany: Vandenhoeck & Ruprecht.

Weinhardt, M., & Kelava, A. (2016). Die performanzorientierte Erfassung psychosozialer Beratungskompetenz. *Neue Praxis, 2016*(4), 363–377.

Welter-Enderlin, R., & Hildenbrand, B. (2004). *Systemische Therapie als Begegnung*. Stuttgart, Germany: Klett Cotta.

Zwicker-Pelzer, R. (2010). Beratung in der sozialen Arbeit. Bad Heilbrunn, Germany: UTB.

Publication in Family Therapy Journals: *Family Process*, *Journal of Family Therapy*, and *Australian and New Zealand Journal of Family Therapy* – A Discussion with Editors

Maria Borcsa ⓘ**, Jay L. Lebow, Reenee Singh, Glenn Larner, and Philip Messent**

Introduction

Scientific journals are activists in the history of ideas by expressing, preserving, or changing academic discourses over time. What is the history behind the three most prominent family therapy journals edited and printed on three different continents? What were – and are – their trends? In what areas would they particularly like to see further articles? How are quantitative and qualitative research valued, and what is the link between research and practice? How do reviewing processes and decisions about articles happen? What are the challenges for authors, and how can they maximize the chances of their papers being accepted? What changes do family therapy journals face in a globalized world? This chapter will shed some light on these facets of the scientific world, usually not discussed.

M. Borcsa (✉)
Institute of Social Medicine, Rehabilitation Sciences and Healthcare Research,
University of Applied Sciences Nordhausen, Nordhausen, Germany
e-mail: Maria.Borcsa@hs-nordhausen.de

J. L. Lebow
Family Institute at Northwestern University, Evanston, IL, USA

R. Singh
Association of Family Therapy and Systemic Practice, Warrington & Child and Family
Practice, London, UK

G. Larner
Riley Street Practice, Surry Hills, Sydney, NSW, Australia

P. Messent
Association of Family Therapy and Systemic Practice, Warrington, UK

© Springer Nature Switzerland AG 2020
M. Ochs et al. (eds.), *Systemic Research in Individual, Couple, and Family Therapy and Counseling*, European Family Therapy Association Series,
https://doi.org/10.1007/978-3-030-36560-8_23

Background and History

The 1960s was a time of social revolt, having its reflections on the psychotherapeutic field. The launch of *Family Process* is grounded in this development: founded in 1961, it was the first journal devoted to family therapy; its inception came in parallel with the beginning of family therapy embedded in the anti-psychiatric movement. Therefore, it is no surprise that almost 2/3 of the articles of the first issue in March 1962 were dedicated to schizophrenia and family therapy, giving protocol of a respective symposium as well as reviewing books on the topic.

Originally, *Family Process* consisted of a combination of cutting-edge articles about the theory and practice of family therapy, coupled with a newsletter for the family therapy community. Jay Haley was its first editor, and he was followed by Don Bloch, Carlos Sluzki, Peter Steinglass, Carol Anderson, and Evan Imber-Black, each of whom significantly advanced the journal. It has evolved into a prominent international journal publishing articles from all around the globe about family therapy, couple therapy, as well as theory and research about family processes. Per year, it publishes approximately 70 articles over 1000 pages, derived from approximately 300 submitted manuscripts. *Family Process* is published today through a collaboration between the Family Process Institute (the organization which published the journal itself over its first 40 years) and John Wiley and Sons. For 2018, it had an impact factor of 3.116. Since 2010, all abstracts are translated into Spanish and Simplified Chinese, which has been also the case for one article per issue. Recent special sections have covered such diverse topics as research and practice with step-families (57(1)), the research base for evidence-based couple and family therapies (55(3)), resilience in families (55(4); Walsh, 2016), and the state of family therapy (53(3)). While remaining solidly based on evidence and the best of clinical practice, *Family Process* promotes an understanding of the importance of social justice (Imber-Black, 2011). The journal has an extensive back catalog of many of the most important articles in the history of family therapy and family science, available online (http://onlinelibrary.wiley.com/journal/10.1111/(ISSN)1545-5300). Groups of these articles about specific topics are gathered together in "virtual" issues on the website. Many of the articles feature in recent years a video abstract, being compiled on YouTube.

The late 1970s saw the founding of several family therapy journals in Europe, e.g., *Familiendynamik* in Germany, *Cahiers critiques de thérapie familiale et de pratiques de réseaux* in Belgium, and *Terapia Familiare* in Italy (see respective entries in Lebow, Chambers, & Breunlin, 2019). To this day, the *Journal of Family Therapy* founded in 1979 in the United Kingdom has been one of the most important representatives of this historical development of growing interest on and implementation of family therapy in the psychotherapeutic arena in Europe. In the run-up to its founding, a group of child psychiatrists and professionals working in child guidance clinics and interested in developing systemic thinking and practice in the United Kingdom got together to form the *Association for Family Therapy*. The association was set up to provide training, accreditation, supervision of clinical practice, and a professional journal; the *Journal of Family Therapy* was born 4 years later, focusing on a variety of practically relevant texts from its beginning. The founding editor was Christopher Dare, and the subsequent editors have been Bryan Lask, John Carpenter and Bebe Speed, Eddy Street, Ivan Eisler, and Mark Rivett. Being a British journal, first and foremost, it has been reflecting the changing zeitgeist of systemic family therapy in the United Kingdom. In recent years, it has become increasingly international, with contributions from the United States, Europe, Australia, and Asia (Singh, 2015), reflected also by the international members of the editorial board and the fact that its abstracts are translated into Mandarin and Spanish. The impact factor of the journal rose to 1.186 in 2018. The journal welcomes and publishes research, both quantitative and qualitative; theoretical expositions; articles based on teaching and learning, e.g., describing practice-based learning; as well as clinical case studies. As the journal of a professional association, all articles need to have clinical relevance, and authors are asked to complete "practice learning points" to help to ensure that they keep this in mind. Podcasts by authors discussing their articles are a regular feature.

In the same founding year, the *Australian and New Zealand Journal of Family Therapy* (ANZJFT) started, reflecting the spread and innovations of systemic approaches all over the world. *ANZJFT* is a signature peer-reviewed quarterly professional journal that publishes original articles on theory, research, teaching, and practice in family therapy. Beginning in 1979 with Michael White as its foundation editor, the journal from "down under" quickly developed an international reputation. Under subsequent editors Max Cornwell (1985–1996) and Hugh and Maureen Crago (1997–2008) and co-editors Paul Rhodes, Alistair Campbell, and Glenn Larner (2009–2010), it evolved into a respected and widely read professional publication. Since 2010, the current editor-in-chief Glenn Larner has directed the development of a contemporary family therapy journal for the twenty-first century with a wide-ranging focus on theoretical, research, practice, and pedagogical issues in the discipline. *ANZJFT* is overseen by an editorial board under the auspices of the *Australian Association for Family Therapy* (AAFT), the national body representing family therapists in Australia. With this background, *ANZJFT* is primarily a journal for practitioners besides scholars or academics, which is reflected on its practice focus and reader-friendly style. The journal's impact factor was 0.575 in 2018. A recent innovation is an *In-Practice* section that invites mini papers on various aspects of family therapy practice. There are plans to develop virtual technology features in the near future including the use of video abstracts and podcasts.

Trends of Publications Reflect Trends in Couple and Family Therapy

With regard to the United States, publications in couple and family therapy have changed a great deal over the years. Early issues of *Family Process* are filled with articles primarily concerned with systemic theory and the beginnings of the application of systemic principles to clinical practice. Writing today in the field has evolved from that early work. All recent publications derive from the basic concepts that were earlier brilliantly described, but are situated now in a literature in which each topic covered in the early volumes of the journal has been extensively explored in over 50 years of investigation and clinical practice. Publication today compared to the early days of the journal tends to be more pragmatic and more specifically focused. There is less speculation with the accrual of evidence over time about areas of content having become much more important. Research occupies a much greater space in *Family Process* today, as it does in the sector of therapy itself. At the outset of the field of family therapy, there was very little family science from which to build those methods. Today relational and family sciences present vast literatures with findings of considerable importance in relation to almost every family dilemma and family form that informs therapists' understandings and clinical practice. The types of couple and family therapy that are written about also have changed decidedly over the years. Some earlier threads of work have been abandoned because they did not fit well with the evidence (e.g., the double bind); other early understandings have evolved in relation to other recent developments, such as feminism and the greater recognition of the importance of cultural context. In the early issues of the journal, articles about treatment were primarily about structural, strategic, and psychodynamic approaches of family therapy. Today, in contrast, articles are largely about integrative, post-modern/post-structural, and cognitive- behavioral therapies and are much more likely to be resilience based than pathology based.

The integrative therapies have particularly grown; often they are not labeled as such, but as therapies for specific difficulties or types of families or therapy for groups of people; or they are described in articles focused on common factors in therapy. A vast literature has emerged about widely disseminated evidence-based treatments for couples and families. These include emotionally focused therapy, Gottman therapy, functional family therapy, multi-systemic therapy, multidimensional family therapy, brief strategic family therapy, psychoeducational-based family therapies, and a variety of cognitive-behavioral models. In earlier times, cognitive- behavioral couple and family therapies were written about almost exclusively in cognitive-behavioral journals. Today, articles about that sort of therapy have migrated to *Family Process* and other prominent family therapy journals. Space in journals has become much more competitive; the most prominent journals have high rejection rates for submissions. In part, this means that the quality of articles has improved considerably.

Also in the United Kingdom, there is a move toward evidence-based practice within the field of family therapy, and this is reflected on the kinds of articles received for submission to the *Journal of Family Therapy* – for example, an entire special issue entitled Adolescent Self Harm and Systemic Practice was published in 2016 (38(2)). This issue was based on the randomized control trial, SHIFT (Self-Harm Intervention Family Therapy), a landmark research study in the United Kingdom and all over the world, which looked at the efficacy of systemic family therapy for deliberate adolescent self-harm. Similarly, the special section on SCORE (Systemic Core Outcome Routine Evaluation) (39(1); see also chapter "The SCORE in Europe: Measuring Effectiveness and Assisting Therapy", Stratton, Carr, and Schepisi in this book) emphasized the importance of this family outcome measure as the only one that originated in Europe, being available on the European Family Therapy Association and the Association for Family Therapy websites (http://www. europeanfamilytherapy.eu/efta-community-news/;   http://www.aft.org.uk/view/ score.html). In recent years, some excellent systematic reviews were published, such as one on parental alienation (Templer, Matthewson, Haines, & Cox, 2017) and functional somatic disorders (Hulgaard, Dehlholm-Lambertsen, & Rask, 2019).

Alongside an increasing trend toward articles that enhance and add to the evidence base in systemic psychotherapy, there is an equal interest in articles on practice-based evidence and on critiquing and questioning the politics of evidence in our field – maybe some "revolutionary" spirit has remained in the field? In recent years, the journal has published original articles on contemporary social and political issues – such as the impact of information communication technologies and digital social media on family relationships and the systemic implications of public debates on assisted dying.

Over the years, *ANZJFT* has attracted contributions from many luminaries in the family therapy community including Michael White, Lyn Hoffman, Harlene Anderson, Harry Goolishian, Tom Andersen, Helm Stierlin, Luigi Boscolo, Carmel Flaskas, Monica McGoldrick, Jaakko Seikkula, Maurizio Andolfi, Paolo Bertrando and Peter Rober. Publications of the first 10 years came 60% from male authors, and 48% were written by a sole author, with a growing tendency toward collaborative authorship over the years (Davis & Lipson, 1996). To date, a broad range of family therapy themes have been covered including training and supervision; reflecting teams; epistemology and family therapy; Milan and post-Milan therapy; brief family therapy; Bowen family systems therapy; feminist family therapy; just therapy; family interventions for mental illness; family therapy with children and adolescents; separation, divorce, and custody issues; culture and gender concerns; family violence; child protection and sexual abuse; serious medical illness; refugee families; and working with Aboriginal peoples and Torres Strait islanders and Maori families. *ANZJFT* regularly brings out special themed issues on key topics in family therapy like research in marital and family therapy, ethics, couple therapy, gay and lesbian relationships, single-session therapy, psychiatric diagnosis, narrative family therapy, and spirituality. Recent special issues have provided a platform for current cutting-edge developments in the discipline such as Dialogical Practices (36(1)), Attachment-Based Family Therapy (ABFT) (37(2)), Relational Trauma (38(4)), and Community, Psychology and Family Therapy (39(3)). The latest special issue on Children, Separation and Divorce in March 2019 includes a groundbreaking article from a Federal Court judge.

All the above has implications for the quantity and type of publications submitted to *ANZJFT* over the last few decades compared to previous submissions under a more generic definition of systemic family therapy. Here there is recognition of the broad range of theory topics and practices that fall under the umbrella term of "family therapy." Articles in *ANZJFT* trend toward being diverse, integrative, and family-focused at the same time as they engage with traditional systemic theory and research and practice developments in the discipline (e.g., supervision or investigations of family therapy process). This is over and above an increasing focus on specialized evidence-based approaches as described earlier.

Publication of Research: Linked to Practice

Family Process emphasizes the connection between research and practice. More specifically, it focuses on a strong connection between the practice of couple and family therapy and knowledge from family and relational science; based on this link, articles also about basic family and relational research are published. In articles with a clinical emphasis, authors are asked to explicate the research foundation for their work. Similarly, authors of research articles are requested to suggest the clinical implications of their article.

The research published is both quantitative and qualitative. A thorough understanding of family processes emerges from a combination of work that explores the phenomenon through quantitative *and* through qualitative methods, i.e., mixed method studies. Overall, research is approached from the perspective that each study further informs knowledge about the field and methods of practice. No single study is definitive; each study is adding to the cumulative base of knowledge. Therefore, authors of research papers are requested to clearly enumerate the strengths of their study but also the threats to the validity of the study and its potential limitations: it is important for both quantitative and qualitative researchers to be aware of and communicate the limits of what can be known through their methods of inquiry.

The *Journal of Family Therapy* has a rich tradition of publishing qualitative, process- and patient-focused research. Publication of research, both qualitative and quantitative, is essential in advancing knowledge in the field of systemic family therapy and supporting the further establishment and impact of the discipline. Quantitative research papers, in the form of articles arising from randomized controlled trials such as SHIFT (Self-Harm Intervention Family Therapy), as well as meta-analysis papers and systematic reviews provide a strong foundation for clinical practice.

ANZJFT also recognizes the importance of both quantitative and qualitative research for the continuing development of the profession in order to enhance its profile in the politics of mental health practice (Larner, 2004). Qualitative research that expounds the minutiae of the relational and dialogic therapeutic process is particularly to be encouraged. Another important topic is practice-based research into the effectiveness of family therapy in practice settings. Also relevant is investigation into integrative family therapy treatment approaches across a range of common mental health issues like depression and anxiety in everyday practice settings.

Reviewing Processes and Decisions about Articles

Family Process has an editor-in-chief and three associate editors, who manage papers and make decisions about them; reviewers are members of the editorial advisory board. *JFT* has approximately 100 peer reviewers, some of whom are editorial board members and associate editors. *ANZJFT* has thematic associate editors (general, research, or in-practice) who select and contact appropriate reviewers.

Having all three journals published by Wiley & Co., the reviewing processes have their similarities. First, all journals offer guidelines and instructions for authors on their respective websites. Papers are required to be submitted through the corresponding ScholarOne online system. The peer-reviewing process is comparable throughout the three journals: submissions are initially screened by the *editor-in-chief* for relevance and a decision made about general suitability for journal publication. Usually, the papers are then assigned to *associate editors* who select and contact at least two expert *peer reviewers*. These are scholars with very diverse backgrounds and expertise, with the general idea to best match reviewers to authors' subjects. The peer reviewers submit their reviews preferably within 4–6 weeks. The decisions fall into the categories of "accept," "accept with minor revisions," "accept with major revisions," and "reject." After reviews are returned, a recommendation is made about publication by the editorial team: the author(s) are notified by email with the reviewer reports compiled and typically allowed 6 weeks for revision. After a revised paper is received, a decision is made about publication or the need for further revision, mostly by sending out for review again to the same reviewers who reviewed the paper the first time (*Family Process*), or the editor-in-chief and/or associate editor checks if it has satisfactorily met the requirements for revision (*JFT, ANZJFT*). Papers under revision may be asked for revision several times. When the reviewers/editors are satisfied with the content of the paper, the paper is accepted for publication. On average, it takes not less than 6 months from the time of submission until papers are published (online on Early View, i.e., not assigned to a certain issue yet). *JFT* and *Family Process* invite authors to provide a video abstract with their final version of the paper.

Challenges for Authors

There are a number of specific problems that emerge frequently in submissions to *Family Process*. For research papers, some research begins with an inadequate methodology; the studies therefore cannot be repaired at the stage of writing. A second problem is that authors fail to shape a focal question in research studies, such that it becomes difficult to determine the purpose and meaning of the investigation. Third, several papers are poorly written. These papers may have excellent content, but it is difficult to discern the value of the study, because that is obscured by the writing. Some of the papers with this problem are written by authors for whom

English is a foreign language: The English verbiage may be sufficient, but the English is not idiomatic. A fourth problem in research papers lies in the use of statistical analyses that are inadequate and, frequently, out of date, given the developments in methods of analysis of family data. Authors of research articles should examine recent examples in *Family Process* and other journals for analyses in the context of the multiple reporters, and often the multiple points in time, involved in family studies.

The most important challenge for authors of *Journal of Family Therapy* is to present something that is original and has clinical relevance to systemic practitioners. Articles are rated by peer reviewers for originality, rigor, and coherence. Postgraduate students of family therapy/systemic psychotherapy often submit articles based on their dissertations; these articles usually need a fair amount of work in order for them to be suitable for publication. *JFT* offers writing workshops that can guide students to revise their dissertations into an appropriate format. As already mentioned, articles from authors whose first language is not English often require significant re-writing before final submission. Authors are also expected to include an element of self-reflexivity, recognizing that their perspective is limited by their context and that they are writing for an international audience who will be reading and making sense of articles from other contexts and perspectives.

Articles submitted to *ANZJFT* should have relevance for theory, practice, research, and training in the discipline with clear links to the family therapy, relational, and family-focused treatment literature. *ANZJFT* contributors should demonstrate clear English expression and good sentence structure and minimize repetition. They are often asked to include practice vignettes to illustrate theory ideas and provide key points that summarize the article in straightforward terms for readers and practitioners. New authors are advised to look at examples of articles in recent issues of *ANZJFT* for guidance on text presentation, referencing, structure, and format and to follow recommendations on the website for reporting research and using case illustrations.

How Does an Author Maximize the Chances of Papers Being Accepted?

Authors maximize their chances for having their work accepted in *Family Process* by beginning with a crisp well-formed idea for their papers. Choosing a topic that is important in the body of work of family science or couple/family therapy is enormously helpful toward papers being responded to positively. They further their chances by following state-of-the-art methods for research papers and conventions for theoretical and clinical papers. Each article needs a clear introduction that sets the frame for what is going to be presented, a section that presents the core of the work, and a discussion section, which speaks about what has been presented (and for research, following the conventions for those papers with all the relevant information needed to evaluate the study). Parsimony is important, and clear logical presentation enables a positive response. If an article is evaluated as suitable for revision, it becomes essential for authors to speak clearly to each of the comments that reviewers offer for changing their text. Most importantly, this should appear prominently in the body of the paper. In addition, the author should include a thorough letter that accompanies their next version, which specifies the changes that have been made and, if there are any modifications suggested that have not been made, the reasons the author has chosen to not follow the suggestions.

The editor and editorial board of *JFT* are open to the idea of previewing articles to assess their suitability for publication. However, all articles have to go through a "blind" peer-review process and are assessed on the basis of the criteria outlined above. Articles that are more likely to increase the impact factor, that have clinical relevance, and that are interesting and well written have a good chance of being accepted. Students and younger, less experienced authors are encouraged to attend the writing workshops offered and to team up with their research supervisors, tutors, and/or more experienced authors. *JFT* has also awarded a *student essay prize* every year, which is 2 years' free membership to the Association for Family Therapy, with a member of the editorial board offering mentorship to the winner of the essay, in order to help publish the article. Along with student representation on the editorial board and special issues of the journal focusing on developments in systemic practitioner research (39(3)), this helps to encourage writing and publication in *JFT* among students and trainees.

An article with relevance to the field of family therapy (as described above), thoughtfully organized, clearly written, having an appropriate introduction and conclusion as well as interesting practice examples, and finally, offering recommendations for practitioners, has a good chance of publication in *ANZJFT*.

Publishing in a Globalized World

Family Process emphasizes that any research, clinical, or theoretical paper can only be considered in the context in which it was developed and implemented. For those parts of the world in which there has been less development of research and less history of exploration of methods of practice, there is a great need for work to help illuminate processes in families and what works best in those contexts. There is much room for developments from these new centers of research and practice, e.g., in replicating studies done elsewhere, helping us understand how culture impacts various findings, and culturally adapting treatment methods to these new contexts developed in a different place on the globe. The principal problem arising in research is that authors are not aware of the relevant studies, and of more recent research methods, and therefore begin their effort without access to the most important body of work. Further, research methods employed might be below the international standards for publication even if large samples can be generated. For research articles, having a consultant well-versed in research methods and the pertinent studies can be an antidote for this problem. For theoretical and clinical articles, the parallel problem that arises is that concepts and theories may be developed which substantially overlap with other work already published. Again, here, it is enormously helpful to have colleagues from other parts of the world read papers before they are submitted to help provide context before articles are written.

Some countries favor a style of academic writing, which is very formal, and from a positivist tradition. In such cases, authors of *JFT* can be mentored to make the links between research, theory, and practice and to write in a more self-reflexive style. Generally, one of the tasks of the editor and editorial board members of *JFT* is to foster links with countries that have shorter histories of publication. This can be done through networking, attending conferences, and developing relationships with senior professionals in such countries, thus creating communities of systemic researchers/practitioners. Such senior members of the community can act as mentors for less experienced authors, in order to promote submission to *JFT*. From time to time, having a special section from another country can also promote publications from that region – for example, *JFT* had a special section on working with Chinese families (39(2)), guest edited by Timothy Sim and Chao Wentao. Last but not least, publishing abstracts in different languages can also encourage publication from other countries.

ANZJFT has offered publication opportunities for authors from South Africa, Indonesia, Iran, Brazil, Chile, Turkey, and Korea and would like to see relevant submissions from more countries in other parts of the world particularly those of the Asian area including China. A major issue for authors in countries where family therapy is an emerging discipline is article relevance, for example, being aware that having the term "family" in the title does not mean an article is suitable for publication in a family *therapy* journal; some authors confuse family research with family therapy.

Areas for Further Publications

Publication about theory has declined over the years in *Family Process*; for this reason, articles, which advance theory, are welcome. Similarly, writing that features an exposition of the systemic understandings is now less frequently encountered. Quality research which examines new family forms and dilemmas of the twenty-first-century life has recently emerged and become a high-priority topic for *Family Process*. Studies that add to the evidence base for couple and family therapy and to the cultural adaption of therapies to new contexts are also prioritized. Exceptional case studies are welcome when focused on innovative methods, but fewer articles are submitted of this type today. Research is often driven by funding, and there is little funding for family issues that are purely about family problems, such as relations with in-laws, step-families, family conflicts, and what makes for satisfying family experiences. More articles on such family-focused issues would balance publication better in relation to the many research articles explicating aspects of psychopathology, such as family contribution to the development and amelioration of depression.

Although the journal prides itself on publishing papers from all over the world, there is still little representation from Asia, Africa, and South America in the *Journal of Family Therapy*; articles from these countries, describing the different ways in which family therapy and systemic ideas have had an impact, could increase the global profile of the journal. Some subjects are transnational, for example, the impact of migration and attitudes to refugees; the journal would be particularly interested in articles on such topics from the perspective of different parts of the world.

A group of scholars, associated with *JFT*, is working on a narrative review of process research; the outputs of this collaborative research endeavor are planned to be published in future issues. In the near future, *JFT* is planning a series of special editions focusing on particular areas of practice. In the United Kingdom, one of the major developments in systemic work and family therapy has been in social care, with many social workers receiving training and support to carry out their duties using a systemic approach, and it is hoped to attract articles, which describe and honor this work. Another series of articles is planned which will revisit key systemic ideas and techniques, tracking their changing use over time and evaluating their status and usefulness in contemporary practice. Again, it is hoped that this will include international perspectives, recognizing the variety of ways in which ideas and techniques have been taken forward in different contexts.

Family therapists remain a relatively small (and sometimes beleaguered!) profession in the United Kingdom, and it is important that *JFT* provides a context which supports their efforts to establish themselves and find their place in the professional field. Articles need to connect with their experience in a way that helps practitioners, supervisors, and managers to feel that both the possibilities and constraints of their working contexts are recognized. The most important and impactful articles published will contain new and inspiring ideas about how, as systemic therapists, they can work effectively with their client families and find their place as a discipline within a world of different and competing discourses, adjusting to the new challenges of a changing political, social, and organizational climate.

ANZJFT accepts submissions across the broad range of relational, systemic, and contextual therapies including family-sensitive practice and family-based interventions. It recognizes the need to present family therapy as an effective and evidence-informed therapeutic discipline with relevance across the spectrum of mental health professions. An integrative ethic of hospitality toward different therapeutic modalities is seen as crucial for the future development of family therapy. To this end, *ANZJFT* invites theory, research, and practice articles that address the intersection between family therapy and a range of approaches in psychiatry, psychology, and mental health. A recent example is a study of the attachment effectiveness of a Circle of Security intervention for parents of children with autism spectrum disorder (Fardoulys & Coyne, 2016). Another is research investigating a family-focused intervention for children affected by parent gambling (von Doussa, Sundbery, Cuff, Jones, & Goodyear, 2016).

One of the measures of the success of family therapy in Australia has paradoxically been a loss of collective identity as its systemic influence has widened and other disciplines increasingly adopt a more relational perspective. Thus, in child and adolescent mental health services, many practitioners acknowledge a relational focus and working with families, but only a minority would identify as "family therapists" per se. Family therapy is not yet accredited as a stand-alone employment qualification in Australia, which presents ongoing challenges for professional membership, attendance at conferences, and pedagogy. In addition, the field has developed many rivulets of specialization over the last two decades, for example, the Maudsley approach for eating disorders (Conti et al., 2017), Open Dialogue for serious mental illness (Brown & Mikes-Liu, 2015), and Attachment-Based Family Therapy (ABFT) for adolescent depression and other mental health issues (Wagner, Levy, & Diamond, 2016). These family-oriented therapy approaches attract a large number of generalist mental health practitioners to their training programs, conferences, and workshops.

Publishing in Family Therapy Journals in the Twenty-First Century: Some Final Remarks

Globalization and digitalization have an impact not only on the families we work with but on family therapy journals as well. Just decades ago, scholars had to visit their university libraries in person to gain access to the printed versions of the abovementioned journals (or to order a paper copy of respective articles). Now, it's primarily a matter of institutional or financial resources having access to each article of interest from almost everywhere on the world. Embedded in these cross-linking developments is the use of English language as lingua franca (with concession to the high number of Spanish-speaking and Chinese colleagues). More and more, family therapists are becoming a global community.

Some common aspects in the developments of the described journals can be observed, e.g., having a respective professional association as foundation and background, offering family therapists with diverse basic disciplines the possibility to unite and exchange. In this context, the issue of the identity as a family therapist, the recognition in the psychosocial and therapeutic field (family therapy as accredited/ not accredited profession), as well as the politics of the profession, all these facets have an impact on the orientation and the function of the journals. In terms of content, there seem to be some common trends: to publish research is regarded as necessary for conveying best practice and proving efficacy. The type of research preferred is embedded in the guiding principles of the respective journal; nevertheless, diversity is generally encouraged: practice-based evidence and randomized controlled trials representing the poles of an entire range.

With regard to the approaches in family therapy, there is a wide variety, e.g., those focusing on specific treatment groups, alongside those employing more or less standardized methodologies, and many others. An integration of theoretical models and methods, transcending traditionally disparate schools of psychotherapy (e.g., cognitive-behavioral models), seems to go hand in hand with the ethics of providing optimum procedures to patients and clients. Being international while accounting for cultural diversity, the three journals reflect furthermore the multiplicity in systemic thinking: both positivist and constructionist epistemologies have their place in each journal.

From the outset of family therapy, one part of the identity of systemic thinkers and practitioners has been a revolutionary attitude, that hasn't lost its significance until today. To honor this legacy, it is worth continuing the discussion: what are the pros and cons of losing a distinct profile and becoming more and more "mainstream"? What are the political challenges we have to face in our profession in the years to come? What are our responsibilities for the twenty-first century, not only as family therapists but also as systemic scholars?

References

Brown, J. M., & Mikes-Liu, K. (2015). Editorial special issue: Dialogical practices. *Australian and New Zealand Journal of Family Therapy, 36*(1), 1–5. https://doi.org/10.1002/anzf.1101

Conti, J., Calder, J., Cibralic, S., Rhodes, P., Meade, T., & Hewson, D. (2017). 'Somebody else's roadmap': Lived experience of Maudsley and family-based therapy for adolescent anorexia nervosa. *Australian and New Zealand Journal of Family Therapy, 38*(3), 405–429. https://doi.org/10.1002/anzf.1229

Davis, M., & Lipson, L. (1996). A contribution to the history of family therapy in Australia and New Zealand: A bibliometric perspective. *Australian and New Zealand Journal of Family Therapy, 17*(1), 9–18. https://doi.org/10.1002/j.1467-8438.1996.tb01067.x

Fardoulys, C., & Coyne, J. (2016). Circle of security intervention for parents of children with autism spectrum disorder. *Australian and New Zealand Journal of Family Therapy, 37*(4), 572–584. https://doi.org/10.1002/anzf.1193

Hulgaard, D., Dehlholm-Lambertsen, G., & Rask, C. U. (2019). Family-based interventions for children and adolescents with functional somatic symptoms: A systematic review. *Journal of Family Therapy, 41*(1), 4–28. https://doi.org/10.1111/1467-6427.12199

Imber-Black, E. (2011). Toward a contemporary social justice agenda in family therapy research and practice. *Family Process, 50*(2), 129–131. https://doi.org/10.1111/j.1545-5300.2011.01350.x

Larner, G. (2004). Family therapy and the politics of evidence. *Journal of Family Therapy, 26*(1), 17–39. https://doi.org/10.1111/j.1467-6427.2004.00265.x

Lebow, J., Chambers, A., & Breunlin, D. C. (Eds.). (2019). *Encyclopedia of Couple and Family Therapy.* Cham: Springer International.

Singh, R. (2015). A journal in time. Past, present and future themes. *Journal of Family Therapy, 37*(4), 407–408. https://doi.org/10.1111/1467-6427.12097

Templer, K., Matthewson, M., Haines, J., & Cox, G. (2017). Recommendations for best practice in response to parental alienation: Findings from a systematic review. *Journal of Family Therapy, 39*(1), 103–122. https://doi.org/10.1111/1467-6427.12137

von Doussa, H., Sundbery, J., Cuff, R., Jones, S., & Goodyear, M. (2016). 'Let's talk about children': Investigating the use of a family-focused intervention in the gambling support services sector. *Australian and New Zealand Journal of Family Therapy, 38*(3), 482–495. https://doi.org/10.1002/anzf.1233

Wagner, W., Levy, S. A., & Diamond, G. S. (2016). Special issue: Attachment based family therapy: Adaptation and dissemination. *Australian and New Zealand Journal of Family Therapy, 37*(2), 141–250. https://doi.org/10.1002/anzf.1148

Walsh, F. (2016). Applying a family resilience framework in training, practice, and research: Mastering the art of the possible. *Family Process, 55*(4), 616–632. https://doi.org/10.1111/famp.12260

Index

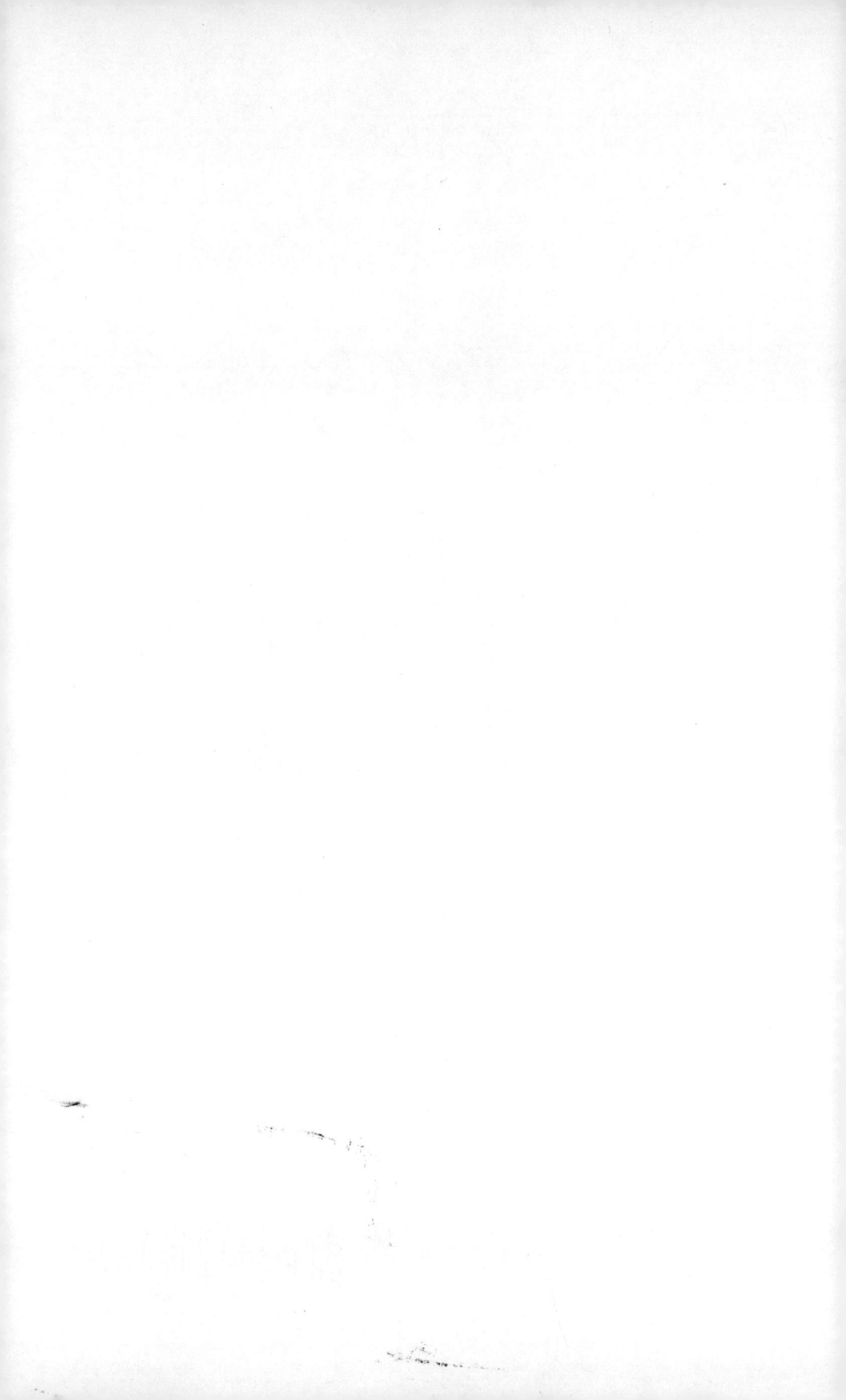

Printed in Great Britain
by Amazon